EVOKED POTENTIALS IN CLINICAL TESTING

CLINICAL NEUROLOGY AND NEUROSURGERY MONOGRAPHS
Volume 3

Titles already published

Benson: *Aphasia, Alexia, and Agraphia*
Fenichel: *Neonatal Neurology*

Forthcoming titles in the series

Rudge: *Clinical Neuro-otology*
Arnason: *Clinical Neuroimmunology*
Glaser: *Temporal Lobe Epilepsy*
Thomas, Stewart & Bundey: *Clinical Neurogenetics*

EVOKED POTENTIALS IN CLINICAL TESTING

EDITED BY

A.M. HALLIDAY BSc MB ChB FBCS

Member of the External Staff of the Medical Research Council;
Consultant in Clinical Neurophysiology,
The National Hospital for Nervous Diseases, London

CHURCHILL LIVINGSTONE
EDINBURGH LONDON MELBOURNE AND NEW YORK   1982

CHURCHILL LIVINGSTONE
Medical Division of Longman Group Limited

Distributed in the United States of America by Churchill Livingstone Inc., 1560 Broadway, New York, N.Y. 10036, and by associated companies, branches and representatives throughout the world.

© Longman Group Limited 1982

First published 1982

ISBN 0 443 01791 3

British Library Cataloguing in Publication Data
Evoked potentials in clinical testing — (Clinical neurology and neurosurgery monographs; v. 3)
1. Evoked potentials (Electrophysiology)
I. Halliday, A.M. II. Series
612'.822   QP461

Library of Congress Catalog Card Number 81-68936

Printed in Great Britain at The Pitman Press, Bath

Preface

The aim of this book has been to provide the sort of information which will be useful to someone who is setting up an evoked potential (EP) service. It is not really intended for the evoked potential specialist, who is already catered for in the large number of research-oriented volumes which have appeared over the last few years. The expert will indeed find much of the contents too simple and well-known to need saying, but the fact remains that much of this common-place lore, which is familiar to everyone who has worked for some time in the field, is not to be found in any of the standard publications.

People enter the field of evoked potentials from many different disciplines. Clinicians, hospital physicists, electronic engineers, electrophysiological technicians and experimental or clinical psychologists are all liable to find themselves involved in the recording of EPs in one way or another. The clinician cannot be expected to be familiar with the well-known principles governing the occurrence of electrical interference or dictating suitable amplifier filter settings to suit the bandwidth of the signal, which are taken as read by every electronic technician or electrical engineer. For this reason, in the first two chapters an attempt has been made to provide as full a description as possible of the basic technical considerations which need to be taken into consideration when setting up a recording laboratory. In the clinical chapters which follow, some account must necessarily be given of the more research-oriented growing points in this rapidly advancing field, but an effort has also been made to include practical guidance for those who simply want to get started on using any of the techniques. For this reason, several of the chapters provide a step-by-step outline of the recording technique used in the authors' own practice.

In each field, the chapters have been written by someone who is familiar with the day-to-day use of EP recording. This inevitably means that the account reflects to some extent the particular approach of one laboratory. When starting out, however, it is much better to have detailed guidance on one tested and tried technique, than a more diffuse survey referring to a confusing variety of alternative (and perhaps mutually incompatible) methods. With experience the adaptable EP worker will soon learn when and how to modify his initial laboratory technique in order to adopt improvements advocated or developed elsewhere.

I am grateful to all the authors for finding the time amidst their busy schedules to complete their contributions, and also to my wife, Elise, for help in preparing the text for publication and for making many of the figures, particularly for the section on the visual and somatosensory evoked responses. It was originally my intention to write the chapters on the visual evoked potential in collaboration with Dr L.D. Blumhardt. Unfortunately, circumstances intervened to make his participation impossible at the time, but these sections of the book, and particularly the account of the visual evoked response in field defects, owes much to our work together. Our own development of the EP technique in clinical testing would have been impossible without the support and encouragement of my clinical colleagues and, in particular, Professor Ian McDonald, and I am glad to have this opportunity to express my gratitude to him for his active and enthusiastic collaboration over more than a decade. Some other early collaborators, among them Dr G.S. Wakefield, Dr W.F. Michael and Dr Joan Mushin, also deserve mention for the valuable contributions they made to the development of this work. I also want to thank Carmel Riley for her careful typing of the manuscript of the book and the list of references and A.H. Prentice and his staff in the Department of Medical Illustration of the Institute of Neurology who photographed many of the figures. The book has benefited from the helpful comments of Dr Geoff Barrett, Keith Cunningham, Lisl Halliday, Dr Tony Kriss, Dr Eva Peringer and Jack Pitman who read it in draft, either in full or in part. Finally my thanks go to the staff of Churchill Livingstone for their patience during the long gestation period, and to Keith Cunningham for his technical help in arranging the transfer of the typescript from word processor via floppy disc to photo-typesetter.

London, 1982   A.M.H.

Contributors

Geoffrey Barrett BSc PhD
Member of the External Staff of the Medical Research Council, The National Hospital for Nervous Diseases, London

W.P.R. Gibson MD FRCS
Consultant Neuro-otologist, The National Hospital for Nervous Diseases; Consultant ENT Surgeon, Royal National Throat, Nose and Ear Hospital, London

A.M. Halliday BSc MB ChB FBCS
Member of the External Staff of the Medical Research Council; Consultant in Clinical Neurophysiology, The National Hospital for Nervous Diseases, London

Hisako Ikeda PhD DSc
Head of Vision Research Unit, The Rayne Institute, St Thomas' Hospital; Senior Lecturer in Physiology, St Thomas' Hospital Medical School, London

S.J. Jones MA PhD
Member of the External Staff of the Medical Research Council, The National Hospital for Nervous Diseases, London

Anthony Kriss BSc MSc PhD
Senior Research Officer, Medical Research Council, The National Hospital for Nervous Diseases, London

Kathleen Robinson BSc
Department of Clinical Neurophysiology, The National Hospital for Nervous Diseases, London

Peter Rudge BSc FRCP
Consultant Neurologist, The National Hospital for Nervous Diseases and Northwick Park Hospital, London

Hiroshi Shibasaki MD DMS
Division of Neurology, Department of Internal Medicine, Saga Medical School, Saga, Japan

Contents

1

Setting up an Evoked Potential (EP) Laboratory

A. Kriss

INTRODUCTION

The kind of evoked potential (EP) with which this book is concerned is the sequence of voltage changes generated in the brain, and in the sense organ and pathway leading to the brain, following the administration of a transient stimulus in any sensory modality. Sensitive amplifying and averaging equipment is required to enhance potentials picked up from skin electrodes, which are inevitably situated at a considerable distance from the generator source, and to discriminate between the evoked response and other, usually larger, potentials of physiological and extrinsic origin with which it is intermixed. In order to establish and run an EP laboratory to satisfactory standards, it is necessary to be able to record the evoked potential faithfully and with minimal adulteration. Only then is one in a position to comment on its clinical significance. Interpretation of the response requires awareness of the effects of many variables including stimulus characteristics, functional properties of recording equipment, and physiological factors operating in health and disease, or drug-induced, all of which may affect its form, timing or scalp distribution.

The present chapter is concerned with technical aspects of recording. It will begin by suggesting ways of ensuring a satisfactory environment for both subject and equipment, and then go on to describe apparatus and methods for acquiring, analyzing and storing EPs. In the following chapter techniques for stimulating in the visual, auditory and somatosensory modalities will be covered. Some common and more unusual recording problems will also be described to emphasize the constant vigilance needed to obtain good quality recordings.

Basic requirements for recording EPs

In order to be recordable evoked potentials have to be constantly related in time to a brusque and physically identifiable event. This 'time-locked' property allows them to be discriminated from the larger intrinsic spontaneous voltage fluctuations of the brain (i.e. the electroencephalogram or EEG) and other sources of electrical 'noise', which do not show a systematic relationship to the stimulating event.

Most current clinical and research interest is focussed on potentials elicited by externally delivered stimuli (so-called exogenous potentials) but potentials time-locked to internal events (endogenous components) such as voluntary or involuntary movements or the moment of decision in a cognitive task, are also included within the wide category of event-related potentials (ERPs) (Hillyard, Picton and Regan, 1978). In general, for the response to be clearly discernible a stimulus has to be somewhat above its subjective detection threshold. It also has to have an abrupt onset and/or offset so that a discrete volley is set up in the afferent pathway, capable of eliciting in turn, distinct cortical potential changes.

It is conceptually useful to distinguish between early (sensory) potentials occurring within the first 150 msec or so after a stimulus from later and slower voltage changes (long latency potentials and slow potential shifts) which occur after this and within a second and a half of the stimulus (Vaughan, 1969). Current knowledge suggests that early potential changes represent neural processing concerned with physical and temporal properties of the stimulus (i.e. exogenous variables) while later potentials tend to be correlated with the endogenous psychological processes associated with assessing the significance of the stimulus. Although the same stimulating and recording equipment can be used to study fast and slow potentials, there are important differences between the two as regards the optimum recording characteristics of electrodes and amplifiers, and the collaborative procedures required from the patient.

In recording event-related potentials to stimuli or responses generated by the subject himself, use can be made of equipment which permits storage of potentials preceding the event. For example, the electromyogram (EMG) associated with voluntary movement of the subject's fingers can be used as a trigger to record the slower and faster cortical voltage changes occurring before and just after the movement (readiness and motor potentials) (Kornhuber and Deecke, 1964; Gilden et al, 1966; Shibasaki et al, 1980a). Interestingly, potential changes have also been recorded to the omission of an expected event (Picton and Hillyard, 1974; Weinberg et al, 1974; Barlow, 1969; Ruchkin et al, 1980).

RECORDING ENVIRONMENT

The location, construction, equipping and layout of an EP laboratory has to be carefully thought out. The advice of colleagues who have already set-up laboratories and of professional experts is well worth seeking. Progress in the implementation of plans should be monitored throughout in order to tackle unforeseen problems at an early stage and ensure a satisfactory end-product. What follows is a general account which attempts to highlight in a practical way the more important factors to be considered when creating an EP laboratory. The experiences of a host of research workers has been distilled by Gale and Smith (1980) to provide a useful description of setting up a psychophysiological laboratory. Lee (1967) reports on the construction of an electrically shielded, sound attenuating chamber.

Extraneous interference

The electrical environment both within and outside an EP laboratory should be controlled as much as possible. The electrical supply and electrically powered equipment are capable of inducing potential changes on human subjects and recording apparatus. These extraneously generated potentials have to be minimized, because, if they are allowed to rise much above the recordable threshold, the detection of an evoked potential can be seriously compromised.

Extraneous interference most commonly arises in the immediate vicinity of the patient and recording equipment as a result of electrostatic and magnetic induction and usually alternates at mains supply frequencies (50 Hz in Europe and 60 Hz in North America). Interference due to electromagnetic radiation alternates at much higher frequencies (radio frequency (RF)) and usually originates from sources outside the recording room.

Electrostatic interference

Electrostatic potentials occur due to the fact that an object charged with static electricity induces a charge of opposite polarity on the surface of another object in close proximity to it. The objects are said to be capacitatively coupled and the potential difference or voltage which exists between them is dependent on the magnitude of the charge and inversely related to the distance between the two objects. As an example, a room may be considered as a large capacitor with lighting and unscreened electrical cables in the ceiling acting as one 'plate' and the floor as the other. Conductors (such as people and the stimulating and recording equipment) will assume an intermediate potential, the magnitude of which depends on the impedance* between the object and ceiling and between object and floor. Electrostatic interference can be effectively overcome by surrounding either the offending source or the recording equipment (or both) with earthed metal shields

---

* Impedance is the resistance (measured in ohms) to varying electrical flow (i.e. AC) which is due to the combined effects of resistive and reactive (i.e. capacitative and/or inductive) elements in a circuit. Alterations in impedance are associated with changes in the rate of current flow.

(e.g. wire netting). In order to efficiently dissipate electrostatic charges and avoid further problems of a similar nature, a good (i.e. low resistance) connection between shield and earth should be ensured. A low resistance contact has also to be present between the subject and the equipment earth. One earthing point common to all equipment should be used, as small differences in potential and current flow (earth loops) can occur between two pieces of equipment connected to independent earthing points. Fluorescent lighting and electrical heaters are particularly potent sources of electrostatic interference. The latter are best avoided while the former should be at least ten feet away from the subject and recording equipment. If nearer, then the light needs to be enclosed by an earthed wire mesh. An electrical cable connected to the mains supply will be electrically charged even though no current is flowing. It is desirable therefore to disconnect unnecessary cables which are not in use. All cables should have an outer metal braid (screen) which is properly earthed.

Magnetic interference

Current flowing through an electrical conductor produces a magnetic field around it. The greater the current the stronger the field. If a conducting loop is placed in the vicinity of a changing magnetic field a voltage will be induced in the loop, the magnitude of which depends on the strength of the field, the rate at which the magnetic field changes and the area of the loop measured in a plane perpendicular to the direction of the field. Thus if a loop, formed by the head, electrode leads and input circuitry of the amplifiers, is subjected to a changing magnetic field, usually alternating at power line frequencies and multiples thereof, then interference potentials at these frequencies will be induced and amplified together with the desired potentials. Keeping the electrode leads close together (e.g. by twisting or bundling them together loosely with a strap) greatly reduces the cross sectional area of the loop and hence minimizes interference of this nature.

Common sources of magnetic interference are electrical devices using relatively heavy currents, such as power transformers and electric motors fitted in nearby lifts, fans and air-conditioning equipment. Moving away from the cause of the trouble greatly reduces contamination. Another effective manoeuvre is to change the relative orientation of the problem source and recording set-up. If it is not possible to increase physical separation, small local sources of interference can be enclosed by an earthed metal shield of high magnetic permeability (e.g. MU metal), although this can be expensive. The magnetic field surrounding electrical supply cables is largely neutralized due to the fact that there are two wires carrying similar currents flowing in opposite directions. It is worth-while, nonetheless, to ensure that any power cables, supplying both lighting and power sockets, are enclosed in properly earthed metal conduits.

In older buildings, water and central heating pipes were commonly used as conductors to earth. These pipes form part of an extensive network and, as they are capable of carrying heavy currents, they can bring about intolerable magnetic fields covering a wide area. In these circumstances an alternative earthing point needs to be found. This is most easily achieved by supplying power and earthing facilities for the laboratory from one distribution point.

Some types of paging system in use within hospitals induce a magnetic field within a wire loop going around the building. These systems normally function at relatively low frequencies (1KHz - 150 KHz) and it is advisable to check and ensure that their operating frequency is well above the frequency range of the recording amplifiers. If the paging frequency cannot be altered then special high frequency filters need to be fitted to the amplifiers (Hospital Technical Memorandum, 14, 1965; Bramslev et al, 1967).

Radio frequency (RF) interference

Electromagnetic radiation (radio frequency, RF) interference arises from the fact that as a radiation field moves through space it induces a small voltage in any conductor which it encounters. Electrodes and their leads can act like antennae and introduce the interference into amplifiers. Radiation fields can also induce voltages in the power lines which then re-radiate the interference round a building via the mains network. Another possibility is for the interference to be injected directly into the equipment power supply.

Diathermy or other electrosurgical equipment which uses high frequency generators and radio frequency (VHF) paging systems are sources of RF interference within hospitals. Sources external to the building include nearby radio or television transmitters (stationary or mobile). The frequencies which interfere with electrophysiological recording are usually the low frequency signals carried by the high frequency transmitting waves. They become a problem due to demodulation brought about by the non-linear behaviour to higher frequencies of the electrode/skin interface and components in the amplifier input circuitry (Carr et al, 1974). It is also possible for rectified interference to fully or partially block the input stages of amplifiers and thus lead to obliteration or distortion of the amplified signal.

Transient or pulse interference is a form of electromagnetic radiation with a broad frequency content which apart from interfering with the detection of physiological signals can cause spurious triggering of stimulating and recording equipment. It commonly arises from sparking contacts in switches, relays or commutators and abrupt changes in power supply due to switching on of equipment requiring heavy currents.

Recording problems associated with radio frequency interference can commonly be overcome by fitting high frequency filters at the inputs to amplifiers and at the power intake of electrical equipment. Where possible, devices liable to cause electromagnetic interference should be suppressed with high frequency filters. Descriptions of filter circuits which include specification of components have been provided by numerous authors, amongst others are Whitfield (1960), Hospital Technical Memorandum, No. 14 (1965), Jasper (1974).

It is always good policy to assess the amount of extraneous interference present in a newly established laboratory and to deal with problems of this nature before routine recording is started. Detection and localization of electrostatic, magnetic and electromagnetic interference can be carried out by connecting appropriate detectors (e.g. Fig. 1.1) to a biological or audio-amplifier and monitoring the

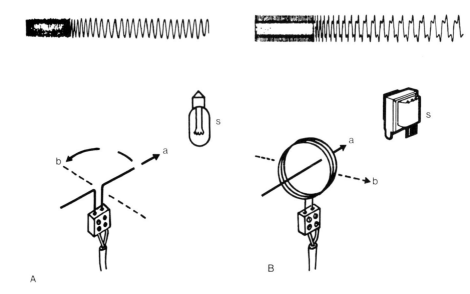

Figure 1.1 *Detection of interference. The top tracings are mains frequency interference as it appears when written out on a chart recorder at increasing paper speed.   A. For detection of electrostatic (capacitative) interference a dipole aerial consisting of two 20 cm lengths of stiff wire mounted in a block connector is connected to the inputs of a biological or audio amplifier, or of an oscilloscope. Maximum interference is obtained when the aerial points to a source(s) as at 'a' and the interference is at a minimum when the source is in direction 'b'.*
B. A wire coil having about 10-20 turns can be used to detect magnetic interference. Maximum and minimum pick-up is obtained in directions 'a' and 'b' respectively. Harmonics arising from induction effects in transformers make the tracing in B more complex. When the interference source is a simple loop, as is often the case when current flows in earth wiring or water pipes, harmonics will not normally be present. (From MacGillivray, 1974.)

output either on an oscilloscope or with high impedance earphones. Interference sources can usually be readily localized by alterations in the magnitude of the interference associated with changes in the orientation of the detector (Hospital Technical Memorandum, No. 14, 1965 and MacGillivray, 1974).

In summary, extraneous interference may normally be reduced below recordable levels by keeping well away from problem sources and by careful screening and suppression. If it is not possible to move away from the origin of the interference, in particular from sources generating electromagnetic radiation, then it becomes necessary to screen the recording room. This requires elaborate techniques and costly materials. Details concerning construction of screened rooms and means of ensuring effective screening are beyond the scope of this chapter. The topic is dealt with in some excellent reviews of methods of reducing extraneous interference in electrophysiological laboratories (Whitfield, 1960; Wolbarsht, 1964; Hospital Technical Memorandum, No. 14, 1965; Leadbitter, 1963; Dobbie, 1965;

Bramslev et al, 1967; Thompson and Yarborough, 1967; Wolbarsht and Spekreijse, 1968; Huhta and Webster, 1974; Lindsley and Wicke, 1974).

Furnishings, fittings and accessories

Some of the more necessary furnishings, fittings and accessories required to equip an EP laboratory will be mentioned. The final choice of items will, of course, depend on individual circumstances such as the size and location of the room(s), the clinical and experimental requirements of the laboratory and, most importantly, the finance available for equipping it.

An EP laboratory should be spacious enough to accommodate a bed, cupboards, work surfaces and a wash-basin as well as all the recording and stimulating equipment. Due allowance has to be made for easy access into the room for wheel-chairs and stretcher trolleys. Within the laboratory, the recordist must be able to reach the patient and equipment easily. In order to ensure a quiet environment for the patient, it may be advantageous to have two rooms, one for the equipment and the other for the patient. As was stressed in the previous section, equipment must always be kept together so that connecting leads are short and common power and earthing facilities can be shared by all stimulating and recording devices.

The lighting level within the laboratory should be good and easily controllable by the recordist. It should be noted, however, that dimming devices (triacs) can be a source of high frequency interference, so it may be better to have several light fittings providing different light levels and to turn them off as required. For auditory and somatosensory stimulation dim lighting is conducive to good relaxation in patients, while for visual stimulation darkness is more appropriate. Care must be taken to mask from the patient any undesirable stimuli, for example, flashing indicator lights from stimulus control devices or sweep monitoring displays, and clicks associated with the operation of relays or photic stimulators.

Comfortable ventilation, temperature and humidity levels are desirable in order to avoid sweating, tension, restlessness or shivering on the part of the patient. If air-conditioning has to be used, this should preferably be baffled to reduce the noise level. It is worth mentioning, however, that some low level continuous noise may serve as a useful mask for distracting sounds such as people talking. If some degree of sound-proofing is needed then this may be achieved by means of heavy doors, double glazing, carpeting, sound absorbing curtains and acoustic tiles. For near perfect sound insulation, required, for example, in routine determination of auditory thresholds, a 'silent' room or anechoic chamber must be used. This can be bought as a prefabricated unit or may be specially constructed (Lee, 1967).

In order to detect poor visual fixation and to reveal, for example, sudden epileptic attacks or accidental alterations of the stimulus, patients should be visually monitored during the recording session either by direct viewing or closed circuit television.

It is useful to have an upright chair with a low back in which a patient can sit while his head is being measured and the electrodes are being applied. For the recording itself, a bed or a reclining chair with a head support will help to reduce contamination of recordings by EMG activity associated with tension in neck muscles.

Every clinical laboratory must have emergency equipment at hand. This should include oxygen, airways, first-aid kit, an eye-wash and a general purpose fire extinguisher. There should be a telephone in the room or nearby, to summon help in case of a cardiac arrest, fire or other emergency.

Mobile surgical trolleys are convenient for holding recording accessories such as electrodes, acetone, swabs, tissues, cotton wool, tape measure, scissors, eye-pads, stimulating electrodes, etc. If collodion is to be used routinely then a small compressor or air-line is very useful. A wash-hand basin is a necessity, not only for cleaning electrodes and washing the hands, but also for providing drinking water. Easily accessible cupboards for storing supplies are important to avoid clutter. Storage cabinets for filing records may be kept in the laboratory, if space permits, or, if not, then nearby, so that past records can be readily retrieved.

Both patients and recordists may apppreciate wall coverings and curtains which are in tasteful and relaxing colours rather than in plain, austere, hospital white. If visual responses are to be recorded then glass partitions in doors and windows must have efficient blackouts fitted. Floors should preferably be covered with a vinyl surface as this withstands acetone spillages better than carpeting. Synthetic floor coverings may lead to problems, however, as they readily give rise to electrostatic charges on people walking round the laboratory and they in turn could capacitatively induce large potential changes when moving near the patient and/or amplifier inputs ('triboelectric' noise, Gordon, 1975). Ensuring moderate humidity levels will help reduce this problem. Special carpeting and spray compounds for reducing the build-up of static are commercially available.

RECORDING ELECTRODES

Electrode characteristics

Electrodes are the metallic conductors by means of which scalp potentials are transferred to the recording amplifiers. A conducting medium such as electrode paste or physiological fluid is needed to transfer the physiological potentials to conventional electrodes. 'Dry' capacitive electrodes which require no electrode paste have been described but as yet their overall performance does not match that of the commonly used 'wet' types (Ko and Hynecek, 1974). The skin/electrolyte/ electrode interface forms the first and in many ways the most vital link for the faithful acquisition of scalp potentials. Neglect in the care of electrodes, and poor application, lead to the most common recording problems.

When an electrode comes in contact with an electrolyte electrochemical changes take place in the immediate vicinity of the electrode with ionic migrations from electrode surface into solution and vice versa. These migrations proceed at different rates and the net result is a local charge distribution known as the electrical double layer in which there is predominance of one charge on the metal surface and an opposite charge in the immediately adjacent electrolyte (Figure 1.2). The electrical

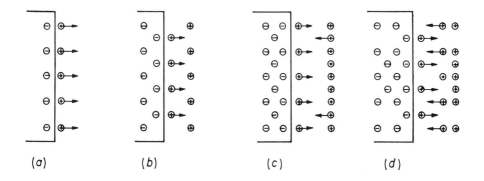

Figure 1.2 *Formation of electrical double layer. a. Ionic flow into solution immediately after immersion. b. Accumulation of ions in solution. c. Ionic flow into and out of solution at different rates. d.equilibrium when rates are equal. Note excess of positive ions in solution giving electrical double layer. (From Cooper et al, 1974.)*

behaviour of the double layer is rather like that of a capacitor and resistor connected in parallel to a voltage source. The values of these components are not constant, however, and depend on such variables as the kind of electrode metal, the nature, concentration and temperature of the electrolyte, and the frequency and density of the current passed (Geddes, 1972; Cooper et al 1974; Neuman, 1978). The skin/electrolyte interface also presents a complex surface, having both capacitative and resistive elements (Montagu and Coles, 1966; Swanson and Webster, 1974; Gatzke, 1974; Neuman, 1978). Figure 1.3 shows an equivalent circuit to the electrode/electrolyte/skin interface.

Two phenomena occur as a consequence of the electrical double layer. The first is the potential difference known as the electrode or half-cell potential which exists between an electrode and the electrolyte with which it makes contact. Differences in the magnitude of these potentials (bias potentials) can occur between electrodes of the same compound, mainly as a result of impurities in the substance of the metal and surface contamination. Bias potentials tend to be very large (1-10 mV) relative to the size of brain potentials (Cooper et al, 1974) and can be minimized by using good quality, well cleaned electrodes and storing them together in a saline bath with their leads electrically shorted (Cooper, 1956). When electrodes are connected to amplifiers they present the relatively large standing potentials arising at the electrode/skin interface as well as the desired physiological signals. Amplifiers designed to respond to alternating potentials (AC amplifiers) will initially be overwhelmed (blocked) by the bias potentials for a period of time determined by the settings which control the effectiveness with which the amplifiers are able to attenuate low frequency signals (i.e. time constant setting). Anti-blocking devices can be fitted to shorten these periods.

Electrode potentials can vary slowly during the course of a recording due mainly to local chemical and temperature changes (Geddes, 1972). Movement of the electrode will affect the electrical double layer and consequently alter the potential

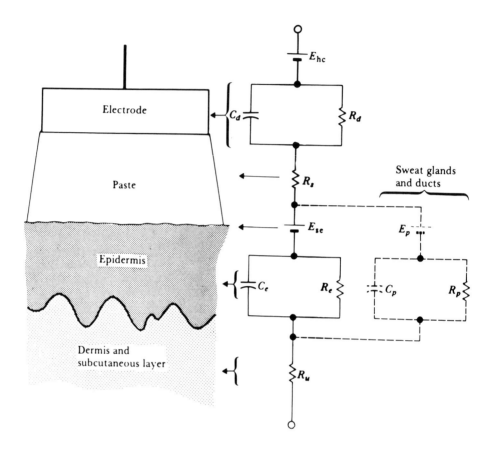

Figure 1.3 *Electrode/electrolyte/skin interface and its equivalent electrical circuit. Elements of the circuit are arranged so as to be at approximately the same level as the physical entity they represent. E_{hc}-electrode or half-cell potential; E_{se} and E_p -potentials generated in epidermis and sweat glands, respectively. Resistive (R_d) and capacitative (C_d) elements which make up the impedance due to the electrical double layer. Resistive and capacitative elements are also associated with the epidermis (C_e and R_e) and sweat glands and their ducts (C_p and R_p). The dermis and subcutaneous layers have purely resistive properties (R_u). (From Neuman, 1978.)*

between electrode and electrolyte. These effects may be particularly troublesome when monitoring slow evoked potentials such as the CNV, Readiness Potential or P300. Special systems have been designed for recording these responses in which the electrode surface is displaced from the skin surface in order to minimize the effects of movement and changes in the chemical and temperature environment (Girton and Kamiya, 1974).

When electrodes are placed in a circuit and a small steady current is passed through them, the ionic distribution of the electrical double layer is altered. Pure noble metals (i.e. gold, silver and platinum) are relatively inert and become polarized as a result of inequalities in the ease with which ions go in and out of solution. After an initial surge these polarizable or non-reversible electrodes pass very little current due to the build-up of a backing potential (i.e. they behave like capacitors). Because of this property they are unsuitable for recording slow evoked potentials like the CNV, as the polarization potential will bias the amplifiers and could lead to distortion of the desired signal.

In non-polarizable or reversible electrodes the ease with which ions go into and out of solution is similar. Reversible electrodes allow relatively unrestricted passage of both fast and slowly changing currents and they are therefore favoured for recording scalp potentials in general. Janz and Ives (1968) provide a detailed description of the physico-chemical properties of silver/silver chloride electrodes.

Types of electrode and their application and care

Evoked potentials are usually recorded using standard EEG electrodes. The most popular type is the disc or stick-on which consists of a cupped disc, about 1 cm in diameter, and made of pure silver, coated with silver chloride. Gold plated electrodes are also available and, though more expensive, are claimed by a manufacturer (Grass Instruments) to be less liable to produce recording problems. A few laboratories use electrodes made from solder (alloy of tin and lead) or just tin.

Disc electrodes are usually attached to the scalp by means of a fast-drying adhesive (collodion) which is applied round the rim of the electrode (Figure 1.4). A jet of air from an air-gun or hair dryer may be used to speed up the setting process. Alternatively, a water-soluble conducting paste such as Bentonite or Grass Cream can be employed (Figure 1.4 H). The paste method is quicker to implement, but electrodes are not attached as securely as with collodion and this method is, therefore, not suitable for recording from restless subjects. Taylor and Abraham (1969) and Cooper et al (1974) give details of how to make Bentonite but it should be noted that, although occurring very rarely, allergic reactions to this substance have been reported (see Taylor and Abraham, 1969).

A common type of disc has a small hole in its centre through which electrode jelly may be injected and the underlying skin scarified with a blunted syringe needle (Figure 1.4 J). When using the paste method of application it is important to thoroughly rub the area of skin on which the electrode will lie with acetone or alcohol. This procedure will remove epidermal substances (surface scales of skin and sebum) which account for high skin impedance. Some prefer to obtain a low impedance by thoroughly rubbing the skin with electrode jelly. These operations are not normally necessary, however, if the skin is to be scarified with a blunted needle. Abrading, scratching or puncturing the skin surface also helps in reducing the size of electrodermal potentials (Picton and Hillyard, 1972; Shackel, 1959). Whichever method is used to lower electrode contact impedances, they should be below 10 KΩ, preferably 5 KΩ or less, and roughly similar for all electrodes.

Double sided adhesive rings (Figure 1.4 I) or hospital adhesive tape (e.g. Micropore) may be used to apply discs to areas with little or no hair. Clips with a cupped section and conductive cloth electrodes which can be attached to the ear lobe are commercially available.

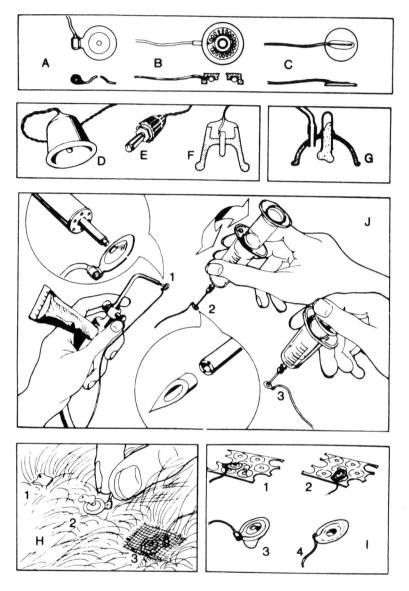

Figure 1.4 *Examples of stick-on disc electrodes and suction type electrodes. A silver disc; B plastic electrode with silver coil insert, C gold or solder solid disc button electrode, D and F rubber cup suction electrode with central silver core, E O/Z plug for connection to headbox, G active suction electrode consisting of soft rubber cup, central silver electrode element with sponge pledget for electrolyte solution and evacuator tube attached to low pressure vacuum pump to hold electrode in place. H, application of disc electrode using bentonite or Grass cream: 1 electrode paste applied to previously cleaned scalp, 2 electrode pressed into position and 3 covered with small gauze square. I, using double-sided adhesive rings: the top protective covering is removed, 1, electrode centred on the exposed tacky surface and the disc removed, 2, 3 and applied to non-hairy skin*

It is sound practice to first measure and mark the scalp in order to accurately determine the sites where electrodes are to be attached. Discrepancies in electrode placement over homologous scalp areas can lead to false interpretation of a record. Wax based pencils (e.g. Chinagraph[R]) will make conspicuous marks on the scalp and are obtainable in a wide range of bright colours. In order to identify electrode leads rapidly and effectively, each may be individually colour-coded by coiling a few turns of fine PVC coated wire of the appropriate colour around the lead at both ends.

Electrodes attached with collodion can be readily removed with acetone. This is a potent solvent and an irritant to the eyes and throat. Great care has to be exercised in its use. It is strongly advisable to shield a patient's clothing by use of a vinyl shoulder cape and to protect his eyes with pads. Following removal of electrodes the hair should be combed through to remove bits of undissolved collodion.

The condition of electrodes and their leads must be checked regularly. For EEG, at least, their useful life has been reported to be about 60-80 recordings (McNie, 1967; George, 1968; Coles and Binnie, 1968). Continuous exposure to acetone tends to harden the PVC insulation at its junction with the electrode. With time the lead becomes brittle and eventually cracks exposing the wires in the core. If the bare wires, which are usually made of copper, and the electrode are bridged by electrode jelly, recording problems will be encountered due to the fact that multi-metal junctions are a source of large and somewhat erratic potential changes (Geddes 1972, Cooper et al, 1974).

Damage to the chloride coating of silver electrodes can also give rise to electrical noise (Geddes 1972) and, if eroded altogether, will result in polarizable electrodes. It is advisable therefore to regularly chloride silver electrodes so as to maintain them in optimum condition. Chloriding is normally done by electrolysis. First, the electrode surface is cleaned thoroughly either with a mild abrasive (fine emery paper or household cleaner) or better still by 'stripping'; that is, by placing the electrode in saline solution and attaching its lead to the cathode of a 9 volt battery. The anode may be another piece of silver, for example, silver wire or an old electrode. There will be vigorous bubbling at the cathode electrode when the circuit is completed. Following removal of any surface coating and ensuring that the electrode to be chlorided is spotlessly clean, both electrodes are now transferred to another beaker containing 5% saline solution (one tablespoonful sodium chloride per pint of distilled water). This time a 1.5 volt battery is used and the battery polarities reversed so that the electrode to be chlorided is attached to the anode. Apparatus is commercially available or may be built (Roberts et al, 1974) which will produce appropriate current densities (2.5 mA/cm) to chloride many electrodes at once. A chloriding time of 30 sec to 1 minute is normally sufficient to produce a mauve or dark brown coating under normal lighting conditions. A very thick chloride layer

after the second protective cover is removed from the under surface. Electrode jelly is inserted through the hole as in J below. J shows the method of attaching disc electrodes with collodion using special air gun. 1, with compressed air for drying; in 2 and 3, electrode jelly is inserted through the hole by means of a syringe with blunted needle (prepared as in inset) which is rotated, 2, to reduce scalp resistance. (From MacGillivray, 1974.)

should be avoided as it may adversely affect recording performance (Geddes, 1972) and tends to peel off easily if attached to adhesive discs. Slower and more elaborate chloriding methods which give greater durability to the chloride coat have been described by Venables and Martin (1967), Geddes (1972) and Coles and Binnie (1968). A method of sterilizing and chloriding electrodes at one go is to immerse them for at least 10 minutes in a concentrated solution of sodium hypochlorite (e.g. the sterilizing and bleaching agent Chloros). After chloriding, care should be taken to thoroughly wash electrodes before use as this chemical is a powerful skin irritant.

Pad electrodes are used less commonly than discs to record evoked potentials. They consist of a threaded silver rod screwed to a plastic frame. The frame is pressed on to the scalp by strong rubber bands which are linked to form a cap. A cotton wool or foam cushion enclosed by gauze and soaked in saline forms the conducting bridge between rod and skin. To ensure a good electrical contact the skin has to be thoroughly rubbed or, better still, abraded. Though quick to apply, pad electrodes are uncomfortable to wear for periods longer than half-an-hour or so and compared to discs are more liable to produce movement artifact. Cooper (1956) describes a method of self-chloriding and equalizing electrode potentials in which pad electrodes are placed in a saline bath and connected to a carbon cathode.

A third type of scalp electrode is the subdermal needle. It is normally made of platinum alloy and inserted tangentially into the skin. This procedure can be made relatively painless by pinching the skin and inserting the needle to about half its length with a quick firm push. Before insertion, the skin surface should be wiped clean with alcohol or any other efficient sterilizing compound. Once in place, electrode leads should be kept together and attached to clothing or skin, for example with tape or a 'crocodile clip', to prevent accidental tugging and electrostatic artifacts resulting from swaying of the thin Teflon-covered leads. Needle tips have to be inspected regularly for sharpness as insertion of a blunt electrode can be painful.

Needles have inter-electrode impedances which are about five to ten times that of stick-ons and because of this are more liable to produce 'noise' contaminated records in electrically hostile environments (see Section IV). Zablow and Goldensohn (1969) compared the recording characteristics of needle and gold-plated disc electrodes and found that the former distorted waveforms below 5 Hz if the input impedance of the amplifiers was less than 1 MΩ. Because of differences in both electrode potential and recording characteristics one should avoid recording scalp activity between electrodes made of different metals.

Rubber suction-cup electrodes have a central chlorided silver element and are normally filled with electrode jelly (Figure 1.4 F). They are only suitable for applying to non-hairy areas where a good seal can be made (Shackel, 1959). Cooper and Walter (1957) devised a special suction electrode attached to a low pressure vacuum pump which was suitable for using on the delicate skin of babies (Figure 1.4 G). There have been a few descriptions of caps, helmets, harnesses and plates with electrodes in prefixed positions but these have not become popular (Dawson, 1954b; Pitman and Whiteside, 1955; Perry and Childers, 1969; Hanley et al, 1974).

Long electrodes designed for insertion into the deep tissues (sphenoidal) or into the nose and pharynx (ethmoidal and nasopharyngeal) have only rarely been used to record evoked potentials. Accounts detailing their method of insertion, and problems which could be encountered in their use, are to be found in Lehtinen and Bergstrom, 1970, Smith et al, 1973, and MacGillivray, 1974.

A transtympanic electrode placed at the promontory of the middle ear and an electrode attached to the cornea of the eye will record large potentials associated with reception of the stimulus by the sensory organ. These specialized electrodes normally require the use of local anaesthesia and considerable skill in application. Details concerning their construction, application and care will be found in Chapters 4 and 8. For auditory stimulation, a smaller, though reliably obtained, auditory nerve potential can be recorded, from a springy V-shaped plastic electrode inserted into the external auditory meatus. A silver ball at the end of one of the electrode limbs presses against the previously cleaned skin of the canal near the tympanic membrane (Coats and Martin, 1977). Alternatively, a needle electrode, such as that used for EEG recording can be inserted into the wall of the external auditory canal (Martin and Coats, 1973; Chiappa, 1981). Arden et al (1979) have described a promising gold foil electrode for recording the electroretinogram. The thin foil is hooked over the lower eyelid and can be worn comfortably for long periods without local anaesthesia. Retinal responses to pattern stimulation recorded with this electrode show interesting results (Arden et al, 1980).

It is essential to wipe clean and sterilize, after every use, both subdermal needle electrodes and the blunted needles used to lower skin resistance. Conn and Neil (1959) pointed out that immersion of needle electrodes in sterilizing solutions or exposure to ultra-violet light was not enough to destroy the hepatitis virus. Until recently steam autoclaving utilizing a pressure of 15-20 psi and a temperature of at least 250°F (121°C) for 5-20 minutes was generally accepted as a safe method of rendering electrodes free from infection. However, Gadjusek et al (1977) have recommended increasing the autoclave time to one hour in order to ensure destruction of the transmissible agent associated with Creutzfeldt-Jakob disease.

The soundness of the contact between electrode and skin is an essential factor in determining the quality of the record which is obtained. If physical contact is poor and the electrode/skin impedance high relative to the input impedance of the amplifiers the desired signals may be attenuated and contaminated by intrusion of extraneous interference and electrode movement artifacts. A DC meter may be used to measure the resistance of reversible electrodes (say 50 µA for full scale deflection from a 1.5 V source), but it is unsuitable for non-reversible electrodes. This is because (1) the electrodes will become polarized, (2) the resistance reading will be misleading due to the polarization backing potential and (3) polarized electrodes will confound recordings of slow potential shifts. It is therefore more appropriate to measure interelectrode impedance using alternating current within the frequency range of the neurophysiological signals (e.g. 20 Hz). AC meters specifically designed for this purpose are commercially available. A few manufacturers incorporate electrode impedance measuring facilities into their recording amplifiers. If a direct current meter has to be used it should be fitted with a reversing switch which will allow reversal of the direction of current flow through the electrode pairs while their resistance is being determined.

Montage

Electrode derivation and placement

The siting of electrodes on the head should be dictated primarily by the expected scalp distribution of the evoked potential which it is intended to record. The choice of electrodes to be connected to each amplifier (channel) needs to be such as to make the response and its distribution readily and easily appreciated.

Differential amplifiers are universally employed to record bioelectric activity primarily because they greatly reduce the effects of widespread interference potentials of extraneous and physiological origin. They achieve this by amplifying only the algebraic difference of voltages presented to their pair of input leads. Electrical activity which is of the same polarity and magnitude at both leads is, within limits, cancelled out (so called "in-phase or common-mode rejection"; see Amplifier Section).

An agreed practice in electroencephalography is to identify the two input leads of a recording amplifier, respectively, as the 'black' lead or Grid 1 (drawn as a solid line in diagrams) and the 'white' lead or Grid 2 (illustrated by a broken line). By convention, an electrode over a presumed active site is connected to the black lead and when it picks up electronegative activity (with respect to the white lead) this is represented as an upward deflection in the output trace. The EEG system is widely adopted when displaying human evoked potentials, although the opposite convention (i.e. positive up) is used by some laboratories. It is important, therefore, to specify which convention is being used, and this can be conveniently indicated by adding a '+' or '-' sign to opposite ends of the calibration on illustrations (e.g. see Figure 1.10).

The pair of electrodes connected to an amplifier is called a derivation and an established pattern of connections involving several electrodes is named a montage. Essentially, there are three ways of displaying electrical activity from an array of electrodes. In the so-called bipolar derivation electrodes are normally connected in chains so that the activity picked up by an electrode within the chain is fed to the black lead of one amplifier and the white of another, usually adjacent, amplifier (Figure 1.5 A). As will be demonstrated later, such an arrangement is useful for locating changes in potential gradient and improving localization, but it is not ideally suited for visualizing the distribution of potentials across the scalp.

The common reference method (also called monopolar or unipolar) uses one electrode as a common input to amplifiers while the other inputs, normally the black leads, are from electrodes over or near an 'active' area (Figure 1. 6 A). It is important that the reference site be judiciously chosen so as not to be influenced by the spatial field of the evoked potential, or at least only minimally so. It should be noted that a single reference electrode feeding many amplifiers will tend to unbalance their input circuits, and make them prone to extraneous electrical interference. This is due to the lowering of input impedance when many inputs are lined-up in parallel. By ensuring that the reference electrode has as low a contact impedance as possible (of the order of 2 KΩ) the imbalance can be partially corrected (Osselton, 1970).

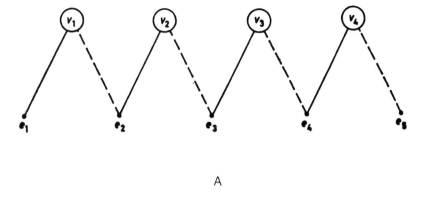

A

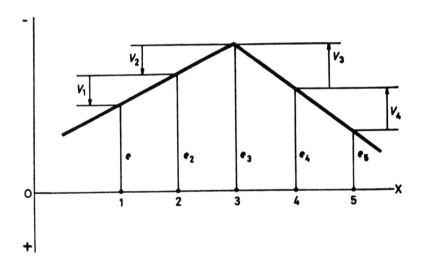

B

Figure 1.5 *Serial bipolar linkage. A. e is the potential at each electrode and V is the difference in potential between adjacent electrodes which is recorded. B. Graph of potential distribution along a row of bipolarly linked electrodes (1-5) having different potentials. The slope of the graph is the potential gradient and this changes sign at the maximum value. The magnitudes and directions of the potential differences recorded are represented by the arrows. Amplifiers fed by V_2 and V_3 will deflect in oposite directions (called phase reversal). (Adapted from Cooper et al, 1974.)*

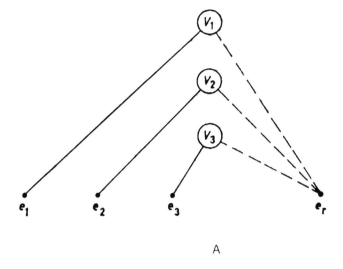

A

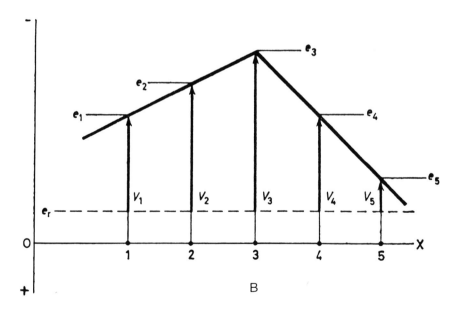

B

Figure 1.6 *Common reference derivations. e represents the potential at the electrode and V indicates the input voltage. B. Graphical illustration of potentials recorded from electrodes having potentials e_1 to e_5 and connected to a common reference electrode with potential er. Channel deflections are represented by V_1 to V_5. (Adapted from Cooper et al, 1974.)*

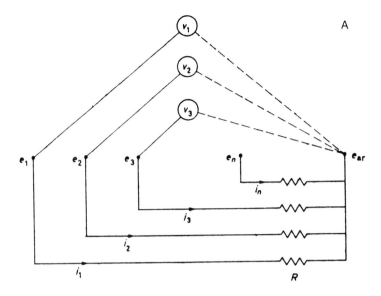

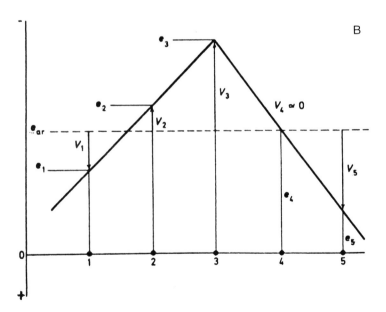

Figure 1.7 A. *Average reference derivation. Electrodes are connected through equal resistors to a single point which is then used as a common reference. The algebraic sum of currents (i) that flow through the resistors (R) and meet at e*ar *will be zero; the potential at this reference point will be the average of potentials recorded from electrodes e*₁ *to e*n. *B. Average reference derivation from electrodes having potentials e*₁ *to e*₅. *The potential distribution is the same as in Figure 1.5. The common average reference has a potential e*ar. *Channel deflections V*₁ *and V*₅ *are of opposite polarity to V*₂ *and V*₃. *(Adapted from Cooper et al, 1974.)*

In the average reference method all active electrodes are connected through resistors of equal value to a single point which is then used as a common reference and connected to the white leads (Figure 1.7 A). The potential at this point of convergence is an algebraic sum and tends towards zero. However, in practice, activity occurring at an appreciable proportion of the electrodes may be injected in reversed phase into 'inactive' channels; thus large amplitude potential changes, such as those associated with eye movements or blinking, tend to break through and appear in all channels (Osselton, 1966). This derivation is rarely used in EP work.

If a laboratory has an averaging computer with fewer than four channels it is all the more important that the restricted number of electrodes in use at any one time be placed in positions where responses will be optimally recorded. This requires knowledge of the form, maximal amplitude and distribution of the response and the use of a derivation which permits easy identification of components. Such knowledge should ideally be established by individual laboratories using their own standard stimulating and recording parameters.

When recording all types of evoked potentials, it is common practice to place electrodes at or near sites determined by the 10-20 system of electrode location. This system was originally designed to standardize placement of electrodes for recording EEGs and makes use of percentage distances (mostly 10 and 20%) to compensate for different head sizes and shapes. Locations are determined by measuring from nasion to inion along the anterior to posterior axis and from pre-auricular points, through the vertex, along the coronal axis (Figure 1.8). Further details on how to

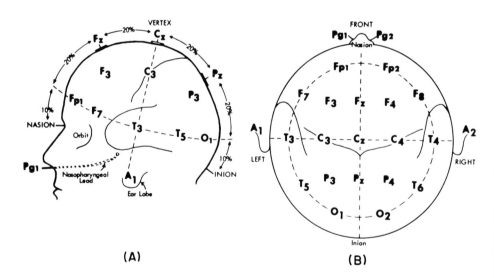

(A)   (B)

Figure 1.8 The 10-20 system of electrode placement is based on percentage distances from four standard points on the head: the nasion, inion, left and right pre-auricular points. In B the positions of electrodes relative to the Rolandic and Sylvian fissures are indicated. (From Stevens, 1974.)

arm length can be eliminated (Jones, 1977).
commonly recorded over cervical spinous p:
scalp an electrode sited 7 cm laterally on a li
vertex to the point immediately anterior to the
opposite to the stimulated hand is well placed
representation in the primary somatosenso
Cracco and Cracco, 1976; Matthews et al, I
Dawson, 1947a). Frontal or contralateral ea
appropriate reference sites for recording som;
al (1969) claim that electrodes at locations P_3
the contralateral earlobe, record all cerebral c
of their maximal scalp amplitude.

Following stimulation of the leg (usually
over the spine are recorded maximally at a
cervical levels, while scalp responses are best s
the lower limb just 1 cm contralateral to the
vertex (Jones and Small, 1978).

The slow potential shift preceding a mo\
around the vertex. The faster scalp potential
contraction (motor potentials) show some
tending to be largest over the contralate
components are also seen ipsilaterally and o
1980a). Thus, to adequately record most
movement, electrodes need to be spaced over
frontal locations at the level of F_z and over t
For hand movements C_3 and C_4 (10-20 sy
contralateral ear lobe or linked ears being a
Kornhuber and Deecke, 1964; Shibasaki et

Goff et al (1969) studied the spatial distrib
flash and found that early components (less t
the inion. Electrodes at O_1, O_z and O_2 (10-20 s
the side contralateral to the eye stimulated w
flash response. Later components were maxin
the pattern EP, however, it is our experience
locations and at the ear are not adequately sit
waveform and spatial distribution of the res

Using a 16° radius field and 50′ checks, th
is the sum of two asymmetric half-field respo
field stimulation, the characteristic prominei
the midline 5 cm above the inion for whole f
side ipsilateral to the half-field stimulus, be
while on the contralateral side there is a pos
between 50-200 msec which tends to be larg

In order to make the distribution clear a s
has been already mentioned, a common refer
for displaying the distribution of potentials a
a suitable site for a reference as it lies with

implement the system and a description of the relative positions of electrodes with respect to neuroanatomical structures are to be found in Jasper (1958) and Cooper et al (1974). A major problem with using the 10-20 electrode placements for recording evoked potentials is that the sites and spacing of electrodes are not optimal for displaying all types of responses. Picton et al (1978c) describe a modification of the 10-20 system which allows one to specify the positions of more closely spaced electrodes (Figure 1.9).

The use of differential amplifiers dictates that the difference between the electrical activity of two electrodes is measured. Consideration has therefore to be given to the siting of *both* electrodes. Some components of evoked potentials are discretely localized on the scalp while others can spread well beyond their presumed area of generation. Indeed, some types of evoked activity such as auditory and somatosensory subcortical potentials can be picked up throughout most of the body.

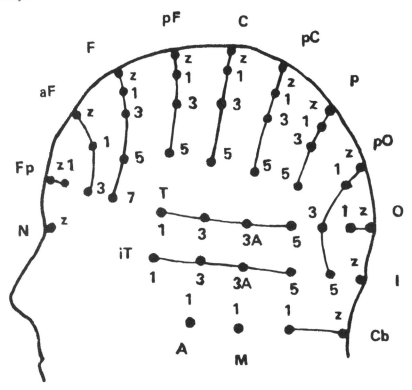

Figure 1.9 *Modificaton of the 10-20 electrode system suggested by Picton et al (1978c) which incorporates and permits specification of closer inter-electrode placements (2 to 4 cm) more appropriate to the recording of evoked potentials. Most additional electrodes are situated half-way between the standard 10-20 positions with new lines of electrodes over anterior frontal (aF), posterior frontal (pF), postcentral (pC), pre-occipital (pO) and inferior temporal (iT) areas. (From Picton et al, 1978c).*

Far-field and near-field record

Jewett and Williston (1971) i
far-field recording into neuroph;
the position of a recording ele
amplitude and waveform of the
many of the potentials generated
over an activated peripheral ner
brain and spinal cord can only
generator. The far-field potential
will only alter relatively little wit
field (of similar shape to the ma;
generation of most (probably all
the size, orientation and depth o
be picked up from electrodes
orientation of the generator in
important determinant of the fo
recorded by any electrode pa
relationship of the generator to
see Goff et al, 1978). The size ol
important determinant of what

Early (brainstem), middle la
potential all tend to be maxima
on topographic studies, Goff et
contralateral to stimulus deliv
components. However, the audi
mastoid ipsilateral to the stim
potentials, being recordable ov
however, subtle differences in t

Late potentials common to
msec), and later task-related co
shifts (e.g. the CNV) also tend
(C_z), frontal (F_z) and parietal (P
in their elicitation. Vertex to lin
potentials in general, primar
contaminate a record with eye
reference it is advisable to mal
impedances for, if not, the ac
impedance will predominate (I

Responses to electrical stir
near-field potentials at various
potentials elsewhere. Followin
sensory action potentials can b
the latter area, Erb's point (C
1977) are appropriate sites, an
marker from which to measure
evoked potentials. By this mea

midfrontal electrode is more apt, as can be seen from Figure 1.10. This figure clearly demonstrates that the relative sizes of ipsilateral and contralateral components to pattern stimulation of the right half-field are affected according to the ear which is being used as a reference. More disturbingly, a comparison of linked ear and

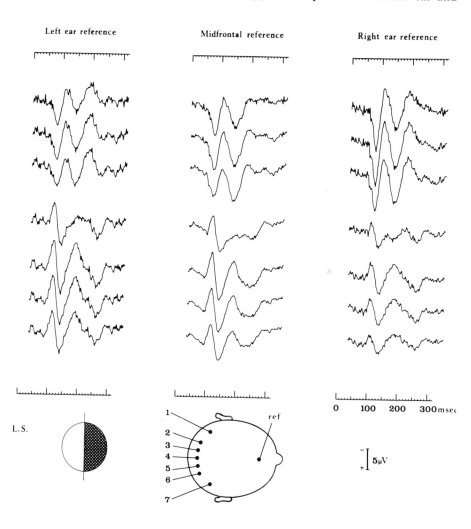

Figure 1.10 *Right half-field response to pattern stimulation recorded with three different references. Electrodes are placed 2.5 cm, 5 cm and 10 cm to the left and right of a midline electrode sited 5 cm above the inion. With the reference on the right ear, the amplitude of the prominent positive peak at 100 msec (and its accompanying negative waves), seen on the side of the head ipsilateral to the half-field stimulated, is greatly attenuated because this activity is also picked up by the reference electrode. Conversely, when the left ear reference is used, the positive-negative-positive complex of waves, on the side of the scalp contralateral to the half-field stimulated, is slightly attenuated, as this activity is picked up at the left ear. (From Halliday et al, 1979a.)*

arm length can be eliminated (Jones, 1977). Spinal and subcortical responses are commonly recorded over cervical spinous processes, Cv2 and Cv7, while on the scalp an electrode sited 7 cm laterally on a line joining a point 2.5 cm behind the vertex to the point immediately anterior to the external auditory meatus on the side opposite to the stimulated hand is well placed for recording activity from the hand representation in the primary somatosensory area of the cortex (Jones, 1977; Cracco and Cracco, 1976; Matthews et al, 1974; Halliday and Wakefield, 1963; Dawson, 1947a). Frontal or contralateral ear locations are found to be the most appropriate reference sites for recording somatosensory evoked potentials. Goff et al (1969) claim that electrodes at locations P_3 and P_4 of the 10-20 system, referred to the contralateral earlobe, record all cerebral components of the SEP to within 75% of their maximal scalp amplitude.

Following stimulation of the leg (usually popliteal or tibial nerves) responses over the spine are recorded maximally at around -T12 and to a lesser extent at cervical levels, while scalp responses are best seen over the cortical representation of the lower limb just 1 cm contralateral to the midline and 2.5 cm posterior to the vertex (Jones and Small, 1978).

The slow potential shift preceding a movement (readiness potential) is largest around the vertex. The faster scalp potentials preceding and following the muscle contraction (motor potentials) show some degree of somatotopic distribution tending to be largest over the contralateral Rolandic area, although some components are also seen ipsilaterally and over the frontal areas (Shibasaki et al, 1980a). Thus, to adequately record most scalp components associated with movement, electrodes need to be spaced over a fairly wide area including the vertex, frontal locations at the level of F_z and over the relevant motor and sensory areas. For hand movements C_3 and C_4 (10-20 system) are appropriate sites, with the contralateral ear lobe or linked ears being a suitable reference (Gilden et al, 1966; Kornhuber and Deecke, 1964; Shibasaki et al, 1980a).

Goff et al (1969) studied the spatial distribution of the visual evoked potential to flash and found that early components (less than 100 msec) were largest just above the inion. Electrodes at O_1, O_z and O_2 (10-20 system) referred to an ear electrode on the side contralateral to the eye stimulated were optimally placed for recording the flash response. Later components were maximal over parietal and central areas. For the pattern EP, however, it is our experience that electrodes at the 10-20 occipital locations and at the ear are not adequately sited for giving a full appreciation of the waveform and spatial distribution of the response to wide field stimulation.

Using a 16° radius field and 50' checks, the whole field pattern reversal response is the sum of two asymmetric half-field responses (Blumhardt et al, 1977). For half-field stimulation, the characteristic prominent positivity ($\overline{P100}$), seen maximally in the midline 5 cm above the inion for whole field stimulation, is distributed on the side ipsilateral to the half-field stimulus, being maximal 5 cm from the midline, while on the contralateral side there is a positive-negative-positive (PNP) complex between 50-200 msec which tends to be largest 10 cm from the midline.

In order to make the distribution clear a suitable montage has to be adopted. As has been already mentioned, a common reference derivation is the most appropriate for displaying the distribution of potentials across the scalp. However, the ear is not a suitable site for a reference as it lies within the spatial field of the response. A midfrontal electrode is more apt, as can be seen from Figure 1.10. This figure clearly demonstrates that the relative sizes of ipsilateral and contralateral components to pattern stimulation of the right half-field are affected according to the ear which is being used as a reference. More disturbingly, a comparison of linked ear and

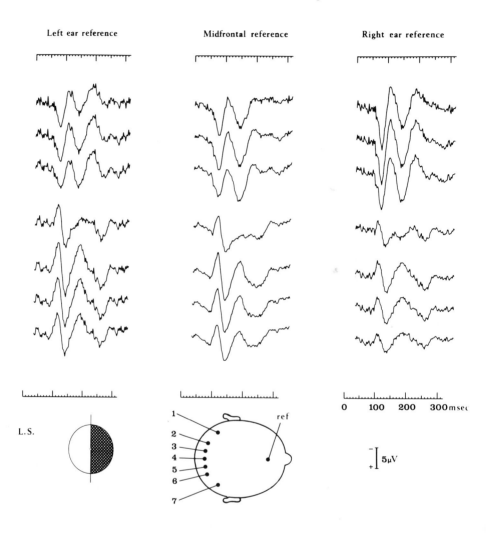

Figure 1.10 *Right half-field response to pattern stimulation recorded with three different references. Electrodes are placed 2.5 cm, 5 cm and 10 cm to the left and right of a midline electrode sited 5 cm above the inion. With the reference on the right ear, the amplitude of the prominent positive peak at 100 msec (and its accompanying negative waves), seen on the side of the head ipsilateral to the half-field stimulated, is greatly attenuated because this activity is also picked up by the reference electrode. Conversely, when the left ear reference is used, the positive-negative-positive complex of waves, on the side of the scalp contralateral to the half-field stimulated, is slightly attenuated, as this activity is picked up at the left ear. (From Halliday et al, 1979a.)*

midfrontal reference sites for stimulation of the upper field (Figure 1.11) may show differences in the polarity of a particular component which is attributable to the activity at the ear reference (Michael and Halliday, 1971).

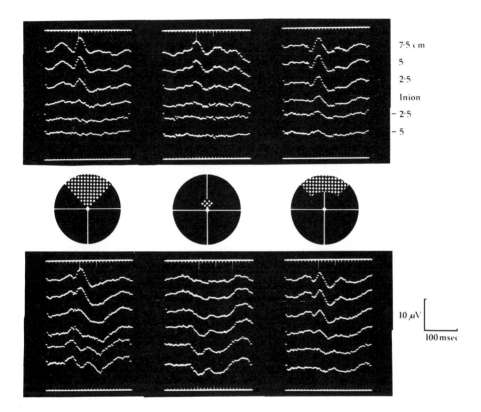

Figure 1.11 *Responses from the same subject to upper field stimuli recorded with a two-ear (above) and midfrontal reference (below). Comparing the two reference recordings, note differences in distribution and polarity for component at 100 msec following stimulation with small central stimulus. (From Michael and Halliday, 1971.)*

The apparent lateralization of left and right half-field responses can be reversed by using a bipolar montage or by the injudicious placement of lateralized references (Halliday et al, 1979a). Figure 1.12 compares common reference and bipolar records for stimulation of the left and right half fields. In the common reference record the prominent positive component ($\overline{P100}$) is seen on the side ipsilateral to the stimulus field and a small PNP complex is present on the contralateral side. In the bipolar record, which reflects changes in potential gradient, the ipsilateral channels show little or no response, while the midline to contralateral channel displays the largest response. The bipolar montage in this case apparently obscures the fact that there is a widespread response of large amplitude over the ipsilateral side of the head

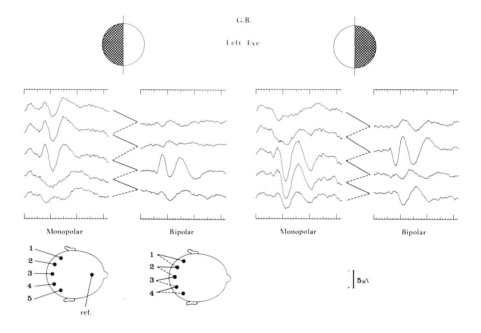

Figure 1.12 *Common reference and bipolar records for stimulation of the two half-fields for the left eye of one subject. In the common reference record the major positive component at 100 msec is seen in the midline and at the electrodes ipsilateral to the stimulated half-field, whereas the contralateral channels are relatively flat. In the bipolar record, which reflects voltage gradient, the ipsilateral channels show little or no response, whereas the midline-contralateral channel shows the maximum response. (From Barrett et al, 1976.)*

and a much smaller response of opposite polarity and more restricted distribution on the contralateral side. It emphasizes clearly, however, the region of maximum gradient between the zones of activity and relative inactivity, but without indicating which is which.

Figure 1.13 demonstrates the combined effects of positioning electrodes too near the midline and of employing lateralized references well within the potential field of the response. The upper row of records are taken from occipital electrodes with a 5 cm spacing referred to a common midfrontal reference, 12 cm above the nasion. These electrodes show an ipsilateral distribution for the $\overline{P100}$ and a contralateral PNP complex. When, as shown in the Figure, occipital electrodes are placed much nearer the midline, as in the left occipital (LO) and right occipital (RO) locations of the Modified Maudsley System (2 cm either side of the midline on a line 2 cm above the inion) and also in the slightly higher and more lateral 10-20 system locations (about 3.5 cm up and out from the inion), the lateralization of the ipsilateral $\overline{P100}$ is less clearly seen due to the spread of this positivity for a short distance across the midline. When the choice of an electrode site too near the midline is further compounded by the use of a reference location on the same side of

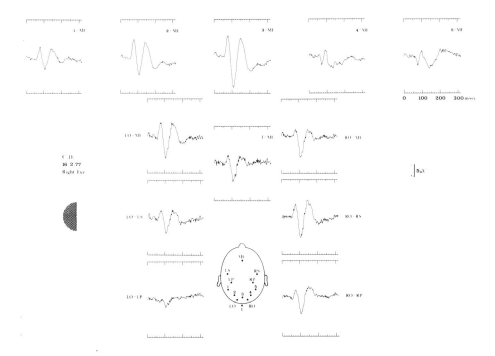

Figure 1.13 *Pattern response from the left half-field of a healthy subject recorded with different electrode montages. The upper five records are from a transverse row of five occipital electrodes, spaced at 5 cm, referred to a common midfrontal reference. Note the distribution of the NPN complex in the midline and ipsilateral channels and the smaller PNP complex seen at the two contralateral electrodes. The lower records are taken with the left occipital (LO) and right occipital (RO) electrode of the modified Maudsley montage referred (from above down) to a common midfrontal reference, to a Sylvian electrode on the same side of the head and to a parietal electrode on the same side of the head. Note that the NPN complex is seen for both channels with the midfrontal reference because the electrodes are only 2 cm from the midline. With the ipsilateral Sylvian or parietal reference the NPN complex is mislateralized, appearing larger in the contralateral channel. This is because the response is picked up and partially cancelled by the Sylvian and parietal reference on the left side of the head, but not on the right. (From Halliday et al, 1979a.)*

the head and within the potential field of the $\overline{\text{P100}}$, for example, in the Sylvian (S) or Parietal (P) areas, then the lateralization becomes apparently reversed. The $\overline{\text{P100}}$ is now smaller on the ipsilateral side because it is being picked up by both the occipital and reference electrode, while on the contralateral side the $\overline{\text{P100}}$ only affects the occipital electrode near the midline.

In general, common reference derivations are preferable because scalp potentials at different electrodes can be directly compared in a more obvious and easily comprehensible manner (Goff et al, 1969; Vaughan, 1969; Barrett et al, 1976). As has been mentioned, it is important to ensure that the site chosen for a reference electrode is the most appropriate with respect to (1) indifference to the evoked potential field and (2) freedom from other physiological potentials liable to introduce excessive interference. Depending on the response being evoked, locations favoured for the reference electrode include earlobe(s), mastoid(s), tip of nose, nasion, midfrontal (F_z), chin and laryngeal prominence (Adam's apple).

The electrical activity present at a reference electrode should be assessed by referring the electrode to other reference sites. An off-the-head location is probably the most appropriate for this purpose. Stephenson and Gibbs (1951) describe a cancellation technique to minimize the large ECG activity picked up by body electrodes. Two electrodes are employed, one over the right sternoclavicular junction and the other over the tip of the 7th cervical spine. Each of these electrode leads incorporates a variable 20 KΩ resistor and the leads are linked to form the body reference. The variable resistors are adjusted so that the ECG, which is of opposite polarity at each electrode, is cancelled out. Lehtonen and Koivikko (1970) employed this technique to study the activity of cephalic reference sites traditionally used to record evoked potentials. They found the earlobe to be very active for flash stimulation. The chin was a more appropriate site as it was less active. The earlobe, however, was an adequate reference location for both auditory and somatosensory stimulation. The effects of the ECG artifact can also be avoided by using the technique described by Jewett (1970a) in which an averaging computer is triggered during the periods between ECG complexes.

Bipolar derivations can be useful in particular instances, for example, to improve resolution of small amplitude components especially if they are associated with larger ones (e.g. Dawson, 1947a; Goff, 1974; Deecke and Kornhuber, 1977). Some investigators use a bipolar derivation to exploit the dipolar properties of some EP components. By this means components are enhanced and made more amenable to measurement (Jones, 1977; Jeffreys, 1977). It is preferable where possible to derive bipolar records from monopolar recordings so that both types of information are available. This can be done by subtracting channels sharing a reference either at the raw data stage, e.g. when using an instrumentation tape recorder, or from the averaged waveforms themselves, a facility which is available in many microprocessor-based averagers and can be readily programmed on a general purpose computer (e.g. Barrett et al, 1976).

There have been several descriptions of methods of displaying the spatial distribution of an evoked potential and its changes with time (Remond, 1964; Lehmann and Skrandies, 1978; Halliday et al, 1977a). These methods are not commonly used for routine clinical assessment as they are time-consuming and require relatively sophisticated computing facilities.

AMPLIFIERS

In order to use differential (recording) amplifiers competently it is necessary to be aware of design features which are important to their optimum performance.

Differential amplifiers are basically voltage multiplying devices. Their functional characteristics are normally specified in terms of the following parameters: input impedance, common mode rejection, sensitivity, gain, noise, frequency response and output impedance.

Input impedance

Efficient amplification requires that, as far as possible, the scalp voltage should be presented to the amplifier without attenuation. For this to occur the impedance of the amplifier input must be very much greater (in practice 100 times or more) than that between the electrodes feeding the amplifier. With an inter-electrode impedance of 10 KΩ and an input impedance of 1 MΩ an input signal is only attenuated by about 1%. Zablow and Goldensohn (1969) demonstrated distortions that could occur to the recorded signal if the input impedance was too low. When platinum needle electrodes with inter-electrode impedances of about 0.1 MΩ were used in conjunction with amplifiers of input impedance 0.6 MΩ signal frequencies of 1 Hz or less were significantly attenuated in comparison with the same frequencies recorded with lower impedance disc electrodes. Nowadays, commercially available biological amplifiers commonly have input impedances of 1 MΩ or more.

If electrostatic interference is particularly troublesome, as, for example, when recording in an Intensive Care Unit, or if the higher frequencies in the recorded signal are being attenuated due to capacitative loss from a long input cable, the quality of records can be improved by having short electrode leads and preamplifiers near the head or, better still, on the head itself (Apple and Burgess, 1976; Quy, 1978). With this system, the common arrangement of a low voltage EEG signal fed into a high input impedance becomes one of a moderate voltage signal from a source with low output impedance. With such an arrangement the signal is less likely to be significantly contaminated by extraneous interference and can be transmitted some distance without degradation.

Discrimination ratio or common-mode rejection ratio

This is an index expressing the effectiveness with which a differential amplifier discriminates between in-phase and out-of-phase signals presented to its two input leads. Modern amplifiers have a common mode rejection in the region of 10,000 to 1 (80 dB)*. This means that an in-phase signal has to be ten thousand times larger than an out-of-phase signal in order for both to be recorded as the same size. The ratio can change with signal frequency and it is useful to know not only what it is for the mains supply frequency, but also for slower and faster frequencies as well. In actual use electrode impedances must be low and well-matched as inequalities in the

---

* Measurements expressed in decibels are commonly used in electronic and sound engineering. Decibels express the logarithmic ratio between two values, one of which is a reference.

For intensity measures,

voltage or sound pressure:

$$dB = 20 \log_{10} \frac{\text{Measured value}}{\text{Reference value}}$$

size of the common mode voltage presented to the two input leads of an amplifier will produce an out-of-phase signal which will be amplified. Some manufacturers incorporate a differential balance control which permits fine adjustment of common mode rejection capabilities.

Sensitivity and gain

Sensitivity specifies the input voltage which gives a designated output voltage. In order to establish the useful working range of an amplifier one has to know both the minimum voltage which will produce a specified output voltage and the largest input voltage producing an undistorted (i.e. linear) output. For a given amplification (gain setting) the ratio between the smallest signal and the largest signal that can be accurately recorded should be of the order of 100 to 1 or better. It is now very common to standardize the magnitude of output voltages to within certain limits (e.g. IRIG standards*). To record evoked potentials the sensitivity of amplifiers is usually set so that 10-20 μV at the input gives an output of ±1 to 2 volts. Outputs of this size can readily be fed into averagers or tape recorders. The sensitivity control is normally continuously adjustable to permit fine setting and equalization of gain between different amplifiers.

The term 'gain' refers to the amount by which an input signal is enlarged. It is expressed as a ratio, usually in decibels, which indicates how many times larger the output is compared to the input. Gain controls, often called attenuators, are normally adjustable in predetermined steps. The most common change per step is 2 or 1.4:1 (3 dB), so that adjustment by two steps (6 dB) results in halving or doubling the size of the signal, as the case may be. For routine use it is best for the gain control to be near the middle of its range so that a signal may be either enhanced or attenuated when required.

Amplifiers must be operated well within their linear range and this depends on the judicious use of gain controls. If an excessively large voltage is applied to the input on too high a gain setting the amplifier will be driven beyond this range into non-linearity and the desired signals will be distorted or obliterated. For a sine wave input, for example, the peaks at the output will be attenuated or may even be flattened (clipped). It is possible to distort the peaks of only one polarity if the signal is biased with a standing potential. An extremely large standing potential, as, for example, the difference between electrode potentials which an AC amplifier encounters on first switching to the record position, will bias the amplifier beyond its operating range and no signals will be recorded. The amplifier is then said to be 'blocked'. It is important to allow sufficient time for a blocked amplifier to return to its linear stage before proceeding to record.

Noise

Amplifiers themselves can generate small random voltage fluctuations, called noise, which can be assessed when there is no input signal and the amplifier inputs

---

* IRIG = The American Inter-Range Instrumentation Group Telemetry Standards (1969).

are cross-connected (i.e. shorted and earthed). Electronic components give rise to noise mainly by two effects. The first is due to thermal agitation of electrons in resistive components (Johnsonian noise). The second is as a result of current flowing through components. In resistive components current noise is directly related to the amount of current passing and inversely proportional to its frequency. In addition, there is also a type of noise consisting of intermittent bursts of larger short duration pulses. Noise is usually specified in terms of an equivalent input voltage (rms or peak voltage*). This is obtained by dividing the size of the noise at the output by the amplifier gain. In practice, noise levels of 1-2 µV are achievable. Discrimination of the evoked potential from amplifier noise is helped by the method of averaging and can be further assisted by restricting the recorded frequencies only to those necessary for faithful reproduction of the desired response. High quality, low noise transistors and resistors should always be used in the initial amplifying stages in order to ensure that noise levels at these critical stages are kept to a minimum.

Instability during recording, and mains frequency interference arising from within an amplifier, can be included under the broader definition of amplifier noise. Only properly designed and carefully built circuits will overcome these deficiencies. Dirty switch contacts on amplifier controls (e.g. attenuators) can also be a cause of noise, particularly where switches have been left in the same position over long periods. This noise problem can often be remedied simply by working the switch several times and/or by careful application of switch cleaning fluid.

Frequency response

An evoked potential may be thought of as a number of peaks or components having various durations. The durations may be thought of as representing, to a rough approximation, the period of one cycle of a sine wave and may be expressed as a corresponding frequency.

Thus
$$\frac{1000}{\text{Period in milliseconds}} = \text{Frequency in c/sec or Hz}$$

Amplifiers should enlarge equally all the composite frequencies which make up the evoked potential being recorded.

In Direct Current (DC) amplifiers the various stages of amplification are directly linked with each other and both sustained and fluctuating potentials are enhanced. Thus these amplifiers are generally favoured for recording the slow event-related shifts in steady potential (e.g. CNV). Alternating current (AC) amplifiers have capacitors coupling each stage of amplification. These capacitors block off large unwanted standing potentials of physiological origin or arising from the recording equipment itself and thus minimize signal distortion due to amplifiers being driven off their linear range.

Amplifiers normally incorporate filter controls which alter the upper and lower limit of their frequency range. The spectrum of frequencies which are freely

---

* The magnitude of alternating signals is commonly described in terms of either root mean square or peak voltage. For a sinusoidal waveform the rms value is 0.707 of the baseline to peak value.

amplified is called the bandpass or bandwidth. Adjustment of the bandwidth may be necessary to minimize the effect of undesirable potentials, such as those arising from amplifier noise, extraneous interference and physiological potentials not generated by the brain. The lower frequency limit of a selected bandwidth is determined by what is normally called the low frequency setting or time-constant, while the upper end is specified by the high frequency setting. Rather confusingly, a few investigators and manufacturers use an apparently converse nomenclature referring to the low frequency filter as the high *pass* filter, as it passes frequencies above that specified and by similar reasoning the high frequency filter is called the low *pass* filter.

Filters do not abruptly exclude frequencies beyond their demarcated limits. Instead, they progressively attenuate them, starting well before the cut-off points. A cut-off point is the frequency at which there is predefined attenuation with respect to the maximal amplitude of frequencies passed (expressed as a percentage or decibel ratio). Thus at the frequency specified as being the -3 dB point the amount of attenuation is such as to be 70.7% of the maximal (i.e. unattenuated) amplitude (e.g. Figure 1.14 A). Other commonly quoted cut off points are 80% (-2 dB voltage attenuation) and 50% (-6 dB voltage attenuation). The term roll-off is used to specify the rate of amplitude decline with respect to frequency. Attenuating characteristics tend to be asymptotic in shape and the rate of attenuation is described in terms of decibels per octave. A common figure, which is characteristic of a single capacitance-resistance filter, is 6 dB per octave, which represents a 50% decrease in amplitude of the input frequency for every doubling or halving of frequency at the upper or lower end of the bandwidth, respectively. With more complex filter designs steeper rates of attenuation can be obtained (see Figure 1.14).

In addition to filter controls for attenuating high and low frequencies at the extremes, many amplifiers have a 'notch filter' which is specifically designed to reduce a particular frequency, e.g. mains frequency interference (50 Hz in Europe, 60 Hz in U.S.A.) or the frequency of a hospital paging system, while frequencies above and below this are allowed to pass. The roll-off of notch filters is usually much steeper than those of filters controlling the high and low frequency limits.

An effect of filters, which has important repercussions for the recording of evoked potentials, is that they alter the time (i.e. phase) relationship between the input and output of attenuated frequencies. As a rule, the greater the attenuation, the greater the phase-shift. Thus, if a selected bandpass is restricted too much, it is possible to distort an evoked potential by altering the relative amplitudes and latencies of short and long duration components.

The effect of using inappropriate filter settings has been lucidly illustrated by Goff (1974) and Desmedt (Desmedt et al 1974, Desmedt 1977b). Figure 1.14 shows comparisons of the cortical somatosensory evoked potential recorded with high frequency filter settings at 3 KHz and 100 Hz (-3 dB cut off points). For the upper pair of traces (B) the filter roll-off was 6 dB/octave, while for the lower traces (C) it was much steeper, being 24 dB/octave. Although the 100 Hz filter gives a smoother trace it attenuates and increases the latency of components, the effect being more marked with a roll-off of 24 dB/octave.

The frequency response of amplifiers has to be selected with due consideration to the duration or frequency of components of the evoked potential to be recorded.

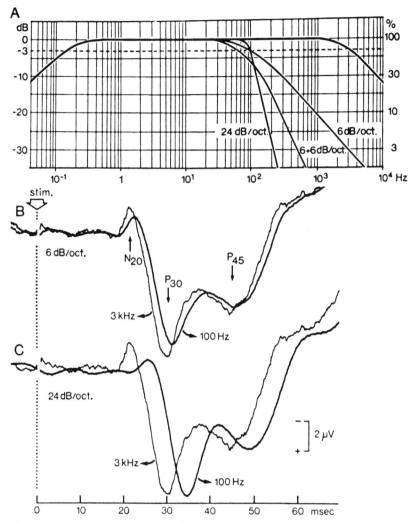

Figure 1.14 *Effect of analogue high frequency filters on the somatosensory evoked potential (SEP). A. Graphical representation of amplifier bandpass as obtained with sinusoidal test signals. Abscissa, frequency of test signal. Ordinate, signal attenuation expressed in dB (left) and as percentage (right) of the unattenuated (i.e. flat) portion of graph. The dotted horizontal line indicates an attenuation of -3 dB or 30% below maximum. The full line showing the most extensive flat response is the bandpass recommended for recording average SEPs in man. In addition the effects of 3 different high frequency filters set to attenuate from about 100 Hz; these are a single resistance-capacitance (RC) filter circuit with 6 dB/octave roll off, two such circuits in series (6 + 6 dB/octave) and the effects of an active Butterworth filter with much sharper roll off (24 dB/octave). Figures B and C present identical SEP data which have been averaged with the wide bandpass or with a frequency cut off at 100 Hz with either 6 or 24 dB/octave roll-off (thicker traces). Note reduction in size of early* $\overline{N20}$ *component and severe phase shift distortion of* $\overline{N20}$, $\overline{P30}$ *and* $\overline{P45}$ *components. (From Desmedt, 1977b.)*

As a guideline, it is best to have generous high and low filter settings with cut-off points at more than half or twice the frequency of components with the shortest and longest duration, respectively.

Many of the disadvantages of the commonly used analogue filters incorporated into amplifiers can be avoided by using a suitably programmed computer to digitally filter the averaged responses. Digital filtering techniques have been devised which do not introduce distortions of phase (latency) of EP components (Dawson and Doddington, 1973; Wastell, 1979; Boston and Ainslie, 1980).

A calibration unit delivering square waves of known voltage and duration is an essential ancillary to recording amplifiers, as its signal serves as a means of routinely checking the relative sensitivity of amplifier and averager channels. Square waves are also useful for gauging the performance of high and low frequency filters, as their sharp rising and falling edges are affected by high frequency filters while the low frequency filters alter the shape of the upper and lower levels following the rising and falling edges (Figure 1.15).

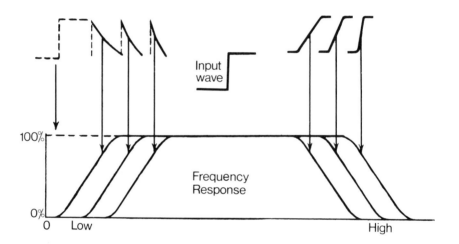

Figure 1.15 *Effect of amplifier filters on the reproduction of a square wave. High frequency filtering will alter the duration of the initial leading edge (as indicated to the right of the Figure), while low frequency filters affect the time taken for the initial deflection to return to the baseline (as indicated to the left of the Figure). (From Geddes and Baker, 1968).*

Output impedance and DC level

Efficient transfer of a signal voltage from an amplifier to another device, such as an averager or tape recorder, requires the output impedance of the amplifier to be low relative to the input impedance of the device receiving the signal. Due consideration has also to be given to the electrical properties of cables connecting different devices. If the output impedance of the amplifier is too high and there is excessive capacitative loss from connecting cables, part of the output voltage will be shunted to earth with consequent distortion (attenuation and loss of high frequency components) of the transmitted signal.

In general, commercial devices are designed to have high input impedances (more than 1 MΩ) and low output impedances (less than 1 KΩ) so that interfacing of equipment is usually accomplished without problems. Care must be taken, however, when connecting an amplifier in parallel to two or more devices with different input impedances. Although each may have a high input impedance with respect to the amplifier output, when connected in parallel the lower impedance device(s) may take a disproportionate amount of the output current resulting in a relative attenuation of the signal fed to the higher impedance device(s). By comparing the relative sizes of calibration signals fed to devices connected in parallel problems of this nature can be readily detected.

The output of amplifiers may have an unwanted DC bias and it is usual to have a variable resistor within the amplifier which enables this output DC level to be adjusted or zeroed.

ANALYSIS AND STORAGE

Averaging

Sensory evoked potentials are generally a fraction of the size of the spontaneous EEG activity (1/5th to 1/100th). Dawson was the first to introduce methods of extracting evoked potentials from the background EEG, initially by means of photographic superimposition (1947a), and later by the technique of averaging (1951, 1954a). The essence of both methods is to systematically reinforce the common features in the scalp potential changes occurring immediately after each of a series of stimuli. The enhanced response stands out well against the random changes of the background activity.

Dawson's first averager was an electromechanical analogue computer which sampled the magnitude of the input voltage at regular predetermined intervals after the stimulus. A rotary switch driven by an electrical motor was used to distribute the information sequentially to a memory consisting of a bank of capacitors. Successive responses added to the charge of the capacitors.

With the development of small digital computers it became technologically more convenient to analyze the input data digitally and store it in magnetic core memory. Digital averagers enormously increased the versatility and flexibility of the averaging technique with regard to such things as variation in sampling rate and data manipulation. Both purpose-built and general purpose digital computers are now universally used for averaging evoked potentials.

In digital averaging the EEG activity of a single channel is sampled sequentially by an analogue-to-digital converter and the amplitude information is stored in the computer memory as a binary number. The input data is thus represented by a series of sampling points or ordinates and the voltage value of each point is stored in a particular location (address) in memory (Figure 1.16). If several channels are averaged at once, the usual way of handling the analysis is for the data to be

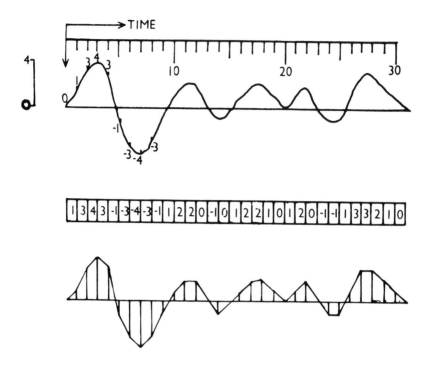

Figure 1.16 *Sampling of EEG activity. The amplitude of the EEG occurring immediately after a stimulus is sampled and measured at regular intervals and the amplitude value is stored as a number (in binary form). The original signal can be reproduced from the numbers (lower trace). (From Cooper, 1975.)*

multiplexed; i.e. at each sampling interval the input of each channel is measured sequentially by the analogue-to-digital converter. At least 8 bits, representing a measuring accuracy of 2^8 voltage (256) levels, are needed for adequate amplitude resolution of the input signal. An 8-10 bit ADC is commonly provided in commercial averagers. The sampled wave can be reconstructed accurately from the digital representation by reading out the stored amplitude values, converting them back to analogue form, and plotting or displaying them.

Figure 1.17 illustrates three records of scalp activity and their numerical representation. The result of summing and averaging these records is shown at the bottom. Some computers give a true average at the end of an averaging run, while others, though still commonly called averagers, simply provide the running sum. By adding many individual responses, called trials, the resulting evoked potential (signal) is rendered clearly discernible from the continuous, random background activity (noise). In fact, the improvement in the signal-to-noise ratio is closely proportional to the square root of the number of added trials. For sporadic transient noise the improvement is greater, being reduced by a factor equal to the number of trials (Cooper et al, 1974). Figure 1.18 shows the enhancement achieved with increasing number of trials for the visual response to pattern reversal

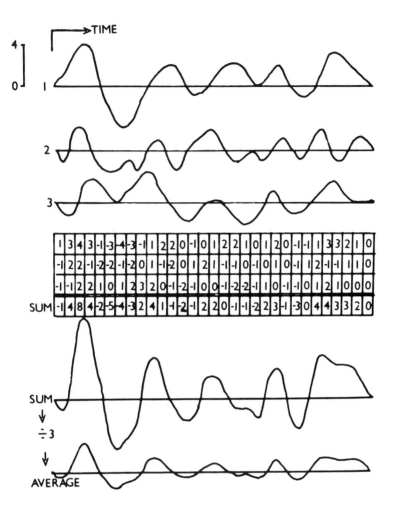

Figure 1.17 *Summation and average of three samples of activity. The amplitudes of the signal are sampled, stored as binary numbers and summated. The lower traces show the sum and average of the sampled activities. (From Cooper, 1975.)*

stimulation. Two features are to be noted. Firstly, the response stays about the same size, while the accompanying noise progressively decreases with increasing trial number (left hand column). Secondly, noise attenuation is greatest at the beginning of the averaging run and a progressively larger number of trials are needed to improve the signal-to-noise ratio by the same proportion.

In practice, under favourable recording conditions between about 10 to several hundred trials are necessary for satisfactory recording of larger (10-50 μV) evoked potentials, such as slow potential shifts (CNV, $\overline{P300}$, etc.) or the visual response, while for the very small (1 μV or less) subcortical potentials evoked from the auditory and somatosensory modalities many hundreds or thousands of trials may

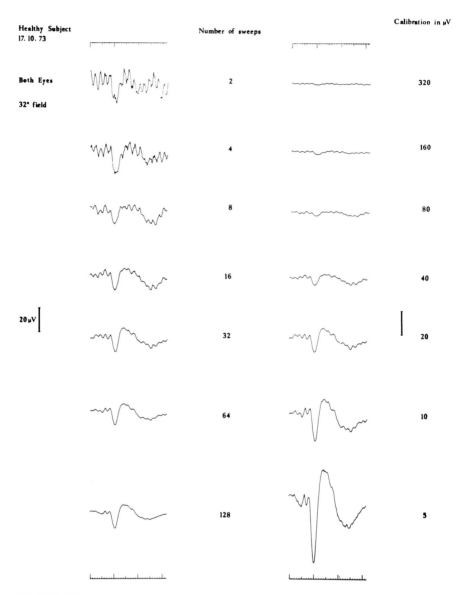

Healthy Subject
17. 10. 73

Number of sweeps

Calibration in μV

Both Eyes

32° field

2

320

4

160

8

80

16

40

20 μV

32

20

64

10

128

5

Midoccipital - Midfrontal

Figure 1.18 *Averaging has the effect of reducing the background noise level (left hand column) or increasing the size of the recorded response (right hand column). The records illustrate the effect of adding together an increasing number of responses evoked by a reversing checkerboard pattern in a healthy individual (number of inputs indicated in the central column), displayed either as a running average (left hand records) or a running sum (right hand records). The average can be obtained from the running sum by adjusting the calibration for the number of inputs, as shown on the right. (From Halliday, 1978a.)*

be needed. Care must be taken to match the sensitivity of the amplifiers to the working range of the ADC at the input of the averager. If the sensitivity is set too low, the signal may fall below the resolving power of the two smallest steps in the input ADC (see Picton and Hink, 1974). Although added noise may help to overcome this problem, there will nonetheless be a danger of reducing the apparent response size in the final average. The signal level should ideally be well within the resolving power of the ADC (e.g. at least twice the smallest step of the ADC).

Purpose-built averagers are usually designed to accept one to four channels of EEG data into a memory containing 1024 addresses (1K memory). All their functions are pre-programmed and alterations to averaging requirements are usually made by means of switches. Sampling rate (i.e. ordinates per millisecond) and number of sample points per channel are normally limited by the number of input channels selected and the duration over which the input signal is to be analyzed (sweep time or window time). For a given sweep time increasing the number of input channels reduces the number of sampled points per channel. It may be necessary in certain circumstances, therefore, to decrease the number of channels to obtain an adequate number of ordinates per channel for satisfactory resolution of the response.

As has been mentioned, the high frequency filter setting of recording amplifiers must be selected with due consideration to the highest frequency present in the evoked potential. The sampling rate of the averager should be governed by the highest frequency likely to be present in the input signal and the accuracy with which it is desired to measure the latency of the recorded waveform. It can be shown that more than two samples are needed to define a sine wave of given frequency. Thus the minimum sampling rate should be more than twice the highest frequency present in the input signal (Nyquist criterion) (see Bendat and Piersol, 1971). If the sampling rate is too low the faster frequencies in the input will not be faithfully represented and undetected distortions, called aliasing errors, can occur. Figure 1.19 shows an example of aliasing where a 40 Hz signal appears as 10 Hz. To be on the safe side, frequencies greater than one quarter the analogue-to-digital conversion rate should be filtered out of the input signal (Picton and Hink, 1974). An anti-aliasing filter of sharper roll-off than the high frequency filter of the recording amplifier may be inserted between amplifier and analogue-to-digital converter in order to further limit the higher frequencies in the input and thus minimize aliasing problems. However, with such an arrangement compensation may have to be made for time-lags introduced by the filter (Buchsbaum and Coppola, 1974).

General purpose computers designed for laboratory use offer greater computing power and larger memories (usually more than 16 K) so that 16 channels or more may be averaged at once. A variety of peripheral devices can be interfaced to the computer to add to its versatility. These include cathode ray displays, teletypes, teleprinters, graphic plotting devices (X-Y plotter or line printer) and magnetic storage media such as tape (industry compatible reels, cartridge or cassette) or disks (fixed head, cartridge or 'floppy' diskette) which will permit bulk storage of digital information at the time it is being acquired (i.e. on-line storage).

A general purpose computer's flexibility is achieved through programming. Programs are usually written by individual users to their own requirements. This,

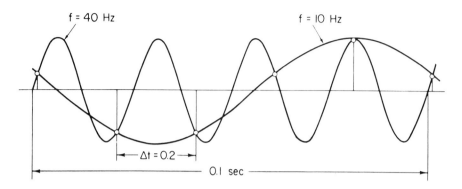

Figure 1.19 *'Aliasing' of a 40 Hz waveform as a 10 Hz fluctuation, due to the use of a sampling rate (50 Hz) less than twice the frequency of the true signal. (From Vaughan, 1974.)*

however, can be time-consuming for the inexperienced, especially if written in machine language. In many cases it is possible to utilize programs developed by other users of the same machine. The computer manufacturer or 'software houses' may also be able to provide a variety of routine laboratory programs, though usually at a price and perhaps not to the full requirements of the buyer. Ideally, averaging programs should offer flexibility in selecting number of channels and sweep duration. Desirable additional features may include display of the input EEG during averaging, rejection of trials in which large voltage artifacts occur, and an assessment of amplitude variability within an averaging run. Programs for manipulating the averaged data can include compensation for interchannel differences in gain and DC levels, digital filtering of high and low frequencies, and addition and subtraction of waveforms. The latter facility can be used, for instance, to make bipolar derivations from a monopolar montage. Measurement of response components may be carried out under operator control or, alternatively, programming techniques are available which will automatically label peaks and measure their amplitude and latency. With larger machines sophisticated statistical techniques may be employed which will identify principal components or show which parts of the response can best discriminate between given experimental or clinical conditions. Alternative forms of analysis, such as Wiener filtering (e.g. see Ungan and Basar, 1976), template matching and Fourier analysis, can also be effected (see Chapter 15). Lastly, a general purpose computer is ideally suited for programming complicated sequences of stimulus delivery and for controlling by means of relays the operation of other pieces of equipment.

Recently, manufacturers of special purpose averagers have adopted a modular design in their equipment and have started to incorporate microprocessors. This has greatly increased their versatility and has made the distinction between general purpose computers and special purpose averagers nebulous. Microprocessor-based averagers usually include features such as artifact rejection, addition and subtraction of waveforms and peak measurements. Many may incorporate storage of data on magnetic media or offer an interface connection for storage devices. Some of these special purpose averagers even permit limited operator programming to cater for more sophisticated analysis and manipulation of data as well as microprocessor control of amplifier and stimulator settings. There is little difference in price between general purpose laboratory computers and fully equipped microprocessor based averagers. The choice of system must therefore depend on individual requirements and the availability of programming expertise. As far as routine clinical use is concerned, microprocessor-based devices offer ease of operation with little or no need to develop programs. Further sophistication in processing is usually obtained by adding plug-in modules. From the research point of view, general purpose computers offer greater computing power and adaptability.

Interfacing

As has been mentioned the power and adaptability of both general purpose computers and microprocessor-based averagers can be extended by interfacing them with peripheral devices. Although interfaces are usually standard on general purpose computers, they are by no means common on processor-based averagers. This can be an important consideration when buying equipment, particularly if data is to be transferred to a central computer for analysis. Generally, the interfacing for large magnetic tape drives, analogue-to-digital converters and disc drives is provided by the manufacturer of these devices. Other types of peripheral equipment can also be interfaced using one of several electronic standards of interfacing. It is well worth deciding which of these standards to adopt when setting up a laboratory.

The common interface standards for information exchange encountered in laboratory peripherals are 20 mA loop, EIA RS232C for serial transmission of data and the IEEE488 for parallel transmission. Physically, interfaces comprise a plug and socket with five or more pins connected to wires which carry the information being transferred. International standards define the function for each pin connection. These functions operate at low voltage logic levels and include signals for initiating the transfer of information as well as carrying the information itself. The coding of the transmitted information depends on the complexity of the device being driven; a simple X-Y plotter only requires signals for pen movement and drum movement whereas a teletypewriter needs codes defining printable and control characters. The teletypewriter is a typical example of a serial device, i.e. data is transferred bit by bit. The rates of transfer can vary from 100 bits/second to 9600 bits/second and faster. For keyboard printers, dividing the bit rate by 10 gives the approximate number of characters that can be printed in a second. The most common rate for serial printers is 30 characters per second although faster rates are possible. The most common communication code is ASCII (American Standard Code for Information Interchange) in which seven bits define the character being transferred, an eighth bit is a parity check and two further bits indicate the beginning and end of a transmitted character. With seven-character bits it is possible to define 128 different combinations each corresponding to a unique character in the ASCII code. The first 32 of these codes are control characters used for such operations as line feed and carriage return on a teletypewriter or setting a cassette or floppy disc drive to record or play back. The next 64 codes are the standard upper case characters, numbers and symbols. The next 31 characters are lower case alphabet and further special characters. The final character has all bits set to one and is defined as the rub-out code. Manufacturers of peripheral equipment are incorporating sufficient intelligence to allow their devices to be driven entirely by ASCII characters. Cassette and floppy disc units, graphics displays and plotters can all be interfaced to the same computer or averager. Thus, even if only a single standard interface port is available a user can display waveforms, plot them and store them permanently on a magnetic medium.

Measurement and write-out

Square-wave calibration pulses are commonly used for determining the amplitude of evoked potentials. The calibration signal can be added to each trial by having the EEG input pass through the secondary winding of a suitable transformer while a correctly synchronized pulse of apropriate size and shape is applied to the primary winding. The calibration pulse is inserted at the beginning or end of the sweep time, where it does not impinge on the response. It is thus averaged for the same number of trials, and ostensibly for the same conditions of background 'noise', as the evoked potential (Emde, 1964; Lindley and Harding, 1974). Disadvantages of this method are (1) that the calibration is not clearly delineated due to its mixing with the background EEG activity and (2) that the presence of the pulse precludes Fourier or correlation analysis of waveforms. An alternative and more widely used approach is to separately average calibration signals for the same number of trials as used for the response. Calibration units are usually incorporated into commercial amplifiers, but, if not, purpose-built units may be purchased.

The simplest and most commonly used method for measuring evoked potentials is to visually identify and measure the timing (latency) and amplitude of particular components according to empirical or pragmatic criteria. In healthy subjects components are usually readily identified by their latency and configuration. In disease, however, responses are often degraded and component identification is made difficult. In such cases strategies which may prove helpful include: studying the scalp distribution of the response (Blumhardt et al, 1978), enhancing particular components by altering stimulation rates (Don et al, 1977; Stockard et al, 1978) and adopting a more favourable montage (Jones, 1977; Jeffreys, 1977). The latency of a component is normally taken as the time, in milliseconds, from the moment the stimulus trigger is delivered to a peak or trough, or less commonly the onset, of a component. The amplitudes of the various peaks in a response may be measured either with respect to the preceding peak of opposite polarity or to a baseline. The baseline is usually taken as the mean amplitude of a portion of the record occurring either shortly before or just after the stimulus (but before the onset of the response). A disadvantage of this technique is that the relationship between peaks and baseline may not always be the same. A component of constant polarity and latency can 'ride' on a neighbouring component or on a slow potential change, which will then alter its amplitude and even polarity with respect to the baseline. This effect is not usually a problem with peak-to-peak measurement, as the amplitude relationship between peaks will usually be maintained in this situation. However, if some components are specifically altered in amplitude by a particular stimulus or task, measurement with respect to a baseline may be more accurate than that between peaks. In experimental situations the two methods should be considered as complementary. For routine clinical applications peak-to-peak measurement offers the advantage of being more easily implemented. Woods et al (1980) have measured slow potentials ($\overline{P300}$) with respect to a sloping baseline derived from the mean response shortly before and after the stimulus.

Averaging devices usually display the analyzed data on a cathode ray screen, enabling an immediate visual assessment of each response to be made. It is almost always advisable to obtain a paper copy (i.e. hard copy) of all responses so that these can be stored for future reference. This may be done by photographing the screen with a Polaroid camera or, more usually, by writing-out the responses using an analogue or digital X-Y plotter. Other devices which may be used include electrostatic copiers, chart recorders using ultra-violet light-sensitive paper, ink writers (e.g. EEG machines), line printers and teletypes. Where a device involves the contact of a pen on paper, it is important to ensure that there is not excessive friction between the two which could result in smearing out of the higher frequencies present in the record. Whatever the write-out medium may be, a time-scale should be provided and the scale of the response should be such as to permit ready identification of components and, if necessary, accurate manual measurement of latency and amplitude. Picton and Hink (1174) suggest the height of an EP be approximately 62% of its width (the 'golden ratio' of Greek aesthetics).

Keeping records

Permanent storage of averaged waveforms on magnetic media is a great advantage, as it permits further manipulation and analysis of data for either planned or unforseen reasons. If possible, information about the patient, recording settings and stimulus parameters should also be included with the waveforms. This facility is now being incorporated in microprocessor based averagers. Large capacity storage devices, such as industry-compatible magnetic tape or cartridge discs, are expensive, but offer the advantage of keeping a lot of data together. On a more modest scale, but offering faster retrieval times than their larger counterparts, are cassette tapes and diskettes (floppy discs). A more cumbersome method is to store waveforms on punched paper-tape. An alternative is to keep the raw EEG and trigger pulses on magnetic tape. This will permit re-averaging of the data using different sweep times and also allows assessment of any evoked potential/EEG relationships.

Paper copies of the responses for each patient can be conveniently kept in folders or envelopes and stored alphabetically in cupboards, filing cabinets or on shelves. With each record there should be details about the patient, including his relevant medical history, the measured values of his EPs and a report of the findings. For rapid reference it is useful also to keep copies of reports separately and to have a record book with entries in chronological order which include a summary of the more important identifying details such as recording date, patient's name, sex, age, hospital number, referring physician, diagnosis and, if relevant, where a record may be found on stored media. It may also be helpful to code each entry and/or record in terms of diagnosis, stimulating procedures and results. This will permit cross-referencing and facilitate retrieval of particular groups of records as well as helping to give a statistical assessment of the department's work-load.

2

Stimulating Techniques and Recording Problems

A. Kriss

STIMULATION

Introduction

Both the physical and temporal features of a stimulus are important in determining the form, size, timing and scalp distribution of the response it evokes. It is vital, therefore, to carefully measure and control stimulus parameters, and to be aware of the evoked potential changes associated with variations in any particular parameter.

As differing stimulating and recording conditions have subtle effects on responses it is important not to rely on the published data from other laboratories when determining the limits of normality. Each laboratory should perform its own 'biological calibration'. This is done by recording from healthy control subjects employing the stimulus and recording parameters selected for routine use. It should be noted that evoked potentials may change with age (Dustman and Beck, 1969; Lueders, 1970; Celesia and Daly, 1977a; Klorman et al, 1978; Shaw and Cant, 1980) and that there are statistically significant differences between the responses of adult males and females (Stockard et al, 1978; Stockard et al, 1979; Michaelewski et al, 1980; Halliday et al, 1982a). In view of this, equal numbers of normal subjects of each sex (for statistical soundness at least 10) should be recorded in the young, middle age and older (over 60) adult age groups. A laboratory mainly concerned with recording from children will need larger representative sampling as children's responses are more variable and change rapidly with age (Ellingson et al, 1973).

In most contexts the mean latency ± more than, say 2.5 times the standard deviation can be used to set the statistical limits of normality for each group (see Chapter 5). There are some EPs, however, for which this type of measure is inappropriate, as its assumption of a normal distribution is not met. An instance of this is the amplitude measurements for components of the auditory brainstem response (BAEP). Between-subject amplitude variability is usually too great to allow similar limits to be set for clinical purposes; however, within subject limits for differences between left and right sides of the body are very useful. Providing a sufficiently large sample of normal subjects is recorded (e.g. more than 20), it may be useful to use the smallest amplitude value of the normal data as the lowest acceptable limit of normal (Jones et al, 1980a; Carroll et al, 1980c).

Although most commercially available stimulating equipment both accepts and delivers single triggering pulses to operate averagers, etc, a 'master' timing device with triggering capability, e.g. a Digitimer, can be a very useful ancillary to any EP laboratory. This equipment permits several trigger pulses, accurately timed to within a millisecond or less, to be given simultaneously or at different intervals. It can also be used to deliver pulse trains for repetitive stimulation. When connecting trigger outputs to other equipment, it is always important to ensure that the voltage, duration and polarity of the trigger pulse meets the input requirements of the device being triggered.

Rates of stimulation

Both stimulus and response characteristics may be considered either as a function of time (time domain) or as a function of frequency (frequency domain). Transient stimuli, well separated in time, will elicit transient responses which may be envisaged as a combination of many components. As described already, these components are usually characterized by their size, polarity and latency, measured from the stimulus onset or offset, as the case may be. Averaging is an appropriate technique for analysing transient responses. When closely-spaced stimuli are repetitively presented in long trains, within certain frequency limits, the evoked response (steady state response) will also be a long train of identical repetitive waveforms, the characteristics of which are most appropriately described in terms of their size and temporal (phase) relationship to the stimuli in the train. For routine application, measurement of the change in response amplitude and phase with change in stimulus frequency is normally carried out. Frequency analysis provides an accurate means of doing this. In order to provide information regarding phase, both sine and cosine spectra must be computed (Fourier analysis).

Transient stimuli are usually administered against a basal level of no stimulation, whereas with steady state stimuli it is quite common to increase and/or decrease (i.e. modulate) stimulus intensity against a constant background level of pre-existing stimulation. With the latter type of stimuli, therefore, both the modulated maxima and minima, and the basal level, have to be controlled and specified.

For transient responses the inter-stimulus interval can have significant effects on the response. Transient responses need time to 'recover' and if responses are repeated just within their recovery period then the later, slower components will usually be attenuated. For slow potentials (e.g. CNV and $\overline{P300}$) inter-stimulus intervals of about 3 seconds are commonly used in order to avoid this effect. For visual stimulation 1 to 2 stimuli per second give satisfactory responses, while for short lasting subcortical potentials following auditory and somatosensory stimulation, rates of about 20/sec and 10/sec, respectively, can be used safely. As a guide, Picton and Hink (1974) suggest having interstimulus intervals of at least two, and preferably four, times the period of time in which the evoked potentials are occurring.

Some of the more common methods of stimulation will be described. At present, there is little or no agreement concerning standardization of stimulus parameters for investigating clinical or experimental problems and this is reflected in the substantial inter-laboratory variability for the flash and late auditory potentials reported by Aunon and Cantor (1977). Thus for a particular modality, the decision as to which method and parameters to employ must be based on such factors as the stimulating and analysing equipment which is available and an appraisal of the effectiveness of the various methods and parameters in bringing out pathological correlates.

Visual stimulation

Methods

In the 1960s most clinical studies concerned with the VEP used an unstructured flash (stroboscopic) stimulus delivered usually from a Xenon gas discharge tube. Nowadays, flash stimulation is chiefly favoured for eliciting evoked potentials from patients with very poor acuity and those unable or unwilling to fixate a stimulus. It is also the most common and effective means of eliciting the electroretinogram. Light-emitting diodes mounted on spectacles (Casler et al, 1973) or attached to contact lenses (Feinsod et al, 1975b) have been used to stimulate comatose patients. Among the disadvantages of standard photic stimulation are: the audible click concurrent with the light discharge, unreliable performance of the lamp at low ambient lighting levels and a decrease of light output at high flicker rates. From the clinical point of view a major drawback is that flash responses are very variable in waveform when comparing different subjects.

Sine wave modulated light generated by means of fluorescent tubes, glow modulator tubes or cathode ray displays has been used successfully by several investigators to evoke steady-state responses (Kamp et al, 1960; van der Tweel and Verduyn Lunel, 1965; Spekreijse, 1966; Regan, 1972a; Townsend, 1973).

A patterned flash stimulus obtained by placing a grid in front of the flash tube is reported to be more effective than unstructured flash in eliciting photo-convulsive responses from patients with photosensitive epilepsy (Jeavons et al, 1972).

At present there is much clinical interest in the use of pattern stimulation without any concomitant change in the overall mean luminance, primarily because this type of stimulus evokes transient responses which show great inter-subject similarity in waveform and latency. There is evidence that different neural systems may subserve responses to luminance and pattern, so that, unlike patterned flash stimuli, 'pure' pattern stimulation will avoid confounding the two types of responses.

When using pattern stimuli the following variables have to be carefully controlled (Arden et al, 1977a). (1) The shape of the pattern elements and their orientation can affect the response waveform (Spekreijse and Estevez, 1972). Regular patterns such as a checkerboard, a sine- or square-wave grating and an array of dots have all been used. For clinical purposes the checkerboard is preferred by most as it tends to evoke larger and clearer responses than other patterns (Spekreijse and Estevez, 1972). (2) The size and sharpness of the pattern elements can have a significant effect on both amplitude and latency. Element size is usually specified in terms of the angle it subtends at the eye. For checkerboard stimuli the angular size of one check is normally described. The most commonly used type of grating is that with a sinusoidal luminance profile. The term *spatial frequency* is used to describe the number of elements per unit width of the grating and is specified in terms of cycles per degree. A cycle is the distance between either luminance maxima or minima for the light or dark elements, respectively. (3) The size of the stimulus field, its shape and position in visual space with respect to the fixation spot affect the distribution of the pattern response (Blumhardt et al 1978, Jeffreys and Axford 1972a, 1972b). The size and position of the stimulus within the visual field are also best expressed in terms of visual angle and angular eccentricity from the fixation spot. (4) The luminance of the pattern is important. In general, response latency increases and amplitude decreases with decrease in stimulus intensity (Halliday et al, 1973b). (5) The contrast between pattern elements also has a significant effect. Low contrast responses are smaller and broader than those elicited from higher contrast patterns (Spekreijse et al, 1973). (6) The method of pattern presentation has to be carefully considered. Responses may be recorded to pattern onset, offset and reversal (Jeffreys, 1977; Spekreijse and Estevez, 1972; Kriss and Halliday, 1980). There are important differences in latency and distribution between onset on the one hand and offset and reversal on the other (Kriss and Halliday, 1980). (7) The timing of the stimulus is important. For pattern onset/offset the presentation rate and the duration of the two phases have been reported to alter response shape and size (Estevez and Spekreijse, 1974; Jeffreys, 1977; Barber and Galloway, 1979). For pattern reversal by movement the speed and duration of the movement critically affects the latency of the response (Halliday et al, 1973a).

Various types of equipment have been used to present pattern stimuli. From the point of view of clinical application the two most popular devices are the slide projector and screen and the television display. Both are commercially available. In the slide projector method, pattern reversal is usually effected by projecting the image of a patterned slide onto a translucent screen by way of a rotatable mirror placed at approximately 45° to the projector lens. The amplitude of the mirror displacement must be accurately controlled and the transducer should include mechanical and/or electronic means of damping the effects of inertia. The mirror movement time has to be standardized as this affects the latency of the response (Halliday et al, 1973a). By alternately projecting two complementary checkerboard slides by means of two projectors fitted with shutters, pattern reversal without movement can be effected; replacement of one slide by a neutral density filter giving the same mean luminance will provide pattern onset/offset stimulation (Halliday and Michael, 1970; Kriss and Halliday, 1980). However, with two projectors, difficulty may be experienced in accurately lining up the images, particularly if a large stimulus field is being used. Another problem with projectors is that with ageing the bulbs tend to alter in brightness (and to some extent in colour) and inconsistencies in the filament brightness can cause luminance differences across the stimulus field.

Domestic TV sets (electromagnetic tubes) are becoming popular as a means of presenting visual stimuli. They offer great flexibility and are easy to use. A wide range of patterns, field sizes and positions can be presented and changes in contrast and even colour can be accomplished at the touch of a switch. In addition it is possible to mix the stimulus pattern with a picture (e.g. derived from a video-cassette) such as a cartoon, thus helping to direct the patient's fixation towards the stimulus. This feature is very useful when testing children. Arden et al (1977b) and Spraker and Arnett (1977) describe checkerboard pattern generators for use with commercial TV sets. In general the luminance levels of television stimulators are lower than those obtained from projectors (about one tenth as bright). Studies which have compared the TV and projector methods have variously found that responses are very similar in waveform and latency (Stockard et al, 1979; Lowitzsch et al, 1980), that TV derived responses are slightly later and smaller (Galvin et al, 1980) or that the TV system gives responses which are more variable in latency (Bartl et al, 1978). With a TV stimulator it takes one cycle of the mains frequency to build up the whole picture. If the pattern change is always started at the same point of the cycle, mains interference is liable to be recorded (Hayward and Mills, 1980). To avoid this it is possible to have triggering randomly related to the mains cycle, i.e. the free-running mode, although this may produce some latency jitter in the response.

A variety of other techniques have also been used to generate pattern stimuli but mainly for research purposes. Oscilloscope (electrostatic) displays offer the same advantages as TV sets but tend to be smaller and less bright (Arden et al, 1977b). Maxwellian view stimulators are efficient at getting most of the light from the stimulus into the eye (Westheimer, 1966). The pattern is viewed through a lens which forms an image of the stimulus field within the pupil (Figure 2.1). An advantage of this method is that the amount of light falling on the retina is not influenced by changes in pupillary size. However, the equipment is complex to construct and requires the subject to use a bite-bar or a chin rest in order to ensure and maintain accurate alignment between eye and optical system (Regan, 1972a; Armington, 1974, 1980). Jeffreys (1977) uses a multi-field tachistoscope to alternate stimuli, while Spekreijse et al (1973) employ two mirrors with their surfaces silvered in a checkerboard pattern to provide transparent and reflecting elements which are independently illuminated by separate high quality fluorescent light sources. Other methods include the use of a matrix of light-emitting diodes (Evans et al, 1974; Purves and Low, 1976; Nilsson, 1978; Stockard et al, 1979), a fibre optic display (Spehlmann and Smathers, 1968) and a rotating polaroid film (Behrman et al, 1972; Regan, 1972a).

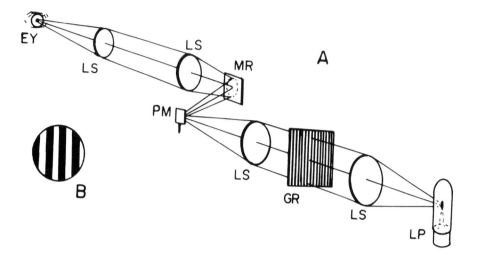

Figure 2.1 *A Maxwellian view stimulator is sketched in section A of this figure. Light from a lamp, LP, is delivered to the eye, EY, by means of lenses, LS, and mirrors, MR and PM. This particular version is designed to present alternating stimuli. The grating, GR, is imaged on the retina. Mirror, PM, is mounted on a pivot. When it turns, the position of the light and dark strips are interchanged. Neutral density filters, not shown in this figure, are usually inserted in the optical path to control luminance, and other components such as shutters, monochromators, etc., are required for specific applications. Insert B shows how the stimulus appears to the subject. (From Armington, 1980.)*

Stimulus measurement

The time-course of a visual stimulus can be assessed by having light from the stimulus impinge on a photo-electric device and feeding the suitably amplified electrical output into an oscilloscope. The photo-electric device and its associated amplifier should have a frequency response adequate for measuring fast voltage changes. For this reason photo-multipliers are more suitable than selenium photocells.

Photometry is the branch of physics concerned with the measurement of light as it affects human vision. Photopic and scotopic viewing conditions are known to alter the spectral sensitivity of the eye and spectral sensitivity curves for the light and dark-adapted eye have been standardized by international agreement. The standard light source for photometry is a black body radiator at the temperature of solidification of platinum (2042°K). The candela (cd) is used to describe luminous intensity, i.e. the strength of a light source, and is defined as 1/60th of the luminous intensity per square centimetre of the standard source. Luminous flux, measured in lumens, represents the light output of a source per unit of time. The light impinging on a given surface (illumination) is described by the luminous flux reaching it per unit area and is measured in lumens per square foot (foot candles), lumens per square centimeter (phots) or lumens per square metre (lux). Illumination is inversely proportional to the square of the distance of the receiving surface from a point source. Luminance (i.e. brightness) is used to describe the luminous intensity of a surface in terms of unit projected area as viewed from a distance perpendicular to the surface. Its value is independent of the distance of the eye or measuring instrument from the source and is measured in candelas per sq. cm (equivalent to one lambert), candelas per sq. metre (nit), candelas per sq. ft or candelas per sq. inch.

The amount of light reaching the retina, which is a determinant of perceived brightness, depends upon the product of the luminance of the surface being viewed and pupillary area. The latter fluctuates due to the influence of several physical and psycho-physiological factors. In order to finely control retinal illumination, as for example when using Maxwellian view stimulation, an artifical pupil is used. The troland is defined as the amount of light falling on the retina when viewing a surface having a luminance of one candela per sq. metre through a pupil with an area of one sq. millimetre. When measuring retinal illumination levels, due allowance has to be made for the fact that light entering through the edge of the pupil is less effective in stimulating the retina than that entering through the centre (Stiles-Crawford effect).

The contrast between pattern elements is an important parameter and is commonly specified as

$$\text{Contrast} = \frac{L\,MAX - L\,MIN}{L\,MAX + L\,MIN}$$

where L MAX and L MIN are the maximum and minimum luminance values of the light and dark pattern elements, respectively. This is known as Michelson's contrast and takes account of the background level of illumination.

In the EP laboratory luminance levels are measured either with photometers which require subjective visual matching or with more expensive photometric devices which have sensitivity characteristics similar to the human eye and automatically measure luminance values. With the former devices measurements are performed by adjusting the brightness of a spot of light until it appears to be the same as that of the surrounding test object. Slight differences in hue between test object and spot can be a source of error and it is best to use the average reading derived from several observers. Standard photometers do not respond fast enough to accurately measure the intensity of a flash stimulus. The intensity of the light discharge is sometimes quoted in terms of the electrical energy stored in the condenser which is used to discharge through the ionized gas of the flash tube. In practice, however, only a small part (about 15%) of this energy is emitted as light. It is more apppropriate and accurate to measure the integrated light output using a vacuum phototube capable of a rapid response time and to compare the output to that of a known light source (Cobb and Morton, 1952; Brunnette and Molotchnikoff, 1970).

More detailed descriptions and discussions of photometric methods, including the measurement of colour are to be found in Riggs (1965), Boynton (1966), Le Grand (1968) and Regan (1972a).

Auditory stimulation

Methods

Clicks are commonly used to test the integrity of the auditory pathway as, in general, they tend to produce larger and consequently better defined evoked potentials than other more frequency specific stimuli such as tone bursts or pips (Picton and Durieux Smith, 1978). The usual method of producing a click is to feed a short duration monophasic square wave into earphones or loudspeakers. The duration of the pulse should be less than 1 msec in order to deliver a clear, crisp stimulus to the subject. With durations longer than a millisecond the click quality is degraded and it is possible to perceive both its onset and offset. Although a square wave signal is fed into the sound transducer, its sound output as viewed on an oscilloscope appears rather like a dampened oscillation, and Fourier analysis of this shows it to have a complex frequency composition, most commonly with a predominant contribution from frequencies in the 2-5 KHz range (Picton et al, 1977; Gibson, 1978). By masking selected frequencies present in click stimuli responses to particular frequency ranges may be derived (Parker and Thornton, 1978a, 1978b; Don and Eggermont, 1978).

In evoked response audiometry an assessment of the range and amount of hearing loss can be made using several fixed frequencies. When using short duration tones of fixed frequency, however, there is the problem that, when the stimulus is turned on and off abruptly, switching transients produce audible onsets and offsets (clicks) which compromise the purity of the tone. Special switching devices or circuits are normally used to provide suitable gradual rise- and fall-times of the order of 2.5 msec to 15 msec. Commercial audiometers designed for evoked potential testing normally incorporate this feature. These devices will also produce masking sounds (tones or noise) which are introduced into the non-stimulated ear to prevent it being significantly affected by the stimulus and will (if desired) invert the polarity of alternate stimuli within an averaging run. The latter technique cancels out cochlear microphonic potentials and stimulus artifacts, as both of these closely follow the phase and polarity of the stimulus. It should be noted, however, that Stockard et al (1980) and Maurer et al (1980) find that clicks which initially move the tympanic membrane outwards (rarefaction) tend to produce better brainstem responses than clicks moving it at first inwards (condensation).

Auditory stimuli may be delivered by means of speakers (free field stimulation) or through earphones. Free field stimulation leaves a patient unrestrained, which may be of particular advantage when recording from children. Its main drawbacks, however, are that the intensity and quality of the emitted sound is greatly affected by the distance and angular relationship between a patient's ears and the speaker, as well as by the acoustic qualities of the testing room. Ideally, if free field stimulation is to be used, it should be done in an anechoic chamber or at least in a silent room. Stereophonic earphones permit monaural stimulation and greatly attenuate conventional environmental noise. Unfortunately, however, they tend to produce a prominent stimulus artifact due to the close proximity of the electromagnetic coils of the earphone to the recording electrodes. Common ways of minimizing the artifact include reversing the polarity of alternate stimuli, attaching an earphone or speaker to one end of a plastic tube, while the other end is inserted in the ear canal, using electromagnetically shielded earphones, and inserting miniature hearing aid earphones into the ear canal. Hughes and Fino (1980) report that piezo-electric earphones produce only a very small stimulus artifact and claim that they are able to record a very early component (1.1 msec) which is not part of the cochlear microphonic and is normally masked by the larger stimulus artifact produced by standard electromagnetic earphones (Figure 2.2).

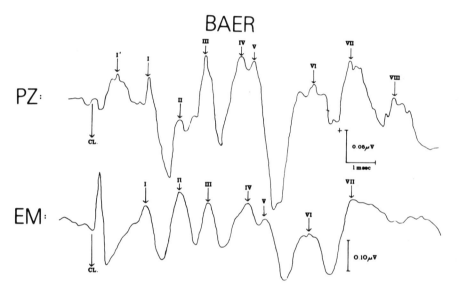

Figure 2.2 *Typical click-evoked brainstem responses elicited by: (a) piezo-electric (PZ) earphones containing a transducer with a Rochelle crystal connected to a diaphragm in a standard head-set mould, and (b) electromagnetic (EM) earphones with magnetic shielding. Note absence of stimulus artifact with PZ earphone and the presence of waves I' and VIII, compared to the prominent stimulus artifact and absence of wave VIII with the EM earphone. The two traces have different write-out gain in order that the stimulus artifact could be adequately viewed with the EM unit. Beginning of the click (CL) is indicated by downward pointing arrow. (From Hughes and Fino, 1980.)*

Stimulus measurement

It is conventional in acoustic measurements to specify the intensity of a sound with respect to its threshold of audibility. Decibels are used to express the magnitude of this ratio (see page 29). Auditory sensitivity is tested with sine waves and varies with the frequency of the sound. The most sensitive range is between 2

KHz and 5 KHz, while the least sensitive regions are at the high and low extremes of the auditory range (20 Hz-20 KHz). An important factor to take account of is that the relative audibility of frequencies above and below a test stimulus (e.g. 1 KHz tone) will change in a non-uniform way when the intensity of the test stimulus is changed. When assessing the intensity of a stimulus in physical terms, i.e. measuring sound pressure level (SPL), reference is most commonly made to 0 dB at 1000 Hz, which represents a sound pressure level of 0.0002 dynes/cm (Weighting Curve A). Other weighting curves (B, C and D) represent frequency/intensity relationships for higher intensity stimuli.

Sound level meters are designed to have similar frequency/intensity characteristics to the human ear. They are used to measure the intensity of pure tones and complex frequencies (e.g. noise), providing that the test sound is not too short-lived. Sounds of very short duration (e.g. clicks) are a problem to measure. This is due both to their transience and multifarious frequency composition. Transient sounds may be measured with impulse meters which will show peak intensity and duration, while a spectrum analyser can be used to indicate the relative intensities of composite frequencies. A complicating factor which has to be taken into account, however, is that a sound of less than 70 msec or so appears to be less loud than when it is of longer duration.

For this reason click stimuli should always be biologically calibrated. This is done by testing a group of normal hearing subjects in their late teens and early twenties who show no signs or symptoms of ear disease, are free of excessive wax in their ears, and have had no history of noise exposure sufficient to be considered a health risk. The mean hearing threshold (i.e. 0 dB) to presentation of the click is thus established and may be referred to as normal hearing level (nHL). Hearing levels (HL) for longer lasting (0.5 sec) pure tones have been similarly derived using standardized earphones and audiometers. These values are formallly published (ISO standards, etc.) and are commonly used to calibrate audiometers. Clicks between 65-100 dB (nHL) are commonly used to elicit brainstem potentials.

A person's own auditory threshold or sensation level (SL) may be used as reference zero, but in clinical assessment it is obviously best to measure with respect to the mean threshold in normals (hearing level).

If a clinical audiometer is not available, it is possible to produce pure tones using a voltage controlled oscillator, while a pulse generator can be used to produce clicks of variable duration. The output frequencies of the oscillator can be checked with an oscilloscope or frequency meter. Stimulus intensity can be accurately varied by means of a calibrated attenuator. For maximum power transfer the impedances of the signal generator and earphones (or speakers) must be correctly matched to the attenuator. Thus, having established threshold, the sound intensity can be increased in accurate steps relative to threshold. However, with such equipment the measurements have still to be related to absolute sound intensity. National Standards Laboratories or University Departments specializing in sound and vibration are usually willing to measure this, but often at a price.

Further details concerning sound measurement and evoked response audiometry are to be found in Hirsh (1966), Picton et al (1977), Picton and Durieux Smith (1978), Davis (1976), Gibson (1978), Stockard et al (1978) and Beagley (1979).

Somatosensory stimulation

Methods

Electrical stimulation of peripheral nerves through skin electrodes (per-cutaneous stimulation) is the most common method of eliciting both cortical and subcortical somatosensory evoked potentials. Unfortunately more natural stimuli are either not sufficiently 'sharp-fronted' to be suitable for averaging (e.g. stroking the skin) or produce a well-defined response, but are difficult to standardize or quantify in terms of threshold or stimulus strength (Halliday and Mason, 1964; Larsson and Prevec, 1970; Nakanishi et al, 1973). However, simultaneous stimulation using electrical and mechanical vibration or stroking appears to show interesting effects (Abbruzzese et al, 1980; Jones, 1980).

Ring electrodes placed on the fingers, or stick-on electrodes sited on the distal phalanges of the thumb, index and/or middle finger, can be used to activate sensory afferents of the median nerve. Ring electrodes on the fifth finger will stimulate afferents in the ulnar nerve. Stimulation of the median or ulnar nerve trunks at the wrist produce larger responses at all levels of the somatosensory pathway but at this site motor fibres and muscle afferents are also activated. In healthy individuals optimal and comfortable stimulation intensities are usually achieved with a stimulus level at twice to three times sensory threshold or, if an objective measure is preferable, the strength may be conveniently set at a level where a muscle twitch is just perceptible in the thumb or fingers, depending on the nerve trunk which is being stimulated (motor threshold).

The areas of skin over which the stimulating electrodes are going to be placed should always be thoroughly rubbed with acetone or an alcohol-impregnated swab in order to ensure a low resistance contact. If necessary the outer layers of the skin can be pierced with a sharp needle. Saline solution, or better still, saline jelly is used to make the conducting connection between electrode and skin. Great care has to be taken to ensure that there is no shunting of the applied current due to bridging between the pair of stimulating electrodes by the saline.

Stick-on electrodes can conveniently be utilized as stimulating electrodes but will have to be chlorided before they can be used for EP recording again. Alternatively, a saddle electrode can be used in which anode and cathode are separated by at least 2 cm (Dawson and Scott, 1949). Ready-made saddle electrodes are commercially available. The usual convention is to place the cathode or both electrodes over the nerve trunk with the cathode being proximal. This theoretically prevents the possibility of anodal hyperpolarization blocking the stimulus volley. In practice, however, it appears to make little difference if cathode is proximal or distal and it may be more convenient when stimulating at the wrist with a saddle electrode to have the cathode distal (see Jones, 1977 and Chapter 12). A stimulating probe can be very useful in helping to locate a particular nerve trunk (see Goff, 1974 for further details). In normal subjects, square wave pulses less than 1 msec in duration and up to 10 mA are commonly used. In the lower limb, stimulation of lateral peroneal and anterior and posterior tibial nerves evokes large cortical potentials, though responses from the spine are smaller and more difficult to discern (Jones and Small, 1978).

Constant current stimulators are preferred by many investigators as their output will hardly be affected by minor variations in electrode/skin impedance. However, the effective current flow at the nerve itself varies with this and other factors, so that constant current stimulators are not obviously superior in performance to constant voltage stimulators. Schwartz et al (1964) compared constant current and constant voltage stimulators and found that both evoked responses which were virtually identical in all aspects. These authors stressed that the constancy of the output was more important than the type of stimulator.

It is desirable to ensure that the output from a stimulator is both resistively and capacitatively isolated from earth. This feature will greatly reduce the stimulus artifact. With mains powered stimulators, the input or output circuitry can be separated from the mains supply by means of a pulse or isolation transformer which has low capacitance between its windings. An alternative approach is to power the stimulator from batteries (Emde and Shipton, 1970). Without isolation there is the risk that if the stimulator malfunctions and the patient is accidentally connected between stimulator and earth, uncomfortable or even dangerous amounts of current could flow through the patient.

Stimulus measurement

A somatosensory stimulator may be calibrated and checked by connecting a resistor of similar value to the skin impedance (e.g. 10 KΩ) across the output leads. An oscilloscope with a differential input is also connected across the resistor and the stimulus voltage read off. Dividing the voltage by the resistor value (in kilohms) gives the current flowing through the resistor (in milliamps). This method presumes that skin impedance is a fixed value which in fact is not necessarily the case. The electrical properties of skin and its interface with an electrode are complex and can be roughly appproximated to the behaviour of capacitances and resistances connected in parallel (see Figure 1.3). The surface epidermal layer offers the highest electrical resistance and behaves non-linearly, while the deeper dermal layers have a lower resistance with linear characteristics. Factors such as electrode area, the size and frequency of applied current, electrolyte concentration, degree to which the epidermis is scarified or penetrated and the emotional (sudomotor) state of the subject all affect the electrode/skin impedance (Montagu and Coles, 1966; Lane, 1970; Swanson and Webster, 1974; Neuman, 1978).

RECORDING PROBLEMS - ARTIFACTS

Artifacts are defined here as potentials not generated by the brain which interfere with the recording and interpretation of evoked potentials. These unwanted potentials can be either continuous or intermittent, and, if the latter, may be either related or unrelated to the delivery of the stimulus. For convenience, artifacts can be categorized into potentials arising at the electrode/skin interface (electrode artifacts), interference of extraneous origin, potentials generated by the patient (physiological artifacts) and artifacts originating from stimulating equipment or associated with the impinging stimulus (stimulus artifacts).

Electrode artifacts and extraneous interference

Causes of extraneous interference and electrode artifacts have already been described in the preceding Chapter. It is worth mentioning here, however, some procedures that may help in both identifying and dealing with electrode artifacts and mains frequency interference in conditions where they are proving unusually troublesome. Continuously monitoring the background EEG during an averaging run can be a very useful way of detecting artifacts, and in some contexts it is essential. If an EEG machine is used to do this a permanent paper copy can be kept. Alternatively an oscilloscope display can be used.

Artifacts can most commonly be ascribed to the electrodes themselves or to the quality of their contact with the skin. Electrode artifacts are characterized by abrupt, large potential swings due to disturbance of the electrode/skin interface by movement of the electrode or by chemical changes in the electrolyte (e.g. blood, sweat, etc.). A corroded connection between an electrode and its lead can also produce recording problems. At the least, these artifacts impose appreciable baseline shifts on the average response and at the worst they may not only distort the response by driving amplifiers outside their linear range, but can also produce spurious components in the recorded response. Electrode artifacts are usually easily localized by noting the channel(s) in which they occur and then deducing from the montage which electrode(s) is giving the problem. A malfunctioning stick-on electrode should be checked for firmness of contact, refilled with saline jelly and the skin scarified further. If this does not improve matters, the electrode must be replaced, making sure that its substitute has a low impedance (less than 10 KΩ). Care has to be taken, however, not to re-scarify the skin too severely as blood in the electrolyte could result in further artifacts.

High inter-electrode impedance will usually result in obtrusive mains interference. If restricted to particular channels then the electrodes connected to these channels should be checked. If interference is seen in all channels, both earth electrode and common reference electrode (if the latter is being used) should be inspected first. Re-scarifying the skin will normally solve the problem, but if it does not, the integrity of the lead and socket should be checked. It is important in this context to make sure that electrode leads are kept bunched together on their way to the headboard in order to minimize electromagnetic pick-up.

If the interference cannot be ascribed to faulty electrodes then the next step is to short and earth the amplifier inputs at the headboard. This manoeuvre will help decide whether the problem is arising from the amplifiers and their interconnections with other equipment or alternatively is due to extraneous interference affecting the input.

Interference persisting after input shorting indicates either a fault within the amplifier or an earth loop problem arising from separate earthing points being used for the various pieces of equipment. If isolated to one amplifier it is likely to be the former, in which case that amplifier should be disconnected. If all amplifiers have interference, then by watching the amplifier outputs while disconnecting the power and earth leads of any interlinked equipment, the device(s) producing the problem should be readily identified.

If the interference is eliminated following shorting of the input, it points to the origin of the problem as being extraneous to the equipment and hence other sources both within and outside the laboratory should be investigated (see Chapter 1). Mains frequency interference may be averaged out to a certain extent by having an inter-trigger time which is a multiple of the period of the mains frequency and adding to it the duration of half a mains cycle (e.g. 10 msec for 50 Hz mains and 8.3 msec for 60 Hz mains). By this means cancellation of the interference by addition of alternate mains cycles of opposite phase occurs throughout the sequence of trials making up the average response. If fine timing control of the interstimulus period is not available (e.g. from a Digitimer), then it is better to trigger randomly with respect to mains frequency rather than to have the trigger phase-locked to the mains (Figure 2.3), or alternatively to try and drift systematically with respect to mains frequency, so that the mains interference does not build up (e.g. Dawson's original averager had a synchronous motor with gear ratio 110:100 to effect this).

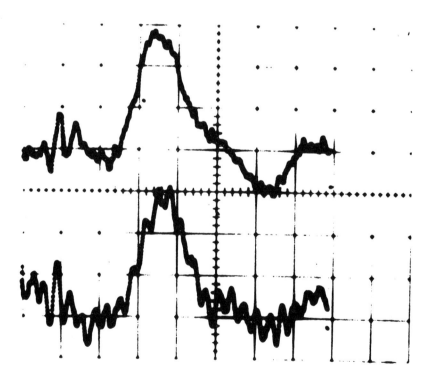

Figure 2.3 *Effect of accidental phase-locking to 60 Hz mains interference on the recording of the click-evoked cortical response. A nominal 4 sec interstimulus interval caused summation of 60 Hz activity (bottom record) compared to recording under identical conditions but with no 60 Hz phase-locking (top record). (From Goff, 1974.)*

Physiological artifacts

Apart from the brain, there are several other structures in the head and body which generate potentials large enough to interfere with the accurate detection of evoked potentials. The most troublesome of these sources are the eyes, the heart and skeletal muscles.

Ocular artifacts

The eye has a standing potential of about 60 mV between the cornea and retina, which is attributable for the most part to the potential across the pigment epithelium (Ikeda, 1976). The cornea is electropositive with respect to the back of the retina. The magnitude of this corneo-retinal potential alters according to the state of light adaptation of the eye (see Chapter 4). Scalp electrodes, particularly those over the frontal regions, will record changes in potential brought about by light stimulation and by alterations of the potential field due to movement of the eyelid and/or eyeball. Voluntarily closing the eyelids produces a large positive - - going potential (200-300 μV) lasting for about a second, whereas in blinking this potential is smaller (100-200 μV) and its duration is a quarter of a second or so. If blinking is reflexly produced by the presentation of a flash the positivity has a peak latency of the order of 200 msec. This reflex artifact is particularly common in children (Eisengart and Symmes, 1971).

Other sources of noise are movements such as lateral nystagmus and flickering of the eyelids. These produce fairly rapid modulations of the electro-oculogram (Figure 2.4).

Ocular artifacts are relatively large compared to evoked responses. They are detectable at the vertex, ears and as far back as the occipital areas (Hillyard, 1974; Eisengart and Symmes, 1971). When recording any type of evoked potential every effort should be made to reduce them, as if they occur too frequently or are systematically related to stimulation, baseline shifts and spurious components may appear or the response may even be totally obliterated (Figure 2.5).

The simplest, and in many ways the most effective, method of reducing electro-ocular artifacts is to instruct patients not to blink excessively and to get them to fixate a spot, or if appropriate, to look at their own eyes in a mirror (Papakostopoulous et al, 1973). If it is not necessary to have the eyes open, it may help to keep them closed, although this may result in other problems such as an increase in alpha activity and drowsiness. In the latter case lateral to-and-fro rolling of the eyeballs can occur. Nowadays, many commercial averagers incorporate some means of artifact rejection whereby if the input voltage exceeds certain pre-specified levels and durations, the averaging trial is rejected.

As ocular artifacts are particularly liable to contaminate the CNV, it is important to devote an averaging channel to monitoring eye movements when recording this response. Electrodes are best placed along the vertical axis just above and below the eye. Techniques are available which to a great extent nullify the adverse effects of eye movements. McCallum and Walter (1968) described a special montage in which reference electrodes were placed on each mastoid, thus reducing potentials due to lateral eye movements. To compensate for vertical eye movements

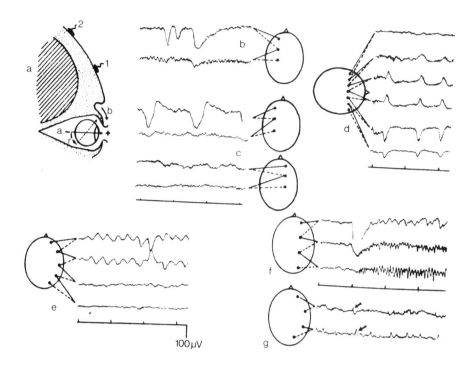

Figure 2.4 *Eye-movement and eye-blink artifacts written out on an EEG machine. (a) schematic drawing of eyeball showing corneo-retinal potential with the cornea being positive with respect to the back of the eye. Rotation of the eyeball, r, or movement of the eyelid across the cornea as in a blink, b, most prominently alters the electrical potentials at frontal electrodes 1 and 2. In recording (b) is shown a typical blink and eye closure potential in frontal leads. (c) eye blink artifact produced artifically by moving left eyelid with a match-stick. There is no eyeball movement and therefore no accompanying artifact. (d) eyeblinks in a subject with the left eye enucleated. The artifact is now lateralized over the surviving right eye. (e) lateral nystagmus. (f) eyelid flutter after eye closure seen in frontal electrodes. More posteriorly the eye closure is associated with the appearance of an alpha rhythm. (g) surface positive wave (lambda wave) in occipital leads preceded by small lateral rectus eye muscle EMG associated with saccadic eye movements in reading. Time scale: 1 second per division. (From MacGillivray, 1974.)*

an electrode just above the nasion is referred to the linked ear lead through a 25 KΩ potentiometer (Figure 2.6). The adjustable centre tap of the potentiometer is set so that a potential is obtained which is equal to that present at the vertex when calibrating eye movements are made (Figure 2.7). However, once set this technique will not compensate for subsequent variation in the speed and extent of actual eye movements which may, in practice, produce a different vertex component. Using similar reasoning some authors have suggested referring the vertex to a temporal electrode which is isopotential to the vertex with respect to vertical eye movement

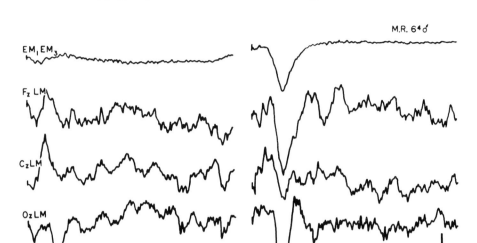

Figure 2.5 *Effect of reflex blinking on the flash evoked response of a 6-year-old boy. EM₁ EM₃ - derivation linking electrodes above and below the left eye. Other channels are from midline electrodes at frontal (Fz), central (Cz) and occipital (Oz) sites connected to a left mastoid reference electrode. Twelve sweeps were averaged for each condition. Calibration: 200 μV for channel 1 and 20 μV for channels 2-4. Time scale 100 msec per division. Responses have been segregated with respect to the absence (left) or presence (right) of reflex blinks. The positive component at approximately 170 msec in the occipital derivation is greatly enhanced during blinking. (From Eisengart and Symmes, 1971.)*

potentials (Straumanis et al, 1969). With general purpose computers it is possible to measure beforehand the magnitude of eye movement potentials present at the vertex and to subtract them from the vertex CNV. The CNV has been found to be typically comprised of 10-50% (mean 23%) ocular artifact (Hillyard and Galambos, 1970).

When the retina is transiently stimulated by a flash it produces a short-lasting well-defined response (the electroretinogram) within the first 40 msec following the stimulus, which also alters with the state of adaptation of the eye (Ikeda, 1976). The ERG is optimally recorded by corneal electrodes, but by the use of averaging can be detected from skin electrodes placed around the eyes even for pattern reversal stimulation (Halliday and Mushin, 1980). The ERG to flash can spread as far back as the vertex (Cobb and Dawson, 1960). Care is needed, therefore, in correctly identifying the source of components in the early part of visual responses recorded from occipital-frontal derivations.

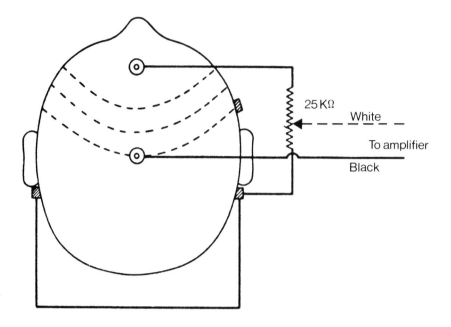

Figure 2.6 *Electrode montage for reduction of artefact due to eye movements. Directly linking electrodes at each mastoid process will much reduce the effect of lateral eye movements, since rotation of the eyes to left or right will increase the potential at one mastoid electrode and reduce it at the other. Vertical eye movements have a transverse equipotential field (dotted lines) and it is possible to choose an electrode position (X, somewhere in the temporal region) that is equipotential with the vertex. The electrode position can be simulated using the moveable arm of a potentiometer. (From Cooper et al, 1974.)*

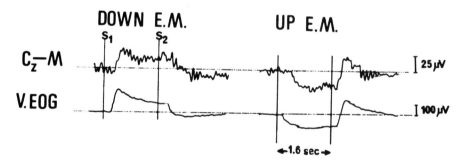

Figure 2.7 *Simultaneous averaged potential shifts induced in vertex-mastoid (C_z-M) channel and pair of electrodes placed above and below eye (vertical electro-oculogram - V.EOG) by downward (left) and upward (right) voluntary eye movements (E.M.). The indicated E.M. (of about 10 degrees) was made in response to S_1 (click), with return E.M. made after S_2 (tone). Recordings were DC with upward deflections signifying negativity in Cz and upper orbital leads. The magnitude of these shifts, measured over 0.3 sec before S_2 relative to the pre-S_1 baseline were: Down E.M., C_z-M = -22.8 μV, V.EOG = -119 μV; Up E.M., C_z-M = 24.8 μV; V.EOG = 132 μV. (From Hillyard, 1974.)*

Auditory and somatosensory responses appear not to be directly affected by whether the eyes are open or closed. For the visual response, however, the position of the eyelids is important as there are significant latency differences between flash responses recorded through the open and closed eyelids (Kriss et al, 1980b). For pattern stimulation it is vital that the eyelid should not droop excessively. We have found that if more than 50% of the pupil is obscured by a drooping eyelid then marked changes in latency and amplitude can occur, which may be sufficient to lead to the mis-categorization of a response as abnormal (Figure 2.8). A decrease in the amount of light entering the eye is most probably responsible for these VEP changes. Thus in the clinical context patients should be encouraged to keep alert and, if ptosis is present, the lid should be held or taped open.

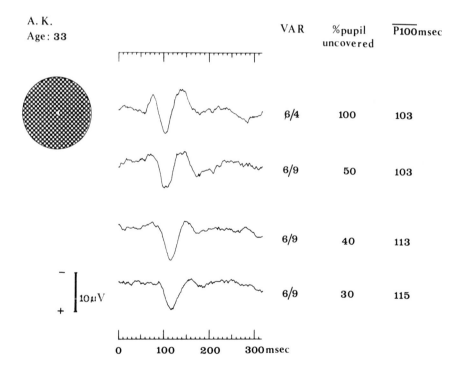

Figure 2.8 *Effect of drooping upper eyelid on the pattern evoked potential to full-field stimulation. The major positive component of the response will increase in latency when more than 50% of the pupil is covered.*

Muscle artifacts

Interference associated with the electrical activity of muscles can be very troublesome when recording any of the evoked potentials. Two types of artifact may be conveniently distinguished according to whether it is or is not contingent on presentation of the stimulus. Continuous EMG activity or non-stimulus - related bursts have large amplitudes, being often in the millivolt range, and have a range of frequencies (20 Hz to 1 KHz) overlapping most types of evoked potential. EMG interference on the head arises mainly from contraction of frontal, temporal, post-auricular, occipital and neck muscles. Movements such as tensing the neck, swallowing, frowning and clenching the jaw are common sources of trouble, which can be reduced dramatically by instructing the patient to relax. Some form of visual or audio feedback to the patient as to when the artifact is occurring may also prove helpful in minimizing EMG activity. In patients who are seated, slight opening of the mouth and repositioning of the head are usually very effective manoeuvres. If the interference persists, then increasing the number of trials per average will usually improve the signal/noise ratio, since the occurrence of the EMG is random with respect to the stimulus. Increasing the number of averaging runs will help in assessing the reproducibility of the response, and, if computing facilities are available, a grand average of the runs can subsequently be obtained. As a last resort the amplifier filters which attenuate high frequencies can be used, but due consideration has to be given to the possibility of introducing attenuation and phase shift of short duration components of the evoked potential. A more desirable alternative, if computing facilities are available, is to use digital filters to 'clean-up' a response. In exceptional circumstances, such as when assessing the auditory responses of restless children, sedation or general anaesthesia can be employed to ensure relaxation (Davis, 1976; Picton et al, 1977; Stockard et al, 1980). However, the slower, later components of evoked potentials are profoundly altered by these procedures.

Involuntary muscle activity in response to stimuli (microreflexes) are less easily recognized in a trace and in many cases difficult to eliminate. These myogenic responses are usually elicited from muscles under tension and are found to be prominent with high intensity stimuli to the visual, auditory or somatosensory modalities (Figure 2.9). Tension of the neck or forehead muscles produces prominent photomotor responses with a positive peak at about 75 msec maximal in size over the tensed muscle (Bickford, 1972). The orbicularis oculi muscle which surrounds the eye also reflexly contracts to a flashing light (photo-palpebral reflex) (Inanaga and Yamagushi, 1969). Somatomotor responses may be recorded at the scalp following median nerve stimulation in 70% of normals (Cracco and Bickford, 1966). These myogenic responses have a prominent positive peak at 40 msec which is largest over the side of the scalp contralateral to the hand stimulated. Its distribution, however, is more widespread than that of the somatosensory response (Calmes and Cracco, 1971). The sonomotor response has several components in the range 8-60 msec which are widely distributed over the scalp. Tensioning of the neck muscles and a high intensity click (>90 dB) produces a particularly prominent response at the inion within the first 50 msec following the stimulus. In the majority of healthy individuals auditory stimulation also produces a prominent response

(8-50 msec) from the post-auricular muscle which, unlike other myogenic responses, is not usually abolished by voluntary relaxation or light sleep and can be elicited even with near-threshold stimuli. This latter feature has practical applications in evoked response audiometry (Dus and Wilson, 1975; Douek et al, 1973; Gibson, 1978).

In general, microreflexes can be eliminated by ensuring that the patient relaxes the offending muscle group. Re-positioning the head and supporting it at the neck may help in reducing neck tension. The post-auricular response can be a problem, however, as in some individuals it is always present, no matter what manoeuvre is performed. If necessary, sedation, local or general anaesthesia can be used to eliminate awkward microreflexes (Picton et al, 1977; Davis, 1976; Gibson, 1978; Stockard et al, 1980).

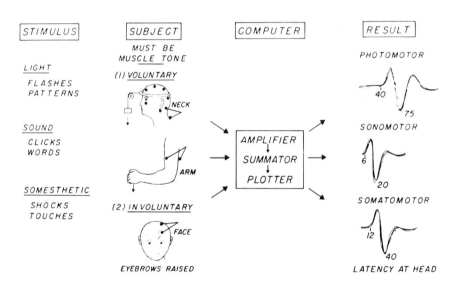

Figure 2.9 *Microreflexes are usually encountered when using intense stimuli and having muscles under tension. The shortest latency response of about 6-8 msec (the sonomotor response) is recorded from neck muscles (and elsewhere at greater latency). Electrical stimuli applied to peripheral nerves will evoke a response with an onset latency of about 12 msec recorded from the scalp and inion regions (somatomotor responses). The response to flash stimuli (photomotor response) has the longest latency of 40-70 msec and can be recorded for a total period of 100-200 msec following the stimulus. (From Bickford, 1972.)*

Cardiac artifacts

In the majority of people, the electrical field of the heart tends to be equipotential over most of the scalp. Thus, when recordings are confined to electrodes on the scalp, the in-phase rejection of differential amplifiers ensures that the ECG is not obtrusive. However, the R wave of the ECG complex is electronegative at the right ear (compared to the left) so that a transauricular derivation is liable to be contaminated by artifact. In plump people and those with short necks the ECG can be prominent at the neck. The disrupting effect of ECG artifact depends very much on the averaging window time. If it is very short, as when recording subcortical auditory or somatosensory responses, then the presence of the

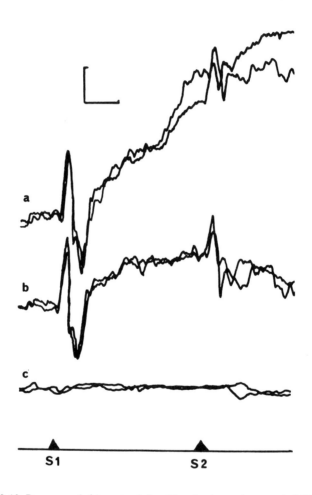

Figure 2.10 *Presence of skin potential artifact in the scalp recorded CNV.*
Replicated superimposed averages (each the sum of 20) of concurrent recordings
from unscratched (a) and scratched (b) vertex-mastoid sites and from upper-lower
orbital ridges (c) Calibrations: 10 μV for CNV channels and 125 μV for ocular
channel, negative up; 0.5 sec. (From Picton and Hillyard, 1972.)

artifact may result in baseline shifts without any severe disruption to the evoked response. However, with longer window times, for example, as used to record the visual response to pattern, the evoked potential may be severely distorted.

Because of the wide scalp distribution of some types of evoked potential, it is on occasions desirable to use a reference off the head. In such circumstances a very large ECG artifact is encountered and its effects may be minimized either by using the cancellation technique of Stephenson and Gibbs (1951) or that of Jewett (1970a), which have been already described (see page 28).

An electrode over an artery can produce rhythmic oscillations in potential which are roughly triangular in shape and synchronous with the heart beat. This artifact is due to movement, with its consequent disturbance of the electrode double layer (Cooper et al, 1974) and re-positioning the electrode a short distance away (about 1 cm) from the offending artery will usually overcome the problem.

Other sources of noise

The skin itself may be a source of artifacts due to differences in potential between two areas and changes in skin resistance resulting from sweat gland activity. Both factors are known to vary under emotional or stressful conditions. Picton and Hillyard (1972) reported skin potentials, measured transcutaneously, to be from +20 to -20 mV depending upon cephalic site and subject. However, when the skin under one electrode was scratched, the potential difference was always negative and of the order of 30 mV. With electrodes over unscratched skin considerable augmentation and distortion of the CNV was seen (Figure 2.10). Pricking or scratching the skin surface was always found to be very effective in reducing skin potentials. In order to minimize this type of artifact it is also important to ensure that the recording room is not so hot that it induces excessive sweating and to relax and reassure patients if they appear anxious.

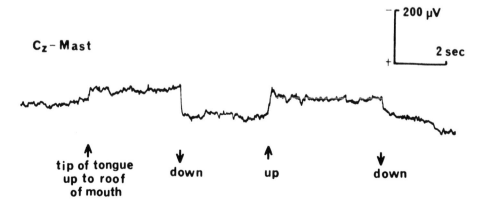

Figure 2.11 *Direct current potential shifts produced in a vertex-mastoid channel as a function of tongue position. Data obtained by Dr T.W. Picton and reproduced from Hillyard (1974).*

Movements of the tongue (glossokinetic artifact) have been reported to produce slow potential changes recordable at the scalp (Figure 2.11). A negativity of up to 100 μV is seen at the vertex when the negatively charged tip of the tongue touches the roof of the mouth (Klass and Bickford 1960). Milnarch et al (1957) describe slow potentials which they attribute to the modulation of a standing potential field generated by dissimilar metals in tooth fillings as a result of mouth and tongue movements.

Stimulus artifact

When recording somatosensory or auditory evoked potentials, it is not uncommon to elicit an artifact coincident with stimulation. Stimulus artifacts are usually due to the stimulus current directly affecting the electrodes and also to capacitative or magnetic coupling between the stimulating equipment and the amplifier input leads. It is important that the magnitude of the stimulus artifact is kept to a minimum as, particularly with short latency evoked potentials, a large artifact can drive the amplifiers beyond their linear range, or even block them, and hence lead to distortion of the early part of the subsequent evoked potential. The presence of a stimulus artifact will also vitiate any form of cross-correlation or frequency analysis. For convenience, it is proposed to deal separately with the various modalities.

For somatosensory stimulation, current from the shock stimulus may spread to recording electrodes through tissue conduction. This effect may be greatly reduced by placing a large, low resistance earth electrode between the stimulating electrode and the recording electrodes but close to the former. This arrangement ensures that most of the stray stimulus current preferentially flows down to earth. If both the subject and stimulus equipment are earthed (either deliberately or by mistake) then currents associated with stimulation can flow through a 'common earth circuit'. An effective way of eliminating this possibility (and also, as has already been stressed, of ensuring that a patient is safeguarded from accidental heavy current flows through his body) is to isolate the stimulator from earth, either by means of an isolation transformer which has low capacitance between its primary and secondary windings (pulse transformer) or by powering the stimulator with batteries. Stimulating and recording leads should always be kept well apart. Stimulus pulses usually have a sharp onset and offset and consequently have a content of high frequency components which easily become capacitatively coupled to nearby input leads or to the equipment earth.

In auditory stimulation, where the stimulus is delivered via earphones, an artifact usually occurs as a result of the activation of the electromagnet operating the earphone diaphragm. This induces a potential electromagnetically on the nearby mastoid or earlobe electrodes. An effective, though expensive, solution to this problem is to utilize earphones which have compensation coils and are enclosed in mu-metal. The latter has high magnetic permeability and virtually eliminates the magnetic field reaching the electrode. Other approaches to reducing the auditory stimulus artifact include using miniature earphones (as used in hearing aids) which are inserted into the external auditory meatus (Goff, 1974). These devices, however, have a much poorer frequency response than standard earphones. Some workers have attached each earphone to the end of a tube which is inserted into the ear. By this means there is minimal sound loss and the effects of the artifact are reduced, firstly, by keeping earphones away from the head and, secondly, by introducing a fixed delay between the delivery of the stimulus and the response. Stimulus artifacts are not normally a problem in visual stimulation. It has been reported, however, that a bright light falling on a silver electrode can produce a highly transient photo-electric artifact. If such an artifact is evident with photic stimulation then the affected electrodes should be masked from the light. It is also worth checking, however, that interference is not a result of electrostatic or electromagnetic pick-up due to amplifiers or their input leads being too close to the stimulating device. In this context it is worth mentioning the usefulness of estimating the effects of stimulus artifacts by performing 'control' averaging runs in which the stimulator is operated in its usual place, but masked from the subject. If the stimulus artifact is of very short duration and is not interfering with the recording of the evoked potential, the artifact may be eliminated from the record by triggering the averaging computer shortly after the stimulus event. Due allowance has, of course, to be made for this delay when computing response latencies. Alternatively, a general purpose computer can be programmed to zero the first few ordinates in which the artifact occurs.

Electronic circuits which suppress the stimulus artifact have been described (Freeman, 1971 Roby and Lettich, 1975). Basically these circuits are incorporated into recording amplifiers and are designed to hold the signal voltage at a specified level (voltage clamp) for the pre-set duration of the artifact.

SUMMARY: SOME RECOMMENDATIONS

1. Ensure that the laboratory is located well away from powerful sources of electromagnetic interference and loud noise. Within the laboratory keep the patient and the recording equipment away from sources of electrostatic and magnetic interference. Shield vulnerable equipment and, where possible, suppress problem sources.

2. Plan the lay-out of the laboratory ergonomically and ensure comfortable, efficient and controllable temperature, ventilation and lighting levels.

3. Good recording technique is essential. Use well-maintained non-polarizable electrodes. Ensure low impedances for skin/electrode contacts (especially for the reference electrode) and adopt a montage appropriate to the full appreciation of the response in the modality being stimulated. Keep electrode leads bunched together to reduce any magnetic pick-up.

4. Recording amplifiers should have high input impedance (>1 MΩ), high discrimination ratio, high gain and low noise. It is vital to select a frequency response which will not distort the signal of interest.

5. It is advisable to have an averaging computer with four or more channels. The sampling rate and sweep time should be suitable for obtaining undistorted and well-resolved responses. Average an adequate number of trials. Repeat averaging runs. Write out responses with good resolution and include a calibration for amplitude and time in each recording.

6. It is an advantage to store responses permanently on magnetic media (disk or tape) and to have copies of all data on paper.

7. Use an efficient stimulating technique. Stimulus parameters should be accurately measured and well controlled. Calibrate biologically using an adequate sample to obtain laboratory norms. Take account of age and sex differences.

8. Minimize artifacts. Reassure and relax patients. Be aware of physiological artifacts. Reduce or prevent stimulus artifacts.

Acknowledgements
I would like to thank Dr A.M. Halliday, Jack Pitman, Dr Geoff Barrett, Keith Cunningham and Dr Eva Peringer for their helpful comments on Chapters 1 and 2.

3

The Visual Evoked Potential in Healthy Subjects

A.M. Halliday

The only firm basis for recognizing abnormalities in the visual evoked potential (VEP) is a thorough understanding of the normal response and a clear delineation of the limits of response variability in the healthy population. Two of the principal causes of the variability encountered in recordings of the normal response are: (1) variations in the character and properties of the stimulus being used; and (2) differences in the anatomical structure of the visual pathways and generators in different individuals. Subjective or behavioural factors, including the quality of cooperation in fixation, accommodation, etc., also play some part in determining the character of the VEP recorded, but given a reasonable degree of cooperation it is less significant than the two factors already mentioned. Nonetheless, all three of these causes of normal response variability must be recognized and allowed for in clinical testing. The large number of different types of visual stimulus employed to produce EPs (e.g. flash, flashed-pattern, pattern-onset, -offset or -reversal) is compounded by further important variables such as the choice of pattern (e.g. checkerboard or grating), and other important stimulus characteristics such as field size, spatial frequency, contrast and mean luminance. The frequency of presentation of the stimulus is also critical, since it determines whether the steady-state or transient response is to be recorded. Differences in stimulating equipment and technique may make it very difficult to compare and equate results from different laboratories.

The various types of stimulus employed in clinical testing have been described in Chapter 2. In the present chapter the character of the responses to the various stimuli in the healthy population and their variability in different individuals will be dealt with, with particular emphasis on the transient response to 2 Hz checkerboard pattern-reversal, which has proved the most widely used stimulus in clinical practice.

THE FLASH RESPONSE IN HEALTHY INDIVIDUALS

Until about 1970, the most frequently recorded visual evoked potential was the response to a diffuse, unstructured stroboscopic flash. At low flash frequencies (e.g. 1-2 Hz) the so-called 'transient response' is recorded, which has a polyphasic waveform. Several systems of labelling the successive positive and negative components have been suggested, but the most commonly used are those due to Cigànek (1961a) and Gastaut et al (1967b), both of which are shown in Figure 3.1.

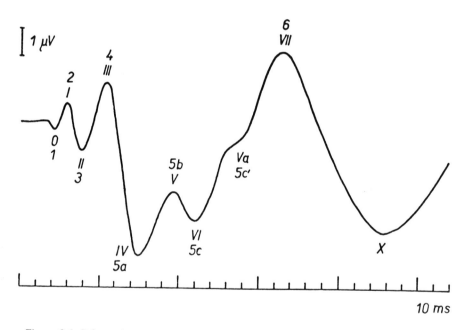

Figure 3.1 *Schematic representation of the flash evoked potential recorded from a mid-occipital electrode, with negative peaks plotted upwards, to show the numbering of the various components used by Ciganek (1961a) in Roman numerals and by Gastaut and Regis (1965) in Arabic numerals. X is the first wave of the rhythmic after-discharge (cf Figure 3.2). (From Ciganek, 1975.)*

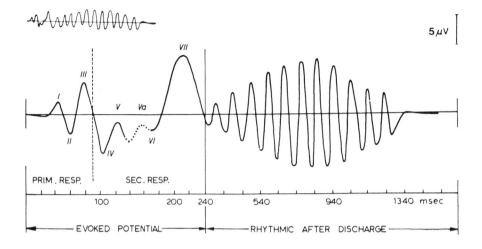

5μV

Figure 3.2 *Schematic representation of the flash EP to show the primary response, secondary response, and rhythmic after-discharge. Note the different time scales. (From Ciganek, 1961b.)*

Cigànek's nomenclature uses Roman numerals and Gastaut's Arabic and both systems resort to subdividing the components further by adding letters. The early occipital EP to flash stimulation is often followed by an after-discharge, consisting of a phase-locked sinusoidal potential in the alpha frequency range (Figure 3.2).

The two main disadvantages of the flash EP in clinical testing are its very large variability in waveform between individuals, which makes the reliable identification of the different subcomponents insecure, and its relative insensitivity to the effect of visual impairment, whether due to opacities of the media or lesions of the retina or visual pathways (see Chapters 5, 6 and 7). The size of the response thus correlates poorly with such things as visual acuity. It is, however, the most robust of the visual EPs and can often be obtained when normal vision is so much impaired that the pattern evoked EPs are unobtainable. Under these circumstances, it can give valuable information about the character of the abnormality present. Flash stimulation is also invaluable for recording the ERG (see Chapter 4).

Mean latency of the components of the flash response

EP components are recognized by their polarity, latency and distribution. All the components of the occipital VEPs to full-field stimulation are recorded with a maximum at the midline, usually about 6 cm above the inion. This is certainly true of the flash response (Cobb and Dawson, 1960; Cigànek, 1961, 1969b). Table 3.1 gives the mean latency and amplitude for the onset and first five subsequent peaks of the flash response from each eye of the 17 healthy subjects comprising the control group in the study by Halliday, McDonald and Mushin (1972). Peak latencies were

Table 3.1. MEAN LATENCY AND AMPLITUDE OF THE COMPONENTS OF THE FLASH IN 17 HEALTHY SUBJECTS

	Flash EP			
	Left eye		Right eye	
	Latency (msec)	Amplitude (V)	Latency (msec)	Amplitude (μV)
Onset	42.9 ± 7.2		43.3 ± 7.0	
P̄6̄0̄	60.8 ± 10.6	+5.52 ± 2.56	59.4 ± 10.8	+6.59 ± 3.59
N̄7̄0̄	72.9 ± 15.8	-5.02 ± 4.20	73.0 ± 14.1	-6.65 ± 5.15
P̄1̄0̄0̄	102.7 ± 15.3	+8.69 ± 4.42	102.3 ± 13.7	+9.99 ± 5.53
N̄1̄2̄5̄	128.2 ± 22.4	-9.18 ± 5.79	125.2 ± 19.6	-8.15 ± 5.75
P̄1̄6̄0̄	162.0 ± 36.1	+7.87 ± 3.85	160.5 ± 36.6	+7.18 ± 3.77

Table 3.2 MEAN LATENCY AND AMPLITUDE OF THE COMPONENTS OF THE PATTERN EP IN 17 HEALTHY SUBJECTS

	Pattern reversal EP			
	Left eye		Right eye	
	Latency (msec)	Amplitude (V)	Latency (msec)	Amplitude (V)
Onset	59.6 ± 5.7	μ	58.9 ± 5.2	
P̄7̄5̄	75.0 ± 2.6	+1.38 ± 0.75	73.3 ± 3.1	+1.54 ± 0.81
N̄9̄0̄	87.0 ± 3.0	-2.01 ± 1.00	88.1 ± 4.2	-2.12 ± 1.08
P̄1̄2̄0̄	119.6 ± 3.4	+7.82 ± 3.13	120.1 ± 4.0	+7.74 ± 3.26
N̄1̄5̄0̄	150.6 ± 8.6	-8.40 ± 4.22	151.4 ± 11.0	-7.87 ± 3.68
P̄1̄9̄0̄	187.9 ± 28.6	+5.45 ± 3.59	190.9 ± 29.5	+5.48 ± 3.33

measured in milliseconds from the flash, and peak amplitudes were measured in microvolts from the immediately preceding peak of opposite polarity (the baseline preceding the onset in the case of P̄6̄0̄).

Inspection of Table 3.1 will show that there is good agreement between the mean latencies of the peaks in the two eyes, with a maximum difference of 3 msec (for the N̄1̄2̄5̄ component). Discrepancies for the peak amplitudes, however, are proportionately much larger, approaching 30% in the case of N̄7̄0̄. Even with latency, the inter-individual variability, indicated by the standard deviation, is large. This has been the invariable finding (Cigànek, 1975).

Although there is some discrepancy in the exact latencies reported by different authors for the components of the flash response (as would be expected from this normal variability combined with differences in the exact stimulus parameters used), there is enough general agreement between the published studies to correlate the different proposed nomenclatures. In addition to the widely used systems of Cigànek and Gastaut et al, Korol and Stangos (1972) have labelled three of the main

Table 3.3 ALTERNATIVE NOMENCLATURES FOR THE COMPONENTS OF THE FLASH RESPONSE

Polarity of peak	N	P	N	P	N	P	N
Cigánek (1961)	I	II	III	IV	V	VI	VII
	40	55	75	95	115	135	190
	39.12	53.4	73.33	94.19	114.0	134.55	
	± 4.18	± 4.42	± 6.36	± 7.13	± 7.41	± 9.92	
Gastaut and	2	3	4	5a	5b	5c	6
Regis (1964)	40	60	80	130	140	160	220
Korol and	—	A	B	C	—	—	
Stangos (1972)		55	80	110			
		53.9 ±	81.8 ±	108 ±			
		3.5	4.3	7.1			
Halliday, Barrett, Halliday and Mushin (1979)	Onset	P60	N70	P100	N125	P160	

The approximate latency in milliseconds is indicated under each component named. For the nomenclature used by Halliday et al (1979b) mean latencies ± SD are given in Table 3.1

early components A, B and C, and this system has been used in the monograph on the ERG, EOG and flash VEP by Babel, Stangos, Korol and Spiritus (1977), which summarizes an extensive experience with these responses in clinical ophthalmology. The various nomenclatures are compared in Table 3.3.

Variability of the flash response

According to Cigànek (1975) most of the trial-by-trial variability of the flash response is contributed by the background activity of the EEG, because the standard deviation of the ongoing activity does not increase significantly with the onset of the VEP itself. There is, indeed, a significant reduction in the variance in about half the healthy subjects tested beginning about 80 msec after the flash. This appears typically in those individuals in whom there is clear-cut blocking of the background activity after the flash in the routine EEG record and appears to be a manifestation of such blocking. The repeatability of the flash response in any one individual from run to run is relatively very good. Contamin and Cathala (1961) found a ± 15% latency variability. This stability of the individual flash EP waveform can be observed over intervals as long as months or years. By contrast there are large differences between the flash VEP waveform in different healthy subjects. As with all the visual EPs, the variability in amplitude is much greater than the variability in the peak latencies of the various components.

The sinusoidal after-discharge to flash stimulation

The relationship of the after-discharge to the resting alpha rhythm is interesting. There is evidence that the after-discharge is less prominent or absent in subjects without alpha, and that it can be reduced by such manoeuvres as opening the eye, which are known to block the alpha rhythm (Cigànek, 1975). With prolonged light stimulation, rather than flash, the after-discharge is evoked only by the 'off' stimulus and not by the 'on' stimulus (Clynes et al, 1964; Efron, 1964). According to Cohn (1964), with 1 Hz flash stimulation the rhythmic after-discharge appears in about one in five individuals with eyes open and in more than four out of five individuals when the eyes are closed. It is not seen in infants and young children until the age is reached when a normal alpha rhythm appears in the EEG.

Photopic and scotopic flash EPs

Reducing the intensity of the flash stimulus leads to a reduction in amplitude of the occipital VEP associated with an increase in the peak latencies of the various components. However, the maximum peak-to-peak amplitude of the early response with the eyes closed is usually somewhat larger than with the eyes open. It is possible that this is because the prestimulus luminance level with eyes closed is further below the intensity level at which the retinal receptors show saturation; increases of stimulus intensity above this saturation level are not accompanied by any further increase in amplitude, and the size of the response may actually decrease somewhat (Cigànek, 1975). At very low stimulus intensities, when the subject is fully dark-adapted, a new positive wave appears at a latency of about 270 msec, corresponding to the photopic wave V which has a normal peak latency more than 100 msec earlier (Gastaut et al, 1966). The change from photopic to scotopic flash responses is discontinuous, and the two types of response are quite distinct, like the corresponding photopic and scotopic ERG components (see Chapter 4, pages 125-6). These two flash responses can therefore be used to discriminate between cone (photopic) and rod (scotopic) vision.

Below the saturation level within the photopic range, the peak latency of the flash response alters with stimulus intensity (Figure 3.3) with an increase in latency over the range 2.5-5.0 log units of approximately 16.5 msec per log unit diminution in brightness (Diamond, 1964; Efron, 1964) and a corresponding reduction in amplitude of 1.72 µV per log unit (Mushin, 1974).

'On' and 'off' responses to an unstructured diffuse light stimulus

The usual flash stimulus, delivered by a xenon flash discharge tube, can be regarded as a mixture of an 'on' and 'off' stimulus, and the 'on' and 'off' responses can be separated by substituting an unstructured light stimulus of longer duration. When this is done the 'on' and 'off' responses can be shown to differ somewhat in waveform (Clynes et al, 1964; Efron, 1964). As has already been mentioned, the after-discharge at alpha frequency is particularly associated with the 'off' response (see Clynes et al, 1964, for further details).

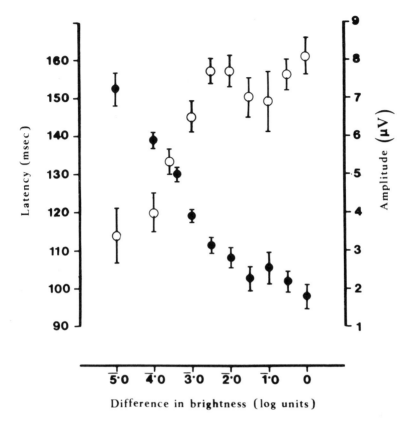

Figure 3.3 *Effect of the intensity of the flash stimulus on the mean amplitude (o) and latency (●) of the major positivity (Ciganek's component IV) ± the standard error of the mean. Data from Mushin (1974.)*

EP amplitude to an unstructured diffuse light stimulus (luminance response) as a function of field size and stimulus frequency

A great deal of experimental work has been carried out on the characteristics of the EP to diffuse light, using not only repetitive flash stimulation, but also light pulses or sinusoidally modulated flicker (van der Tweel and Verduyn Lunel, 1965; Regan, 1972a; Desmedt, 1977a). It can be shown that the amplitude of the so-called steady-state response to sinusoidally modulated light depends, among other things, upon the modulation depth, the stimulus frequency and the field size. With increasing modulation depth, the EP amplitude rises linearly to a maximum and then saturates.

Above stimulus frequencies of 8 Hz the separate components of the transient flash EP are no longer seen and the waveform of the response takes on the character of a quasi-sinusoidal train of waves (Cigànek, 1975). However, the waveform of the transient response may still be reproduced to the first stimulus of the train, when this is initially turned on (Cigànek, 1975). The advantage of the steady-state EP to faster stimulus rates is that, since the individual components are no longer visible, measurement is simplified to a determination of changes in peak-to-peak amplitude or phase. Since both stimulus and response trains are repetitive and on-going, latency measurements can only be made indirectly in terms of changes of phase. Flicker responses of this kind have been quite widely used for clinical testing (e.g. Milner et al, 1974; Regan et al, 1976; Celesia and Daly, 1977b; Cohen et al, 1980).

PATTERNED FLASH EP

If a patterned grid is placed in front of the strobe tube, giving a structured flash stimulus, the character of the occipital EP is altered. Commonly used transparencies have been black-and-white checkerboards or gratings (Spehlmann, 1965; Rietveld et al, 1967). Such flashed pattern EPs, which are a mixture of the responses to luminance and contrast changes, show a much closer correlation between the amplitude and the visual acuity level, and have been used to study the changes in VEPs with uncorrected and corrected refractive errors (Harter and White, 1968, 1969). Jeavons and Harding (1975) have found this response to be particularly valuable in the study of photosensitive epilepsy.

Jeffreys (1968) used the subtraction method on the patterned flash EP to separate the response to the unpatterned luminance onset from the pattern response. The pattern specific responses are clearly dependent on stimulation of the central region of the retina and are reduced or abolished in patients with amblyopia (Duffy et al, 1967; Lombroso et al, 1969).

The pattern specific responses are sensitive to a variety of stimulus parameters (contrast, field size and eccentricity, spatial frequency, etc.). These will be considered further in the following sections.

PATTERN CHANGE EPs

Evoked responses to changes in the pattern of a stimulus, unaccompanied by luminance responses, can be recorded if it is arranged that the change in contour takes place within a stimulus field of constant mean luminance. This can be effected by arranging that the total areas of black and white in the pattern remain unchanged, as in the reversal of a black-and-white checkerboard, or by presenting the black-and-white pattern in place of a neutral grey background of equal mean luminance. The former is termed a *pattern reversal response*, the latter a *pattern appearance response*. Like flash, pattern appearance has both an 'on' and an 'off' stimulus implicit in it. The responses to these two will be separated if the pattern appearance (onset) and disappearance (offset) are sufficiently far apart in time (e.g. 600 msec), but in a short duration pattern appearance (e.g. 25 msec) the 'on' and 'off' responses are superimposed. The most commonly used stimulus in clinical testing is the reversal of a black-and-white checkerboard. Again, like the flash stimulus, this can be presented at relatively slow stimulus rates, producing the so-called transient pattern-reversal response, or at faster rates above 8 Hz, when a quasi-sinusoidal steady-state pattern-reversal response is produced (see Figure 3.4).

When the checkerboard reversal response is compared with the corresponding pattern onset and offset responses (Estevez and Spekreijse, 1974; Kriss and Halliday, 1980) it is found that the waveform of the pattern reversal response corresponds much more closely to the pattern offset than to the pattern onset response (Figure 3.5).

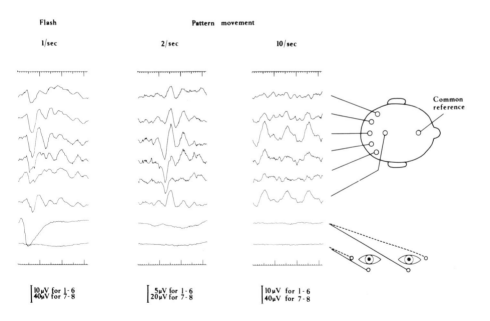

Figure 3.4 *Averaged VEPs recorded from the left eye of a healthy subject to (1) 100 flash stimuli at 1 Hz (left hand record); (2) 200 checkerboard pattern reversals at 2 Hz (middle record); and (3) 100 checkerboard pattern reversals at 10 Hz. Time base 320 msec, marked in 10, 50 and 100 msec intervals. Note the large flash ERG accompanying the luminance response and the quasi-sinusoidal form of the steady-state pattern EP as compared with the well-defined components of the transient response to 2/second pattern reversal. (From Halliday, 1972.)*

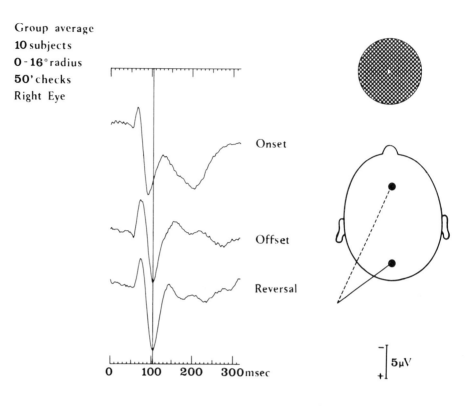

Group average
10 subjects
0 - 16° radius
50' checks
Right Eye

Onset

Offset

Reversal

0   100   200   300 msec

5μV

Figure 3.5 *Group average responses from the right eye of 10 healthy individuals to pattern onset, pattern offset and pattern reversal. (From Kriss and Halliday, 1980.)*

Waveform of the normal checkerboard reversal EP

The checkerboard reversal EP has a somewhat different waveform from the flash EP, as can be seen from Figure 3.4, which compares the flash response with the transient and steady-state responses to 2 Hz and 10 Hz checkerboard reversal, all recorded from the left eye of the same healthy subject. The mean latency and amplitude of the first five component peaks of the 2 Hz reversal response are shown in Table 3.2 on page 74 for the same control group of 17 healthy subjects included in the 1972 study by Halliday et al. It can be seen that the peak latency values show substantially less variability for the earlier peaks, the standard deviation being very much smaller than for the corresponding components of the flash response (Table 3.1). The amplitude variability is, however, about the same for both responses.

Such control values are important in determining the limits of normal. The exact values depend on a large number of stimulus variables, including the mean luminance of the stimulus and the speed of the pattern reversal ('transition time'). For this reason each laboratory must determine its own control values, using the equipment which is to be employed in clinical testing.

Table 3.4 THE EFFECT OF THE SPEED OF PATTERN MOVEMENT ('TRANSITION TIME') ON THE MEAN LATENCY AND AMPLITUDE OF THE COMPONENTS OF THE PATTERN EP IN 18 HEALTHY INDIVIDUALS

35 msec pattern movement

Right eye				Left eye			
Latency (msec)		Amplitude (μV)		Latency (msec)		Amplitude (μV)	
Mean	SD	Mean	SD	Mean	SD	Mean	SD
54.0	2.1			53.3	2.6		
64.3	3.5	+ 1.17	1.08	63.6	4.2	+ 1.09	0.71
81.5	5.3	- 2.94	2.79	80.7	5.8	- 3.06	2.50
118.9	4.4	+10.81	4.17	118.1	4.6	+10.13	3.81
153.9	9.0	- 11.29	5.40	154.0	9.5	- 10.18	5.05
202.2	31.3	+ 6.65	6.57	203.1	32.7	+ 6.64	6.27

10 msec pattern movement

Right eye				Left eye			
Latency (msec)		Amplitude (μV)		Latency (msec)		Amplitude (μV)	
Mean	SD	Mean	SD	Mean	SD	Mean	SD
49 .8	2.9			49.7	2.4		
58.2	3.6	+ 1.17	0.87	58.3	2.8	+ 1.43	0.97
74.9	4.9	- 4.00	2.60	75.1	5.4	- 3.87	2.20
103.9	4.5	+14.63	4.62	103.3	4.3	+14.59	4.60
140.9	9.6	- 13.42	6.70	139.2	9.6	- 13.05	6.67
179.5	31.7	+ 6.30	6.68	179.1	33.7	+ 6.01	6.41

(Data from Mushin, 1974)

This point can be underlined by the data in Table 3.4, which also illustrates the effect of transition time on the mean latency of the checkerboard reversal response. Following the original study (Halliday et al, 1972) a new improved stimulator was built, employing a lighter mirror capable of faster movement and therefore of shorter transition times. Slower transition times could be accurately reproduced, however, by adjusting the timing of the ramp waveform driving the mirror movement. A different control group of 18 healthy subjects was run on this new stimulator and an attempt was made to reproduce exactly the speed of the original stimulator. Nonetheless, a comparison of the mean latencies for the 35 msec pattern reversal in Table 3.4 with those for the same response in Table 3.1 will show that there are some significant discrepancies, particularly in the latency of the earlier components. Furthermore, decreasing the transition time of the mirror to 10 msec reduced the mean latency of the major positive component by 15 msec from 118 msec to 103 msec.

With TV stimulators, where the pattern reversal has to be built up over the time taken to completely scan one frame, there is an effect analogous to the transition time of the projection and rotating mirror method. Furthermore, in the commonly adopted desynchronized mode, where the instant of commencing the reversed pattern is allowed to occur randomly at any point in the frame in order to avoid averaging hum from mains artifact, a latency 'jitter' is introduced which degrades the response, increasing the intratrial variance, broadening the peak of the $\overline{P100}$ component, and leading to a mean amplitude reduction of approximately 25% (Stockard et al, 1979; Galvin et al, 1980; van Lith et al, 1978; Lowitzsch et al, 1980). This does not necessarily increase the intertrial variance, however, at least for averages of 200 or more responses. Stockard et al (1979) found the mean peak latency of the $\overline{P100}$ to be extremely consistent in any given individual for either the TV or the LED display stimulus with a test-retest reliability within 1-2 msec even over a period of some months. The mean latencies produced by the two stimulators nonetheless differed by 10-15 msec in the same individual. Galvin et al (1980), who compared the free-running TV stimulus with the mirror/projector stimulus in 22 healthy eyes, found a mean latency increase of 4.2 msec for the TV method; but the responses from 23 patients with suspected or established multiple sclerosis were similar for both stimuli.

It is thus clear that small, and sometimes undetermined, differences in the stimulus parameters used in different laboratories will render invalid any attempt to produce any generally acceptable standardized 'normal latency range'. Each laboratory must determine its own norms. One of the first tasks, therefore, facing anyone who wishes to use pattern EPs in clinical testing is to run their own series of control recordings. A corollary to this is that much of the normal data given in this book, which is derived from the authors' own laboratory experience, can only be taken as a representative guide to the kind of results to be expected. Exact values will depend on the design and performance of the stimulator in each laboratory.

Distribution of the normal 'full-field' checkerboard pattern response

The mean values given in Tables 3.1 and 3.2 are for the response recorded at the mid-occipital electrode (with reference to a mid-frontal indifferent electrode). With a stimulus field which is symmetrical about the fixation point, this is generally the point of maximum response over the head. As can be seen from Figure 3.4, however, the response spreads laterally and can be picked up at reduced amplitude at the electrodes 5 and 10 cm out on each side. The flash EP has a less well localized maximum than the pattern response, although the earliest components are again recorded best at a point about 6 cm above the inion (Cobb and Dawson, 1960).

Figure 3.6 shows the mean response waveform for a centrally fixated 0-16°. circular checkerboard field, reversed at 2 Hz, recorded from the standard montage used in the author's laboratory, consisting of a transverse row of five electrodes placed 5 cm apart across the back of the head, with the middle electrode 5 cm directly above the inion. The record is a grand average from 50 healthy subjects, and the standard deviation is indicated above and below the mean. The almost identical waveform of the responses from each eye is to be noted. The large amplitude mid-

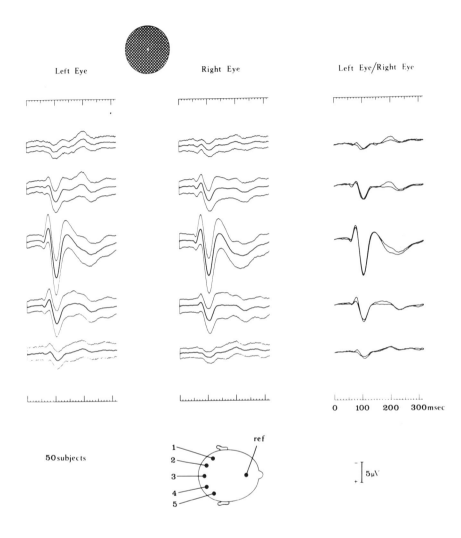

Figure 3.6 *Group average pattern reversal EPs from each eye of 50 healthy individuals, plotted with the standard deviation. The mean waveforms from each eye are superimposed in the right hand column. The stimulus is a circular checkerboard subtending 32°, made up of 50′ checks. (From Blumhardt and Halliday, 1979.)*

occipital response falls off rapidly at the electrodes 5 and 10 cm out on each side, but this, although characteristic of the 'full-field' response, is somewhat misleading, as it can be shown to be an artifact of the cancellation of sub-components from the two half fields at the lateral electrodes (see below). Essentially the same features may be

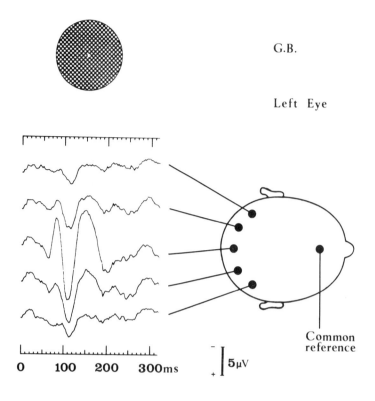

G.B.

Left Eye

Figure 3.7 *Pattern reversal EP to a 0-16° checkerboard recorded from the left eye of a healthy individual. (From Barrett et al, 1976.)*

seen in the record from an individual healthy subject (Figure 3.7). Its main feature is a triphasic negative-positive-negative complex in which the major positive component ($\overline{P100}$) is preceded and followed by smaller negative peaks ($\overline{N75}$ and $\overline{N145}$). Detailed tabulated values for these components in the group of 50 healthy subjects is given in Blumhardt and Halliday (1979), but, as has been made clear, the exact values obtained depend critically on stimulus parameters and cannot be extrapolated to other control groups. The main peaks of the pattern reversal response, however, are much more consistent than those of the flash response and it is precisely this constancy which has provided a firm basis for its use in clinical testing.

Comparison of pattern reversal responses from the two eyes

In spite of the relatively large variance in amplitude between the pattern reversal EPs from different healthy individuals, the amplitude and waveform of the response from each eye of a given individual is very similar. As can be seen from Figure 3.6 the responses from the two eyes are almost identical. This is valuable in the context of clinical testing, because many pathological lesions associated with alteration of the VEP are uniocular or affect only one optic nerve. A comparison of the latency or amplitude of the major positive component of the response from each eye may therefore provide significant evidence of an abnormality, even where the absolute values are not beyond the normal range. Figures 3.8 and 3.9 show the distributions of the latencies and amplitudes for the $\overline{P100}$ component in a group of 50 healthy individuals, with the value for the right eye plotted along the ordinate and that from the left eye along the abscissa. The mean for the group has an origin close to, but not quite identical with, zero. This represents a small absolute difference in the mean latency or amplitude of the response from the two eyes. The upper and lower lines in each graph are the 99% confidence limits for the regression line computed for the data points. As can be seen, an absolute difference of 8 msec between the mid-occipital P100 peaks from each eye is invariably abnormal, as is an absolute amplitude difference of 7 μV. It must be remembered, however, that amplitude

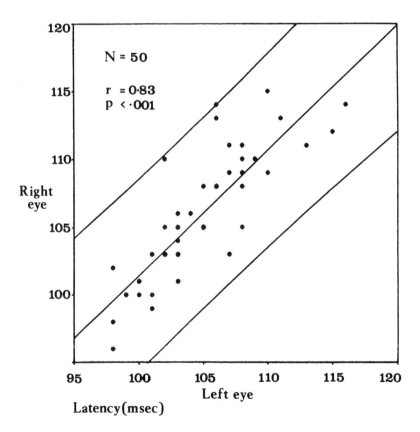

Figure 3.8 *Latency of the $\overline{P100}$ component of the checkerboard reversal response from each eye of 50 healthy individuals. Note the small range (25 msec) of the scales used on the ordinate and abscissa. The upper and lower lines are the 99% confidence limits. The correlation coefficient for the interocular latency is high (r = 0.83) and the values for the healthy population fall within less than 8 msec of the mean.*

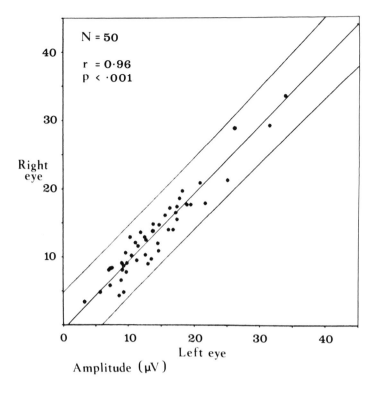

Figure 3.9 *Amplitude of the* $\overline{P100}$ *component in the left and right eyes of 50 healthy individuals, plotted with the 99% confidence limits. In spite of the wide difference in amplitudes between individuals, the correlation coefficient is very high (0.96) and the interocular difference falls within 7 μV.*

changes can also be induced by poor fixation and the use of this amplitude difference criterion presupposes a careful monitoring and control of the subject's fixation during the test.

While accepting that many factors alter the normal latency of the pattern reversal response, it is equally clear that the range of latencies encountered in responses from the healthy population to a checkerboard of reasonably large squares (30′-70′) and field size (>10°) covers not more than 20-35 msec for any one method. This has been the consistent finding since the earliest studies with the mirror and projector stimulator (Halliday et al, 1972, 1973a, 1973b) and has been confirmed by Stockard et al (1979) for both TV and LED stimulators on a large control population. Stockard suggests that for adequately large control groups, the normal latency is best expressed in percentiles, rather than in terms of standard deviations of the mean, since the distribution of response latency appears to depart somewhat from a normal distribution, particularly as regards the incidence of elderly outliers with increased latency. Within the age range 15-50 years, however, the use of the standard deviation measure is not likely to lead to any appreciable error and separate age control data for the two sexes is needed to adequately deal with the elderly population.

Effect of mean stimulus intensity on pattern reversal EP

Reduction in the mean brightness of the checkerboard stimulus results in a decrease in amplitude and an increase in latency, as in the case of the flash response. Figures 3.10 and 3.11 show the effect upon the mean latency and amplitude of the major positivity of the pattern reversal response of introducing neutral density filters into the projector beam (Halliday et al, 1973b). There is an increase in latency of 15 msec per log unit and a corresponding reduction in amplitude of 18 per cent per log unit. These are very comparable to the slopes for the flash EP (see above).

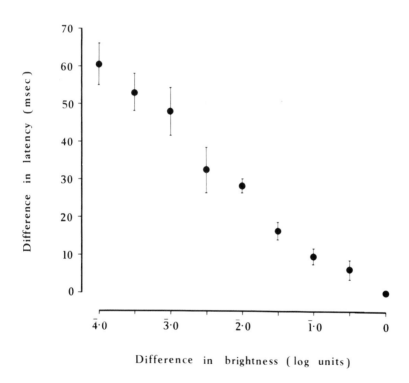

Figure 3.10 Change in the mean latency of the $\overline{P100}$ component of the pattern evoked potential with decrease in brightness of the checkerboard stimulus. The mean data for 5 healthy individuals is plotted with the standard deviation. (From Halliday, McDonald and Mushin, 1973b.)

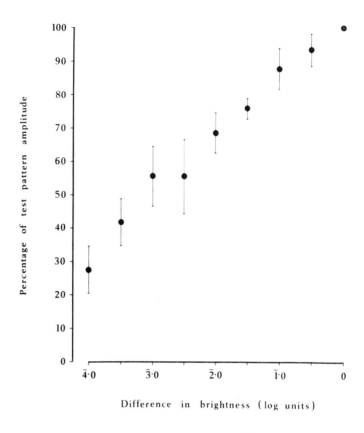

Figure 3.11 *Mean change in the amplitude of the $\overline{P100}$ component of the pattern evoked potential with change in brightness of the checkerboard stimulus. The mean data for 5 healthy individuals plotted with the standard deviation.*

SEX DIFFERENCES IN THE NORMAL VEP

Stockard et al (1979) have drawn attention to the small, but significant, differences between the two sexes in the mean latency of the checkerboard pattern reversal EP. Using a TV pattern stimulator to compare the responses in 50 age-matched men and women, they recorded mean latencies for the major positivity of 98.80 ± 5.78 msec for the women and 101.49 ± 6.21 msec for the men. These means, which were for the responses from the right eye, were significantly different at the $p = 0.03$ level. There was no sex difference in the interocular latency difference which was less than 5 msec for over 90% of the subjects, less than 6 msec for 95% and less than 9 msec for 99%.

Data from the author's own laboratory, obtained with a projector and mirror pattern stimulator, have confirmed these latency differences between the sexes at a much higher level of significance and have also demonstrated that the mean amplitude of the response is several microvolts larger in women. The mean values

Table 3.5 DIFFERENCES IN THE MEAN LATENCY AND AMPLITUDE OF THE $\overline{P100}$ COMPONENT OF THE CHECKERBOARD REVERSAL RESPONSE IN THE TWO SEXES

	N	Latency (msec)		Amplitude (μV)	
		Left eye	**Right eye**	**Left eye**	**Right eye**
Men.	65	107.7 ± 4.55	108.2 ± 4.95	11.5 ± 4.28	10.9 ± 4.52
Women	69	103.8 ± 4.19	104.7 ± 4.95	16.1 ± 5.71	15.8 ± 5.85
Difference		-3.9	-3.5	+4.6	+4.9
		p<0.001	p<0.001	p<0.001	p<0.001

are given in Table 3.5 for a comparison group of 69 healthy women and 65 healthy men with normal vision. Although not age-matched, both amplitude and latency effects are consistently present from the second to the fifth decade. The reason for these differences has not been established, although it may be related to the greater head size and skull thickness in men (Parsons and Keene, 1919; Johnston and Whillis, 1938) and possibly also to the higher deep body temperature in women

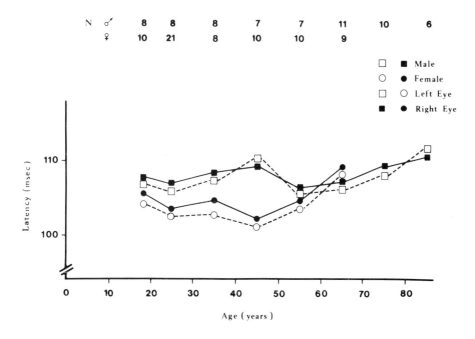

Figure 3.12 *The effect of age and sex on mean latency of the* $\overline{P100}$ *component of the pattern reversal EP, plotted separately for the left and right eye of healthy men and women falling in each decade (from 15-19 years for the earliest group). The numbers contributing to each mean are shown above. Note the shorter mean latency for the responses in women up till the age of 50 and the increase in latency in the female subjects between 50 and 70 years. (From Halliday, Barrett, Carroll and Kriss, 1982a.)*

(Stockard et al, 1979; Christie and McCreartey, 1977). Comparable sex differences have also been reported for the brainstem and somatosensory responses, the shorter latency being found in women in each case (Stockard et al, 1978; Michalewski et al, 1980; Shagass, 1972). There are small differences in the latency of the response from the left and right eye, with the mean right eye latency consistently 0.5 to 0.9 msec longer. Although small, this interocular difference is seen for the sub-groups at all ages (see Figure 3.12). The explanation for this difference is not clear. Small sex differences in the flash response have also been reported (Beaumont and Mayes, 1977; Buchsbaum et al, 1974; Rodin et al, 1965; Shagass and Schwartz, 1965).

THE EFFECT OF AGE ON THE NORMAL VEP

There have been a number of studies of the effect of age on the pattern-reversal EP. There is general agreement in the published literature that the $\overline{\text{P100}}$ latency increases in the elderly, but the form of the age/latency function is a matter of debate. Celesia and Daly (1977a), who used a TV pattern display of low luminance (10 foot lamberts), small field size (9.3°) and small checks (15.5') in a study of 74 volunteers, reported a linear increase in mean latency with age, which was significant at the p < 0.001 level. The regression line fitting the data had a slope of approximately 0.18 msec per annum over the age range from 15 to 70, increasing from 93 to 103 msec over that period. The data collected by Allison et al (1979), on the other hand, suggested little or no increase in latency until the age of 50 with a progressive increase thereafter, which agrees with our own earlier conclusions (Halliday et al, 1973a). Faust et al (1978) reached a similar conclusion in their study of 60 healthy individuals between 10 and 69 years of age; those under 15 years and over 65 showed a significantly longer $\overline{\text{P100}}$ latency. In a subsequent study they also report higher $\overline{\text{P100}}$ amplitudes in individuals under 25 years and over 55. The study by Stockard et al (1979), which was the first published series to separate out the sex differences, dealt only with latency and reported no significant age effect on latency between 20 and 55 years of age. In the sixth decade, they found an increase in the variance, but not in the mean latency, of the $\overline{\text{P100}}$, which required an increase of 5 msec in the normal limits. In the over 60s, they noted an increase in the mean latency as well, although no formal data for this age group is presented. The sex differences in latency were seen within each age group. This effect is also very clearly evident in our own data (see Figure 3.12) (Halliday et al, 1982a). In addition, the sex difference in mean amplitude, which we had noted, was also clearly seen at all ages (Figure 3.13). Our own study strongly suggested, however, that the increase in mean latency from the age of 50 onwards may be seen only for the female group. In the male group it either does not occur or occurs much later; the data are inconclusive. Clearly, further studies of these sex and age differences are needed.

It is worth pointing out that elderly patients need very careful screening for minor visual defects. Slight opacities, discolouration of the lens and retinal lesions become more frequent in the elderly and may easily pass unnoticed unless a careful clinical ophthalmological screening is carried out. We also eliminated a number of individuals with unexplained increases of interocular latency difference clearly exceeding the normal limit from our control groups. The discrepancy between the data of Celesia and Daly (1977a) and the other studies may also be partly explained by differences in the luminance of the pattern stimulator used in these studies. Shaw and Cant (1980) have shown that the function relating mean latency to age in healthy subjects alters its slope with changes in the mean luminance of the stimulus. Data on maturational changes in the pattern reversal response have been published by Hoffman (1978) and Allison et al (1979).

Data on the effect of ageing on the flash response amplitude and latency are given by Dustman et al (1977). Studies on the maturational changes of the flash EP have been published by Hrbek and Mares (1964), Weinmann et al (1965), Ellingson (1958, 1964, 1968, 1970), Ellingson et al, (1973), Watanabe et al (1972, 1973), Hrbek et al (1973), Hrbek et al, (1977), Laget et al, (1977, 1978), Marcus (1977), Ferris et al, (1967), Blom et al (1980), Gambi et al, (1980) and Barnet et al, (1980).

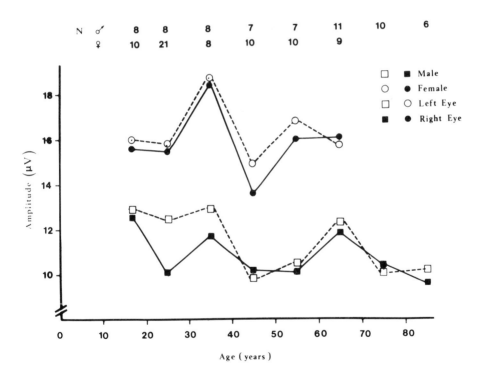

Figure 3.13 *Mean $\overline{P100}$ amplitude of the left and right eye responses in healthy men and women at different ages. Note the larger amplitude of the responses in women. There is no significant effect of age on amplitude. (From Halliday et al, 1982a.)*

VEPs TO HALF FIELD STIMULATION

If instead of presenting a centrally fixated visual stimulus, the stimulus is presented in one half field, a striking asymmetry appears in the pattern reversal response. The midline triphasic NPN complex, encompassing the major positivity and composed of three distinct peaks ($\overline{N75}$, $\overline{P100}$ and $\overline{N145}$), becomes markedly asymmetrical in distribution across the head, being recorded at the midline and ipsilateral electrodes of the transverse occipital chain (Figure 3.14). Furthermore, the response no longer has the marked midline localization characteristic of the full field stimulus and decrements far less steeply at the lateral electrodes (compare Figure 3.7). All these features can be clearly seen in the grand average responses to half-field stimulation from 50 healthy individuals (Figure 3.15). The group averages demonstrate clearly another feature of the responses. In addition to the midline and ipsilateral NPN complex containing the major positive component, there is also a smaller triphasic complex of approximately the same latency but opposite polarity, recorded from the contralateral side of the head. This phase-reversed PNP complex has maximal amplitude, not near the midline, but at the most lateral electrode, 10 cm out from the midline. At the 5 cm electrode contralateral to the half field stimulated the response has a 'transitional' form, somewhere between the ipsilateral

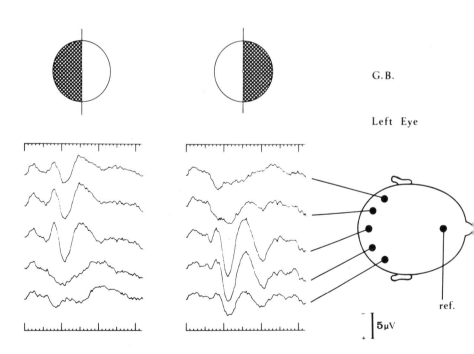

Figure 3.14 *Responses to left and right half-field stimulation from the left eye of the healthy individual whose full-field responses are shown in Figure 3.7.*

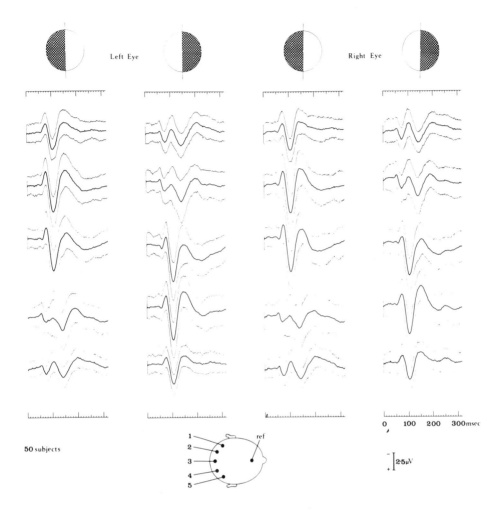

Figure 3.15 *Group average waveforms and standard deviation of the pattern reversal EPs to half-field stimulation in 50 healthy individuals. Note the NPN complex at midline and ipsilateral electrodes, corresponding to the $\overline{P100}$ component of the full-field response and the smaller, more variable components of reversed polarity at the contralateral electrodes. (From Blumhardt and Halliday, 1979.)*

and contralateral waveforms. The variability is also considerably greater at this electrode, as is shown by the increased standard deviation.

It can be shown that the full-field response approximates very closely to an algebraic summation of the responses from each half-field (Figure 3.16). It then becomes clear that the midline maximum of the full-field response is due simply to the summation of the NPN complexes from each half-field. The major positivity is particularly large at this electrode because it is composite, being made up of the

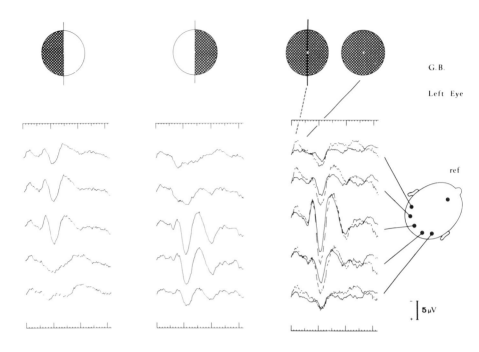

Figure 3.16 *Comparison of the monocular full-field pattern EP with the summated half-field EPs in the same healthy individual as in Figures 3.7 and 3.14. The algebraic summation of the two half-field responses is shown on the right (dotted line) superimposed on the separately recorded full-field response (solid line). (From Blumhardt, Barrett and Halliday, 1977.)*

major component from each half field. The explanation of the lateral decrement in the response lies in a similar combination of the contributions from each half field. Each ipsilateral NPN component is, in fact, recorded over a wide area of the back of the head ipsilateral to the half field stimulated, but in the full-field response it is 'cancelled' at the more lateral electrodes by the phase-reversed contralateral PNP component occurring at the same latency. It therefore appears smaller than it really is. These features can be easily seen by comparing the grand averages of the full-field (Figure 3.6) and half-field (Figure 3.15) responses from the same 50 healthy individuals.

Some of the same asymmetrical features can be detected in the responses to diffuse flash stimulation presented in each half field, but the asymmetry is far less marked and the full-field response shows much greater divergence from the response computed by half field summation (Figures 3.17 and 3.18). In the case of the pattern reversal response, on the other hand, the size of the major positivity of the full-field response closely approximates the predicted sum of the half-field positivities in every case (Figure 3.19) (Blumhardt and Halliday, 1979).

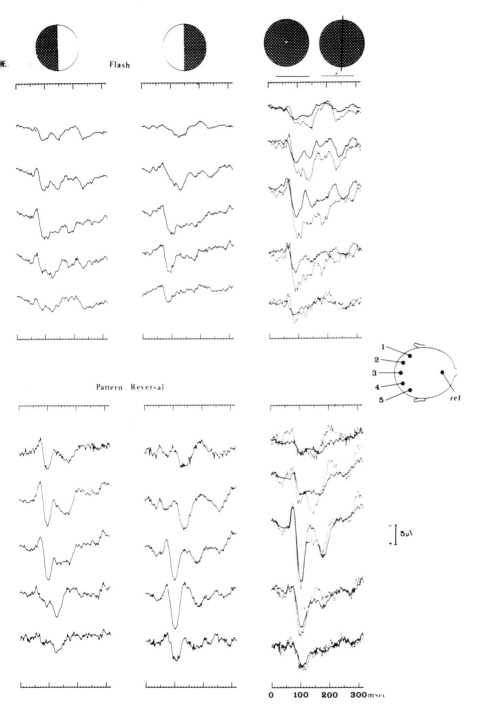

Figure 3.17 *Flash (above) and pattern reversal EPs (below) to half-field stimulation recorded from the same healthy individual. The records on the right show the summated half-field responses compared with the separately recorded full-field response in each case.*

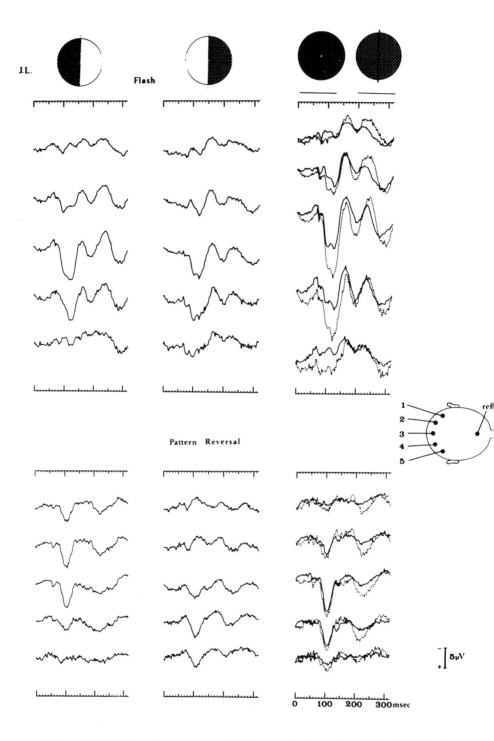

Figure 3.18 *Flash and pattern reversal EPs recorded in another healthy individual, as in Figure 3.17.*

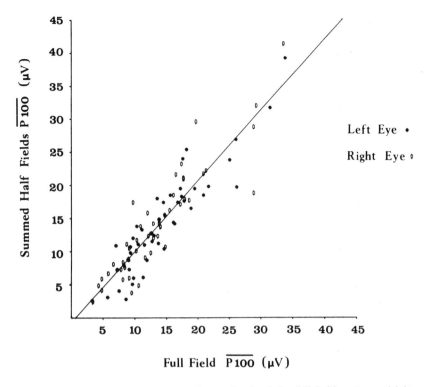

Figure 3.19 *Relationship between the amplitude of the full-field major positivity and the sum of the half-field $\overline{P100}$ components in 50 healthy individuals. Amplitudes measured peak-to-peak from the preceding surface negative wave ($\overline{N75}$) at the midline electrode. (From Blumhardt and Halliday, 1979.)*

Hemisphere contributions to the pattern evoked potential waveform

The resort to half-field stimulation is one approach towards separating out the responses from the visual generator areas in the left and right hemispheres, since the retinocortical pathways from each half field terminate in the visual cortex of the opposite occipital lobe. It would, however, be naive to equate the left half-field response with the visual EP from the right hemisphere and vice versa without further evidence, because there are important transcallosal connections, concerned with the representation of a vertical strip of the visual field up to 2° out on either side of the fixation point (Myers, 1962; Hubel and Wiesel, 1967; Blakemore, 1969; Mitchell and Blakemore, 1970). It is therefore perfectly reasonable to suggest that part of the responses from each half field come from the ipsilateral occipital lobe (Beauchamp et al, 1976). There is, however, decisive evidence that all the components of the normal half-field response, including both the ipsilateral NPN and contralateral PNP complexes, can be obtained from stimulation of the preserved half-field in patients who have had one whole hemisphere removed (Blumhardt and Halliday, 1979, 1981; Blumhardt et al, 1982b). In these cases it is clear that no part of the response from the intact half-field can be generated anywhere but in the contralateral hemisphere (see Figures 7.1-3, on pages 237-240).

How is the ipsilateral half-field response produced?

The records obtained following hemispherectomy make it clear that the whole of the typical half-field response is generated in the hemisphere contralateral to the half-field. This is in line with the anatomy of the retinocortical pathways, in which the fibres from the nasal hemiretina of each eye decussate in the optic chiasma to reach the striate area in the contralateral occipital lobe (Figure 3.20).

The arrangement of the retinotopic projection onto the striate cortex was first fully worked out by Gordon Holmes (1918, 1945) by studying the field defects produced by penetrating missile wounds in the 1914-18 war. He showed that the opposite half-field is represented with the fixation point and foveal projection at the occipital pole and the more peripheral parts of the field placed anteriorly on the medial surface of the hemisphere. The horizontal meridian of the contralateral half-field is represented along the base of the calcarine sulcus with the lower quadrant of the visual field above and the upper quadrant below. The vertical meridian is thus

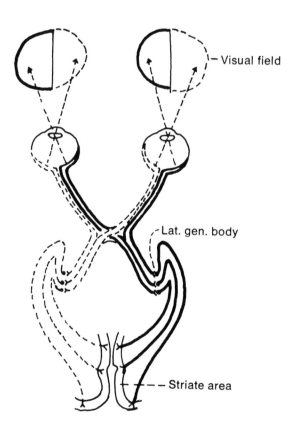

Figure 3.20 *Schematic representation of the projection of the homonymous half-fields to the generator areas in the contralateral occipital lobe (from Brodal, 1981.)*

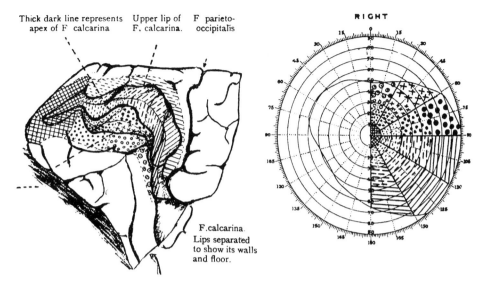

Thick dark line represents apex of F calcarina

Upper lip of F. calcarina.

F parieto-occipitalis

RIGHT

F.calcarina.
Lips separated
to show its walls
and floor.

Figure 3.21 *Gordon Holmes' schematic representation of the retino-cortical projection of the contralateral half-field on the striate area. The horizontal meridian is shown positioned at the base of the opened-out calcarine sulcus with the upper quadrant represented below and the lower quadrant above. The foveal representation is at the occipital pole with the peripheral representation more anterior. Something approaching one-third of the cortical representation is devoted to the central 10° of the visual field. (From Holmes, 1918.)*

represented along the upper and lower border of the striate area (Figure 3.21). Spalding (1952), who confirmed this general arrangement in a similar study of head injuries from the 1939-45 war, added some important details. He found that approximately 8° of the central field is represented on the postero-medial surface of the occipital lobe behind the level of the calcarine fissure and that for the more peripheral parts of the visual field represented more anteriorly, a segment of the half-field about 30° out from the vertical meridian is represented outside the calcarine fissure on the medial surface of the occipital lobe (Figure 3.22). Evidence from the distribution of phosphenes, produced by a stimulating prosthesis implanted over one occipital pole in a blind subject, confirms the general arrangement of the cortical representation suggested by the lesion data (Brindley and Lewin, 1968). Within the striate representation of each half-field there is a far larger area of cortex devoted to central vision than to peripheral vision. This can be expressed in terms of the magnification factor, specified as the millimetres of cortex per degree of the visual field, at different eccentricities from the fixation point. The data for the monkey has been accurately worked out by Daniel and Whitteridge (1961) and shows magnification factors ranging from 6.4 mm/degree at the fovea, reduced tenfold at an eccentricity of 15° and approximately a hundredfold at 65°. Cowey, who has produced similar data using behavioural perimetry in the squirrel monkey (Cowey, 1964) has also looked at the phosphene data on the patient with the stimulating prosthesis studied by Brindley and Lewin (Cowey, 1973). He found a magnification factor of 5 mm/degree in the parafoveal region, declining tenfold to 0.5 mm/degree at an eccentricity of 20-30°. There is thus surprisingly good agreement between the data on monkey and man. Further discussion of the factors relevant to the topography of the pattern EP will be found in Halliday et al (1977).

Since the scalp-recorded pattern evoked potential appears to come predominantly from the central part of the visual field, it is clear that the most important cortical areas for generating this response are represented at or near the occipital pole, where the striate representation at least is made up of neurones oriented with their apical dendrites facing posteromedially, as can be seen in Figure 3.22 from Spalding's paper. In our original report of the 'paradoxical' lateralization of the half-field pattern response (Barrett et al, 1976) we suggested that the major positivity appears at the midline and ipsilateral electrodes because these are best placed to see the surface end of the generator neurones in relation to the midfrontal reference, whereas the contralateral electrodes are oriented transversely across the long axis of the neurones in relation to the reference electrode (Figure 3.23). The position of the reference is, of course, critical and must be taken into account in interpreting the distribution of the response. It is perfectly possible to record what appears to be a contralateral response by the use of a non-indifferent electrode or by the adoption of a bipolar montage (see Chapter 1, page 25, and Halliday et al, 1979a, Halliday, 1980b). In *Nature* in 1976 we pointed out that the *ipsilateral* distribution of the NPN response to half field stimulation was typical for a 0-16°

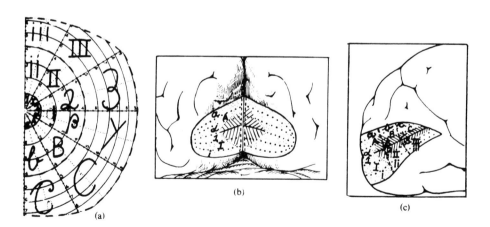

(b)

(c)

(a)

Figure 3.22 *Spalding's schematic representation of the retinotopic projection of the contralateral half-field onto the striate area, showing in (b) that the central 0-8° of the visual field is represented on the postero-medial aspect of the occipital pole before the representation enters the calcarine sulcus (cross hatched area). This data is based on a study of field defects from penetrating head wounds in the 1939-45 war. (From Spalding, 1952.)*

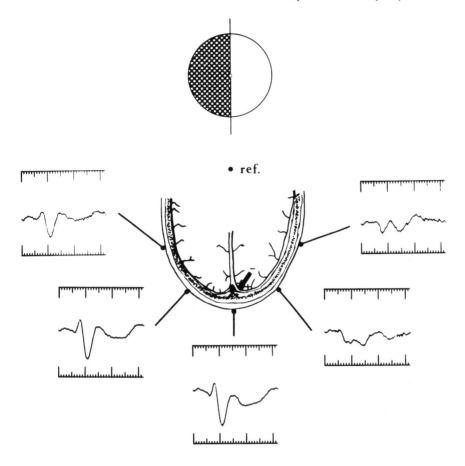

Figure 3.23 *Schematic representation of the relationship between the generator areas of the pattern EP from the left half-field and the scalp electrodes, to explain the ipsilateral distribution of the P100 component of the half-field response. For explanation see text. (From Barrett et al, 1976.)*

stimulus and was still clearly seen even when the stimulus was confined to the central 0-4°. However, when the stimulus is still further reduced to the macular area itself (0-2°), the response becomes markedly less well lateralized and may even have a contralateral predominance. This is precisely what one would expect from the schema proposed in Figure 3.23, because the cortical representation of the fovea may extend round onto the convexity of the occipital lobe at the posterior pole and the generator neurones will then be facing posteriorly rather than medially. The relationship of the striate representation to the occipital pole is rather variable from individual to individual, and even on the two sides in the same individual (see, for example, Polyak, 1957; Brindley, 1972; Stensaas et al, 1974).

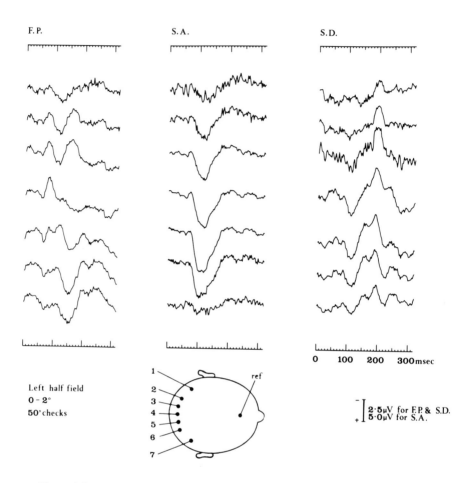

Figure 3.24 *Pattern reversal EPs evoked by a small semicircular checkerboard stimulus of 50' checks presented within the central 2° of the left half-field. The records are from 3 different healthy individuals, chosen to illustrate the variability in the distribution of the foveal $\overline{P100}$ component. The left hand record is from an individual who has a purely ipsilateral $\overline{P100}$ component, while the right hand record exhibits a midline and contralateral distribution for the same component. The second record shows a $\overline{P100}$ in another individual which straddles the midline, but with a slightly contralateral predominance. All three subjects had a normal ipsilateral distribution for the $\overline{P100}$ for the larger 0-16° half-field stimulus. (From Halliday, 1980b.)*

In line with what one would expect from this marked intra-individual anatomical variability, the half-field response to the central 2° of the visual field varies greatly in different individuals. Figure 3.24 illustrates this variability in the central left half-field response from three different individuals. In subject FP, whose 0-2° left half-field response is shown in the left hand column, the NPN complex containing the major positivity ($\overline{P100}$) appears at the ipsilateral electrodes, with the phase reversed PNP complex appearing contralaterally. This individual therefore has a foveal response demonstrating the same lateralization as for the larger 0-16° stimulus field. Subject SA, whose responses are shown in the central column, has a major positivity ($\overline{P100}$) straddling the midline, but slightly larger at the contralateral electrodes. Subject SD, whose responses are shown in the right hand column, has a major positivity ($\overline{P100}$) appearing only at the midline and contralateral electrodes. On the schema shown in Figure 3.23 it would be postulated that the last two subjects (SA and SD) had their foveal reresentations extending progressively further onto the lateral convexity of the occipital pole, so that the generator neurones had their apical dendrites oriented posteriorly and even postero-laterally, facing towards the contralateral recording electrodes (Barrett et al, 1976; Halliday, 1980b).

It can be shown by recordings on hemispherectomised patients that the change from a predominantly ipsilateral distribution for the wider 0-16° half-field stimulus to a predominantly contralateral distribution for the 0-2° foveal stimulus is characteristic of the responses from the contralateral hemisphere itself and does not involve any transcallosal conduction of the response in the central 2° across to the other hemisphere. Figure 3.25 shows the left half-field response recorded from the

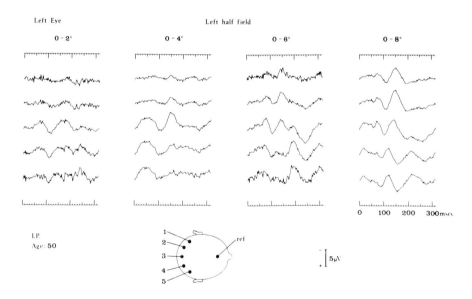

Figure 3.25 *Responses evoked by a semicircular left half-field stimulus of increasing radius in a patient who had previously undergone a left hemispherectomy. Note that the $\overline{P100}$ component is contralateral in distribution for the foveal response but becomes ipsilateral when the radius of the area stimulated is increased to 6° or 8°. This shows that both the ipsilateral response characteristic of a larger half-field stimulus and the contralateral response seen in some individuals with foveal stimulation are generated in the hemisphere contralateral to the stimulated half-field. (From Halliday, 1980b.)*

hemispherectomized patient whose 0-16° response is shown in Figure 7.1 on page 237 for checkerboard stimuli subtending fields of 0-2°, 0-4°, 0-6° and 0-8°. All the stimuli were made up of 50′ checks. The major positivity for the two smaller field sizes has a definitely contralateral distribution which switches to a midline and ipsilateral distribution for the stimuli extending out to 6° or more. By 8° both the ipsilateral NPN and contralateral PNP complexes of the wide-field response are clearly seen.

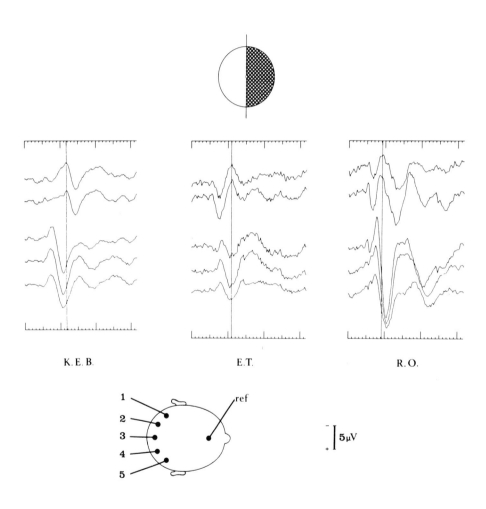

Figure 3.26 *Right half-field pattern EPs from 3 healthy individuals. The vertical lines drawn through the peak of the contralateral N105 component show that this peak may, in different individuals, occur later, simultaneously with, or earlier than the the ipsilateral P100. (From Blumhardt et al, 1978.)*

Components of the half-field response

Examination of the grand average data for the half-field response in 50 healthy subjects in Figure 3.15 will show that the earlier responses on the ipsilateral and contralateral sides of the head are both triphasic, although the components of roughly corresponding latency are of opposite polarity. The mean latencies of the three ipsilateral components ($\overline{N75}$, $\overline{P100}$ and $\overline{N145}$) are shown for each half-field of each eye in a small group of 20 healthy subjects in Table 3.6 and the mean latency for the corresponding contralateral components from the same group of individuals is shown in Table 3.7. It is at once apparent that the mean latency of the two earlier pairs of components is almost the same: 77.4-78.0 for $\overline{N75}$ and 76.5-78.4 for $\overline{P75}$, 104.9-106.2 for $\overline{P100}$ and 103.7-106.3 for $\overline{N105}$. The third pair of components, however, show a discrepancy approaching 10 msec between their peak latencies: 143.6-145.4 for $\overline{N145}$ and 134.6-137.5 for $\overline{P135}$. The standard deviation of the latency of these two later components is also almost twice as great (Blumhardt et al, 1978). However, the averaging process tends to obscure some of the latency variability in individual records, and examination of these shows that even for the earlier components, there is often a marked discrepancy in the latency of the 'corresponding' ipsilateral and contralateral component peaks (Figure 3.26). This suggests that the ipsilateral and contralateral complexes are not, as might at first be thought, simply a reflection of the same triphasic response recorded at opposite ends of the cortical generators, but that they are, on the contrary, to some extent independent of each other in their timing and occurrence. This does indeed appear to be the case.

Table 3.6 MEAN LATENCY AND S.D. OF THE MAJOR IPSILATERAL COMPONENTS OF THE HALF FIELD RESPONSE

Eye	Half field	Onset	$\overline{N75}$	$\overline{P100}$	$\overline{N145}$
Left	Left	58.8 ± 3.5	78.0 ± 4.1	104.9 ± 4.2	144.0 ± 10.7
	Right	60.6 ± 3.9	77.4 ± 4.2	106.2 ± 3.3	144.5 ± 10.5
Right	Left	61.0 ± 4.9	77.4 ± 5.1	105.1 ± 4.1	145.4 ± 9.7
	Right	60.3 ± 5.8	78.0 ± 4.6	105.4 ± 4.0	143.6 ± 9.2

Electrode 10 cm lateral to midline: 20 subjects

Table 3.7 MEAN LATENCY AND S.D. OF THE MAJOR CONTRALATERAL COMPONENTS OF THE HALF FIELD RESPONSE

Eye	Half field	Onset	$\overline{P75}$	$\overline{N105}$	$\overline{P135}$
Left	Left	59.5 ± 6.0	78.1 ± 8.7	105.1 ± 7.5	137.2 ± 8.7
	Right	59.4 ± 4.6	77.6 ± 5.1	103.7 ± 6.8	134.6 ± 14.5
Right	Left	60.9 ± 4.7	78.4 ± 5.3	106.3 ± 8.2	137.5 ± 12.7
	Right	58.7 ± 4.5	76.5 ± 4.6	104.4 ± 7.7	136.2 ± 10.1

Electrode 10 cm lateral to midline: 20 subjects

Variability in the half-field response

In order to understand the variability of the waveform of the pattern EP in the healthy individual, it is essential to grasp three main principles:

(1) The run-to-run variability of the response in any one individual is low and test-retest reliability high, provided that the recording conditions are adequately controlled. Such variability as occurs can usually be put down to poor cooperation on the part of the subject, resulting in wandering fixation, partial eye closure or contamination by excessive muscle artifact, or high voltage alpha due to poor relaxation or drowsiness. Figure 3.27 shows the run-to-run variability of the left half-field response over 11 consecutive averages of 200 pattern reversals each

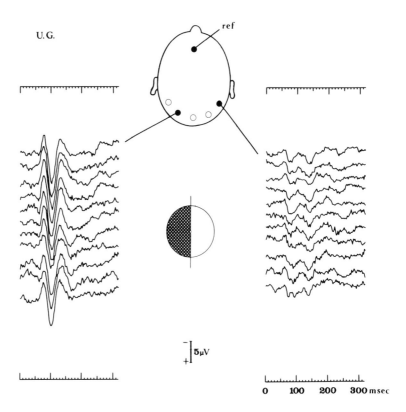

Figure 3.27 *Eleven consecutive VEPs evoked by a 0-16° checkerboard of 50′ checks presented in the left half-field to show the consistency of both the ipsilateral NPN and contralateral PNP complexes in any one subject. (From Blumhardt, 1980.)*

(Blumhardt, 1980). Both the ipsilateral NPN complex and the much smaller contralateral PNP are clearly delineated in each run and even the smaller contralateral complex is not greatly obscured by variation in the background activity.

(2) Inter-individual variability is much greater for the contralateral PNP components than for the ipsilateral NPN and some of these components of the typical half-field response may not be recognizable in the records from some individuals. This virtually never appplies to the major positivity ($\overline{\text{P100}}$) of the ipsilateral complex. Figure 3.28 shows the ipsilateral and contralateral responses at the electrodes 10 cm out in eight healthy subjects, chosen to show the variability of the contralateral components. In some individuals none of the three waves of the

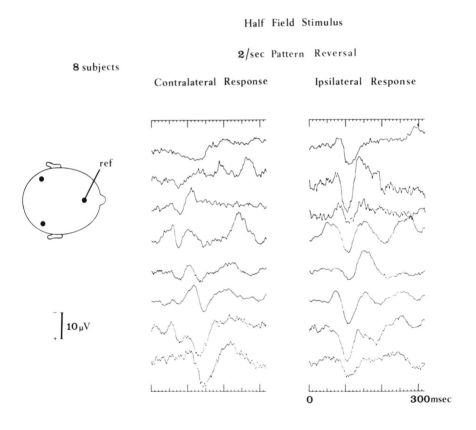

Half Field Stimulus

2/sec Pattern Reversal

8 subjects

Contralateral Response   Ipsilateral Response

ref

10 μV

0   300msec

Figure 3.28 *Simultaneously recorded contralateral and ipsilateral responses from the lateral channels (10 cm from the midline) in 8 healthy individuals. Note the marked variability of the triphasic contralateral waveform (PNP) between subjects. Compare the latency and morphology of the $\overline{\text{P135}}$ and $\underline{\text{N105}}$ components in the different individuals with the more consistent ipsilateral $\overline{\text{P100}}$. (From Blumhardt et al, 1978.)*

contralateral PNP complex are clearly defined, as in the first two records in Figure 3.28. In others only the first two are clearly seen, as in the third and fourth record. In yet others all three are clearly delineated, as in the fifth and seventh record, and in some only the $\overline{P135}$ component is clearly seen, as in the last example. These inter-subject differences are quite consistent in any one individual, provided that the stimulus conditions are not changed. They presumably represent a reflection of significant variations in the detailed anatomy of the cortical generator areas in relation to the overlying scalp electrodes.

(3) The principle of algebraic summation, by which the full-field response is apparently made up of the simple addition of the half field responses (see above, page 93), can be extended to the constituent parts of the half-field response. Thus it can be shown that each half-field response appproximates closely to the computed

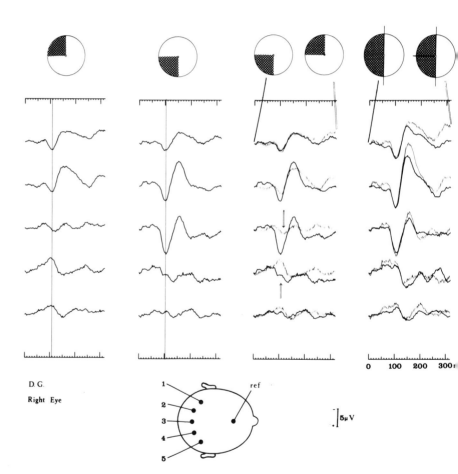

Figure 3.29 *Pattern reversal responses for upper and lower quadrant stimulation of the left half-field in a healthy individual. Note the larger contralateral components on stimulation of the upper quadrant. On the right can be seen the similarity of the summated responses from the two quadrants and the separately recorded response from the whole half-field.*

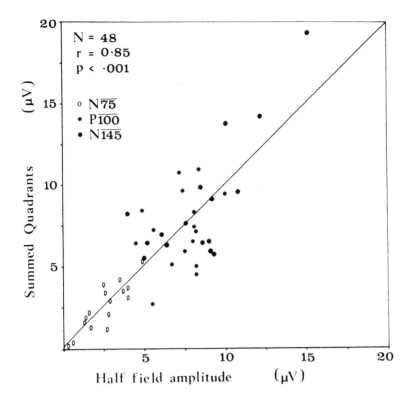

Figure 3.30 *Relationship between the half-field $\overline{N75}$, $\overline{P100}$ and $\overline{N145}$ components and the sum of the constituent upper and lower quadrant components in 50 healthy individuals. Amplitudes of these three ipsilateral components are measured peak-to-peak from the preceding wave of opposite polarity at the electrode 5 cm out from the midline. (From Blumhardt and Halliday, 1979.)*

sum of the constituent upper and lower quadrants (Blumhardt and Halliday, 1979). An example of this is shown in Figure 3.29. The left upper and lower quadrant responses shown here do not approximate nearly so closely to each other in general waveform as do the responses from the left and right half-fields. This no doubt reflects the closer relationship to the recording electrodes of the lower field representation on the upper part of the occipital lobe, as compared with the upper field representation which lies inferiorly in the occipital lobe. Even so, the half-field response corresponds well with the computed sum of the quadrants. Figure 3.30 shows that this relationship holds up well for all three components of the ipsilateral response in a group of 16 healthy individuals. The principle that the whole is equal to the sum of the parts appears to be in good agreement with the experimental data even down to quite small parts of the half-field (e.g. octants or annuli), but the reduction in the size of the response with smaller stimulus fields, particularly when these are at any considerable eccentricity from the fovea, makes it increasingly difficult to observe, as the response is often obscured by the variability of the background noise. Recording responses from small fields is thus rather tedious and demands a large number of trials if it is to produce reliable results. For this reason, it is more practical in clinical testing to stick to fairly large stimulus fields (e.g. half-fields or quadrants). It must be remembered, however, that when larger stimuli are used, some of the important constituent components may actually be obscured by cancellation (see, for example, Figure 3.25 and Figures 3.31-3.36 below). Under these circumstances, one may increase the value of the test by the intelligent adoption of a smaller stimulus. This principle particularly applies to the use of half-field rather than full-field stimulation.

Limits of normal variability in the full-field and half-field response

The principle of summation and of the clarification of the constituent components which can come from resort to analysis of the half-field responses can be well illustrated from the normal variance in the symmetry of the whole-field response in the healthy population (Blumhardt and Halliday, 1979, 1981; Blumhardt et al, 1982b). This becomes of importance clinically in the determination of the limits of normal. Hemianopic patients characteristically produce a response to a full-field stimulus resembling that to the preserved half-field in a healthy individual (see Chapter 7). Less complete field defects in one half-field (e.g. quadrantanopia) will produce a correspondingly smaller degree of asymmetry. If the pattern EP is to be used to distinguish the abnormal from the normal response in such cases, it is necessary to define accurately the limit of normal asymmetry. There are, however, quite marked asymmetries occurring in different individuals in the healthy population. These are almost invariably due to a difference in the waveform of either the ipsilateral or contralateral components of the constituent half-field responses in heteronymous half-fields. These lead to summation or cancellation of complementary components at the electrodes on each side. Where cancellation occurs equally on both sides of the head, another normal variant is produced in which the full-field response is symmetric, but apparently localized to the electrode near the midline.

Figure 3.31 shows full-field responses to a 0-16° checkerboard reversal from six healthy individuals. These examples have been chosen to illustrate the types of variation in distribution and symmetry encountered in the healthy population. In every case the responses from the left and right eye, which are superimposed in Figure 3.31, are extremely similar, but this does not preclude marked asymmetries in the distribution of the responses, as is evident from examples 4-6 (lower records). The first three examples (upper records) show symmetrical responses which vary widely in their lateral spread across the back of the head. As compared with the typical response, shown in example 1, where the major positivity, maximal at the midoccipital electrode, falls off progressively at the 5 and 10 cm electrodes, example 2 shows the response sharply localized at the midline, whereas example 3 shows a more gradual decrement. It can be demonstrated (Blumhardt et al, 1982b) that these differences in lateral spread are all produced by differences in the degree of cancellation of the major NPN complex at the lateral electrodes by the contralateral PNP response. The asymmetries shown in the lower records are produced in the same way, where these complexes are of different amplitude for the two half-fields. It is, particularly, variations in the size of the contralateral PNP complex which contribute towards producing these normal asymmetries (Blumhardt et al, 1982b).

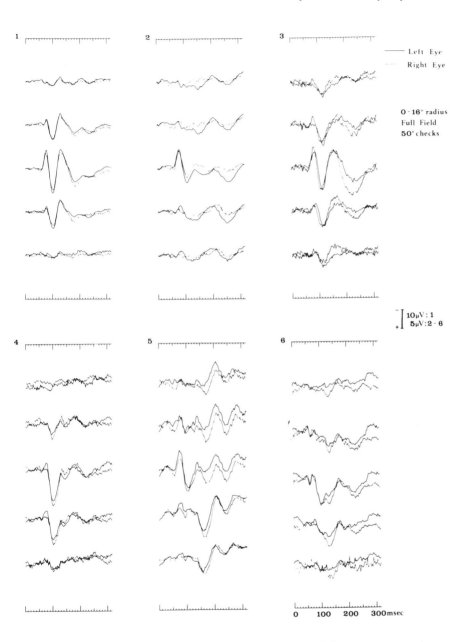

Figure 3.31 *Variation in the topographical distribution of the pattern reversal response to a full-field 0-16° checkerboard stimulus of 50' checks, illustrated by the records from 6 healthy individuals. Montage as in Figures 3.6 and 3.7, etc. The monocular responses to stimulation of the left and right eye are superimposed in each record. Note (1) the variation in the apparent distribution of the $\overline{P100}$ component around the midline; (2) the incidence in these normal individuals of both symmetrical and asymmetrical responses; (3) the occasional occurrence of complex bifid positivities at the midline, as in Case 6. (From Blumhardt et al, 1982b.)*

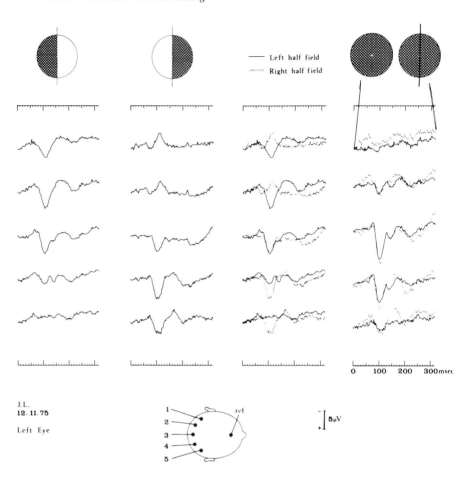

Figure 3.32 *Half-field pattern responses from the left eye of the individual whose full-field responses are shown as example 4 in Figure 3.31. The two half-field responses are superimposed in the third column and are summated and compared with the separately recorded full-field response in the fourth column. Note that the apparent asymmetry of the full-field responses, with its right-sided predominance, is due to partial cancellation of the ipsilateral positivity from the left half-field by the contralateral negativity from the right half-field, resulting in relative flattening of the left-sided channels in the full-field response. (From Blumhardt et al, 1982b.)*

Since the cancellation occurring in the full-field response obscures the relative contribution of the components from the two half-fields, one is in a much stronger position to analyse the responses if one can record and measure each half-field response separately. The full-field response will then be easily predictable, since it is equivalent to a summation of the two. This is well illustrated by Figure 3.32. In this individual the ipsilateral NPN complex from each half-field is very similar and shows the expected complementary asymmetry characteristic of half-field responses. The contralateral PNP complex, on the other hand, is well developed only for the right half-field. As a result the full-field response shows a marked asymmetry in the distribution of the major positivity, which has a midline and right-sided predominance. The full-field response corresponds exactly to the computed sum of the half-field responses, showing that the relative absence of the major positivity on the left side of the head is due to cancellation by the contralateral PNP from the right half-field.

Blumhardt and Halliday (1981) have shown that, using the full-field response alone, the mean amplitude asymmetry for the $\overline{P100}$ component measured at the lateral electrode 5 cm out to either side of the midline in 50 healthy subjects was 1:1.6. The standard deviation was ± 0.56. Taking an upper limit of 2.5 standard deviations above the mean, one therefore has to have an amplitude asymmetry of more than 3:1 between these two lateral electrodes before one can say that it is definitely abnormal. In contrast to this, the corresponding mean asymmetry for the ipsilateral $\overline{P100}$ of the two half-fields was less than 1.36 with a standard deviation of 0.331. In half-field responses, therefore, an asymmetry of appreciably more than 2.2:1 can be regarded as definitely abnormal. In a series of 26 patients with homonymous hemianopia, abnormal asymmetries were found in only 62% of the patients for the full-field response but in 81% for the half-field responses (Blumhardt and Halliday, 1981). This underlines the advantage of using half-field stimulation in clinical testing.

Another benefit of the half-field stimulation technique is that it can often clarify the normal waveforms in which the midline positivity has more than one peak — the so-called 'W-waveform' problem mentioned by Picton (1979), Stockard et al (1979), Shahrokhi et al (1978) and Lueders et al (1980). The bifid positivity can be produced by the incursion of an unusually large $\overline{P135}$ or $\overline{P75}$ into the midline channel or alternately by slight differences in the peak latency of the $\overline{P100}$ from the two hemispheres. In either case the identity of the 'true' $\overline{P100}$ is usually settled by determining which of the positive peaks is ipsilaterally lateralized on half-field stimulation (Blumhardt et al, 1982b).

Macular and paramacular components of the half-field response

It has already been emphasized that the size of the six components of the half-field response shows considerable individual variability, and that this is particularly true of the contralateral PNP complex. Since the summation principle holds even within a single half-field, the question arises as to whether some of this variation within the half-field is also due to cancellation of the pairs of components with similar latency and opposite polarity derived from different parts of the half-field. This does indeed appear to be the case (Blumhardt et al, 1978; Halliday et al, 1979a). By progressive occlusion of the central part of the 0-16° half-field checkerboard stimulus, we found that the ipsilateral NPN complex was increasingly attenuated in size, and that this change was accompanied by a progressive enhancement of the contralateral PNP complex. It therefore appears that the two triphasic complexes depend to some extent upon stimulation of different areas of the half-field and that the contralateral components can be masked by the ipsilateral ones. Figure 3.33 shows the half-field response in a healthy individual in whom almost no contralateral complex can be seen in the response to the complete 0-16° right half-

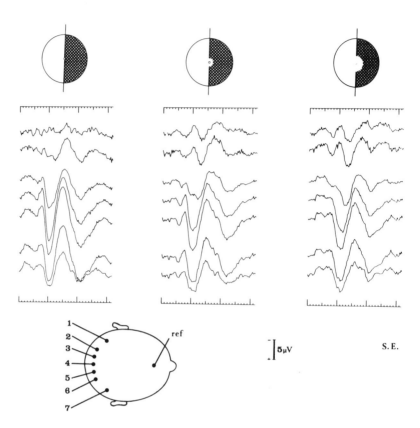

Figure 3.33 *Effect of progressive occlusion of the central stimulus area on the right half-field response from a healthy individual. Note the montage, with additional intermediate electrodes (channels 3 and 5) half-way between the mid-occipital electrode and the lateral electrode 5 cm out on each side, adopted in this case to show the exact distribution of the response waveform about the midline. The records from left to right show: (1) the response to the normal 0-16° half-field stimulus, showing a clear ipsilateral NPN complex but (in this particular healthy individual) no overt contralateral PNP complex; (2) the appearance of the contralateral PNP complex in channels 1 and 2 when a 1.5° central 'scotoma' is introduced into the stimulus; there is also a slight reduction of amplitude in the accompanying ipsilateral NPN complex; (3) increased amplitude and definition of the PNP complex with increase of the occluding 'scotoma' to 2.5°. Note also the accompanying further slight attenuation and loss of definition of the ipsilateral NPN complex and the shift of the 'transitional' channel towards the midline. (From Blumhardt et al, 1978.)*

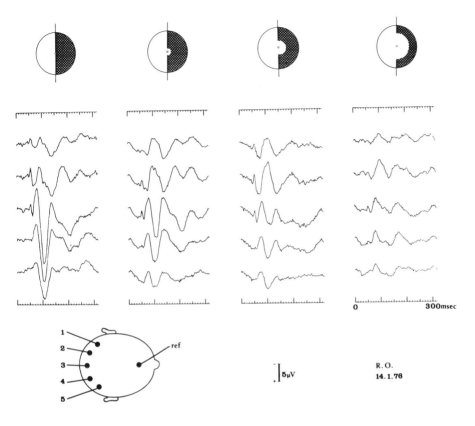

Figure 3.34 *The effect of a series of 'scotomata' of increasing radius on the right half-field response of another healthy individual. The ipsilateral P100 is progressively attenuated, while the contralateral components, particularly the N105, are initially enhanced. From left to right: intact half-field response, and responses with 2.5°, 5.0° and 10.0° 'scotomata' in the central field. (From Blumhardt et al, 1978.)*

field stimulus (left hand record). The occlusion of the central 1.5° and 2.5° of the stimulus field reduces the amplitude of the ipsilateral NPN and a contralateral PNP complex appears out of the background which increases in size as the stimulus becomes increasingly restricted to the paramacular field. Figure 3.34 shows exactly the same effect for another healthy individual with experimental 'scotomata' of 2.5°, 5° and 10°. The ipsilateral NPN complex is rapidly attenuated when the central stimulus is removed, whereas the contralateral PNP complex is enhanced for the 2.5° and 5° scotomata and only begins to decrease in size when the stimulus is restricted to the outer 10-16°. Figure 3.35, which plots the reduction in amplitude of the ipsilateral P100 component against the radius of the experimental 'scotoma' occluding the pattern stimulus from the central field, shows that the slope of attenuation is roughly linear.

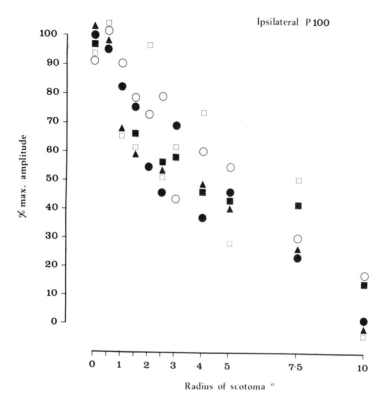

Figure 3.35 *Relationship between the amplitude of the ipsilateral $\overline{P100}$ component (in terms of the percentage of the maximum amplitude) and the radius of the central 'scotoma' occluding the stimulus for 5 healthy individuals. With a 10° radius 'scotoma' the major positivity is completely abolished in 3 individuals and is reduced to less than 16% of its maximum amplitude in the other 2. (From Blumhardt et al, 1978.)*

The much smaller contralateral $\overline{N105}$ component, on the other hand, shows a less consistent pattern, reflecting its variability in the initial half-field response in different individuals. It appears to be simply 'unmasked' by the occlusion of the stimulus from the macular field. Conversely, however, it can be attenuated without affecting the size of the ipsilateral NPN complex, by occlusion of the paramacular portion of the half-field stimulus. Figure 3.36 shows the progressive attenuation of the contralateral PNP, unaccompanied by any change in the ipsilateral NPN complex, by reducing the radius of the pattern stimulus from 16° to 5°. This is from the grand average response of five subjects, in whom the contralateral PNP could be clearly seen in the full half-field response. These results from healthy individuals help to explain the characteristic changes in the pattern response which are encountered in patients with central scotomata (Halliday, 1976; Halliday et al, 1979a; Kriss et al, 1982. See also Chapter 7, page 262). The correct lateralization of the components is important for the interpretation of these results, and due regard must be paid to the selection of a suitable electrode montage and to the choice of a truly indifferent electrode (see Chapter 1, page 23).

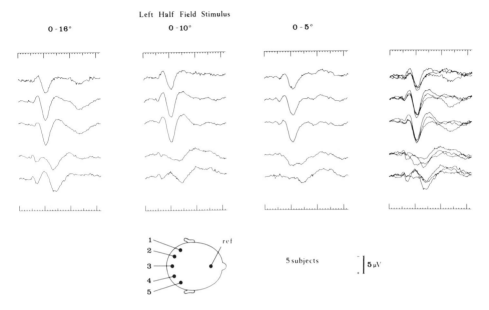

Figure 3.36 *Grand average of the left half-field responses of 5 healthy individuals to show the effect of a reduction of the size of the stimulus field. In the right-hand column the 3 responses are superimposed. The ipsilateral P100 is relatively unaffected by reducing the field radius from 16° to 5°, while the contralateral response (channels 4 and 5) is attenuated. This demonstrates clearly the importance of stimulation of the paramacular areas in producing the contralateral PNP complex. (From Blumhardt et al, 1978.)*

The principle of summation

It has been emphasized that, with regard to the pattern reversal responses from different parts of the visual field, the general principle holds that *the whole is equivalent to the sum of the parts*, i.e. the responses to any particular sectors of the field will summate to produce a combined response which is not significantly different from the response recorded to a stimulus covering all the combined sectors. This implies that there is simple algebraic summation at the scalp of the responses from different areas of the field, and that there is not any major interaction between the adjoining cortical generator areas, such as to produce occlusion or enhancement of the combined response. It is to be noted that this is *not* equivalent to saying that the responses from two homologous areas necessarily have the same or similar waveforms and distributions at the scalp electrodes. The left and right half-field responses in a healthy individual, for instance, are not simply exact mirror images of each other and may show significant 'incongruencies' in their asymmetry. These differences are less marked for homonymous half-fields as compared to heteronymous half-fields, but still not entirely negligible. They are very marked for the upper and lower half-field responses which have entirely different waveforms and distributions at the scalp, but still summate to reproduce the full-field response.

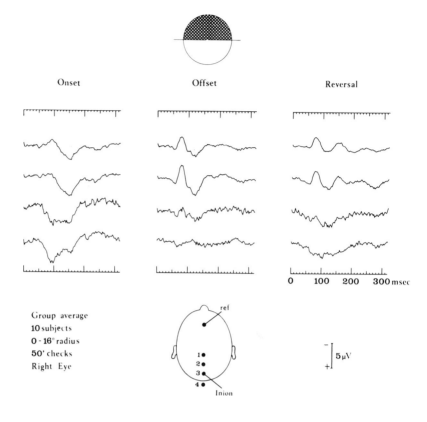

Figure 3.37 *Grand average of the upper field response from the right eye of 10 healthy individuals to (from left to right) pattern onset, pattern offset and pattern reversal stimuli. Note the montage with a sagittal row of occipital electrodes, spaced 5 cm apart. Compare the lower half-field response in Figure 3.38. (From Kriss and Halliday, 1980.)*

Upper and lower field responses

As is evident from Figure 3.29 these important differences between the responses from the upper and lower half-field are evident in the responses from the two quadrants of each half-field. Unlike the left and right half-field responses, these upper and lower field responses are not complementary 'mirror images' of each other when recorded from a row of electrodes in the corresponding plane. This is equally true of the pattern reversal and the pattern onset and offset EPs, if the upper and lower field responses (Figures 3.37 and 3.38) are compared with the left and right half-field responses (Figures 3.39, 3.40). This is, no doubt, largely due to the difference in the spatial relationship between the array of surface electrodes on the back of the head and the two sets of cortical generator areas producing the

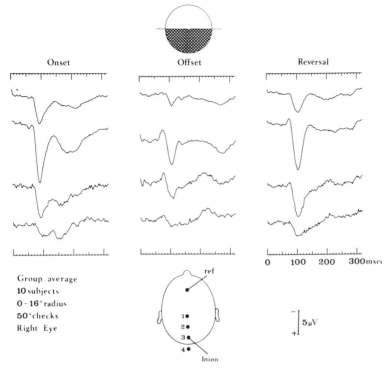

Figure 3.38 *Grand average response to lower half-field stimulation of the right eye in 10 healthy individuals for pattern onset, offset and reversal stimulation, recorded as in Figure 3.37. (From Kriss and Halliday, 1980.)*

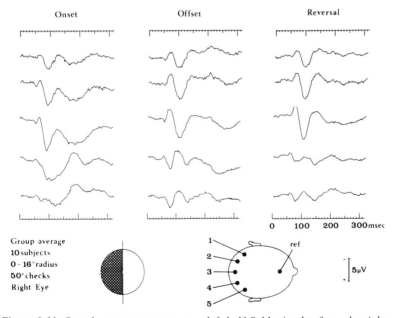

Figure 3.39 *Grand average response to a left half-field stimulus from the right eye of 10 healthy individuals to (left to right) pattern onset, pattern offset and pattern reversal stimulation. Note the standard montage of a transverse occipital chain of electrodes spaced 5 cm apart. (From Kriss and Halliday, 1980.)*

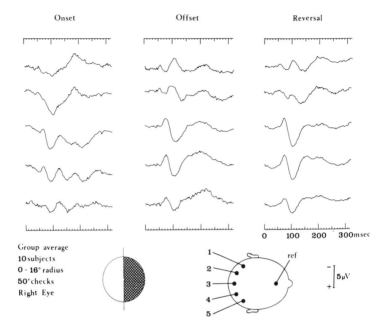

Figure 3.40 *Grand average response to right half-field stimulation of the right eye in the same 10 healthy individuals, whose other responses are shown in Figures 3.37-39. (From Kriss and Halliday, 1980.)*

responses. The upper field response, whether coming from the striate representation or from the parastriate areas, V2 and V3, originates largely from the projection areas on or near the inferior surface of the occipital lobe, which are in general pointing away from the surface electrodes, whereas the lower field response is generated from areas situated much nearer the scalp electrodes. Examination of the quadrant responses (Figure 3.29) shows that the contralateral PNP is preferentially related to the upper field, while the converse is true of the ipsilateral NPN. Furthermore the contralateral $\overline{P135}$, which is clearly seen for both quadrants, has a more lateral distribution for the upper field. Further consideration of the quadrant and octant responses is, however, beyond the scope of this book and the interested reader must refer to studies published elsewhere (Halliday and Michael, 1970; Michael and Halliday, 1971; Halliday et al, 1977a; Blumhardt and Halliday, 1979; Kriss and Halliday, 1980; Blumhardt et al, 1982b).

4

Clinical Electroretinography

H. Ikeda

INTRODUCTION

The possibility of recording the electroretinogram (ERG) from the human eye was shown as long ago as 1865 (Holmgren, 1865). However, the development of the technique into a clinically applicable method seems to have taken an astonishingly long time if one considers the fact that, even today, only a limited number of the major hospitals in the world have facilities for recording the ERG. One of the reasons for the considerable delay in development was the technical difficulty in recording a small electrical response from a mobile structure, i.e. the eyeball, in the conscious human subject. Meanwhile, intense studies on the mode and site of generation of the ERG in the eyes of different anaesthetized animals or in isolated retinae had made immense progress in providing knowledge on the electrical activities of the cells in the retina and their relation to the ERG. This was of great advantage in interpreting the human ERG, since before the technique came to be appplied clinically we knew more or less what we were recording and what to expect the ERG of a normal eye to be.

The development of ERG recording from the eyes of conscious human subjects was due in great part to Riggs (1941), who introduced an electrode embedded in a contact lens, and Karpe (1945) who pioneered the ERG technique using a contact lens electrode as a diagnostic tool in ophthalmology, and became the first president of the International Society for Clinical Electroretinography (ISCERG) in 1958. The ISCERG, now renamed ISCEV (International Society for Clinical Electrophysiology of Vision), publishes the proceedings of the meetings held each year as a separate booklet in the series of Documenta Ophthalmologica (published by Dr W. Junk b.v. Publishers, The Hague, The Netherlands). For those who wish to enter into the field, the booklets of ISCEV would give an overall picture of the capability and limitations of the clinical ERG.

A further, though slow, advance in the clinical ERG since the 1950s was due to two factors. Firstly, to rapid developments in electronics and bioengineering, which have made the recordings easier and simpler. Secondly, and more importantly, to the increasing clinical demand for ERG recording. This is due to a gradual realization amongst ophthalmologists that the ERG can detect biochemical and functional abnormalities of the retina before a pathological change can be seen by ophthalmology or fluorescein angiography.

Initially, it was thought that the clinical ERG had to be correlated with the ophthalmoscopic change, i.e. a degenerative change of the retina, in order to prove that the clinical ERG represented the functional state of the retina. An irony of this approach is that if an ophthalmoscope can diagnose the disease, why should one submit the patients to the ordeal of the ERG recording? This argument can indeed be justified, and is still true at present. Many significant contributions, however, have repeatedly indicated that the abnormality of the ERGs in patients with a minor degree of visual loss could occur without any detectable ophthalmoscopic abnormality of the retina. Furthermore, the ERGs have proved useful in very young children or mentally handicapped patients, in whom the taking of reliable clinical notes or the performance of visual function tests are practically impossible. In cases where the clarity of the ocular media is lost due to cataract or vitreous haemorrhages, so that a satisfactory view of the fundi is impossible, the ERGs have also proved useful in assessing the functional state of the retina and thus they can give some prognosis to the subsequent operations. In my experience, however, the ERGs are more often used to decide whether or not to *do* the operation, rather than to know how the operation will turn out, if performed.

The clinical ERG has also begun to play a rôle in patients with no apparent visual loss but who suffer from neurological diseases, neuromuscular disease or metabolic diseases. The ERG answers the question whether or not the retinal biochemistry is involved in the disease process, even if the patient claims to be visually normal, and this in turn throws light on the mechanism of the disease. It is my belief that in these fields the clinical ERG has an important rôle to play in the future.

THE ANATOMY OF THE RETINA

The retina is a highly complex nervous tissue containing two stages of synaptic layers and at least five types of cells, photoreceptors (rods and cones), horizontal cells, bipolar cells, amacrine cells and ganglion cells, as shown schematically in Figure 4.1.

Although the retina is a continuous tissue, it is not a uniform structure and the distribution of each cell type differs throughout the retina. Thus, the most different parts, i.e. the macula and the periphery are shown separately in Figure 4.1. The macula is an area of central retina 5 mm in diameter, surrounding the fovea (not shown in Figure 4.1). The fovea is an area with no blood vessels and no higher order neurones beyond the specialized thin cones which number 110,000. At the macula, the photoreceptors are mainly cones (650,000) which synapse with bipolar cells and the bipolar cells with the ganglion cells in a one-to-one ratio. Approximately 50% of the optic nerve fibres carry information arising from the macular cones. However, in the peripheral retina, the photoreceptors are a mixture of rods and cones (75,000 rods and 5,000 cones per square millimeter) which converge on a smaller number of bipolar cells and an even smaller number of retinal ganglion cells.

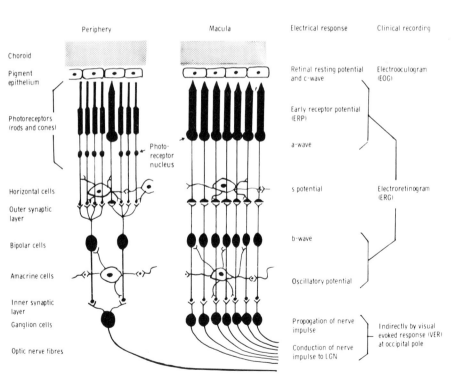

Figure 4.1. *Schematic cross-section of the central retina (the macula) and peripheral retina, indicating the electrical potentials generated at each cell layer and the three types of clinical recording.*

These hierarchical connections receive lateral influences from two groups of interneurones, the horizontal cells of the outer synaptic layer and the amacrine cells of the inner synaptic zone. Recent neuroanatomical, neurophysiological and neurochemical studies have revealed important functional rôles played by these interneurones.

THE ELECTRICAL RESPONSES OF THE RETINA AND THE ERG

The electrical response of the retina reflects the complexity of the anatomical connections in the retina. The electrical responses produced by each class of retinal cell are now well known and these are indicated in Figure 4.1. Although the light enters from the retinal ganglion cell side, the initiation of electrical activity begins, of course, from the deepest layer.

Firstly, an electrical potential is generated at the junction between the photoreceptors and the pigment epithelium. This steady DC potential of about 60 mV is called the retinal resting potential, since it is present even when the retina is not being stimulated by light. The effect of steady light and dark adaptation of the eye on the retinal resting potential is a measure of the functional integrity of these deepest layers of the retina. This effect can be determined clinically using the electro-oculographic technique (EOG) as indicated in Figure 4.1. If the junction between the photoreceptor and the pigment epithelium is separated, as in retinal detachment, the photoreceptors show no response to light and vision is not possible. The importance of the retinal-pigment epithelium interface and the ERG is discussed elegantly by Foulds (1979).

As long as the pigment epithelium, the photoreceptor outer tips, and the choroid which supplies nutrition to these structures, are healthy, the ERG can be recorded as a change from the retinal resting potential. When a flash of light falls on the retina, rapid and well defined electrical responses occur in each cell layer before the final retinal excitation leaves the eye as nerve impulses or action potentials along the optic nerve fibres, i.e. the axons of the retinal ganglion cells.

The photoreceptors, horizontal cells and bipolar cells do not generate action potentials, but generate a slow, smooth change in potential, i.e. in technical terms, the cell membrane becomes either hyperpolarized or depolarized. These slow potentials (graded electrical response) are produced by electrical and chemical coupling between cells which allows the transfer of continuously changing levels of electrical potential from the photoreceptors to the bipolar cells. The response of the bipolar cells is modified by excitation of the horizontal and amacrine cells. The amplitude of the graded response of the photoreceptors, horizontal cells and bipolar cells increases with increase in strength of the stimulus. The amacrine cells, which make three types of synaptic contact, i.e. to other amacrine cells, to ganglion cells and back onto bipolar cells (reciprocal synapse), produce an intermediate response between the slow graded potential and the action potential. The amacrine cells generate depolarizing potentials with limited neural impulse-generating properties, and it has been suggested that they feed back inhibition onto the bipolar cells via lateral spread through their dendrites. (Readers who are interested in the details of the generation of the electrical responses of each type of cell in the retina should read Dowling, 1970, Shepherd, 1974, or Ripps, 1978).

In Figure 4.1 on the right of the schematic diagram of the cross section of the retina, I have indicated the names of the electrical responses arising from different layers. These are:

1. The c-wave representing the extra-cellular current arising from the apical face of the pigment epithelium.

2. Early receptor potential (ERP) at the outer segment of the photoreceptors.

3. Later receptor potential generated at the photoreceptors - the a-wave

4. A slow widespread potential at the horizontal cells - the S-potential.

5. A well defined potential at the inner nuclear layer - the b-wave.

6. Transient on and off potentials with a few spiky oscillations superimposed at the amacrine cells - (probably the oscillatory potential).

7. The action potentials (nerve impulses or spikes) at the retinal ganglion cells.

The clinical ERG is the recording of electrical potentials evoked by a flash of light and picked up at a distance, i.e. at the cornea. It consists of various components (wavelets) which arise in different layers of the retina. Of the seven responses listed above, only five at the most are recordable, i.e. the ERP, the a-wave, the b-wave, the oscillatory potential, and the c-wave, as indicated in Figure 4.2. The waveform of an ERG and the components it reveals, however, exhibit changes depending on the intensity and wavelength of the stimulating flash used and also on the recording system which is used to amplify the response. The ERG illustrated in Figure 4.2 (schematic) is a response recorded using a recording system with a wide frequency range, and evoked by a very bright flash in order to record all five components. (Those readers who are interested in further details of the mode of generation and the component analysis of the ERG can refer to Chapter 18 of the book by Rodieck, 1973).

1. The early receptor potential (ERP) is a rapid discharge only recordable with an extremely high intensity flash in a well dark-adapted eye using high frequency amplifiers, and, as I explain at the end of this chapter, it cannot be considered as an important component of the clinical ERG.

2. The a-wave is sometimes called the PIII component of the ERG after Granit (1933). It is generated extracellularly along a radial path from the cell body of the photoreceptors into the membrane of the outer segments and is an important component of the clinical ERG as a measure of photoreceptor activity. The a-wave consists of two components, i.e. a_1 and a_2 arising from the cones and rods respectively.

3. The b-wave is sometimes called the PII component of the ERG after Granit (1933). It has long been believed to be generated by the cells in the inner nuclear layer, particularly the bipolar cells (Brown, 1968). Of course, the bipolar cell response is modified by the horizontal and amacrine cells. However, recently, several authors (see Miller and Dowling, 1970; Kline et al, 1978; Dick and Miller, 1978; and Ripps, 1978, for a review) have suggested that the b-wave originates in Müller cells (glia) which reflect extracellular current spread due probably to potassium concentration change caused by depolarising activity, probably of the bipolar cells. Regardless of whether the b-wave is generated at the bipolar cells or by the Müller cells, the b-wave is the most readily recordable and the major component

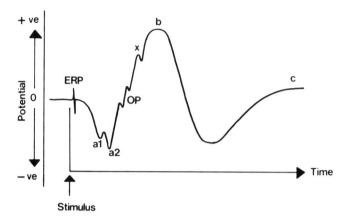

Key	Full name of component	Generator
ERP	early receptor potential	Outer segments of photoreceptors
a1, a2	a - wave	a1 - cones a2 - rods
OP	oscillatory potentials	*amacrine cells ?
x	x - wave or b1	*cells in the inner nuclear layer
b	b - wave or b2	(b - wave)
c	c - wave	*pigment epithelium

* see text

Figure 4.2. Components of an ERG (schematic) evoked by a high intensity white flash in a dark adapted normal eye, using amplifiers with a wide frequency band and recorded with an oscilloscope.

of the clinical ERG. It reflects the post-synaptic summed neuronal activities of the inner nuclear layer and thus is an important measure.

4. The oscillatory potential has been identified as due to amacrine cell activity and apppears as a rapid oscillation on the rising phase of the b-wave of the human ERG evoked by a bright flash. The last oscillation is relatively well defined and can be recorded on a pen recorder and is called the x-wave or b_1. Like the a-wave, the b-wave consists of two components, i.e. b_1 and b_2 representing the cone-mediated and rod-mediated responses respectively. Although the oscillatory potential is discussed in a later section, a recent study on mud puppy retina suggests that it may

represent inhibitory feedback loops within the retina (Wachtmeister and Dowling, 1978).

5. The c-wave is the extra-cellular current arising from a hyperpolarization of the apical face of the pigment epithelium in response to a decrease in extra-cellular potassium in the region of the inner segment of the photoreceptor layer (Oakley and Green, 1976). It can only be seen as a small, slow, positive deflection after the b-wave, although it starts slowly from the beginning of light stimulation. This is the wave representing the PI component of the ERG (Granit, 1933). The integrity of the pigment epithelium and photoreceptors is an essential factor for the generation of the c-wave, and indeed the generation of the ERG as a whole. However, in order to record the c-wave satisfactorily, the base-line of the recording needs to be maintained very steady for at least one or two seconds after stimulation. Since this is difficult, measurements of the c-wave are not very reliable clinically. Fortunately, we can obtain some information on the functional integrity of the pigment epithelium and the photoreceptors by recording the EOG (see Figure 4.1). The technique of recording the EOG has been described, and its clinical significance discussed, by Ikeda (1976).

The s-potential (horizontal cell response) does not appear in the ERG, but the b-wave recorded in the ERG probably represents the extra-cellular activities of the bipolar cells (or Müller cells) after modification by the horizontal cell response.

Unfortunately, the nerve impulses generated by the retinal ganglion cells are not recorded by the clinical ERG. The optic nerve fibres carry the message of the retinal ganglion cells to the lateral geniculate nucleus which relays this message to the visual cortex. The visual evoked responses (VER) can be used to determine whether the propagation of the nerve impulses from the retinal ganglion cells has reached the cerebral cortex, as indicated in Figure 4.1. However, since 50% of the optic nerve fibres arise from the macula, an area of the central retina only 5 mm in diameter, and there is a further cortical magnification factor of this small central retinal region, the VER is largely a measure of macular function.

RECORDING THE CLINICAL ERG

The recording of the clinical ERG is made between an active electrode on the cornea and a reference electrode on the forehead. The response, which occurs when the retina is stimulated by a flash of light, is amplified and recorded on an oscilloscope or by a pen recorder. This is shown in Figure 4.3

The following notes may be helpful for readers who wish to record the ERG.

FACILITIES REQUIRED

1. Air conditioned dark room

This is an essential requirement. The ERG is a function of dark adaptation, so to obtain a reasonably sized ERG, the patients must be dark-adapted and their rod sensitivity increased (see Figure 4.6). The room should be located in a reasonably

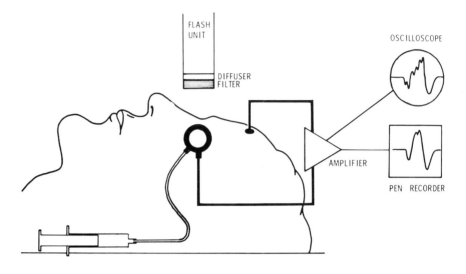

Figure 4.3. *A diagram showing the recording system of the clinical ERG. The patient is wearing a contact lens electrode (see Figure 4.4). The flash unit is a commercially available photic stimulator.*

quiet part of the building, and away from machinery or equipment which produce electrical interference (e.g. lift motors, autoclaves, etc.).

Ideally, you may be advised to have the room electrically screened, or to obtain an isolated power supply for the ERG room in order to eliminate all electrical interference from external sources. However, these are extremely expensive requirements and are not necessary. The most important requirement is that all equipment and the patient are earthed to a common ground. As long as the earthing of the room is carefully and correctly carried out, a quite satisfactory recording of the ERG is possible.

2. A bed or a dental chair for the patient

The ERG can be recorded with a patient sitting up in a dental chair with a firm head support or alternatively lying down. One can obtain a better base-line on which the ERG is recorded if the patient is comfortable and reasonably relaxed. For this a couch or bed with a good head support is preferable.

3. Stimulator

(a) A commercially available flash unit with various filters

A commercially available flash unit or photic stimulator consists of a xenon-filled gas discharge tube mounted with a reflector and a diffusing screen. The flash produced is very short (about 25 microseconds) and this is an advantage in clinical recording. The maximum light intensity produced by such a flash is usually over

2×10^6 candelas/sq. metre. The distance between the flash tube and the patient's eye must be strictly controlled, so that at least 40°-60° of the central retina is stimulated by the flash.

Filters required are a set of neutral density filters in 0.5 log unit steps from 0 log unit to 5 or 6 log units. For a routine clinic, two colour filters would be useful for differentiating the rod and cone components of the ERG. These are Kodak Wratten Filters 47B (scotopic blue) and 29 (photopic red). Of course, for a research project investigating the spectral sensitivity of patients using the ERG, expensive narrow band spectral filters (interference filters) covering from 400 nm to 680 nm are necessary.

(b) Ganzfeld (full-field) stimulation technique

This is a technique used to stimulate as large a retinal area as possible in order to minimize errors caused by the eye movements of the patient (Berson et al, 1968). A stroboscope in a diffusing sphere is used to illuminate the inner white surface of a dome (resembling a perimeter sphere) producing a homogenous full field. The patient with a contact lens electrode in place sits with his head supported by a chin rest looking into the dome. Additional small bulbs recessed above and behind the patient's field-of-view can produce a steady adapting light, which may be altered to give different levels of adapting illumination, i.e. background illumination, on which is superimposed the stimulating flash, lighting up the whole dome.

A combination of neutral density filters and colour filters, interposed between the stroboscope and the diffusing sphere, is used to produce either scotopically balanced or photopically balanced flashes. This stimulator appears to be favoured by the ERG clinics in the United States.

(c) Stimulator-ophthalmoscope

This is principally an ophthalmoscope modified to produce a time-modulated stimulus beam of variable dimension, intensity and wavelength entering the eye in Maxwellian view. It was devised by Sandberg and Ariel (1977), and is not commercially available. It allows one to record ERGs evoked by stimulating a small area at different parts of the retina. Such an ERG is called the focal or local ERG.

The ERG evoked by stimulation of this small area of the retina is, furthermore, very small, so many responses need to be averaged using an averaging computer. Averaging many responses means that the ERGs which are recorded are light adapted, i.e. cone-mediated retinal responses. At present, this stimulator is a research tool rather than a clinical testing technique, but it holds promise of being clinically useful, particularly for studying the function or sensitivity of the macula.

(d) Pattern stimulator

The time locked pattern stimulator which is used for recording the visual evoked potential (VEP) may also be employed for simultaneous recording of the ERG and the VEP. As with the focal (or local) ERG evoked by the stimulator-ophthalmoscope, the pattern-evoked VEP requires an averaging technique, and reflects the cone-mediated retinal response only. So far we know little about the averaged ERGs recorded by these newer stimulators, e.g. their reproducibility, intensity or contrast functions, latency, waveform and components. However, if checkerboard patterns or grating patterns can be used to evoke reliable ERGs, we are at last in a position to assess the contrast function of the distal retina in clinical conditions. Indeed the recent work of Arden et al (1980) on human strabismic amblyopes used the pattern evoked ERGs and showed that the ERG contrast function is already reduced in amblyopic eyes.

Electrodes and the method of application

The reference and ground electrodes

Two electrodes are usually placed on the forehead, one being a reference electrode paired with the corneal active electrode, and the other, a ground electrode close to this, so that the reference electrode is practically earthed. The reference and ground electrodes are commercial EEG disc electrodes fastened by adhesive tape. The forehead must be cleaned with acetone and the electrode filled with an electrode jelly to ensure good contact. Careful appplication of these electrodes is important for a good ERG recording.

The corneal electrode

(a) **Contact lens electrode.** I recommend a Henkes type contact lens electrode, since it is the best electrode for ensuring the success of the ERG recording, and also since it has been tested and used internationally. Figure 4.4 shows photographs of such a contact lens electrode. Two sizes are available; one for adults and the other for children. As shown in Figure 4.4B, a silver wire in ring form is embedded just inside the black artificial pupil. The edge of the artificial pupil forms a kind of speculum to keep the upper and the lower lids apart all the time. The lens is filled with sterile normal saline from a 2 ml syringe via a length of thin polythene tubing as shown in Figure 4.4A.

After making sure that the lens is centred on the dilated pupil of the patient, and that there are no air bubbles between the lens and the cornea, suction is applied to the syringe, and the lens is held firmly on the sclera. Even if the patient blinks or moves the eye, the relative position of the electrode and the retina remains fixed. This is an important requirement for satisfactory recording. The electrode resistance when firmly placed on the eye should be between $2K\Omega$-$3K\Omega$. The artificial pupil prevents the photoelectric artefact, and also controls the amount of light entering the eye so that it is constant for all patients. These controls are all very important for achieving a high reproducibility of response, and obtaining satisfactory limits for the normal ERG.

The contact lens must be thoroughly sterilized by sterile phenyl mercuric borate solution (Merfen), and rinsed in sterile normal saline for each patient. The cornea must be anaesthetized with local anaesthetic eye drops. After the recording, the pupil must be constricted with physostigmine and plenty of ointment (Chloromycetin ophthalmic ointment 1%) should be put into the eye before patching. The patient should be warned of the danger of dust entering the anaesthetized eye and rubbing causing abrasion of the cornea. The patient is asked to arrange to be accompanied by a normal-sighted person for the ERG examination. Although ERG investigators fear that corneal abrasion might occur after ERG recording using a contact lens electrode, having routinely adopted the above mentioned procedure of pre- and post-examination care, we have not experienced a single incident of corneal abrasion over the past 10 years.

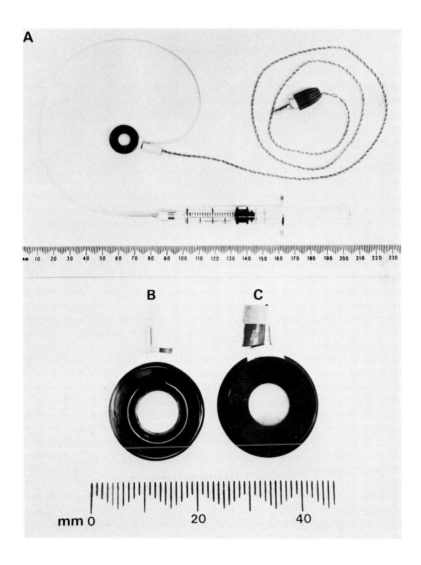

Figure 4.4. *An ERG contact lens (Henkes' type - from Medical Workshop, Groningen, Holland). A: Whole lens assembly. B: Inner side of the lens with a silver ring electrode. C: Outer side of the contact lens with an artificial pupil and speculum.*

However, if one is interested in a research project in which ERGs need to be recorded repeatedly from a normal subject or from a patient, and the recording period must be longer than 30-40 minutes at a time, the contact lens electrode would not be suitable. The following two possibilities (b) and (c) are suggested in such circumstances.

(b) Gold foil electrode. This is a thin film of plastic coated with gold inserted in the lower eyelid fornix without anaesthetic eye drops. Details of its construction and the method of application are described fully by Arden et al (1979) who designed and tested the electrode, and stated that it is satisfactory in recording ERGs which are comparable to those recorded with the contact lens electrode. The idea of inserting a hook-shaped small metal electrode in the lower eyelid or conjunctival sac is a very old one, and such an electrode was used during the 1930s and '40s, before the contact lens electrode had been devised. The design and the material used for the new gold foil electrode are, however, considerably superior to the old types, which never proved to be suitable as clinical ERG electrodes. Arden et al (1979) emphasize that the patient's comfort and the reduced cost of the new gold foil electrode would be a great advantage for the clinical ERG.

However, the gold foil electrode cannot control for the difference in the patient's pupil size; the position of the electrode with respect to the retina may change, and there may be greater interference from blinks. The electrode has to be renewed from time to time, since it has a limited life. As with any new device, judgement on the electrode must wait until the technique has been thoroughly tested for reproducibility of results.

(c) Skin electrode. EEG disc electrodes, fastened on the lateral or medial canthi, are the cheapest and easiest electrodes, but these record the retinal response at a distance, and so are only useful when one is using an averager to record the averaged light-adapted ERG. This method of recording would show interference due to tension in the facial muscles, eye movements, and blinks, but the idea is that these artefacts would be cancelled out in the course of averaging, and only the response of the retina evoked by the time-locked flash or pattern would be summed to produce a sizeable ERG. This method is often used for simultaneous recording of the visual evoked responses and the ERG. This may, however, be replaced by the gold foil electrode, if it can be worn by inexperienced patients without anaesthetic for a considerable time.

Amplifiers and recorders

As Figure 4.5 shows, the ERG waveform and amplitude are greatly influenced by the frequency band-width of the amplifiers and recorders used. If one wants to examine all components of the ERG, as shown in Figure 4.2, one has to use an amplifier of wide frequency range, i.e. 0.5 Hz to 10 KHz, and to record the responses with an oscilloscope and a camera. But one also has to remember that the more sensitive the amplifier and the wider the frequency band-width, the greater the chance of recording noise. Even if one succeeded in recording an ideal response as shown in Figure 4.2 and Figure 4.5 A, the oscillatory potential would appear as a very small oscillation on the rapidly rising slow b-wave. The ERP would also appear as just a small, fast response at the stimulation point in the trace when the oscilloscope time base is set to encompass a full ERG response.

On the other hand, if one is interested in the two major components, i.e. the a-wave and b-wave (and possibly the x-wave), which are due to the pre- and post-synaptic elements of the ERG, commercial EEG amplifiers and pen recorders are quite adequate. This system has a frequency response from 0.5 Hz to 100 Hz. Thus it is possible to record ERGs evoked by a flickering light at up to 30-50 Hz without any reduction in amplitude. A pen recorder has the advantage of immediate results, permanent records and ease of operation compared with an oscilloscope and camera. The response obtained with amplifiers for this frequency range and recorded on a pen recorder, is like that shown in Figure 4.5 B. Here the ERP and the oscillatory potentials are not recorded.

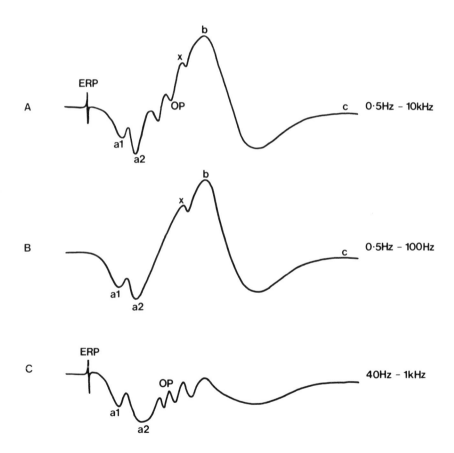

Figure 4.5. *The changes in the waveform and recorded components of the ERG that are found by using amplifiers of different frequency characteristics. The frequency range of the amplifiers is shown on the right. The responses A and C can only be recorded on an oscilloscope, but B can also be recorded on a commercial EEG pen recorder. The responses for all are evoked by a high intensity white flash in a dark adapted normal eye.*

If one is interested in the oscillatory potential of the ERG, the slow components should be eliminated by changing the frequency response of the amplifiers to the fast (high pass) end, i.e. from 40 Hz - 1 KHz. Then, the ERG consists of the fast but reduced ERP and the oscillatory potential superimposed upon an extremely reduced b-wave, as shown in Figure 4.5 C. Although not shown in Figure 4.5, if one is interested in the ERP alone, the response should be recorded setting the frequency response of the amplifiers from 100 Hz - 10 KHz and displaying it with an extremely fast time base, so that the oscillatory potential would not appear on the trace.

A RECOMMENDED RECORDING PROCEDURE FOR ROUTINE CLINICAL ERG

In the previous section I have listed advantages and disadvantages of more elaborate measurements of the human ERG using various types of electrodes, stimulators and recording systems. Here, however, I wish to define a recommended procedure using the contact lens electrode (Henkes type), a commercial flashing unit (Digitimer Photic Stimulator, 3182) and a commercial EEG recorder, which reveals considerable information on the retinal function of a patient within half an hour of recording time:

1. Dilate the pupil by Mydrilate 1% eye drops (cyclopentolate hydrochloride BP) while the patient is still in the waiting room.

2. Get the patient to lie on the bed and explain what is going to happen.

3. Apply the local anaesthetic eye drops (Amethocain 1%).

4. Apply the two reference and ground electrodes to the forehead after cleaning the skin with acetone.

5. Apply the contact lens electrode as described in the previous section. This is the most important factor which decides whether the recording will be successful or not. Do not hurry this procedure and make certain that no air bubbles are present between the cornea and the lens, that the lens is precisely centred and that all eyelashes are free from the contact lens. If necessary, reapply the contact lens until you are quite satisfied.

6. Check the stability of the base-line while encouraging the patient to relax and keep the eye as still as possible. If the base-line is not stable or if it is noisy, this may be due to bad contact of the contact lens, or to air bubbles floating between the lens and the cornea, or to the forehead reference electrode picking up muscle activity of the patient, who may be frowning or very tense. If the patient has nystagmus or the eye wanders, one cannot control this except by encouragement and guidance as to where the eye should be looking, but the majority of patients are able to keep the eye steady.

7. Place the stimulator in position. Measure precisely the distance between the eye and the stimulator (6 cm is the distance we use).

8. Record the ERG using the brightest flashes: a small and fast, light-adapted response should be obtained. Then put a 2.0 log unit filter in the stimulator and record the light-adapted ERG (a minute response as shown in the topmost ERG

record on the left of Figure 4.6 should be obtained from the normal eye, but no response may be obtained in some patients who have low retinal sensitivity).

9. Switch off the room lights to produce complete darkness. Thereafter a red torch is essential for checking the patient's eye position and changing the filters.

10. Follow the b-wave increase with dark adaptation every 2 minutes using a 2 log unit filter. It is important not to give more than two flashes for each measurement during the dark adaptation period, or the dark adaptation will be destroyed. Do not panic even if the records have been contaminated by the patient's eye movements or a blink, but wait for the next chance after a further 2 minutes.

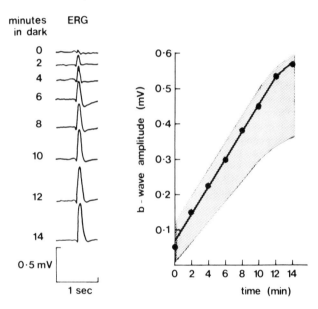

Figure 4.6. *The ERG b-wave as a function of dark adaptation with the normal response illustrated on the left. The shaded band is the normal range. The curve plotted is based on the amplitude measurements of the illustrated responses. All responses were evoked with a 2.0 log unit filter interposed between the flash unit and the eye.*

11. One observes a dramatic increase of the b-wave with dark adaptation (see Figure 4.6). After 12-14 minutes, the rate of increase should become relatively small.

12. Now decrease the intensity of the flash by increasing the value of the neutral density filter step-wise (in 0.5 log units steps starting from 2.5 log units), recording two ERGs at each intensity level. (Two ERGs are recommended for checking the reproducibility. If the two responses are not nearly identical, your records are not reliable). Observe that the response gradually decreases and finally disappears into the base-line. This is the threshold for the scotopic b-wave. During this procedure, one does not have to wait between flashes. Under no circumstances should one give an intense flash (without any filter in). (Each time the distance between the patient's eye and the flash tube, and the eye position should be checked quickly beforehand).

By this time, the patient should have been dark adapted for about 17 minutes; thus the b-wave threshold indicates the retinal sensitivity at about 15-20 minutes of dark adaptation.

13. Record the ERG using the filter 47B (scotopic blue filter, or this blue filter combined with 0.3 log unit neutral density filter to ensure the scotopic response — see Figure 4.9).

14. Record the ERG using the filter 29 (red filter). In the normal eye a distinct x-wave should be seen (see Figure 4.9).

15. Now complete the measurements of the top end of the ERG/intensity function by progressively increasing the intensity of the flash in steps of 0.5 log unit, starting from 1.5 log unit to maximum intensity, i.e. 0 log unit. Observe that the response increases with the intensity of the flash as shown on the left of Figure 4.7.

16. Now that the patient's eye has received the high intensity flash under fairly dark-adapted conditions, one can then study the photopic elements of the ERG, i.e. the cone-mediated retinal response. Use the red filter 29 and increase the flash rate in steps of 5 Hz up to 30 Hz. The normal eye is capable of producing flicker ERG wavelets of over 100 µV at 30 Hz (see Figure 4.8).

17. Lastly, the maximal white flash is used to record the flicker ERG, again increasing the flashing rate in steps of 5 Hz up to 30 Hz. The normal eye is capable of responding with a distinct oscillation with an amplitude of over 150 µV at 30 Hz.

18. Switch on the room light.

19. Remove the contact lens from the patient.

20. Apply physostigmine 0.25% in the recorded eye to hasten the constriction of the pupil.

21. Apply eye ointment (Nivemycin eye ointment 0.5% or Chloromycetin ophthalmic ointment 1%). Chloromycetin is safe even for the patients who are allergic to penicillin, and thus preferable to Nivemycin.

22. Patch the recorded eye and ask the patient not to touch the eye for at least several hours. Also it is important to warn the patient of strange sensations in the eye associated with the gradual recovery from the local anaesthetic and from the pupil dilatation.

ESTABLISHMENT OF THE NORMAL LIMITS OF THE ERG FUNCTION AND QUANTITATIVE ASSESSMENT OF RETINAL FUNCTION IN PATIENTS

Following the procedure described in the previous section, three basic ERG functions are determined for each patient, i.e. the b-wave increase with dark adaptation, the b-wave and a-wave amplitude as a function of stimulus intensity and the cone flicker ERG response as a function of stimulation rate.

The clinical ERG is a measure of the functional state of the retina as a whole. The aim of recording the ERG from a patient is to see: (a) whether there is any reduction in retinal function and (b) whether the loss is more in the rod-mediated or in the cone-mediated retinal function. However, these questions can only be answered if one knows the normal limits of ERG function determined by the particular technique and the particular procedure adopted by the laboratory concerned.

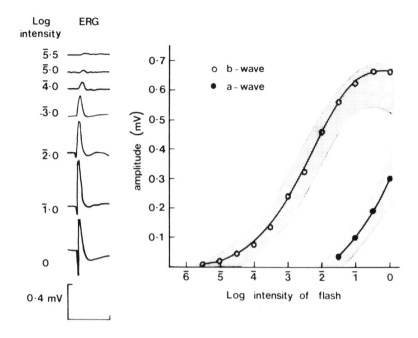

Figure 4.7. Amplitudes of the a- and b-wave of the ERG as a function of the log intensity of the flash. 0 log unit corresponds to 2 x 10 candelas per square metre. The responses shown on the left illustrate the increase in the amplitude of the ERG obtained from a normal eye. The shaded bands indicate the normal ranges for a- and b-wave functions. The curves are obtained from amplitude measurements of the illustrated responses.

The three figures - Figures 4.6, 4.7 and 4.8 - show the normal limits of ERG functions determined in our clinic. Each function is illustrated by records of ERGs obtained from a patient who had normal retinal function. This patient showed severe bone disease and the Gastrointestinal Unit of the hospital felt that she might show symptoms of Vitamin A deficiency and, therefore, reduced rod function. The ERGs suggested that the retina was not involved in the disease.

Figure 4.6 shows the increase in the b-wave amplitude with dark adaptation. The shaded band is our normal range. The slope of the increase and the final amplitude of the b-wave can be used to describe each patient's ERG dark adaptation function, compared with the normal limits. The curve of this patient falls within the shaded band. Vitamin A deficiency, night blindness, retinitis pigmentosa, tapetoretinal degeneration, diabetic retinopathy, choroidaemia or choroiditis, and retinal vascular diseases all show subnormality of this function. In many cases, the loss of rod function is not noticed by the patients, nor detected by assessment of visual field loss but the ERG can detect such minor abnormalities.

Figure 4.7 shows the amplitude of the a-wave and the b-wave as a function of flash intensity. The a-wave appears at higher intensities. This does not mean that the

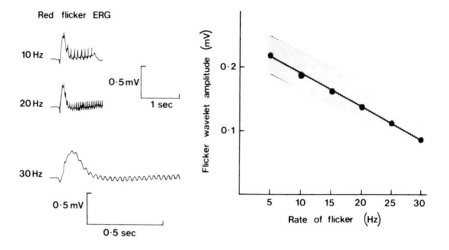

Figure 4.8. *Flicker ERGs evoked by red light as a function of flicker rate. The shaded band indicates the normal range. The normal flicker ERGs illustrated for 30 Hz are recorded on a faster time-base than those for 10 and 20 Hz. Note that the first flash always evokes a large response suppressing the immediately following few wavelet responses, although eventually flicker wavelets of equal amplitude are seen. The measurements of the flicker ERG wavelets are carried out on these later wavelets of equal amplitude and plotted in the graph.*

a-wave receptor potential is non-existent at low intensity levels. Each ERG is a summed response of mainly the a-wave and the b-wave which have opposite polarity. The negative a-wave is cancelled out by the relatively large b-wave at the low intensities.

The relative proportion of the a-wave and b-wave amplitudes is also a useful indicator for isolating the presynaptic retinal response from the post-synaptic retinal response. In normal subjects, the b-wave should be at least twice the size of the a-wave at the highest intensity (2×10^6 candelas/sq. metre) level. In cases of minor retinal vascular disease, and in cases of toxic amblyopia, the proportion is disturbed and the a-wave begins to exceed the b-wave, suggesting a loss of post-synaptic activity. In cases of optic nerve disease where retrograde trans-synaptic degeneration is suspected, the b-wave is reduced and the b-wave to a-wave ratio is usually reduced.

The relationship between b-wave amplitude and intensity of the stimulation flash is a most important function in the clinical ERG, since a major law of the visual system is that the visual threshold, or level of visual excitation, increases linearly (within limits) with the logarithmic increase of the intensity (or contrast) of stimulation. This law is applicable at each cellular level throughout the afferent visual nervous system. Figure 4.7 shows that the human ERG recorded from the cornea reveals such a relationship and suggests that this basic visual function is determined already at the inner nuclear layer of the retina. At higher intensities the b-wave has a small kink near its peak. This is the x-wave.

The waveform of the ERG shown in Figure 4.7 (or 4.6) appears quite different from that of the ERGs shown in Figures 4.2 and 4.5. This is because the time base used for recording the ERG for the two figures was different. The ERGs shown in Figures 4.2 and 4.5 were recorded with a faster time base than those shown in Figures 4.6 and 4.7. The waveform of the ERGs obtained with the same intensity of flash is the same. If one is interested in the amplitude of the a-wave and the b-wave, one does not want to record ERGs with a very fast time base. However, if one wants to study the latency of the response, then a faster time base should be used. Indeed the latency of the ERG is inversely related to the intensity of the flash. The latency of the b-wave is longer for low intensities and becomes progressively shorter for higher intensities. The parameter of latency can also be used as a sensitive indicator of very early retinal disease (Berson and Howard, 1971).

The amplitude of the a-wave is measured from the base-line to the negative peak, whereas that of the b-wave is measured from the trough of the a-wave to the peak of the b-wave. The amplitudes of the responses illustrated fall inside the shaded zones of the graph of Figure 4.7. The shaded zones are again our normal range, so that any patient whose ERG function falls below the lowest limit of the shaded zone has a significant loss of basic retinal function. Again, the curve obtained from each patient can be described quantitatively by three parameters, the threshold intensity, i.e. the lowest intensity at which the b-wave just appears, the maximal amplitude of the a-wave and the b-wave, and the slope of the curve.

The b-wave/intensity function is an extremely sensitive measure, and subnormal visual function may be detected long before any abnormality of the fundi becomes apparent. We found that patients with alcohol and tobacco amblyopia, advanced cases of optic neuritis, sarcoidosis, external or internal ophthalmoplegia and dystrophia myotonica without an obvious fundus abnormality, show some reduction in ERG function. Needless to say all those patients who suffer from primary retinal degeneration show an extremely reduced ERG/intensity function. The ERG function is, however, normal in acute quinine poisoning or in early cerebroretinal lipidosis (the cherry red spot/ganglion cell disease), early demyelinating disease, cone dysfunction, achromatopsia or cerebral disease.

Figure 4.8 shows the ERG wavelets evoked by different rates of flickering light of long wavelength (i.e. with Kodak Wratten filter 29 which has a peak transmission at 640 nm). The ERGs evoked by a rapidly flickering red light measure the response produced by the cones. This is because the broad-band spectral sensitivity of the cones encompasses 430 nm to 700 nm, peaking at 550 nm, whereas that of the rods covers 350 nm to 650 nm, peaking at 500 nm. Thus cones are more sensitive to red than rods. Furthermore, high temporal resolution is a property of cones rather than rods. The amplitude of the flicker ERG decreases with increase in the frequency of stimulation. The flicker frequency at which the wavelets submerge into the baseline is the ERG flicker fusion frequency. Unfortunately, our flash units do not operate beyond 30 Hz, thus the fusion frequencies for normal subjects are not obtainable. However, many patients whose cone retinal functions are reduced show early fusion below 30 Hz.

Again, if a patient's flicker ERG function falls below the normal limit (shaded band), we can say the photopic retinal function of the patient is significantly reduced. This is the function which is reduced in very early cases of cone dystrophy, cone dysfunction, many forms of macular diseases (such as Stargardt's disease, fundus flavimaculitis, macular drusen, vitelliform macular dystrophy), choroidal diseases and dystrophia myotonica. This is also the measure which shows the first signs of reduction in patients with optic neuritis, or other optic nerve disease. Presumably, because 50% of the optic nerve fibres arise from the macula, where the major proportion of cones is situated, if any retrograde trans-synaptic degeneration occurs, it depresses the ERGs mediated by the macular cones. Conversely, with macular disease showing abolition or significant reduction of the flicker ERG, optic atrophy often results due to orthograde trans-synaptic degeneration.

In those patients who show subnormal flicker ERG function, the visual evoked responses obtained at the occipital pole are usually subnormal in amplitude. Thus, a reduction in the VER amplitude may not be entirely due to the loss of optic nerve or cerebral function but may well be due to the fact that the retinal output is already reduced significantly without any ophthalmoscopic change. This is an often neglected factor.

ILLUSTRATED ERG RESPONSES OF ROD AND CONE ABNORMALITIES

Although it is possible to assess the degree of loss of retinal function in a variety of cases, using the normal limits established for the above three major ERG functions (Figures 4.6, 4.7 and 4.8), in some cases, single ERG responses clearly reveal whether the rods or the cones have become affected. This is illustrated in two cases in Figure 4.9. One is an early Stargardt's type maculopathy with vision bilaterally down to 6/12, no known family history and no visual field loss. The patient was a 16-year-old girl, and since the fundi change was too minor to confirm the diagnosis, she was sent to us for electrodiagnosis.

Figure 4.9 B shows the ERG responses of this patient to stimulation with a white, blue and red flash after 18-20 minutes dark adaptation, and the ERG response to red flicker at 30 Hz. These responses are compared with those of another young girl also aged 16 (Figure 4.9 A). This girl showed no visual loss, but came for a check-up, since her maternal uncle appeared to suffer from a hereditary macular degeneration: she was diagnosed as 'unaffected', and all psychophysical investigations and clinical investigations were normal for this girl.

ERGs evoked by white and blue flashes after 18-20 minutes of dark adaptation in the patient with suspected early Stargardt's maculopathy show that the amplitudes of the b-wave are quite normal, except that the x-wave is missing from the response evoked by the white flash. But the ERG evoked by a red flash shows a lack of x-wave, and a reduction in amplitude of the b-wave. The ERG, evoked by 30 Hz red flicker, is practically smooth (flicker fusion). The results thus suggest that the rod retinal responses are normal, but the cone retinal responses are reduced.

It is often said that unless one uses localized stimulation and averaging techniques, a minor localized macular abnormality cannot be shown by the clinical

ERG, but this is not true. As long as the normal limit is clearly set under well controlled conditions, a loss of the macular function should rarely be missed.

The second case, illustrated in Figure 9 C, is a selective loss of rod retinal function. This patient was a male, aged 40, with a family history of retinitis pigmentosa. The fundi appeared quite normal, but he had difficulty in the dark, and his visual fields showed a mild, widespread reduction in visual thresholds in the periphery; however, the visual acuity was 6/6 in both eyes.

The ERGs evoked by white and blue flashes after 18-20 minutes of dark adaptation show a reduction in amplitude of the b-wave. Also note that the b-wave is fast (narrow wave-width), suggesting that the slower rod-mediated component of the b-wave is reduced. The ratio of b-wave to a-wave amplitude is less than 2.0. The increase in b-wave with dark adaptation was poor, and the response curve plotted in the same form as in Figure 4.6 fell below the normal limit. The dark adapted b-wave threshold plotted as in Figure 4.7, also, was 1.5 log units above the normal limit, and the entire curve fell below the shaded normal range. All these observations suggest the loss of retinal sensitivity lacking a contribution from the rods.

In contrast the responses to the red flash are normal in amplitude, but the x-wave is absent. The flicker ERG wavelets plotted as in Figure 4.8 for this patient fell within the normal range, suggesting the cone-mediated retinal response is intact.

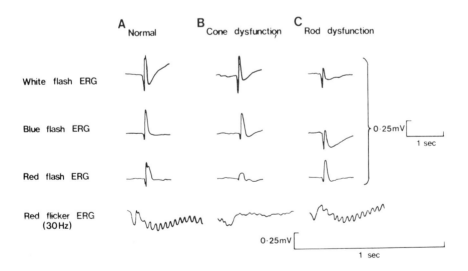

Figure 4.9. *The ERGs evoked by a single white (intensity 0 log unit), blue (with Wratten filter 47B) and red (with Wratten filter 29) flash and the flicker ERG evoked by 30 Hz red light from: A: a normal subject; B: a patient with early Stargardt's disease; and C: a patient with mild retinitis pigmentosa.*

Selective abolition of the b-wave

In most clinical cases of retinal degeneration, diabetic retinopathy, toxic retinopathies, or toxic amblyopia, both the a-wave and the b-wave of the ERG are reduced. However, in some patients we may see, almost unexpectedly, a beautiful demonstration of the selective abolition of the b-wave.

Acute central retinal artery occlusion, for example, provides a classical demonstration of the fact that the b-wave arises from the inner nuclear layer rather than from the receptors (Brown and Watanabe, l962). This is because the central retinal artery supplies the inner nuclear and ganglion cell layers, but the receptors are supplied mainly by the choroid. If the retinal circulation is stopped, the inner retina, of course, becomes anoxic, but the receptors may remain functional as long as the choroidal circulation is maintained. The ERGs recorded under such circumstances show only a large negative potential. This negative potential is the a-wave, the receptor potential without contamination by the b-wave, which is abolished by the anoxia imposed on the inner nuclear layer. Since such cases require immediate medical attention rather than ERG recording, clinically we are not sent

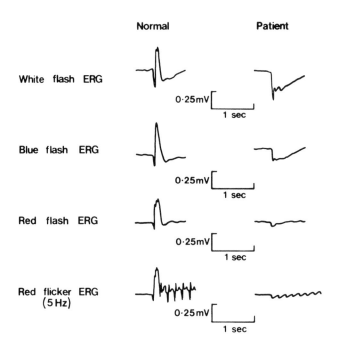

Figure 4.10. *A demonstration of the selective loss of the b-wave in the clinical ERG. Normal ERGs evoked by a single white (intensity 0 log unit), blue (with Wratten filter 47B) and red (with Wratten filter 29) flash and normal flicker ERGs evoked by a red light of 5 Hz are compared with those from a patient who became blind suddenly, after an overdose of various tablets (see text). Note that the patient's ERGs are virtually negative in polarity.*

such patients. But I would like to illustrate a case (Figure 4.10) in which the b-wave of the ERG was found to be virtually extinguished, suggesting a major lesion at the b-wave level, i.e. the inner nuclear layer.

Figure 4.10 shows the ERGs obtained from a patient, aged 27 — a Mandrax addict — who claimed sudden total loss of vision after consuming a large amount of alcohol and taking an overdose of various tablets including flurazepam and codeine! The fundi were completely normal, various investigations including CSF were normal, and the case was diagnosed as hysteria. However, during the following two months the patient's acuity gradually returned to 6/9 in each eye, but the peripheral vision was still lost. At this stage the discs appeared pale, and the retinal blood vessels were thought to be constricted, although the ophthalmologists were sure that there was no pigmentary retinopathy. The patient was sent for ERG examination at this time. As can be seen (Figure 4.10) the responses obtained from this patient were largely negative a-waves and even the flicker ERG consisted of negative wavelets.

The ERG of this patient shows a selective loss of the b-wave suggesting a major reduction in the post-synaptic function of the retina, although the cause for this is still uncertain. The attenuation of retinal blood vessels — presumably causing a deficiency of nutrition of the inner retinal layers — is consistent with the ERG findings. However, selective abolition of the b-wave has also been shown in retinae treated with high concentrations of magnesium (Dowling and Ripps, 1976), sodium aspartate (Yonemura and Kawasaki, 1978), or l-glutamate (Potts et al, 1960). Thus whether an overdose of the drugs taken by the patient together with alcohol resulted in toxic effects similar to those seen with substances which have been shown to abolish the b-wave, remains to be determined.

Selective abolition of the b-wave has also been reported in night-blind patients by Dowling and Ripps (1976), who emphasised the similarity of the ERG changes with those observed in magnesium-treated skate retina. Since magnesium inhibits the release of transmitter agents at nerve terminals, these authors suggested that the lesion in the night-blind subjects is at the terminals of the photoreceptors, impeding the transfer of information from the receptors to the bipolar cells, without destroying the integrity of the receptors themselves. We have also recently investigated a patient with night-blindness associated with severe zinc deficiency. Is it possible that the lack of zinc, which combines with magnesium, leaves an excess of magnesium affecting the transmission of the receptor potential to the bipolar cells, or is zinc associated with rod function in some other way? Further clinical investigations into this particular field would undoubtedly benefit from the use of the ERG. Some forms of night-blindness thus appear to be due to a fault in synaptic transmission within the retina.

Early diagnosis of inner retinal abnormality by the use of the oscillatory potentials

So far I have described the clinical ERGs and their diagnostic value based on the two major components — the a- and b-waves — which can be recorded with conventional EEG amplifiers and a pen recorder. However, the oscillatory potential, which can only be seen in responses evoked by high intensity flashes in dark-adapted eyes recorded on an oscilloscope, may play a rôle in the early diagnosis of inner retinal dysfunction.

It has been suggested that the oscillatory potential is generated by the amacrine cells, or the inner plexiform synaptic activity of the retina involved in inhibitory feed-back circuits (Werblin, 1977; Wachtmeister and Dowling, 1978), although a recent study by Yonemura and Kawasaki (1978) showed that some of the optic nerve fibres produce grouped discharges, which are synchronous with the oscillatory potential of the ERG. Intensive studies on the oscillatory potential of the clinical ERG have been made almost exclusively by Japanese workers, and have been reviewed thoroughly by Yonemura and Kawasaki (1978). These workers have shown that the oscillatory potential is selectively delayed, abolished or reduced *without reducing the b-wave of the ERG* by pentobarbital, glycine, reduced inspired oxygen consumption, quinaldic acid, monoiodoacetic acid, kynurenic acid or picrotoxin. Wachtmeister and Dowling (1978) included GABA, glutamate and dopamine as further substances which selectively abolish the oscillatory potential.

Such findings suggest that the outer plexiform synapses and inner plexiform synapses may use different transmitters, or that the bipolar cells and amacrine cells have different susceptibilities to different chemical agents. These are serious claims, and it would be desirable for these results to be confirmed by other workers. Many other drugs have also been shown to abolish the oscillatory potential, but they have been shown to abolish the b-wave as well.

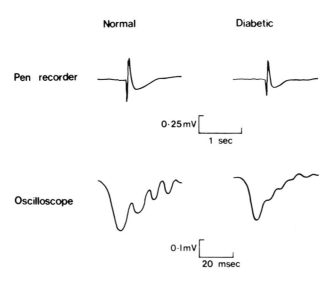

Figure 4.11. *A relatively normal a-wave and b-wave obtained from a diabetic patient compared with those from a normal subject (upper traces recorded on a pen recorder); and a reduced oscillatory potential obtained from the same patient compared with the oscillatory potential from the normal subject (lower traces recorded on an oscilloscope with a fast time base). All responses are evoked by a white flash of high intensity in the dark adapted eye.*

Clinically, the oscillatory potential has been shown to be extremely vulnerable to interference with the retinal circulation by, for example, capillary closure, microaneurysms, arteriovenous anastomoses and neo-vascularization as in mild diabetic retinopathy. However, in our experience it is extremely rare to come across patients with diabetic retinopathy or retinal vascular abnormalities, who do not show any deficits in the a- or b-waves. So far, the use of the oscillatory potential seems, therefore, to be limited to the demonstration of very early cases of neural retinal involvement in the disease process.

A simulated effect of very early diabetes mellitus on the ERG, showing a delay in the oscillatory potential, has been observed following an intravitreal injection of quinaldic acid, one of the metabolites of tryptophan which is suspected of being involved in the generation of the pathological condition of diabetes mellitus (Yonemura and Kawasaki, 1978).

I shall illustrate only one case out of about 200 patients with diabetic retinopathies from whom ERGs have been recorded, to demonstrate the selective abolition of the oscillatory potential (Figure 4.11). This patient showed no fundus abnormalities or visual defects, but had been recently found to be diabetic. All ERG functions measured were near the lower limit of normal (see the ERG recorded on a pen recorder in Figure 4.11) but the lack of an oscillatory potential on the early rising phases of the b-wave may be noted (the lower traces in Figure 4.11). In all other diabetic patients ERG functions (and also EOG light rise) were found to be subnormal.

A NOTE ON THE EARLY RECEPTOR POTENTIAL - ERP

The ERP is generated at the point of light absorption. Its mode of generation, and its relationship to the thermal decay of photo-products of bleached pigments have been studied extensively by many scientists during the 1960s, after its discovery (Brown and Murakami, 1964). They showed how the photochemical reaction of the receptors was converted to the rapid positive and negative charge displacement. However, its mode of generation is fundamentally different from other bioelectric potentials, since it can be recorded in an isolated anoxic eye as long as there are oriented photoreceptor outer segments and unbleached pigments in the eye.

The ERP has been reported to be completely normal in cases of long-standing optic nerve atrophy, or complete central retinal artery occlusion, but absent in total retinal detachment, pigmentary degeneration and phthisis bulbi. But, of course, in the cases in which the ERP is absent the ERG is completely abolished.

Although it may be of academic interest to know whether blindness is caused by a lack of photopigments or orientated photoreceptors, in my opinion, it has only limited clinical application.

COMBINED ASSESSMENT OF THE ERG AND VEP

There is an increasing realization that for accurate diagnosis of CNS disease both the ERG and the VEP must be assessed. The retina is embryologically a part of the forebrain, and its structure is very similar to other parts of the central nervous system. Its oxygen consumption, metabolism, the existence of the blood-brain barrier and many other fundamental similarities could be listed.

Many systemic diseases can affect the retina, even though they do not produce symptoms or fundus changes. Many diseases which were previously thought, or assumed, to be primarily diseases of the optic nerve fibres have also been shown to affect retinal function (Ikeda et al, 1978).

The ERGs were found to be completely normal in the case of *acute* quinine poisoning and in early cases of cherry red spot (ganglion cell death due to lipid disease), whereas the VEPs were reduced or abolished. But when these cases are investigated at a later stage the ERG functions are reduced. In cases of toxic amblyopia, due to consumption of alcohol, tobacco and cassava, retinal involvement is also suggested (Ikeda et al, 1978), and this is perhaps not surprising, since any substance which is toxic for the brain is also likely to be toxic for the retina.

On the other hand, if the ERG is quite normal, but the VEP is reduced or delayed, this suggests that the primary lesion is beyond the retinal ganglion cells. In cases where the scotopic ERG only is affected, the VEP may be normal, since the VEP reveals the functioning of the macular cone projection to the occipital pole, whereas the VEP must be reduced in cases in which the photopic ERG is significantly reduced. Of course, a normal ERG and VEP would suggest a diagnosis of hysterical blindness, but one must note that patients claiming a reduced visual field or difficulty in darkness should be investigated by the ERG as well as the VEP, since the VEP reveals mainly cone-mediated macular function.

FINAL NOTES

This chapter is written in the hope that it covers some of the difficulties which are seldom discussed in publications, and thus may be of help to readers who enter the field of clinical ERG recording. In clinical recordings, unlike research work, each patient gives the examiner a *single* opportunity to obtain the required information. Because of this, it is important to establish normal limits for the measurements. Confidence in the result does not arise from using expensive and modern techniques, but is acquired by perseverance with one particular technique, under carefully controlled recording conditions.

Over the past 10 years, we have recorded ERGs from over 2000 patients in response to requests from Consultants in St Thomas' Hospital and elsewhere. Although it is satisfying to be able to pin-point abnormalities to specific layers of the retina by the ERG, I am always saddened by the thought that for those patients who suffer from degenerative retinal disease, no treatment is available. It is my conviction that future developments in the clinical ERG will depend on our rapidly advancing knowledge of the complex synaptic organization in the retina, and of the neurotransmitters used by different classes of cells, and on an increasing knowledge of how biochemical changes and pharmacological interference in the retina can influence the electrical activities of the retina and hence the ERG. There is still much more to be done before the clinical ERG may play a rôle in the very early diagnosis of neurotransmitter deficiency, such that possible treatment may be suggested before degeneration is too far advanced.

Acknowledgements

Finally, I would like to thank all the ophthalmologists, neurologists and Consultants in other fields of medicine who have shown interest and encouragement in our electrodiagnostic service. I am grateful for the support received in the past from the Godfrey Robinson Fund of the Royal College of Surgeons of England and more recently from the Prevention of Blindness Research Funds, the Royal National Institute for the Blind and St Thomas' Hospital Research Endowment Funds. I thank the members of my unit who are interested in the success of the clinical services the unit renders to hospitals, and particularly I would like to thank Dr Keith Tremain, who assisted in the recordings and drew the Figures in this Chapter.

5

The VEP in the Investigation of Diseases of the Eye

A.M. Halliday

ABNORMALITIES OF THE VISUAL EVOKED RESPONSE

In disease affecting the visual pathways the VEP may show changes in (1) amplitude, (2) latency and (3) waveform in one or more of its components, but the changes can only be of help to the clinician in an individual patient if they are clearly beyond the limits of normal variability. This variability has been considered at length in Chapter 3. The major advantage of the pattern reversal EP over the flash EP lies in the much smaller variability in the waveform and latency of its components in the healthy population (see Table 3.1). This superior consistency of the pattern EP is reinforced by the fact that this response is more sensitive to pathological changes than the flash EP and shows a greater degree of alteration in latency or amplitude for the same degree of damage. This is well illustrated by recordings of both responses in the same group of patients with optic neuritis (see Figure 6.11). Conversely, because it is less sensitive, the flash response is more robust and can often be recorded at a time when, owing to gross visual impairment, the pattern EP can no longer be obtained (see, for example, Figure 6.25). The flash EP is therefore particularly useful to the clinician in severe lesions associated with gross visual impairment. Since the ERG to pattern is very small and largely macular in origin, while the flash ERG is relatively large and is derived from a much wider area of the retina, flash stimulation is also valuable for the detection of changes in the electroretinogram (see Chapter 4 and below). In the author's own laboratory, flash EPs are routinely recorded (in addition to pattern reversal EPs) wherever the visual acuity is 6/36 or worse or in any case where there is a question of retinopathy.

The criteria for regarding any visual EP as abnormal depend on the accepted limits of normality. Assuming that the spread of $\overline{P100}$ latencies and amplitudes in the healthy population have a normal distribution, which is probably legitimate for adults between the ages of 15 and 50 years, there will be a definite false positive rate associated with the choice of 2.0, 2.5 or 3.0 standard deviations of the normal mean as the limit of normality. Since the direction of abnormal change is usually predictable (an increase in latency and/or a reduction in amplitude, except in the well-recognized case of photosensitive epilepsy where an increase in amplitude may be the expected change), the false positive rates can be calculated on the basis of a one-tailed test as approximately 1 in 40, 1 in 160, and 1 in 770 for 2.0, 2.5 and 3.0 standard deviations respectively.

The variation in VEP amplitude and latency between different individuals in the healthy population is very much larger than that between the responses from each eye of a given individual (see Chapter 3). It is therefore possible to characterize much smaller differences between the latency and amplitude of the responses from the left and right eye as abnormal. This can be particularly valuable in unilateral disease of the eye or anterior visual pathways, or in bilateral disease where the two sides are unequally affected. Waveform changes are also more easily recognized when they are more marked in one eye than the other, and, although difficult to quantify, they may provide a valuable early sign of pathology (see, for example, Figure 6.23).

As has already been stressed (Chapter 2) the parameters of the normal response depend critically on a large number of stimulus characteristics. For this reason it is essential for each laboratory to establish its own normal values on a healthy control group, employing, as far as possible, exactly the same equipment and recording conditions as it is intended to use in clinical testing. Published studies show an extremely wide choice of stimulus parameters (Halliday, 1980c) and this is inevitably associated with a considerable variation in the mean normal values (e.g. $\overline{P100}$ latency). There is also little agreement in the published studies on the choice of a criterion for the limit of normal. In the author's own laboratory 2.5 standard deviations has been the accepted criterion for a delayed $\overline{P100}$ in the pattern EP (Halliday et al, 1972, 1973a).

A SUGGESTED ROUTINE FOR CLINICAL VEP TESTING

The following is a brief description of the standard routine VEP examination currently used in the author's own department.

1. On arrival the patient's name, age (including date of birth), address or ward if an in-patient, and referring physician are noted on a protocol, together with the date. The case notes or physician's letter are referred to, to assess the diagnostic problem.

2. The patient's visual acuity in each eye is tested with a Snellen Card. This is done with glasses (if worn). Where the patient has a refractive error but has left their glasses behind, this is noted. Where vision is impaired, this is retested with a pinhole to differentiate refractive errors from neuroretinal lesions.

3. Silver-silver chloride disc electrodes are applied in a standard montage (see page 82), including a midfrontal reference and an earth electrode. Electrode jelly is applied after scarifying the skin and the resistance is measured between electrode pairs. Only a resistance of less than 5 kilohms is acceptable, and further scarification is employed where necessary to achieve this. Resistance is tested with a low-current meter (FSD 50 μA). Electrodes are then plugged into the head board.

4. Before the patient is connected to the amplifiers, these are invariably calibrated on each occasion with a 10 μV square wave. A hundred calibration pulses are averaged and recorded. In the author's laboratory, in order to save time, this calibration is stored digitally on tape or floppy disc, for subsequent write-out when the patient has gone. This calibration serves as a useful check of the filter settings and of the equality of gain between the different channels, and allows any unnoticed variation in amplifier gain to be subsequently identified and allowed for. Furthermore, if any subsequent misbehaviour of an amplifier occurs during the recording session a repeat calibration can be carried out at the end of the session for comparison.

5. Checkerboard reversal responses are recorded for each eye separately, using the standard full-field (0-16°) stimulus. In each run 200 pattern reversals are averaged at a frequency of 1.7 Hz (the actual stimulus interval is 605 msec). As a test of consistency the response from each eye is recorded at least twice using a left-right-right-left design for the four runs. If the two averaged responses from either eye show markedly inconsistent features, or are obscured by muscle or movement artifact, further runs are recorded. While one eye is being stimulated, the other eye is covered with an eye pad.

6. Responses to pattern-reversal presented in each half-field are then recorded from each eye separately. As this involves four further runs, these runs are only individually repeated if the results appear anomalous, technically unsatisfactory or difficult to interpret, or if the progress of a chiasmal lesion is being serially assessed.

7. Following half-field stimulation, the usual practice is to record responses to a checkerboard presented in the central 0-4° field for each eye.

8. Various further runs may be recorded, depending on the initial findings or the clinical features of the case. Among these possibilities are the following.

9. Flash responses are not recorded routinely in every case, where the visual acuity in each eye is better than 6/24. They are invariably recorded, with a pair of peri-orbital electrodes round each eye to detect the ERG, where the visual acuity is equal to or worse than 6/36 or where there is any question of retinopathy. For the flash VEP a hundred flashes are delivered to each eye at 1 Hz with the other eye covered, not only by an eye patch, but also with the hand of the subject held over it. The xenon flash tube, with a 29 cm diameter circular diffusing screen is placed about 30 cm in front of the subject's closed eyes. A repeat run, with eyes open, is also recorded.

10. Where the pattern reversal responses are absent or too small to be clearly differentiated from the background noise, the responses to checkerboard onset and

offset on a blank background of equal mean luminance are often measured, as the onset response in particular is more robust and may still be present when the pattern reversal response is abolished.

11. Where small field defects, e.g. scotomata or quadrantanopias, are at issue the pattern reversal EP may be recorded in response to stimulation of smaller selected areas of the retina (e.g. quadrants or octants). This, however, is time-consuming and is seldom justified unless there is already clinical evidence (e.g. from perimetry) to guide the choice of stimuli (cf Figure 7.20).

12. Throughout the recording, fixation must be carefully monitored, particularly if asymmetric stimulation of portions of the field is being carried out. It is also important to make sure that the patient's eyes are kept fully open and that there is no excessive lid droop or ptosis (see page 63). Where necessary, the upper lids can be taped open gently with Micropore before the run is commenced, or can even be held open by the experimenter or by the patient himself, if appropriate.

PROBLEMS IN RECORDING

Among the problems which may prove troublesome in recording VEPs are poor or wandering fixation, or excessive drowsiness leading to partial eye closure, and the obscuring of the response by bursts of muscle or movement artifact. With regard to muscle artifact, it is especially the facial and neck muscles which produce high voltage noise on the record. It is important for success, therefore, to ensure that the head is resting comfortably backwards in the chair. It is often helpful to have a small pillow or pad behind the nape of the neck, but the patient must be induced not to press backwards against this or the back of the chair, or high voltage EMG activity will appear at the occipital electrodes. Temporalis activity is also troublesome, and it is often helpful to instruct the patient not to clench the jaw and, if necessary, to open the mouth slightly. It is seldom necessary to resort to artifact rejection, although this can be helpful if available (see page 491). With good technique, the EMG activity is usually only noticeable in the first run or so in most subjects. There may be special problems in dealing with patients with pathologically increased muscle activity (e.g. in Parkinsonism). Where this proves troublesome, resort can be made to recording the patients lying down, but this is usually inconvenient to do with the standard visual stimulators. If necessary, a 45° mirror can be helpful in these circumstances, as, suitably placed above the couch, it allows the supine patient to look upwards at the image of a checkerboard stimulus situated on one side. It is, of course, important to adapt the field size or length of the light path to maintain the dimensions of the stimulus.

Interpreting 'difficult' VEP records

Some of the main causes of difficulty encountered in the clinical use of the pattern EP are (1) a poorly defined $\overline{P100}$ component in which the latency cannot be accurately determined; (2) confusion in identifying the $\overline{P100}$ where more than one positive peak is present; (3) a much altered waveform with no positivity; (4) a response so small or ill-defined as to be hardly above the noise level.

There are a number of tips or useful stratagems which can be employed under favourable circumstances to minimize or get over these difficulties. With regard to measuring the peak latency of a poorly defined $\overline{P100}$ component, it may be possible where there is no clear peak to estimate the peak latency by taking a point half-way between the steepest part of the positive-going and negative-going limbs of the wave. Since these are the areas of maximum potential change, they are often still accurately determinable when the peak itself is distorted by superimposed noise or blunted by pathological waveform changes. However, some judgement must be used in applying this technique, and it is only legitimate where the two limbs of the component are still clearly defined and symmetrical. Where this is not the case, and the issue is one of whether there is a delayed latency in only one eye, resort can be taken to cross-correlation, which is both objective and will provide a sensitive method of detecting a relative shift in the whole waveform (see Chapter 15 and Halliday et al, 1979b). This technique is obviously of little use when the responses from both eyes are equally delayed. A less drastic computational technique, which will improve the resolution of the waveform where it is obscured by superimposed higher frequency noise components, is to smooth the response curve by averaging consecutive overlapping sets of two, three, four or even five ordinates at one ordinate interval. Where the facilities are available digital filtering may provide an even better alternative (see Chapter 1).

Where more than one positive component is present, half-field stimulation will often help to identify and distinguish the ipsilateral $\overline{N75}$, $\overline{P100}$ and $\overline{N145}$ components from the contralateral $\overline{P75}$, $\overline{N105}$ and $\overline{P135}$ components (see page 105). Since the $\overline{P135}$ component is a frequent cause of confusion, being mistaken for a delayed $\overline{P100}$, this can be an extremely useful technique, particularly where there is a central scotoma. Stimulation of the central field itself (e.g. 0-4°) will serve to further confirm the loss of the $\overline{P100}$ component from the central field in the presence of a central scotoma.

Half-field stimulation can also be of value in elucidating an altered waveform with no surviving $\overline{P100}$. It can, for instance, clearly identify a prominent negative wave as the contralateral $\overline{N105}$ (see, for example, Figure 7.23).

Where the pattern reversal response is much attenuated or absent, due to the lowered acuity level, the pattern appearance or flash EPs may still be clearly obtained and may reveal a delay in the presence of demyelination.

RELATIVE SENSITIVITY OF THE FLASH EP TO VISUAL IMPAIRMENT FROM REFRACTIVE ERRORS, OPACITIES AND NEURORETINAL LESIONS

In one of the early studies of the use of the flash EP in clinical neuro-ophthalmology Copenhaver and Perry (1964) recorded the occipital responses to a foveally situated stroboscopic flash stimulus subtending a visual angle of 2.5° presented at 3.8 Hz. They compared the findings in a healthy control group (18 subjects) and three other groups, representing refractive errors (9 subjects with otherwise normal eyes), opacities of the mediae (11 subjects with cataract, corneal opacity or vitreous opacity in only one eye) and 'neural' lesions (18 patients with uniocular pre-chiasmal lesions, including macular scars, tumours and degenera-tions, retinal detachment with macular involvement, or optic nerve lesions associated with a central scotoma). They found the inter-individual variability of the flash response in the healthy control group to be too large to allow any correlation between the absolute amplitude of the flash EP and the visual acuity in inter-subject comparisons. However, the left eye/right eye amplitude ratio in the controls was 0.88 (s.d. 0.23), which allowed a more useful comparison between the ratio of the responses between the good and bad eye in the patient groups. For the group with refractive errors, a similar comparison was made between the uncorrected and corrected response from each eye. Using this method, these authors were able to show that for a given level of impairment of the visual acuity the flash EP was significantly smaller in amplitude for the group of patients with neuroretinal lesions than for the group with refractive errors, and that the slope of the regression line of visual acuity against VEP amplitude was steeper for the former group, indicating a progressively more severe impairment of response at lower acuity levels secondary to neuroretinal lesions. In spite of the relative insensitivity of the flash response, these conclusions are important and have remained valid. They also apply with equal or greater force to the pattern reversal EP.

Among the other observations made by Copenhaver and Perry (1964) was that the flash EP amplitude could be significantly increased by dilating the pupil with mydriatics or by recording the response with artificial pupils of larger diameter. Doubling the pupil size produced an increase of approximately one-fifth in the EP amplitude. However, larger responses obtained in this way differed little with regard to the ratio of the responses from the two eyes. A further point was that artificially induced refractive errors produced no significant reduction in the flash EP until the induced error approached 10 dioptres. The authors draw attention to the importance of unsuspected amblyopia in increasing the apparent effect of refractive errors. In the 64 normal eyes tested there was some decrement in response size with increasing age. With the small size of stimulus used, fixation was important and the response amplitude was reduced to a quarter of the size if the 2.5° stimulus field was located only 2.5° off the visual axis. The authors point out that the relative insensitivity of the response amplitude to the effect of opacities is advantageous if the test is to be used for the investigation of preserved retinal function behind a cataract.

REFRACTIVE ERRORS AND VEP REFRACTOMETRY

Not surprisingly, the effect of defocussing on the VEP is best detected with a patterned stimulus. Even the introduction of a static pattern into the flash stimulus greatly increases the sensitivity of the response to the acuity level. Harter and White (1968) used a flashed checkerboard pattern, with checks subtending 12′, 20′ and 46′, to study the effect on EP amplitude of degrading the stimulus image by up to ±6 dioptres. They found two components of the patterned flash EP particularly sensitive to the sharpness of focus, $\overline{N95}$ and $\overline{P190}$, but the effect was much less marked for the large 46′ checks than for the two smaller checks of 20′ and 12′. Examination of the individual subjects showed that their peak EP amplitudes were reached at lens settings which deviated from zero when the subject was either myopic or hypermetropic. In testing subjects with more severe refractive errors, the lens producing the largest EP agreed well with those producing the best subjective acuity.

In another study of the flashed pattern EP in 15 undergraduates with uncorrected vision ranging from 20/9 to 20/400, using a stimulus of small dots of varying diameter (0.75'-19' subtense), Towle and Harter (1977) found a high correlation between subjective visual acuity and the VEP pattern threshold, measured as the smallest stimulus which would evoke a VEP. Purely objective measures of the amplitude of pattern-sensitive response components ($\overline{N120}$ and $\overline{P220}$ for this stimulus) were not quite as effective as visual inspection of the VEP record in detecting the EP threshold, and the EP technique appeared to systematically underestimate perceptual visual acuity, but the correlation coefficient (r) between Jaeger acuity scores and VEP thresholds were as high as 0.85 for objective $\overline{N120}$ measurement and 0.86 for visual inspection (p < 0.001 for both correlations).

The patterned flash EP has the disadvantage of being contaminated by luminance components and the pattern reversal EP should be even more favourable for acuity testing. The use of small checks (subtending 20' or less) is necessary to get the optimal results. Indeed, defocussing checks larger than this may actually increase the amplitude of the pattern EP (Regan and Richards, 1973; Halliday et al, unpublished).

The possible use of the pattern reversal response in refractometry has been explored (Millodot and Riggs, 1970; Ludlam and Meyers, 1972; McCormack and Marg, 1973; Millodot, 1977; Regan, 1977b). The advantage of an entirely objective method of refractometry is that it would avoid the discrepancy of half a dioptre or less which commonly occurs between subjective correction and the use of retinoscopy. However, in spite of the increased sensitivity of pattern reversal over patterned flash, the technique is not yet equal to that obtained psychophysically and it does not appear that it has yet reached the stage at which it can be adopted as a routine procedure. It can, however, allow refractometry to be carried out in infants. Regan (1977b) has suggested a number of ingenious modifications for speeding up the test in EP refractometry. As well as the use of the steady state response with its shorter response time, he has advocated the use of periodically varying check size (produced by a motorized zoom lens) and Fourier analysis of the response. Sinusoidally modulated correcting lenses can also be employed. Further details will be found in Regan (1977b).

Similar results have been obtained on patients with astigmatism, where the refractive defect is limited to one visual axis. Ludlam and Meyers (1972) and McCormack and Marg (1973) recorded EPs to gratings in different orientations and found the orientations which gave the responses of maximum and minimum amplitude. Cylindrical correcting lenses were then used and those giving the largest EP for each axis were determined. This is the simplest method for dealing with refractive astigmatism and can provide an estimate of correction to within 0.5-1 dioptre for the power and 10° for the axis. As Regan (1973, 1977b) has pointed out, a more sophisticated and faster method of carrying out this test is to use a con-tinuously rotating grating pattern, and to Fourier analyse the steady state VEP. In cases of astigmatic amblyopia, the test will still serve to determine the maximum and minimum visual axes, but will show no response to correction of the refractive error. Fiorentini and Maffei (1974) recorded the steady state EPs to reversing sine wave gratings of three cycles/degree in 23 astigmatic subjects, whose refractive error had been fully corrected. They found a persistent asymmetry in VEP amplitude in the two principal meridians of the astigmatic eye in the seven subjects who had a high degree of astigmatism (3-4 dioptres in both eyes), but did not find any significant differences between the amplitude of the VEP to the stimulus grating in the two principal orientations in the other 16 subjects who had only a small degree of astigmatism (0.5-1.5 dioptres in one or both eyes). Since the astigmatic error had been corrected in all the subjects this suggests that the seven more severely astigmatic subjects had a super-added astigmatic amblyopia of neural origin.

From the point of view of routine clinical testing, it is important to know that for the larger check sizes (e.g. 50′) moderate defocussing of the checkerboard stimulus has little or no effect on the $\overline{P100}$ latency. The amplitude, however, decreases in parallel with the reduction in the acuity level. It must be made clear that this result applies only to black and white checkerboard stimuli where the contrast is well over the saturation level (say, at least, 50%) and for relatively large field sizes in which the stimulus is not restricted to the foveal area. Collins et al, (1979) have shown that a foveal checkerboard stimulus made up of 12′ checks is much more sensitive to refractive errors and shows significant changes both in latency and amplitude with defocussing. Spekreijse and Duwaer give examples of changes of checkerboard EP latency with defocussing, lowered contrast and alteration in check size and field size (Spekreijse et al, 1979; Duwaer and Spekreijse, 1978). Carroll and Kriss (1981) have demonstrated similar changes and have also emphasized the additional factors of pupil size and lid-droop or ptosis (see also Halliday et al, 1982a). These observations underline the importance of using well validated controls obtained on the stimuli used for clinical testing and of being aware of the possible significance of variations in these stimulus and response parameters.

Examples of responses recorded in patients with uncorrected and corrected refractive errors from the author's own laboratory are shown in Figures 5.1 and 5.2. The stimulus here was the standard 0-16° checkerboard made up of 50′ black and white checks used for routine clinical testing. Both responses illustrate the lowered amplitude of the pattern reversal EP from the eye with the poor acuity, which is increased after correction. In neither case, however, is there any appreciable change in the latency of the response.

In contrast to this, the pattern reversal EPs shown in Figure 5.3 are recorded with a smaller stimulus field and smaller checks from a 30-year-old myope. Without correction the visual acuity dropped from 6/6 to 6/60. For the response to a 4° radius stimulus of 20′ checks there is only a 2 msec increase in the $\overline{P100}$ latency, but for a 2° radius stimulus of 10′ checks, preferentially stimulating the pattern receptors (sustained X cells) at the fovea, the response latency becomes much more sensitive to the refractive error, with an increase of 16 msec from 108 msec to 124 msec.

If an induced refractive error is sufficiently large, an *apparent* increase in $\overline{P100}$ latency can be produced even with a large checkerboard stimulus of large checks. Figure 5.4 shows (above) the effect of introducing strong lenses of up to + 11 dioptres on the response of a healthy subject to the standard 16° radius

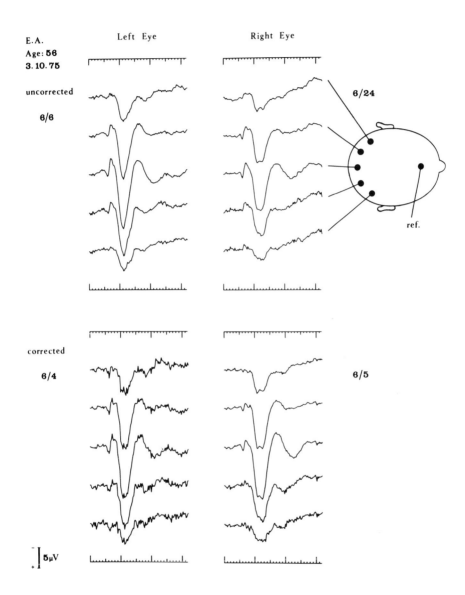

Figure 5.1 *Monocular responses to pattern stimulation with a 0-16° checkerboard of 50' checks in a 56-year-old woman with a refractive error of the right eye. The upper records show the responses obtained with uncorrected vision (VAL 6/6, VAR 6/24) and the lower records with corrected vision (VAL 6/4, VAR 6/5). Note the slightly reduced amplitude of the response from the uncorrected eye with 6/24 vision, increasing in size with correction without change of latency. (From Halliday and Mushin, 1980.)*

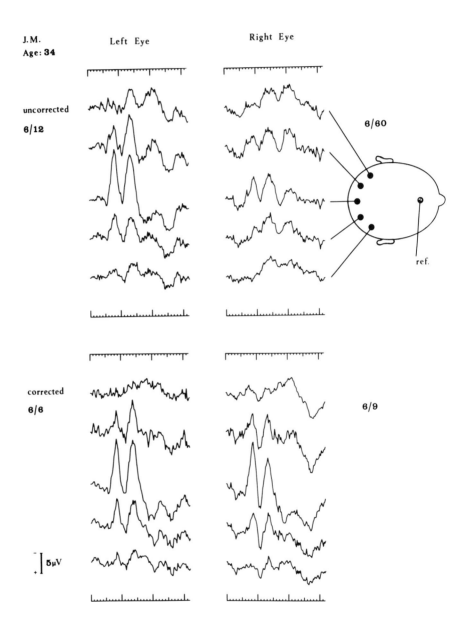

Figure 5.2 *Responses with uncorrected and corrected vision in a 34-year-old woman with more severe myopia. Compare Figure 5.1. (From Halliday and Mushin, 1980.)*

checkerboard stimulus of 50′ checks. The apparent latency of the peak positivity increases from 108 msec to 115 msec (+ 6 D), 139 msec (+ 9 D) and 125 msec (+ 11 D) for the full-field response. Half-field stimulation (lower records) shows that the positivity has changed sides for the defocussed condition. The ipsilateral $\overline{P100}$ component of the corrected response has been partly replaced by the contralateral $\overline{P135}$ component in the defocussed response. The relative contributions from these macular and paramacular components varies with the degree of defocussing. Note that much more information is provided by the multichannel electrode array shown in the lower records than by the single midline channel shown above.

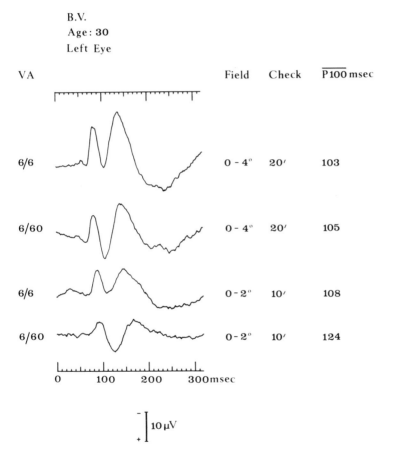

Figure 5.3 *The effect of reduced stimulus field size and check size on the sensitivity of pattern EP latency to refractive errors. Responses from the left eye of a 30-year-old myope with corrected (6/6) and uncorrected (6/60) vision for a 0-4° checkerboard of 20′ checks and a 0-2° checkerboard of 10′ checks. Note the change in $\overline{P100}$ latency with uncorrected vision which is greatly increased for the smaller stimulus field and check size. (From Carroll and Kriss, 1981.)*

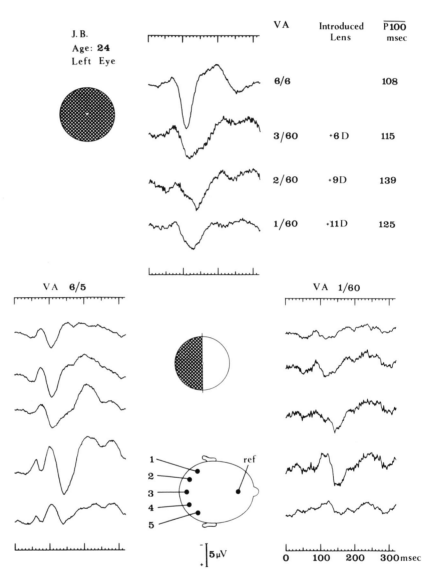

Figure 5.4 *(Upper record) Midline responses recorded from the left eye of a healthy individual with uncorrected 6/6 vision before and after the defocussing of the stimulus by the introduction of an increasingly strong convex lens. The appparent changes in peak latency of the major positivity, together with the power of the introduced lens in dioptres and the resulting visual acuity, are shown to the right of each record. (Lower 2 records) Left half-field responses recorded from a transverse row of 5 electrodes with normal vision (left hand record) and with a + 11 dioptre lens (right hand record). The lower records demonstrate that with severe defocussing, the macular $\overline{P100}$ is attenuated and partially replaced by the paramacular $\overline{P135}$. This effect accounts for much of the apparent change of latency in the major positivity of the whole-field response. (From Carroll and Kriss, 1981.)*

CATARACT AND OPACITIES OF THE CORNEA, LENS AND VITREOUS

Reference has already been made to the study by Copenhaver and Perry (1964) who demonstrated the reduction in the amplitude of the flash EP in a group of patients with opacities of the lens or mediae. Although there was a trend for this reduction to follow the visual acuity level the correlation did not reach statistical significance, unlike that for the comparable group of patients with refractive errors or neuroretinal lesions. This reflects the relative insensitivity of the flash response to even quite gross visual impairment. Ebe et al (1964) included four patients with a total of five cataractacous eyes in their study of the flash response. All the patients were subsequently shown post-operatively to have normal retinal function and visual acuity was fully restored. Pre-operatively the flash EP was normal from all five eyes with cataracts, and in only one case was the flash ERG abnormal. The relative insensitivity of the flash EP to the effect of even a severe opacity is well illustrated in Figure 5.5. The visual acuity in the right eye of this 57-year-old woman was reduced to the perception of light by a dense cataract, but neither the flash ERG nor the occipital EP are very different from those obtained from the good eye, in which visual acuity was 6/6. The responses to checkerboard reversal, on the other hand, are, as would be expected, very sensitive to the reduction in acuity, and the pattern response from the right eye is almost abolished (Figure 5.6). It is notable that even the macular ERG to pattern stimulation is also absent in the right eye, although the ERG channels show a later eye movement artifact, no doubt related to the inability to fixate with this eye.

With less dense opacities, causing a less severe loss of acuity, the pattern EP may be still present but reduced in amplitude. Figure 5.7 shows the checkerboard reversal EPs from a 61-year-old woman, referred because of suspected multiple sclerosis, but also suffering from multiple lens opacities. The visual acuity was 6/60 in the more severely affected right eye and 6/24 in the left eye. Paralleling this difference, the amplitude of the pattern EP from the right eye is about half the size of that from the left.

As with refractive errors the sensitivity of the pattern response to less dense opacities may be increased by resort to smaller field and check sizes and reduced stimulus intensity (Carroll and Kriss, 1981). Figure 5.8 shows the checkerboard reversal EPs from a 31-year-old patient with a moderate right central cataract. With the standard 16° radius stimulus of 50′ checks the response from the affected eye had a P100 latency of only 8 msec more than the normal eye, which is at the upper limit of the normal range. With a 4° radius stimulus the amplitude was reduced and the peak less well defined but with little significant change in latency. However, with a change to smaller 20′ checks the interocular latency difference increases to 12 msec and when the intensity is further reduced by a 1 log unit neutral density filter the difference increases to 18 msec.

It is not absolutely clear which are the most important factors operating to increase the latency of the macular response to small checks when these are defocussed. Probably there is a complex interaction of the effects of brightness, contrast and contour sharpness. We know that the latency of the pattern response becomes sensitive to contrast when this is below saturation level and opacities may well operate by reducing contrast below the critical level, as well as by diminishing mean luminance and defocussing sharp edges. Changes in pupil size and lid-droop may also affect the response in the same three ways (Carroll and Kriss, 1981).

The cases illustrated in Figures 5.5-8 demonstrate the much greater sensitivity of the pattern EP latency to acuity level in the presence of opacities. Conversely, the very insensitivity of the flash response in this respect makes it potentially useful in testing for the function of the retina behind a dense opacity, and this can be of considerable prognostic value in assessing the probable outcome of surgery (Fricker, 1971; Arnal et al, 1972a; Thompson and Harding, 1978; Babel et al, 1977).

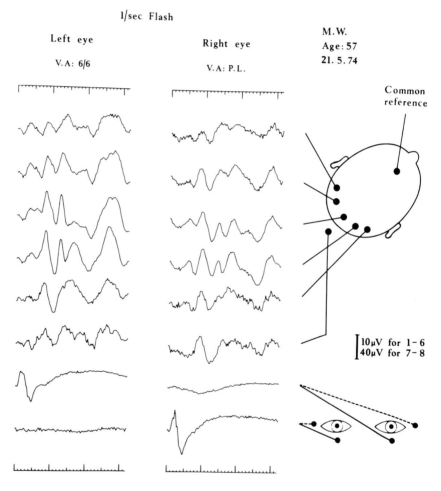

Figure 5.5 *Flash evoked potential from each eye of a 57-year-old woman with a dense cataract in the right eye. In spite of the fact that visual acuity was reduced to the perception of light in this eye, the occipital flash responses is still of only slightly smaller amplitude to that of the eye with 6/6 vision. The accompanying flash ERGs, recorded from peri-orbital skin electrodes, are also very similar for the two eyes. Compare the pattern responses from the same patient shown in Figure 5.6. (From Halliday, 1978b.)*

Thompson and Harding (1978) report a study of the predictive value of the flash EP in 21 patients with dense unilateral cataracts, 20 of whom eventually came to surgery. The EPs were assessed by two observers, one of whom had no knowledge of the clinical history, age or post-operative acuity. Comparing the affected with the normal eye and using a criterion of abnormality of 2 s.d. of their normal mean amplitude or latency difference (33% and 12 msec respectively) and also a measure of the lateral asymmetry of the response at the occiput, the flash EPs were rated into three grades. Grade 1 EPs with little or no difference in the waveform or amplitude from the two eyes predicted a good acuity, Grade 3 EPs with a noticeable reduction

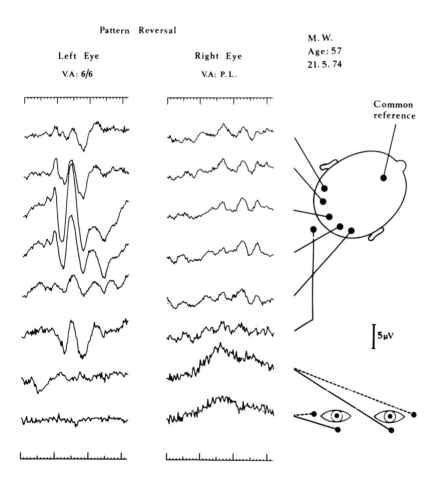

Figure 5.6 *Pattern reversal responses from the same patient whose flash responses are shown in Figure 5.5. Note the almost abolished response from the eye with the dense cataract. A clear pattern ERG is seen in the record from the normal eye, but not from the affected eye. The peri-orbital channels for the latter response show a large eye movement artifact. Compare Figure 5.5. (From Halliday, 1978b.)*

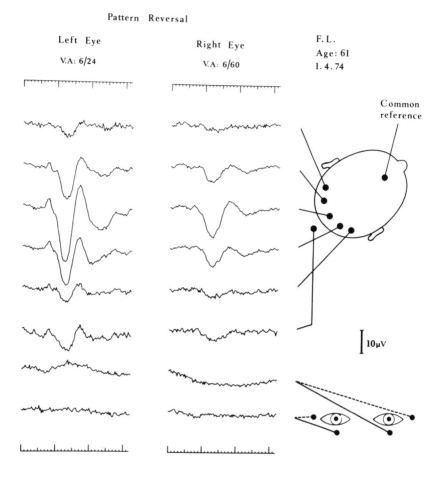

Figure 5.7 *Pattern reversal responses from a 61-year-old woman with reduced visual acuity secondary to multiple lens opacities. The response amplitude parallels the acuity level, being about half the size from the more severely affected right eye. (From Halliday and Mushin, 1980.)*

in amplitude in the affected eye and no clear localization of the major components at the right or left occiput, predicted poor post-operative vision. An intermediate Grade 2 EP was used to categorize responses where judgement was difficult and questionable. Baseline-to-peak amplitude measures of the 'P2' component were the most valuable predictive measure. The authors also found it useful to test the flash EP at more than one stimulus intensity and to note the change in amplitude. Twelve patients had Grade 1 EPs, 3 patients Grade 2, and 5 patients Grade 3. Within the Grade 1 group, 5 had larger 'P2' components from the affected eye, possibly due to the diffusing effect of the cataract. Another 4 showed an amplitude reduction of around 50% in the affected eye, which was beyond the criterion for exclusion from

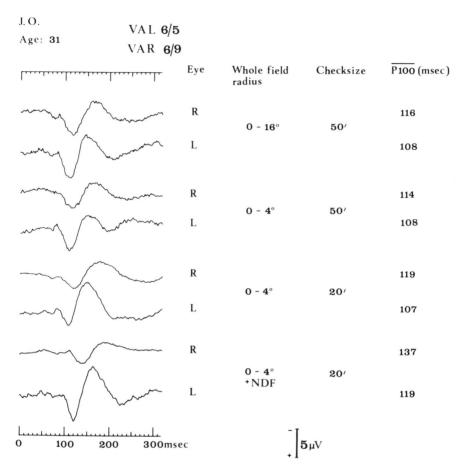

J.O.
Age: 31

VAL 6/5
VAR 6/9

Eye	Whole field radius	Checksize	$\overline{P100}$ (msec)
R			116
	0 - 16°	50′	
L			108
R			114
	0 - 4°	50′	
L			108
R			119
	0 - 4°	20′	
L			107
R			137
	0 - 4° +NDF	20′	
L			119

0   100   200   300 msec

5 μV

Figure 5.8 *Midline pattern reversal EPs, recorded from each eye of a 31-year-old patient with a moderate right central cataract, to a checkerboard stimulus of varying field size, check size and brightness (as indicated on the right). Note that the latency of the major positive peak from the eye with cataract is very much more sensitive to reductions in field size, check size and brightness than is the response from the normal eye. (From Carroll and Kriss, 1981.)*

this group, but this reduction was only seen at the lower stimulus intensity (68 nit/second as against 96 nit/second), and was less marked with the stronger stimulus. Four of the 5 patients with Grade 3 EPs showed an amplitude reduction of more than 45% in the affected eye, even with the dimmer flash, and this difference increased with the higher intensity stimulus. The 12 msec latency difference criterion did not in general correlate with post-operative visual acuity, while the amplitude criterion alone failed in 7 of the 20 patients (one of the original 21 refused surgery). Twelve of the 14 patients who had good post-operative vision (6/12 or better) had Grade 1 EPs. The two others who did well had Grade 2 EPs. They were aged 78 and 87 and one also had early lens opacities and senile macular degeneration in the 'good eye'. Five of the six patients with poor post-operative vision (6/24 or worse) had Grade 3 EPs.

Babel et al (1977) emphasize the good operative prognosis associated with a normal amplitude and waveform of the ERG to a red flash combined with the presence of the oscillatory potentials in the eye with cataract. They recommend the simultaneous recording of both flicker ERG and flash EP and stress the importance of the measures correlating with macular function.

Green (1970) introduced the use of laser-generated interference fringes to test the visual acuity of cataract patients pre-operatively. These fringes are not degraded by ordinary optical aberrations and can be generated at the level of the retina behind the opaque medium. He was able to show good agreement between the subjective pre-operative acuity measured in this way (the fineness of grating the patient could resolve) and the subsequent acuity level achieved after surgery. Some check on the patients' ability to see the gratings could be made by seeing if he could correctly report the orientation. In order to see the fringes the patients had to learn to ignore a changing disordered pattern of jumbled shapes which appeared at the same time in front of the striped pattern of interference fringes.

Arden and Sheorey (1977) have applied the same stimulating technique to record pattern EPs behind a cataract. The EP method has the advantage of being objective and not requiring the use of fine gratings, where the presence of high frequency noise causing laser speckling is particularly troublesome. They report the results of a study of this technique on 15 patients with cataracts, six with vitreous haemorrhages and three with corneal opacities. In only one of the patients was it impossible to obtain reliable VEPs. Four of the patients with cataract had a much reduced or absent EP from the affected eye, while in tèn others it was either equal to or greater than the response from the unaffected eye. In two of the four former cases the cataract was post-traumatic, in one it was associated with diabetic neuropathy, and in the fourth it was in a patient with congenital cataract who was likely to have had amblyopia. In the six patients with vitreous haemorrhages, all due to diabetic retinopathy, the EPs were very small. These results are encouraging, but the technique is a sophisticated one and requires the use of a polarization interferometer, the Moiré fringes being generated by modulating the phase of two orthogonally polarized light beams, derived from a single point source (a helium neon laser) by means of a Wollaston prism. Technical details are given by Arden and Sheorey (1977). Some difficulty was encountered with elderly patients who, because of a variety of disabilities such as spinal arthritis, were unable to sit comfortably at the slit lamp. For all these reasons it seems doubtful whether this technique will gain wide application in a clinical setting.

AMBLYOPIA

Amblyopia, which means literally 'blunt eye', is a permanent loss of visual acuity secondary to a variety of childhood disorders, such as squint, cataract, or a severe refractive error or astigmatism. It can be distinguished from the blurred vision secondary to a refractive error by the fact that it is not reversible by correcting lenses, nor by testing vision through a pinhole. In the case of astigmatism it may be limited to the visual acuity in one visual axis, so-called meridional amblyopia. Meridional amblyopia can be distinguished from simple astigmatism by viewing a fixed pattern through a narrow slit, placed immediately in front of the cornea. In astigmatism, where the cornea is not perfectly spherical, the sharpness of focus of the pattern will vary with the orientation of the slit and the orientation at which maximum blurring or sharpness occurs indicates the principal axes of the cornea (Ludlam and Myers, 1972). In meridional amblyopia, on the other hand, it is the orientation of the viewed grating pattern which is critical, and not that of the slit through which it is viewed (see the discussion by Regan, 1977b).

The underlying defect in amblyopia is therefore neuroretinal rather than refractive, which adds a particular interest to the EP findings, as both flash and pattern EPs are more sensitive to a reduction of visual acuity of neural origin, even where the acuity level itself is the same. Experimental work in animals has suggested that there are specific defects associated with amblyopia recordable at both the cortical and retinal levels (Hubel and Wiesel, 1965; Wiesel and Hubel, 1965a, 1965b; Ikeda, 1980). According to Ikeda (1980) the essential condition for producing this defect is a lack of properly focussed images on the macular area of one eye during the sensitive period in early development when the X cells of the central retina have their receptive fields 'sharpened up' to the adult form as a result of the experience of patterned vision. The defect can be demonstrated in cats reared with an artificial convergent squint as a failure of the X cells of the area centralis to develop the normal sensitivity to gratings of fine spatial frequency in the affected eye. Blakemore and Cooper (1970) have shown that kittens reared without experience of either vertical or horizontal contours may develop a comparable inability to respond behaviourally or electrophysiologically to stimulation by gratings in that particular orientation, the electrophysiological deficit being shown in recordings from the cells of their visual cortex. This appears to be a parallel deficit of the kind that may underlie meridional amblyopia, although in this case the phenomenon has been demonstrated by recordings of cortical, rather than retinal, cells. The sensitive period for the cat is between 3 and 16 weeks.

The defect in retinal X cells observed by Ikeda (1980) is found only for the area of retina around the fixation point. This defect exists independently of, and irrespectively of, any defect in the binocular driving of the cortical cells of the kind found by Hubel and Wiesel. Only those cats who fail to show fixation with the affected eye (even alternate fixation) develop this amblyopic defect. The time-course of development of the normal adult visual acuity in kittens corresponds well with the sensitive period and also follows the curve of myelination of visual pathways (Ikeda, 1980). By analogy, human myelination is known to be complete by the age of two years, so that this perhaps may be the sensitive period for the development of amblyopia in man. Ikeda's recordings show the significant reduction in cellular visual acuity for the pattern-sensitive X cells of the area centralis in the squinting eye as compared with the normal visual acuity for the cat's normal eye. The defect is limited to the cells in the central area of the retina near the fixation point and is not seen more peripherally. Moreover the impaired function in the central X cells is only seen where the squint has been present since before or during the sensitive period. These findings would lead one to expect a deficit in the

VEP in amblyopia particularly associated with the foveal response and with the pattern EP rather than the flash EP.

There is an extensive literature on the recording of EPs in amblyopia which confirms this expectation, but abnormalities have also been reported in the responses to unpatterned flash stimuli. Perry and Childers (1968) found that the flash EP to small foveal targets was reduced in size in amblyopia, but that there was no similar effect for large 20° stimulus fields. Babel et al (1977) studied the flash EP in 29 cases of amblyopia, ranging in age from 3-12 years. Twenty of these cases showed no improvement after orthoptic treatment and 15 of these had an abnormal flash EP on the amblyopic side. Three of the five ERGs recorded were also abnormal. In the second group of nine cases who showed improvement after orthoptic treatment the flash EP was normal in all, except for one case with a subnormal response. All five ERGs recorded in this group were normal. The stimulus in these studies was a diffuse flash and the field size was not therefore controlled.

Using the pattern reversal EP, Spekreijse et al (1972) found that for a 3° stimulus field, the maximum EP amplitude of the normal eye was recorded with check sizes of 10'-20', whereas in the amblyopic eye it was at much larger check sizes. Furthermore, the parafoveal responses were less affected than the foveal responses, as would be expected from the nature of the central defect in amblyopia. Arden (1977) found that removing the central 1° of a 14° checkerboard stimulus of 23' squares reduced the response by more than half in a normal adult, whereas removal of the central 4° made little difference to the response from an amblyopic eye. Sokol (1977) has recorded the steady state checkerboard pattern reversal response, generated by a rotating polaroid stimulator, with a reversal rate of 12 Hz. Changing the check size produced responses from the normal eye with a maximum EP amplitude at 15' for field sizes of 6° and 12°, whereas an amblyopic eye gave peak responses at 60' and 30' respectively. For a 3° field, however, both normal and amblyopic eyes give a maximum EP amplitude for a check size of 15'. This suggested that the amblyopic eye gave a *greater* response than the normal to large checks from the parafoveal region. Further recordings with experimental scotomata showed that the greatest response for the amblyopic eye was coming from the retinal region which lay between 1.5° and 3° out from the fixation point. There was also an interesting phase difference in the response of the normal eye to increasing check sizes presented in a 6° field, which was not seen in the amblyopic eye. Sokol found that in three children with strabismic amblyopia, the maximum EP amplitude for a 12° field was achieved with 15' checks (or in one case 7.5' checks) in the normal eye and 30' checks in the amblyopic eye.

Wanger and Nilsson (1978) recorded the EPs to checkerboard reversal with a stimulus field subtending 8.8° of 23' checks at 98% contrast in ten cases with amblyopia. Both monocular and binocular stimulation were carried out and the two responses were compared. Four of the patients showed an abnormal difference in the amplitude of the response from the two eyes on monocular stimulation (more than 30% where the 2 s.d. limit of normal was 27%) and in four more the normal increase in amplitude with binocular stimulation (usually 12%) was greatly reduced (one patient) or actually reversed (three patients). They also noted an abnormal difference in latency between the monocular responses from the two eyes in two patients (11 and 13 msec respectively as against 5 msec in normals).

Arden (1977) demonstrated a difference in the contrast saturation level in amblyopes. Whereas in normal subjects the maximum EP amplitude is reached with contrasts of 20% or more, Arden confirmed a very large increase in EP amplitudes with stimulus contrast increases of 20-50% in some amblyopes. The peak latency was also reduced at higher contrast. Further, Arden reports that amblyopes show an even more dramatic suppression of the EP from the non-dominant eye during retinal rivalry than normal subjects. He has noted that in his amblyopic patients undergoing therapy by 'penalization' of the good eye by occlusion, the pattern EP from the good eye is consistently small or even absent when recorded soon after the period of ocular occlusion. At this stage it may only be possible to record an EP from the amblyopic eye. This is in spite of the fact that the child can see perfectly well with the originally normal eye. These intriguing phenomena are certainly worth further study.

Arden et al (1980) have recently provided electrophysiological evidence in man that the pattern-evoked ERG is reduced in the amblyopic area of the retina. They recorded the ERG to a 22° x 16° checkerboard field of checks subtending 1° or less in 9 children and 3 adults with amblyopia. Whereas the amplitude asymmetry between the pattern ERG of each eye did not exceed about 10% in a group of 14 controls, the response from 10 of the 12 amblyopic eyes was reduced to between 33% and 77% of that from its fellow eye. All 10 of these cases failed to respond to treatment, while normal pattern ERGs were recorded in the other 2 cases who showed improvement with therapy. These results confirm Ikeda's conclusion that there is a peripheral retinal defect in amblyopia, and suggest that clinical testing of the pattern ERG may prove to be a useful prognostic aid.

The pattern ERG is of much smaller voltage than the ERG recorded following flash stimulation, partly, no doubt, due to the much smaller change in local luminance associated with the checkerboard reversal stimulus. Recorded with peri-orbital electrodes, using the method routinely adopted in the author's laboratory, the peak-to-peak amplitude of the pattern ERG to the standard 0–16° black-and-white checkerboard, made up of 50' checks, does not exceed 1–2 μV. Even so, a clear difference in the amplitude of the ERG from the normal (left) and amblyopic (right) eye is evident in Figure 5.9, and can also just be discerned (although obscured by background muscle) in Figure 5.10.

Arden's study, which clearly established this reduction in the pattern ERG from the amblyopic eye, was carried out using a gold-foil electrode (see page 132) in the conjunctival sac, which provides a larger signal than the peri-orbital electrodes. It is, therefore, clearly not necessary to resort to anaesthetic drops and a contact lens electrode in order to record this effect of amblyopia on the pattern ERG. Where the background noise level is low (as in the record shown in Figure 5.9) a clearer idea of the pattern ERG amplitude from each eye, even where this is recorded with peri-orbital electrodes, can be achieved by doubling the gain of the two ERG channels (7 and 8), but this is unlikely to be helpful where the background is obscured by obtrusive muscle artifact, as in Figure 5.10.

Amblyopia may present itself as a complicating problem in clinical EP testing for demyelinating disease or other lesions of the visual pathways. In the author's experience most amblyopic patients tested with the standard 32° checkerboard of 50' checks show only a reduction in amplitude of the $\overline{P100}$ from the affected eye without any significant change in latency (Figure 5.9). This allows one to clearly differentiate the presence of a delayed response following optic neuritis from a response associated with reduced visual acuity secondary to amblyopia (Figure

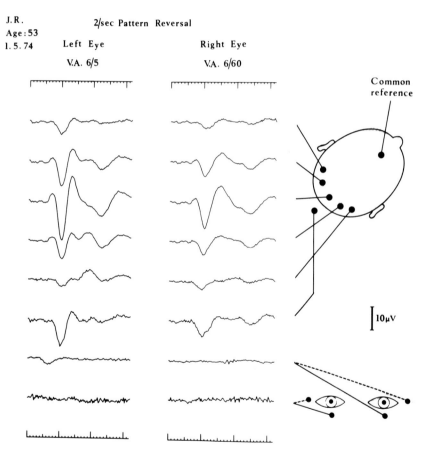

Figure 5.9 *Pattern reversal EPs from each eye of a 53-year-old man with amblyopia of the right eye. Note the smaller amplitude of the response from the affected eye, which nonetheless has a normal latency. The pattern ERG is also significantly smaller from this eye.*

5.10). Occasionally, however, there are problems where the amblyopia manifests itself as a dense central scotomatous defect when the $\overline{P100}$ may be replaced by a $\overline{P135}$ component giving the appearance of a delayed response (Figure 5.11). This problem can be resolved by half-field stimulation, when the positivity will be revealed to have a contralateral, and not an ipsilateral, distribution (see page 105).

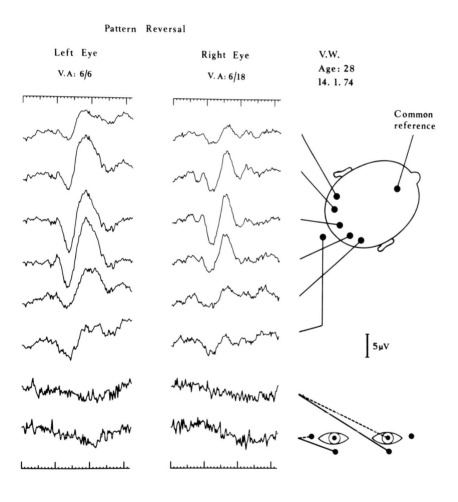

Figure 5.10 Monocular pattern responses from a 28-year-old woman who had recovered from an attack of retrobulbar neuritis in the left eye (visual acuity 6/6), but had a life-long amblyopia in the right eye (6/18). Note the delay of the response from the left eye and the slightly smaller amplitude of the response from the right eye.

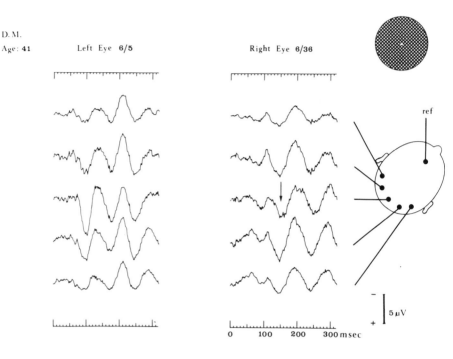

Figure 5.11 *Monocular pattern responses from a 41-year-old woman with right strabismic amblyopia and an associated central scotoma. In contrast to the macular-derived $\overline{P100}$ recorded from the unaffected left eye, the midline channel shows an apparently delayed major positivity from the amplyopic eye, which was identified by half-field stimulation as a $\overline{P135}$ derived from paramacular stimulation. Where the normal NPN complex is replaced by a PNP complex in association with a central scotoma, the appearance may suggest a delayed $\overline{P100}$. Half-field stimulation, however, clarifies the situation, identifying it as a $\overline{P135}$ component. (From Carroll and Kriss, 1981.)*

GLAUCOMA

Cappin and Nissim (1975) used a rotating polaroid stimulator to study the steady-state checkerboard reversal EP in 21 patients with field defects associated with glaucoma, comparing them with 11 cases with ocular hypertension but no field defects and 10 healthy controls. They presented the monocular stimulus, made up of a 22° field of 35′ checks, to each of the four quadrants and compared each response with that from the homonymous quadrant of the other eye. The responses from the quadrants affected by field defects invariably showed a phase shift (lag) of the sinusoidal response compared with the unaffected quadrant, except where the defect was so severe that no response could be obtained. The occurrence of these abnormal phase-shifts correlated perfectly with the incidence of field defects without either false-positive or false-negative results, except for patients with unilateral cataract, which was also associated with a phase-change. All save one of the 21 cases had predominantly upper field defects. The mean phase shift from the affected quadrants in those cases without cataract was 79.8° ± 30.6° as against 13.40° ± 10.74° for the unaffected upper quadrants. The latter figure was not significantly different from that obtained in the healthy control group (11.68° ± 8.48°) and in the patients with ocular hypertension (6.54° ± 7.35°). Twenty of the patients showed good test-retest repeatability in their responses when recorded again within 8 months, while 3 developed phase-shifts correlating with the extension of field defects into previously normal quadrants.

The authors point out that their quadrant comparison technique is not suitable for the study of bilateral field defects, nor for patients with greatly reduced visual acuity (worse than 6/24) or opacities of lens or cornea. There also remains some question as to how these phase changes should be interpreted. They have been widely regarded as representing changes in 'relative latency' but it appears possible that they may equally represent changes in the topography of the pattern EP associated with changes in the cortical generator areas corresponding to the preserved field (see Chapter 3). Cappin and Nissim themselves noted that changing the electrode position resulted in changes in phase, although they report that the presence or absence of phase shift still clearly distinguished the affected or unaffected homonymous fields. This question merits further investigation.

However, Huber and Wagner (1978) have established that there are also clear delays in the latency of the $\overline{P100}$ component of the transient checkerboard reversal EP to 2 Hz stimulation. Using a TV stimulator to present a 14° x 10° stimulus of mean luminance 90 cd/m^2 and 50% contrast with check sizes of 38', 18' and 9', they recorded $\overline{P100}$ latencies of up to 157 msec in studying 39 glaucomatous eyes in 27 patients, while the normal mean for their stimulus was 102.6 ± 6.4 msec. All the patients had a corrected vision of 6/18 or better. Twenty-nine of the 39 glaucomatous eyes gave $\overline{P100}$ latencies of more than 115 msec, and 23 had marked field defects. Although the longest delays occurred in eyes with large field defects, there was no direct relationship between the two and delays were associated with eyes in which the visual fields were nearly intact. The authors suggest that EP testing may be useful in monitoring the progress of optic nerve pathology in glaucoma, particularly where subjective perimetry is difficult to carry out.

Two years later, Huber (1981) re-examined 21 of the glaucomatous eyes in 16 patients of the original group, using static automated perimetry to study the accompanying field defect. The number of eyes recorded on both occasions with $\overline{P100}$ latencies >115 msec had increased from 11 to 13, and 7 eyes showed an increase of over 10 msec in latency over the two year period. The delays appeared to be particularly related to perimetric evidence of subjective visual impairment affecting the most central field; marked impairment could be found at an eccentricity of only 6° with no delay in the accompanying pattern EP. On the other hand, where a generalized reduction in sensitivity (rise in threshold) was present, the PEP could be delayed in the presence of normal acuity. Huber points out that this is an important finding in relation to the differential diagnosis of neurological disease, since glaucoma could be missed in such a patient if he was referred to a neurologist. The delays in the $\overline{P100}$ component of the pattern reversal response in some glaucomatous eyes have been comfirmed in the study by Sokol et al (1981), but these authors stress the importance of monitoring and controlling for other relevant variables such as pupil diameter in interpreting the results of the test, while Huber (1981) concludes that the subjective information provided by automated perimetry is more relevant and more sensitive than the objective measure of pattern EP latency in the management of glaucoma.

A number of studies have been carried out on the reversible depression of the VEP produced by an acute experimentally induced rise in intraocular pressure (Fox et al, 1973; Bartl et al, 1975; Ulrich et al, 1980).

HEREDITARY RETINAL DEGENERATIONS

Retinitis pigmentosa

Müller (1963) recorded the flash evoked response by photographic superimposition in ten patients with tapeto-retinal degeneration and retinitis pigmentosa, with an age range of 18-63 years. In spite of the fact that the flash ERG was abolished in all ten, the occipital EP was still present and unaltered in all except two patients, who showed an increase in the peak latency. Ebe et al (1964) recorded 11 further patients with retinitis pigmentosa by the same superimposition method. Visual acuity was impaired in all 22 eyes, with a restriction of the visual field in ten, lowered visual acuity in six, and a combination of both in six. The flash ERG was undetectable in 18 responses (eyes) and abnormal in four, whereas the occipital EPs were undetectable in seven, abnormal in 12 and normal in three. Where present, the field defect consisted of a peripheral restriction, usually at 20-30°, and there were no central scotomata. Jacobson et al (1968) recorded the flash responses in eight patients with retinitis pigmentosa, all of whom had an unrecordable ERG. Two advanced cases, both showing optic atrophy, also had unrecordable occipital responses, while the other six showed EPs with a reduced amplitude of all waves from one to five without marked change of latency. Several had a loss of all but the later components.

Babel et al (1977) reported the flash ERG as absent in 71% of a large series of patients with pigmentary retinopathy. It was present in the other 29% but invariably pathological, and scotopic activity, reflecting rod function, was completely abolished, except in one patient where it showed diminution. They found that in the dominantly transmitted pigmentary retinopathy, which made up only about 3-4% of the total, the ERG was often still present, whereas it was generally abolished in the autosomal or sex-linked recessive forms, confirming the findings of Berson et al (1969). The a-wave was particularly affected, indicating a disturbance originating in the photoreceptor layer. The b-wave was also altered, but the oscillatory potentials, which are thought to originate in the amacrine cells, often persisted.

The EOG was also invariably abnormal in retinitis pigmentosa. The corneo-retinal potential is a standing potential actually developed across the basement membrane of the pigment epithelium layer in the retina, and the baseline value of the resting potential was abnormal in 83% of the 30 eyes examined, while the change in potential produced by 12 minutes dark adaptation (dark trough) followed by 12 minutes intense photic stimulation (light peak), expressed as the light peak/dark trough percentage ratio, was also abnormal in 96% of eyes. There was an absence of the normal decrease in the EOG on dark adaptation in 53%.

These authors felt that the occipital EP was of definite use as an adjunct to the flash ERG in the study of corneo-retinal disease, particularly where the ERG was abolished, where it was sometimes possible to record responses, undetected at the retina, which nonetheless produced a cortical EP. It also enabled an additional optic nerve lesion to be detected in some cases. The occipital flash EP was abolished in 21 out of 73 patients with pigmentary retinopathy (29%). In the other 52 patients, in whom it could still be recorded, 34 had an abnormal amplitude (47%) and 18 (25%) an abnormal latency. The existence of a significant number of patients in whom the flash VEP is not only preserved, but of normal amplitude and latency, underlines the fact that the EP, even to flash, is particularly dependent on macular function which is relatively spared in retinitis pigmentosa.

MACULOPATHY

Since the pattern reversal EP is largely dependent on the stimulation of the central areas of the field, it is particularly severely affected in lesions of the macula. The flash response is less sensitive, because it includes a much larger contribution from the peripheral retina. Ebe et al (1964) found the flash EPs to be abnormal in one out of five patients with macular atrophy, while the ERG was abnormal in two of the patients. In 53 eyes with macular degeneration Babel et al (1977) found the flash EP to be absent in 9 (17%) and of reduced amplitude in 35 (66%), while in 14 (26%) it had an abnormal latency. This compares with the high percentage of pathological ERGs (79%) recorded by the same authors in 184 patients with macular dystrophy and the 51% of abnormal responses in 31 patients with central serous retinitis. Both juvenile and senile macular degenerations were associated with the 77% of abnormal ERGs. A disturbance in the oscillatory potential of the ERG, particularly after red flash stimuli, was a characteristic change. Borda (1977) reports a total absence of the short latency flash EP components in patients with degeneration of the macula, accompanied by a normal flash ERG. He points out that this is the converse finding to that seen in retinitis pigmentosa, where the ERG is grossly abnormal and the VEP often unchanged. Harding (1977) found a generally reduced major positivity in the flash EPs of patients with macular degeneration. He also found that the normal phase reversal of the occipital response may be lost from the eye with disciform degeneration.

VASCULAR RETINOPATHY

Central retinal artery occlusion

The flash EP can be informative in cases of occlusion of the central retinal artery. One of the first published cases was a patient studied by Jacobson et al (1968) with bilateral occlusion, who was recorded 23 days after acute loss of vision in the right eye and 10 days after the left eye was affected. Visual acuity was reduced to the perception of light in the left eye and to the detection of hand movements in the temporal field of the right eye. The flash ERG, recorded with a contact lens electrode, showed the characteristic depression of the b-wave with a well preserved a-wave. The b-wave was less severely depressed in the right eye than the left eye, paralleling the difference in visual acuity level. The occipital flash EP was also more affected from the left eye, with reduction and delay of waves I, II and III, while right eye stimulation gave an asymmetric response of almost normal amplitude, but with reduction and slight delay of the early components at the right occipital electrode. Vaughan and Katzman (1964) describe another single case in a 55-year-old man with transient ischaemic episodes and stenosis of the right internal carotid artery, who became blind in the right eye and developed a left hemiplegia following attempted endarterectomy. Both ERG and occipital EP were abolished from this eye. Babel et al (1977) describe the flash ERG in 17 cases with occlusion of the central retinal artery, 11 further cases of occlusion of a branch and one case of central artery spasm. The ERG showed a well preserved a-wave, but the b-wave was generally depressed or absent in the severe cases. The oscillatory potentials, which are very sensitive to anoxia, tend to disappear early, but may reappear with revascularization, especially in young patients, and slight reduction in the b-wave amplitude was noted in two patients who had had emboli of the central retinal artery within the previous two years, although the oscillatory potentials were still present. A 54-year-old patient with classical signs of central artery spasm, including macular oedema, had a persistently abnormal ERG, with diminished b-wave and absent oscillatory potentials, even three days after the clinical signs had disappeared following intensive treatment. Fifteen months later, however, the ERG was normal, with well marked oscillatory potentials. In three of the 29 cases, there was also noticed a decrease in the amplitude of the a-wave together with an increase in its latency. These changes were thought to be due to secondary disturbances in the choroidal irrigation.

Figures 5.12 and 5.13 illustrate the flash and pattern responses recorded in a personally observed case, a 53-year-old woman with occlusion of the left central retinal artery. In spite of the greatly impaired visual acuity in the affected eye, which was reduced to the perception of hand movements, the occipital flash EP is only moderately reduced in amplitude. The polyphasic character of the flash response makes it difficult to be certain about latency changes, but there appears to be no marked increase. The flash ERG, recorded in this case by peri-orbital skin electrodes, shows the preservation of the a-wave (an up-going negativity at about 15 msec) and the abolition of the succeeding b-wave (a down-going positivity at about 45 msec) in the response from the left eye. The explanation for this characteristic finding is that the a-wave is produced by the late receptor potential in the outer layer of the retina, which depends for its blood supply on the choroidal circulation, while the b-wave is generated by the Müller cells following the discharge of the bipolar cells of the retina, which receive their blood supply from the central retinal artery.

The pattern reversal EPs recorded in the same patient show, as usual, a much greater sensitivity to the visual impairment (Figure 5.13). The response from the affected left eye is almost abolished with only a small asymmetrical positivity at normal latency for the $\overline{\text{P100}}$ detectable in the midline and left sided channels, while the contralateral channel 5 cm to the right of the midline shows the trace of a negative component at the same latency (Figure 5.13). This therefore appears to be a much reduced response coming only from a presumed island of preserved vision in the more central part of the temporal half field.

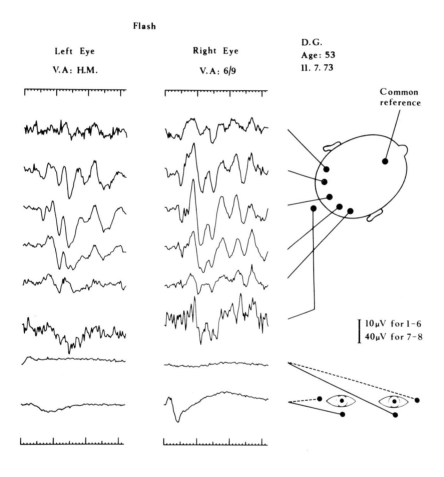

Figure 5.12 *Monocular flash responses from a 53-year-old woman with occlusion of the left central retinal artery. The occipital flash response from the affected eye is only slightly reduced in amplitude, in spite of the reduction in acuity to the perception of hand movements. The flash ERG is of normal waveform from the right eye, with a negative (up-going) a-wave and a positive (down-going) b-wave at peak latencies of 15 msec and 45 msec respectively. The flash ERG from the left eye shows only the a-wave, the b-wave being completely abolished. Compare Figure 5.13.*

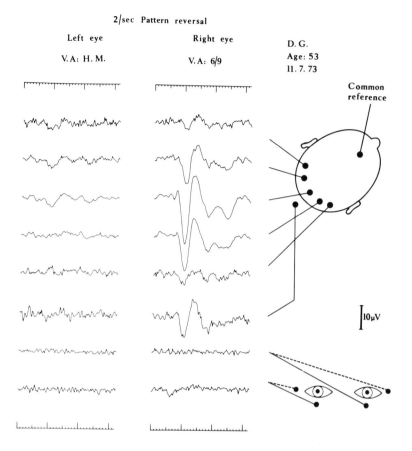

2/sec Pattern reversal

Left eye
V. A: H. M.

Right eye
V. A: 6/9

D. G.
Age: 53
11. 7. 73

Common reference

10μV

Figure 5.13 Monocular pattern reversal responses from the patient with left central retinal artery occlusion whose flash responses are shown in Figure 5.12. The occipital response from the left eye is almost completely abolished, showing only a small asymmetrical positive component at normal latency with a left-sided distribution. There is no evidence of a pattern ERG from this eye. The right eye shows a normal occipital response, and a clear pattern ERG is also evident.

Central retinal vein thrombosis

Babel et al (1977) studied the flash ERG in 94 cases and reported a diminution in the b-wave amplitude, with an unchanged a-wave, giving a diminished b/a ratio. The onset latency of the b-wave was also increased, leading to a considerable apparent increase in the peak latency of the a-wave, which is normally cut short by the developing negativity. The oscillatory potentials are particularly impaired and may be absent, even where the b-wave amplitude is unchanged in some cases of central vein or branch thrombosis. Very rarely an entirely normal recording has been obtained in cases of branch thrombosis, usually where the patients were very young and the condition was secondary to an inflammatory process.

Retinal embolism

Figure 5.14 shows the pattern reversal EPs to a standard 32° diameter checkerboard stimulus with 50′ checks in a 64-year-old hypertensive woman with a history of transient ischaemic attacks, who had a macular hole in the right eye, secondary to a small embolism. She had mild atheroma of the carotid arteries and a small branch occlusion in the region of the angular artery on the right. Visual acuity in the right eye was reduced to counting fingers, but the pattern EP is still of large amplitude and the waveform is only slightly altered (Figure 5.14). It is notable also

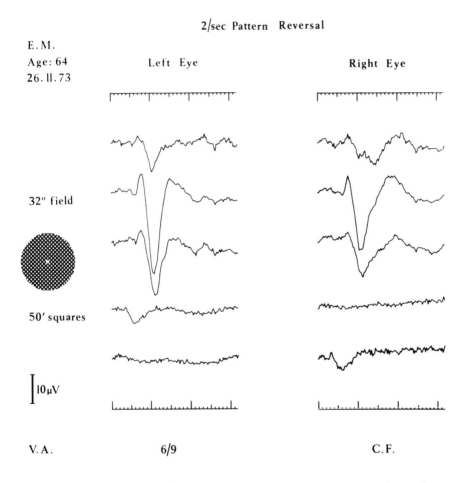

Figure 5.14 *Monocular responses to the standard 0-16° pattern reversal stimulus of 50′ checks in a 64-year-old hypertensive woman with a right macular hole. Visual acuity was reduced to counting fingers in the right eye. Note the normal pattern ERG from each eye and the relatively insignificant reduction and broadening of the waveform of the pattern response from the affected eye. Only the 3 central occipital records are shown (corresponding to channels 2 to 4 in previous figures). The responses to smaller checks and a reduced field size are shown in Figures 5.15 and 5.16 respectively. (From Halliday and Mushin, 1980.)*

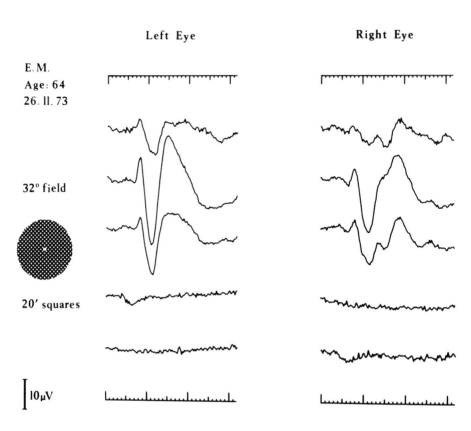

Figure 5.15 *Monocular responses to a 0-16° checkerboard of smaller 20' checks in the patient with the right macular hole whose responses to the standard checkerboard stimulus are shown in Figure 5.14. (From Halliday and Mushin, 1980.)*

that the pattern ERG, which comes mainly from the macular area of the retina, is well preserved in the right eye. More marked abnormalities of the pattern EP could be revealed by switching to a checkerboard stimulus with smaller 20' checks, which preferentially stimulate the area round the fixation point, where the receptive fields of the retinal units are smaller (Figure 5.15). The detection of the pattern EP abnormality for this very small discrete retinal lesion only becomes really clear, however, when the relevant area of the retina is stimulated on its own (Figure 5.16). This is because the normal response from the preserved areas of retina included in the stimulus swamp the abnormal response from the scotomatous zone. These records illustrate well one limitation of the pattern EP method and emphasize that one may miss small subtle changes with a crude clinical screening test unless the test procedure is specifically adapted to investigate particular cases in the appropriate way. This may involve a more sophisticated approach to clinical EP investigation than is usually adopted towards EEG recording, comparable to that often required in the investigation of the EMG.

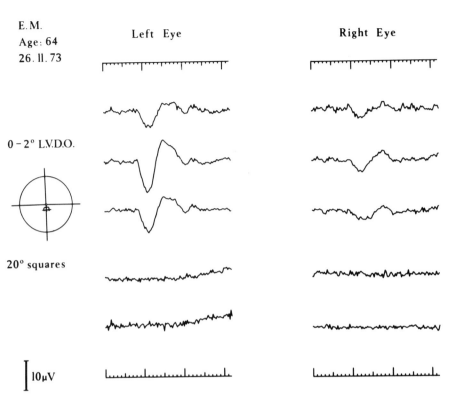

E.M.
Age: 64
26. ll. 73

Left Eye

Right Eye

0 - 2° L.V.D.O.

20° squares

10μV

Figure 5.16 *Monocular responses to a small pattern stimulus of 20' squares, presented only in the central 2° of the visual field immediately below the fixation point to the same patient with a right macular hole whose other responses are illustrated in Figures 5.14 and 5.15. (From Halliday and Mushin, 1980.)*

Diabetic retinopathy

Babel et al (1977) report the flash ERG findings in 98 patients (188 eyes) with diabetic retinopathy. The oscillatory potentials disappear early, even before there are any ophthalmoscopic signs. In more severe cases there are changes in the b-wave, the first sign being an increase in the onset and peak latencies of this component. In 33 eyes, these latency changes were seen with a normal b-wave amplitude. Later in the disease the amplitude of the wave is reduced and the b/a ratio is correspondingly diminished. Only in the late stages, when photoreceptor function is impaired, is there also a decrease in the amplitude of the a-wave. Changes in the occipital EP are similar to those encountered in ischaemic optic neuropathy.

Ischaemic optic neuropathy

Rouher et al (1969) recorded the flash EP in nine cases with vascular lesions of the optic nerve. They found very variable responses, paralleling the polymorphic clinical features, and emphasize the value of the responses recorded to a monochromatic red flash stimulus in correlating with the lesions of the macular bundle. Babel et al (1977) stress the value of recording the ERG and EOG, as well as the occipital EP. Depression of the oscillatory potentials of the flash ERG is a particularly sensitive sign of retinal involvement, whereas, with pure optic nerve lesions, the ERG is normal. Two clinical sub-groups are distinguished by these authors: (1) a predominantly younger group of patients in which the perivascular inflammatory process pursues a long course, presenting a variety of troubles ranging from trivial campimetric deficits to amaurosis; and (2) a group of older patients, often over 60, with an ischaemic papillitis of very brutal onset, usually due to arteriosclerosis, although giant cell arteritis is present in 20% of the cases. Both ERG and VEP responses were very variable, showing a large range of abnormalities. In mild cases the flash EPs may be of normal latency but with diminished amplitude and altered waveform, while in severe cases they may be so diminished as to be virtually abolished. Delayed latencies are encountered but are not very marked and are often a secondary result of the waveform changes, the onset latency of the major positivity being little delayed. Recovery of the response may accompany clinical improvement.

Ellenberger and Ziegler (1977) found delayed flash EPs in 8 of 15 affected eyes, all of which showed stable arcuate field defects, and also, unexpectedly, in 2 of 9 unaffected eyes. In 6 of the 9 patients in whom only one eye was affected the relative amplitude was significantly smaller on the affected side. The mean latency of the initial positivity was increased from 52.8 ± 4.0 msec in the 50 controls to 65.7 ± 10.7 msec in the 12 patients with ischaemic optic neuropathy. Comparable mean latencies for 2 comparison groups of MS patients, with and without a history of retrobulbar neuritis, were 80.5 ± 13.7 msec and 62.5 ± 11.5 msec respectively. The study by Harding et al (1980a), who recorded the flash EP in 8 elderly patients (11 eyes) with ischaemic optic neuropathy, confirms the markedly reduced amplitude and delayed latency of the response from the affected eyes. These authors also draw attention to the fact that many of these patients showed a triphasic PNP complex at around 100 msec with the usual major positivity either being replaced by a negative component or being delayed relatively to it.

The pattern reversal EP frequently shows quite marked abnormalities in association with ischaemic optic neuritis, as has been reported by a number of different laboratories (Asselman et al, 1975; Halliday et al, 1977b; Hennerici et al, 1977; Wilson, 1978). Figure 5.17 shows an example of the type of pattern EP which may be recorded. This 63-year-old woman exhibited a gross alteration in the waveform of the response from the affected eye. The amplitude of the major positivity is reduced by about a half, when compared with the normal eye. The major positive component has a near-normal onset latency, but a prolonged positive-going phase culminating in a delayed peak. The incidence of abnormalities in ischaemic optic neuropathy is high. Delayed pattern EPs were found in all the cases studied by Asselman et al (three patients) and Hennerici et al (five patients). In

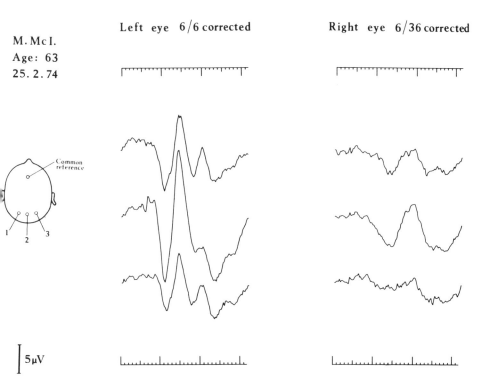

Left eye 6/6 corrected   Right eye 6/36 corrected

M. Mc I.
Age: 63
25. 2. 74

Common
reference

1   3
  2

5μV

Figure 5.17 *Monocular pattern reversal EPs from a 63-year-old woman with right ischaemic papillopathy. Note the reduced amplitude, altered waveform and delayed peak latency of the response from the affected eye. (From Halliday and Mushin, 1980.)*

the author's own series, the alterations in the waveform have sometimes made it difficult to decide whether or not there is a delay, but the incidence of abnormal responses has been equally high.

Wilson (1978) recorded both the flash and pattern reversal EPs in 15 patients with unilateral ischaemic optic neuritis, comparing them with a group of 50 healthy subjects. Adopting a conservative 3 s.d. criterion of normal latency he found that 4 out of the 15 patients showed *minor* increases in response latency. All 15 showed a reduction in amplitude and in 13 this was to less than 50% of the normal mean. The amplitude reduction correlated with both the degree of involvement of central vision and with the area of the visual field involved. Unlike the situation in MS (and in the flash EP study of Ellenberger and Ziegler mentioned above) the responses from the unaffected eye were invariably normal. Another feature which distinguished these responses from those in demyelinating disease was that the amplitude reduction was more marked than the latency increase.

EYE INJURY

Ebe et al (1964) recorded the flash EP in nine patients with unilateral optic atrophy following trauma and found that, while the flash ERG was almost invariably normal, the occipital EP was altered in parallel with the impairment of visual acuity, and was undetectable from the four blind eyes and from one other with impaired acuity. Two other cases had abnormal occipital responses accompanying lowered visual acuity. Rouher et al (1969) recorded the EP to white, red and blue flashes in 17 post-traumatic cases and confirmed these findings, although they found that the flash ERG could be altered where there was severe retinal disturbance. In what appeared physiologically to be complete lesions of the optic nerve, the occipital EP was lost to all forms of stimulation, white, red and blue, while in partial sections the alterations in the flash EP paralleled the severity of the lesion. Central lesions were characterized by a reduction in the amplitude of the response to the white flash stimulus, an abolition of the response to the red flash stimulus and a virtually normal response to the blue flash. Conversely a peripheral constriction of the fields without central deficit gave normal responses to the red and white flash, but abolished the response to the blue flash. They emphasize the particular value of this investigation in comatose patients following trauma, where a persistent occipital response, even if impaired, gives firm grounds for optimism in the prognosis for the recovery of vision. Vaughan and Katzman (1964) recorded a 29-year-old male whose complete blindness was associated with bilateral orbital frontal fractures after having been pushed down a flight of stairs during a fight. The ERG was normal but no VER could be recorded. He subsequently developed definite optic atrophy.

Babel et al (1977) recommend the flash ERG as an indicator of the dysfunction associated with traumatic retinal oedema following a violent contusion of the eyeball. The oscillatory potentials are particularly sensitive to such disturbance, but may return as the oedema subsides.

Crews et al (1978) recorded the flash ERG and EP in 60 patients (64 eyes) within one month of a severe perforating or blunt eye injury, following which the opacity of the media prevented examination of the posterior segment. Clinical assessment at this stage is important, because of the risk of sympathetic ophthalmia or the chances of a blind painful eye, which have to be offset against the prognosis for the recovery of vision. This assessment is critical because upon it may have to be based an early decision on whether to enucleate. Furthermore, the planning of major reconstructive surgery in the early post-operative stage after primary repair demands a detailed and reliable clinical assessment.

Using the b-wave amplitude of the flash ERG as a criterion and comparing it in the injured eye and its fellow (or, where both eyes were injured, with the mean normal value), 22 out of 30 eyes (73%) with a b-wave amplitude from the injured eye of more than 50% at the initial assessment eventually achieved a vision of 6/60 or better, while 13 (43%) achieved 6/12 or better. Only one of the 34 eyes where the b-wave amplitude was reduced by more than 50% achieved useful vision, and the vast majority went blind or were enucleated.

The 'P2 or $\overline{P100}$ component' of the occipital flash EP gave similar results. Of the

33 eyes with a reduction in amplitude of less than 50% and no marked delay, 22 (67%) achieved a final acuity of 6/60 or better, and 12 (36%) an acuity of 6/12 or better. By 'a marked delay' the authors meant a delay of more than 30 msec, which is a large shift for the flash response. Of the 31 eyes with a marked delay of this kind, or a reduction in the amplitude of the positivity of more than 50%, only one achieved an acuity better than 6/60 and the vast majority (94%) went blind or were enucleated. The latency of the flash EP did not clearly differentiate between the degree of ultimate visual recovery in those patients where there was some persistence of accurate projection even with acuity worse than 6/60, but a marked delay in the flash response distinguished clearly at this early stage in the clinical management those cases which would ultimately do worse than this.

Combining the results of the flash ERG and EP recordings improved the predictive power of the tests, correctly identifying all the patients with visual potential and 91% of the patients with a poor visual outcome. Of the 21 enucleated eyes, 16 were found to have the retina detached and all these had had flash ERGs with a b-wave amplitude of less than 25%. All but two had had an absent flash VEP (less than 1.5 μV) and the other two a markedly delayed occipital response reduced to less than 50% of the control amplitude. These results appear to establish the predictive value of the flash ERG following an injury.

6

The Visual Evoked Potential in the Investigation of Diseases of the Optic Nerve

A.M. Halliday

OPTIC NEURITIS

One of the most clear-cut and easily recognized abnormalities of the pattern reversal response can be seen after a clinical attack of retrobulbar neuritis (Halliday et al, 1972). In the acute attack, where visual acuity is greatly reduced, the amplitude of the pattern response is correspondingly diminished, and the response may indeed be unobtainable at this stage if the acuity is reduced to counting fingers or to the perception of light. In the typical case this acute stage lasts only for a day or two and is followed by rapid improvement in the visual acuity, often with complete restoration of normal vision within a month. The pattern reversal EP returns to near normal amplitudes in parallel with the recovering vision. Figure 6.1 shows the pattern reversal EPs recorded in each eye four days and ten days after the onset of acute bilateral optic neuritis in a 14-year-old girl. At the time of the first record visual acuity was reduced to counting fingers in each eye and the pattern EP was unobtainable from the left eye and of very small amplitude from the right eye. Seven days later, the responses had returned and had an absolute amplitude within the normal range, although the response from the left eye was smaller than that from the right eye, paralleling the lower visual acuity (6/12 as against 6/9) (Halliday and McDonald, 1977). In the group data from a study of 53 patients recovering from an attack of optic neuritis, the amplitude of the pattern EP was significantly correlated with the visual acuity level at the time of the recording (Figure 6.2) and had almost returned to the normal mean for the healthy population in those patients with a visual acuity of 6/6 or better (Halliday et al, 1973b). The amplitude of the pattern EP thus appears to follow closely the visual acuity level in demyelinating disease.

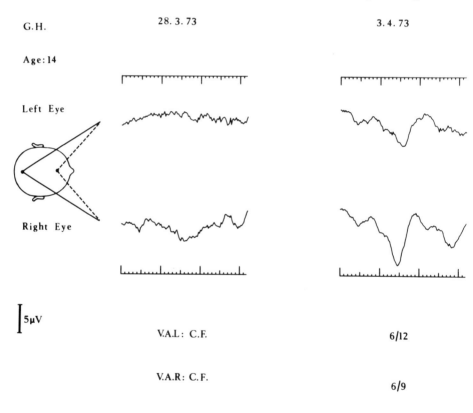

Figure 6.1 *Pattern reversal responses from each eye of a 14-year-old girl with acute bilateral optic neuritis. The left-hand pair of records were recorded 4 days after the onset of visual failure when visual acuity was reduced to counting fingers in both eyes. Note that the normal pattern responses are almost completely abolished, but that there is a trace of the major positivity at a much delayed latency in the response from the right eye. Six days later (right-hand pair of records) the amplitude of the pattern responses has greatly increased, paralleling the improvement in the acuity level, but both responses are grossly delayed. (From Halliday and McDonald, 1977.)*

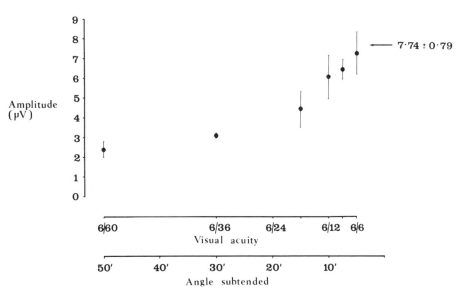

Figure 6.2   *Mean amplitude ± s.d. from 69 records on 53 patients recovering from optic neuritis, to show the significant correlation between the amplitude during recovery and the acuity level (p <0.01). The data at 6/60 includes those cases with visual acuity of 6/60 or less. The mean normal amplitude in a healthy control group is indicated on the right. (From Halliday et al, 1973b.)*

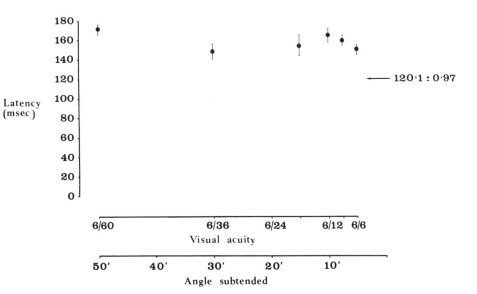

Figure 6.3   *Mean latency of the pattern response ± s.d. in the same group of patients with optic neuritis as in Figure 6.2. The mean normal latency in a healthy control group for the stimulus used in this study is indicated on the right. There is no correlation between latency and acuity level. (From Halliday et al, 1973b.)*

The outstanding change in the pattern EP is, however, in the latency of the major positivity following the attack. Figure 6.4 shows the pattern reversal EP from each eye recorded in a 42-year-old woman one month after an attack of acute left optic neuritis. Visual acuity in the affected eye had returned from counting fingers almost to normal, being 6/9 at the time of the recording; the amplitude of the response differs little in the two eyes. The major positive component is, however, delayed by about 45 msec in the response from the affected left eye. The normal triphasic waveform of the response is well preserved, with the major positivity preceded and followed by smaller negative peaks (see Chapter 3, page 84). Moreover there is no lateral asymmetry in the response. The whole waveform has simply been delayed by 45 msec. In the quasi-sinusoidal steady state response to 10 Hz pattern reversal, shown on the right of Figure 6.4, this delay is manifest in the form of a phase shift,

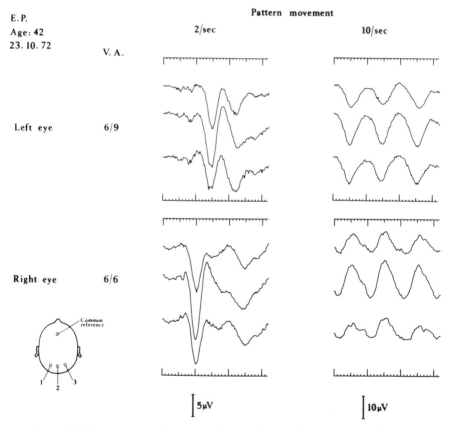

Figure 6.4 *Pattern reversal responses from each eye of a patient recorded one month after an attack of acute left optic neuritis. The transient response to 2 Hz stimulation and the steady-state response to 10 Hz stimulation are each shown. The responses from the right eye are of normal waveform and latency, while the transient response from the affected left eye is delayed by 45 msec. The steady-state response from this eye shows a corresponding phase-lag. (From Halliday, 1976.)*

the positive peak of the sinusoid occurring with the same latency as the delayed $\overline{P100}$ component of the transient 2 Hz response.

A similar delay can be seen in the records taken 10 days after the onset of acute bilateral optic neuritis in the 14-year-old girl, whose VEPs are shown in Figure 6.1. It is also noticeable that even in the acute phase of the attack, only four days after the onset of symptoms, the vestigial response recorded from the right eye is already showing clear evidence of the delayed positive peak. It appears, therefore, that the change in latency must occur early in the acute attack, and it is notable that the recovering positivity recorded in this eye six days later shows no further change in its latency. The recovery of the pattern EP amplitude with recovering visual acuity, demonstrated in the group data shown in Figure 6.2, is not accompanied by any change in the latency of the major positivity. As can be seen in Figure 6.3, the mean latency at all acuities is increased above the normal level, but the amount of the increase shows no correlation with the acuity level. There is thus a dissociation between the amplitude and latency changes following an acute demyelinating lesion of the optic nerve, as originally pointed out by Halliday et al (1973b).

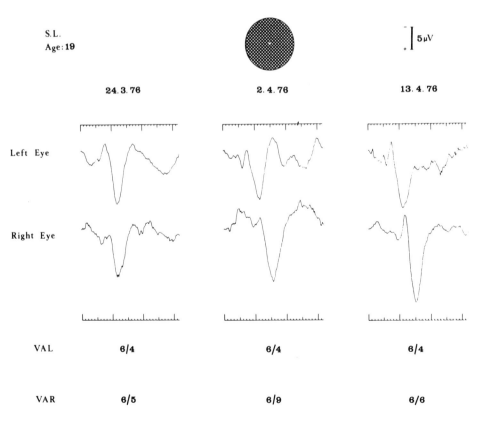

Figure 6.5 *Sudden step-wise increase in the latency of the pattern response from the right eye in a 19-year-old girl undergoing an attack of right optic neuritis. The latency has increased by over 30 msec between the records on 24.3.76 and 2.4.76, but thereafter remains unchanged in the record of 13.4.76.*

The step-like character of the increase in latency in demyelination of the optic nerve can be observed particularly well if the change in latency is unaccompanied by a reduction in the amplitude of the pattern EP. This was the case in a 19-year-old woman who was recorded on three occasions 9 and 11 days apart. Her records are shown in Figure 6.5. On the first occasion, when acuity was normal in both eyes, she had pattern EPs with a major positivity of similar latency from each eye, both within the normal latency range. Some visual impairment in the right eye over the next few days was associated with a marked increase in the latency of the response from this eye, clearly seen in the second record; the amplitude of the response, however, is still large and the acuity has only been reduced from 6/5 to 6/9. On the occasion of the third record, 11 days later, the increased latency of the response from the right eye had remained unchanged.

The magnitude of the delay in the $\overline{P100}$ component of the pattern response, established soon after the onset of an attack of optic neuritis, thereafter remains characteristic of a particular patient. In general, it appears to alter only if a further attack supervenes, when it may increase, or, in a minority of patients, where, owing to some reparative process, it may revert after some time to normal or near normal latencies (see below). Delays can be recorded in patients many years after a clinical attack of optic neuritis (Halliday et al, 1972, 1973a). Serial studies on patients with demyelinating disease have shown that, in the visual modality at least, increases in EP latency are usually associated with clinical episodes of visual impairment (Matthews and Small, 1979), although clinically 'silent' episodes undoubtedly occur and account for the incidence of delays in patients with no history of visual disturbance. The evidence from serial studies has been discussed by the author elsewhere (Halliday, 1980c).

Percentage of abnormally delayed pattern reversal responses after optic neuritis

It was established in an early study by Halliday et al (1972) that after an acute attack of unilateral optic neuritis 17 out of 18 patients had pattern reversal responses with a $\overline{P100}$ latency beyond the upper limit of the normal range. In a subsequent study of a larger group (Halliday et al, 1973b) 50 out of 53 patients had abnormally delayed responses. From this data, therefore, it appears that the latency of the $\overline{P100}$ component will distinguish all but 5-6% of those patients who have suffered a clinically overt acute demyelinating lesion of the optic nerve. In the 1972 study, 17 of the 19 clinically unaffected other eyes had a latency within the normal range; the two others had a marginally increased latency (see Figure 6.6). One of the 19 patients presenting in the acute phase of retrobulbar neuritis had no recordable pattern response from the affected eye, and did not attend subsequently for re-examination. Comparable studies have been made by Bornstein (1975), Matthews et al (1977) and Shahrokhi et al (1978) (see Table 6.1). The study by Matthews et al (1977) included 24 patients with recent retrobulbar neuritis and four patients with exclusively visual symptoms resulting from past episodes of retrobulbar neuritis. Thirty-one of the 38 affected eyes (82%) had delayed responses, but there was no increase in the abnormality rate on including the left eye/right eye differences, and only one patient with normal latency responses had a significantly reduced amplitude. Shahrokhi et al (1978) found delayed responses in 49 out of 59 affected eyes in 51 patients with a history of clinically pure optic neuritis, while 8 other affected eyes showed no recordable response. The mean latency of the patient group was 132.3 msec (range 89-192 msec) as against 103.4 msec for the healthy control group. The criterion of a delayed latency was set at 116 msec, $+2.5$ s.d. above the normal mean. Of the 59 affected eyes, four had responses with latencies within the normal range, two of which could nonetheless be classified as abnormal, because of a significant latency difference between the two eyes in one individual (8 msec), while another eye was classified as abnormal because of an interocular amplitude difference (6 μV). Three of the 59 eyes had completely normal responses as regards

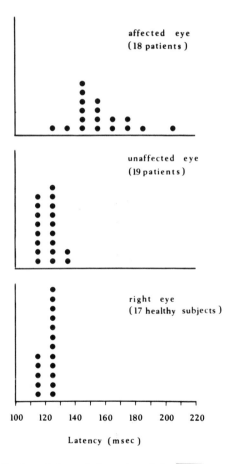

Figure 6.6 *Distribution of the peak latencies of the $\overline{P100}$ component of the pattern reversal EP from the affected eye of 18 patients with acute unilateral optic neuritis (upper histogram), from the unaffected eye of the same 18 patients and from one additional patient who had no measurable response from the affected eye when seen in the acute stage (middle histogram), and from the right eye of 17 healthy subjects (lower histogram). (From Halliday et al, 1972.)*

Table 6.1 INCIDENCE OF DELAYED $\overline{\text{P100}}$ COMPONENTS IN THE PATTERN REVERSAL RESPONSE FOLLOWING A CLINICAL ATTACK OF OPTIC NEURITIS

Reference	Number of patients	Number of affected eyes	Number of measurable responses	Number of delayed $\overline{\text{P100}}$s	Percentage of delayed responses
Halliday, McDonald and Mushin, 1972	19	19	18	17	94
Halliday, McDonald and Mushin, 1973b	53	53	53	50	94
Milner, Regan and Heron, 1974	5	5	3	3	100
Wildberger and van Lith, 1976	17				
11 acute phase		12	6 (11)*	6 (11)*	100
16 chronic phase		20	19	18	95
Mathews, Small, Small and Pountney, 1977	28	38	38	31	82
Shahrokhi, Chiappa and Young, 1978	51	59	51	49	96
Rosén, Bynke and Sandberg, 1980	42	42	42	9	21

*Responses were initially absent in 5 patients, but returned on subsequent recording

latency, despite a clear history of optic neuritis. The false negative rate is thus very comparable to that in the earlier studies (Table 6.1).

Similar results have been obtained in studies of multiple sclerosis patients with a history of optic neuritis (see Table 6.3 on page 210).

The study by Rosén et al (1980), who found only 9 patients with abnormally delayed pattern responses out of 42 patients with unilateral optic neuritis, is puzzling and difficult to reconcile with the results reported elsewhere. In spite of an unusually thorough clinical examination, including CSF electrophoresis and HLA typing, the technique used to record the EPs is open to some question. A LED stimulator of 3.3° with 23′ element-spacing was employed to record the pattern reversal response from only one channel with a pair of midline electrodes placed on the vertex and inion. This C_z to O_z montage must have maximised the possibility of waveform distortion by cancellation, since the normal maximum response is situated about half-way between the two. This interpretation of these anomalous results seems to be borne out by the representative records illustrated. The results of this study therefore need to be treated with caution, but certainly deserve further investigation.

It can be concluded that, adopting the criterion for increased latency of + 2.5 s.d. of the normal mean, about one in 20 patients with definite optic neuritis will be missed. The rates can be improved slightly by including additional criteria, such as the discrepancy between latency or amplitude values for the two eyes in any one individual and the reduction in the response to high frequency flicker stimulation (see page 212). The + 2.5 s.d. criterion itself implies a small but definite false positive rate, approximately one in every 160 healthy individuals being mis-classified as abnormal.

Relative sensitivity of the flash and pattern EPs in optic neuritis

A number of earlier studies had established delays in the mean latency of the flash EP following demyelinating lesions affecting the optic nerves (e.g. Rouher et al, 1969; Richey et al, 1971; Namerow and Enns, 1972; Ellenberger and Ziegler, 1977). Halliday et al (1972) recorded both flash and pattern reversal EPs in their original study of a group of patients with acute unilateral optic neuritis. They found, however, that the flash response was much less sensitive to the effects of demyelinating lesions. In a given patient, the flash EP might be undelayed or delayed only by a few milliseconds, where the pattern EP was markedly increased in latency (See Figures 6.7, 6.8, 6.9 and 6.10). This relative insensitivity of the flash EP to the effects of demyelinating lesions is compounded with the greater variability of

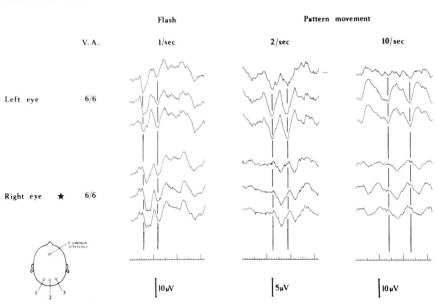

Figure 6.7 *Flash and pattern EPs from each eye of a patient recovering from right optic neuritis, recorded 5 months after the onset of the attack. Visual acuity in the affected eye had returned to normal by the time of the recording. Note the marked delay (about 40 msec) in both the transient and steady-state pattern reversal responses from the affected eye and the relatively small delay in the flash response from this eye. (From Halliday et al, 1979b.)*

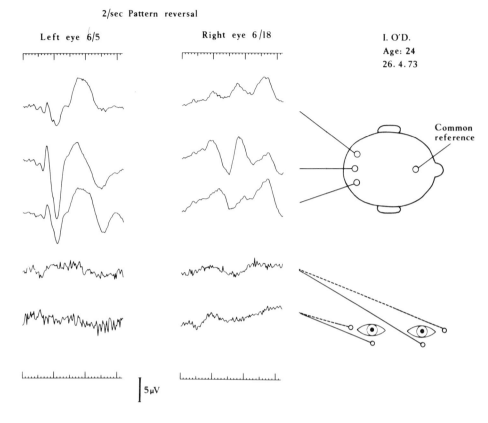

2/sec Pattern reversal

Left eye 6/5   Right eye 6/18

I. O'D.
Age: 24
26. 4. 73

Common reference

5 μV

Figure 6.8 *Monocular pattern reversal EP recorded 4 weeks after the onset of optic neuritis of the right eye in a 24-year-old woman. Visual acuity, originally counting fingers, had improved to 6/18 in the affected eye. Note the delayed major positive component of reduced amplitude from the right eye, accompanied by a normal pattern ERG. Compare Figure 6.9, 6.10 and 6.14. (From Halliday et al, 1977b.)*

the flash response in the healthy population (see Tables 3.1 and 3.2) to render the flash response much less useful in clinical testing (Halliday et al, 1979b; Halliday and Mushin, 1980).

This is illustrated graphically in Figure 6.11 which shows the idealized normal curves corresponding to the mean latency and standard deviation for the flash response (above) and the pattern response (below) for the healthy controls and the affected and unaffected eyes of the patients in the 1972 study. The mean latency of the flash response is 10.2 msec longer in the affected than the unaffected eyes of the patient group, but the corresponding increase in latency for the pattern response is 34.0 msec, more than three times greater. The greater variability of the flash EP latency in the normal population is indicated both by the wider spread of latencies in the control group and by the difference between the healthy controls and the

10/sec Pattern reversal

Left eye   Right eye

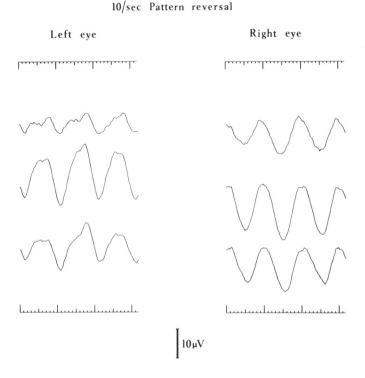

10μV

Figure 6.9 Steady-state response to 10 Hz pattern reversal stimulation in the patient whose transient pattern reversal responses are shown in Figure 6.8. Note the phase-lag in the response from the right eye, corresponding in magnitude to the delay in the transient response. (From Halliday et al, 1977b.)

unaffected eyes, which is not statistically significant but represents the kind of sampling error to be expected in dealing with the flash response. By contrast the mean latency of the pattern evoked potential in the unaffected eye of the patients (121.1 msec) is close to that in the normal controls (119.9 msec) and the spread of latencies is much narrower. As a result there is much less overlap of the abnormal and control groups. The superiority of the pattern response in detecting abnormalities in an individual case is clearly shown in Figure 6.12 in which the dotted line indicates the particularly conservative criterion of 3 standard deviations of the normal latency (implying a one in a thousand false positive rate for the healthy population). All except one of the patients have pattern EPs which are delayed on this criterion, whereas none of the flash responses are so delayed.

One of the problems of the flash response, with its variable waveform, is to be sure that one is accurately measuring the change in latency in the affected eye. The data here was also analysed by an alternative method, using a cross-correlation technique to detect the shift in latency between the response in the affected and unaffected eyes by a purely objective method (see page 492). The interrupted

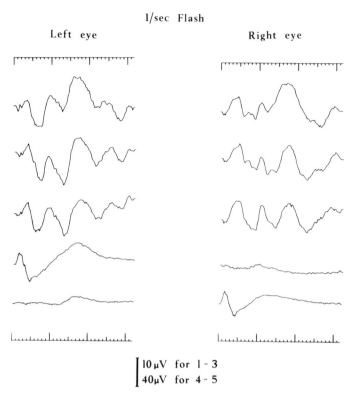

1/sec Flash

Left eye   Right eye

$$\begin{array}{l} 10\,\mu V \quad \text{for} \quad 1\text{-}3 \\ 40\mu V \quad \text{for} \quad 4\text{-}5 \end{array}$$

Figure 6.10 *Flash EPs from the same patient as in Figure 6.8 and 6.9. Note the absence of any delay in the flash EP from the right eye comparable to that in the pattern EP. The ERG to flash is shown at reduced gain. Montage as in Figure 6.8. (From Halliday et al, 1977b.)*

vertical lines in Figure 6.12 indicate the values obtained by this technique and show that, in general, there is good agreement between the results obtained by visual inspection and by cross-correlation. Unfortunately the cross-correlation technique is only applicable where a normal waveform is available, as in the case of uniocular disease, and is not so suitable where there is binocular involvement.

Feinsod and Hoyt (1975), who reported 100% of abnormalities in the flash response studied in 25 patients with multiple sclerosis, lay additional stress on the break-up of the first negative component of the flash response into multiple subcomponents, usually 2-4 in number. We therefore re-examined the data from our optic neuritis study and carried out a blind rating of the flash responses from the patient and control groups, examining them for the break up of the early negativity (Halliday et al, 1982). We found no difference between the affected and unaffected eyes in terms of the proportion of normal to abnormal judgements. With the flash stimulus used in this particular laboratory, therefore, there was no significant association of the early waveform changes in the flash response with the affected eye.

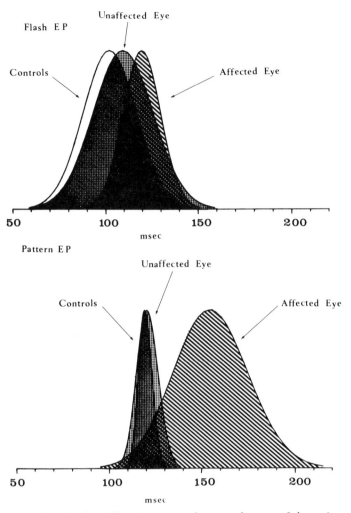

Figure 6.11 *Standardized Gaussian curves for mean latency of the major positivity of the flash and pattern EP in the healthy controls and the affected and unaffected eyes of the patients with acute unilateral optic neuritis from the study by Halliday et al (1972). Note that the spread of latencies in the control group is much smaller for the pattern EP than for the flash EP and that the mean delay in the affected eye is much larger for the pattern response than for flash. (From Halliday et al, 1979b.)*

There have been a number of other studies comparing the flash and pattern EP in the same group of patients with demyelinating disease (Wildberger et al, 1976a; Duwaer and Spekreijse, 1978; Mauguière et al, 1979; Harding et al, 1980a; Lowitzsch et al, 1980; Wilson and Keyser, 1980). They have invariably confirmed the significantly smaller delays in the flash response with demyelinating lesions of the optic nerve and, where the variance has been recorded, the greater overlap with the normal response range due to the greater variability of the flash response latency and waveform in the healthy population.

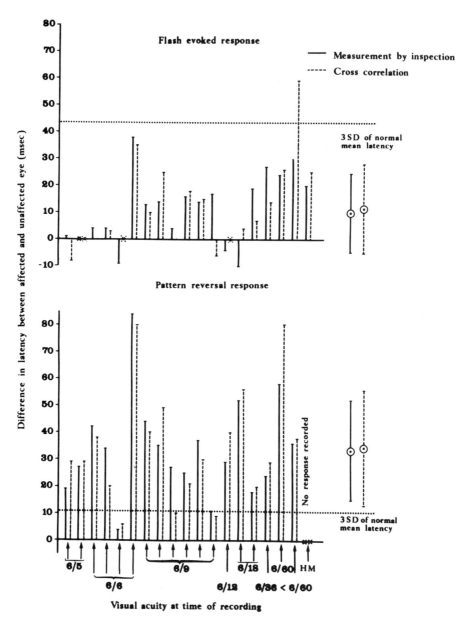

Figure 6.12 *Difference in latency between the affected and unaffected eye of the 19 patients with unilateral optic neuritis for the flash EP (above) and the pattern EP (below). The means for the whole group ± s.d. are shown on the right. For each patient the value obtained by manual measurement (solid line) is followed by the delay calculated by cross correlating the responses from the two eyes (interrupted line). The patients have been ranked according to their visual acuity level at the time of the recording, as indicated below the graph. The horizontal dotted line marks the 3 standard deviation limits of the normal mean latency for the flash and pattern response respectively. (Halliday et al, 1979b.)*

Mechanism of EP abnormalities in demyelinating disease

In focal demyelinating lesions experimentally induced by the direct microinjection of diphtheria toxin into the spinal cord of the cat (McDonald and Sears, 1970) it has been shown that large areas of myelin loss in central nerve fibres produce complete conduction block over the demyelinated zone, whereas normal conduction at an unreduced velocity persists in the still myelinated portions of the nerve to either side of the lesion (see McDonald 1977). In smaller or less complete lesions, conduction persists in many fibres and recording has established that the conduction velocity of the impulse is reduced as it traverses a partially demyelinated zone, but is normal in histologically normal portions of the same fibres. There is also a reduction in the ability of partially demyelinated fibres to conduct high frequency trains of impulses in the normal way, which is an effect of the prolongation of the refractory period in the damaged nerve. These three defects (1) conduction block, (2) slowed conduction, and (3) a reduced high frequency response are reflected in the EP abnormalities encountered in demyelinating disease (Halliday and McDonald, 1977). As has already been emphasized, the sudden step-like increase in latency, apparently established within the first few days of the attack of acute optic neuritis and thereafter persisting unchanged for months or years, suggests a long-standing structural anatomical change in the nerve fibres. It is therefore plausible to correlate the delay with the length of the plaque or plaques in the afferent pathway. If this is the case the range and scatter of latencies shown in Figures 6.6 and 6.17 presumably represent the variation in the mean length of demyelinated fibres in the visual pathways. The unusually short latencies, lying within the limits of the normal latency range, would then be due to the incidence of unusually short plaques in these particular patients.

The discrepancy between the magnitude of the delay in the pattern and flash EPs suggests that these two responses must be transmitted centrally in separate groups of afferent fibres in the visual pathway. From the character of the stimuli it seems plausible to correlate these with the X and Y systems, which are well adapted to detect the changes in relatively persistent pattern contours and rapid fluxes of luminance respectively (Mushin, 1974; Halliday, 1981). Since the Y system is subserved by somewhat larger and faster fibres than the X system, the more delayed pattern EPs may reflect the increased conduction time in the smaller fibres traversing a demyelinated plaque of fixed length. This difference between larger and smaller fibres would be expected, whether conduction over the abnormal zone is saltatory or continuous (Halliday, 1981).

Many of the patients with unilaterally delayed pattern responses are completely unaware of the fact, and it does not appear that the increase in latency in itself is associated with any overt clinical symptomatology (Halliday and McDonald, 1977). The amplitude of the pattern EP, on the other hand, closely parallels the onset and subsequent recovery of the visual impairment at the time of the attack. This effect appears to be a reflection of the degree of conduction block of the afferent fibres. It is well established that partially demyelinated fibres are particularly vulnerable to small changes in temperature or electrolyte balance, which can rapidly lead to a complete failure in impulse transmission in fibres which were previously conducting (Schauf and Davis, 1974; Davis and Schauf, 1975). It appears that most of the clinical deficits in demyelinating disease can be related to the effect of conduction block in the fibres traversing the plaques (Halliday and McDonald, 1977). The sensitivity of the partially demyelinated fibres to small changes in temperature no doubt accounts for the exacerbation of symptoms reported by many patients following hot baths or exercise (see Davis and Schauf, 1975 for a review). Persson and Sachs (1978, 1980) have studied the pattern reversal

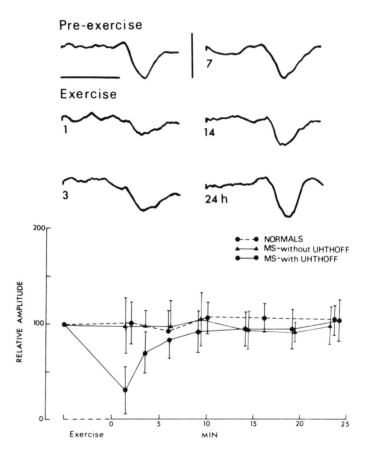

Figure 6.13 *(Above) Pattern reversal EPs recorded from a patient exhibiting Uhthoff's phenomenon. Before exercise, the visual acuity was 6/6, but after 10 minutes work on the bicycle ergometer, it fell, this subjective change being accompanied by a marked decrease in the amplitude of the pattern EP. The pre-exercise control level in amplitude was not reached until 7 minutes after the end of exercise, when the patient reported the return of normal vision. Note that there is no significant alteration in $\overline{P100}$ latency accompanying the amplitude change. The numbers below each response represent the time in minutes or hours (h) after exercise. Horizontal calibration 100 msec; vertical calibration 10 μV. (Below) Changes in mean relative pattern EP amplitude ± s.d. at various time intervals after exercise in the 3 examined groups. 100 represents the mean amplitude of each person's VEP obtained at the pre-exercise control recording and the changes are expressed in relation to that value. (From Persson and Sachs, 1980.)*

EP in seven patients showing a transient reduction in visual acuity after exercise, the phenomenon first described by Uhthoff (1889). This phenomenon was found to occur in 11% of 125 patients with demyelinating optic neuritis studied by Perkin and Rose (1976). As shown in Figure 6.13 the visual impairment on exercise was observed to be accompanied by a transient 60% decrease in the mean amplitude of the major positivity of the pattern EP, unaccompanied by any change in latency (Persson and Sachs, 1978, 1980). No such change was seen in a group of MS patients with delayed $\overline{P100}$s not showing Uhthoff's phenomenon, nor by a group of healthy controls. This result, which agrees with other unpublished observations by the present author, thus follows the predicted pattern, with amplitude and latency effects on the pattern EP dissociated and therefore due to distinct pathophysiological effects of the demyelinating lesion. It appears that the reversible visual impairment occurring at the onset of an attack of optic neuritis closely parallels the period during which the nerve head appears swollen and oedematous. In the patient with acute bilateral optic neuritis whose pattern EPs are shown in Figure 6.1, the fundi were examined and photographed at the time of both the first and second recordings. On the first occasion, when the responses were almost abolished and visual acuity was reduced to counting fingers, both discs showed gross swelling, whereas a week later, when visual acuity had returned to near normal levels and the VEPs were of almost normal amplitude, the swelling had completely subsided. It appears that local compression may be in itself sufficient to cause reversible conduction block in partially demyelinated fibres. Similar amplitude changes, with rapid recovery on decompression, can be observed in the pattern EPs associated with some compressive lesions (see page 225).

The inability to transmit fast trains of impulses is a distinct defect associated with demyelination. This also is reflected in the EP changes recorded in patients. In the somatosensory modality, Sclabassi et al (1974) have demonstrated a highly significant reduction in the SEP to high frequency trains of electrical stimuli in patients with multiple sclerosis, correlating with the severity of the disease. Milner et al (1974) have reported abnormalities in the VEPs to medium and high frequency flicker, which they found to be particularly characteristic of patients presenting with the spinal form of multiple sclerosis. These defects in high frequency following were seen in many patients who had no delays in their pattern reversal EPs. The two defects therefore apppear to be due to different causes. Celesia and Daly (1977b) and Cohen et al (1980) have also reported that the ability to evoke flicker EP following at high frequencies is reduced in a high proportion of patients with demyelinating disease, but that these are not necessarily the same as those showing delayed $\overline{P100}$ components.

Recovery of normal latency after having a delayed VEP

In a minority of patients, recorded serially over some years, a previously delayed pattern reversal response from one eye has been observed to return to normal or near normal latencies (Figure 6.14). This suggests the possibility of some reparative process, such as remyelination. Remyelination of demyelinated fibres in the central nervous system, with restoration of normal conduction, has been shown to occur

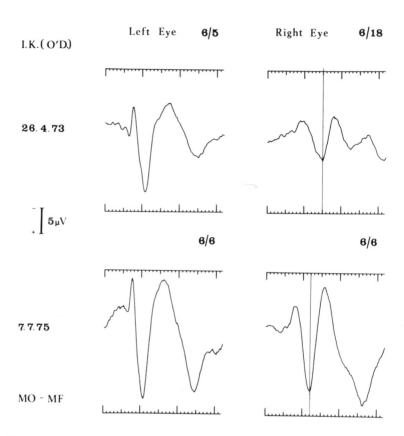

Figure 6.14 *Monocular pattern reversal responses, recorded from a mid-occipital electrode from the same patient as in Figures 6.8-10, one month after an attack of optic neuritis in the right eye (above) and 2 years later (below). The first record shows a much delayed response of reduced amplitude from the right eye, but this has not only increased in size by the time of the second record, paralleling the improvement in visual acuity, but has also regained a peak latency almost within the normal range. (From Halliday and McDonald, 1977.)*

experimentally (Smith et al, 1979). Matthews and Small (1979) recorded the return of a delayed pattern response to normal latencies in 9 out of 51 patients who were recorded on two or more occasions at varying intervals. This is a higher percentage than the earlier literature would suggest. Asselman, Chadwick and Marsden (1975) encountered 2 out of 51 patients with multiple sclerosis who had an initially delayed pattern response following an attack of acute retrobulbar neuritis which later returned to normal latency. Halliday and McDonald (1977) had seen only 2 cases, but more recently, the present author recorded 4 out of 31 patients showing similar improvement on serial recording (Carroll and Halliday, unpublished). In the EPs to stimulation in other modalities, return of a delayed response to normal latency seems even more common (Namerow, 1968; Kimura, 1975).

Apart from such changes, which clearly reflect a significant change in the underlying deficit, the test-retest reliability of the pattern EP on serial recording is good (Matthews and Small, 1979; Stockard et al, 1979). Increases in latency are, in general, related to the clinical attacks of visual impairment. The more labile latency variations observed in the case of the short latency brainstem EP to auditory stimulation (Robinson and Rudge, 1978) and the subcortical somatosensory response (Matthews and Small, 1979), are not encountered in the behaviour of the visual EP (see Halliday, 1980c). Matthews and Small (1979) did, however, observe a gradual decline in the amplitude of the response, irrespective of changes in latency or visual acuity, over the period of 18 months during which they intensively studied seven patients with demyelinating disease. The mean amplitude of the pattern EP from the 14 eyes decreased from 7 ± 2.5 μV in the first recording to 3.6 ± 2.2 μV in the last recording. The difference was significant at the $p < 0.001$ level. In their larger group of 51 patients in whom the VEP was recorded at least twice, there was a similar reduction in the amplitude of the $\overline{P100}$, from a mean of 7.7 ± 4.2 μV at the first recording to 6.2 ± 3.9 μV at the final recording. This difference was significant at the $p < 0.01$ level.

Central scotomata simulating delayed EPs in optic neuritis

In some patients with demyelinating disease an apparently delayed major positivity may be simulated by the replacement of the $\overline{P100}$ component, derived from the macula, by the paramacular $\overline{P135}$ component. Where conduction block of the fibres of the papillomacular bundle subserving central vision has resulted in a dense central scotoma, this change can be readily explained. Figure 6.15 illustrates such a response in a 47-year-old patient with definite MS. Half-field stimulation shows that the large 'delayed' positivity seen in the response to the full-field $16°$ checkerboard stimulus is formed by the summation of contralateral $\overline{P135}$ components within the normal latency range contributed by each half-field response. Strictly speaking, therefore, the response is not 'delayed' and the abnormality is typical of that associated with a dense central scotoma. Although central scotomata are not uncommon in optic neuritis, the routine use of half-field stimulation shows that this variant is relatively uncommon compared with delayed responses.

MULTIPLE SCLEROSIS

Delayed pattern EPs in patients with no history of optic neuritis

Delayed pattern responses are frequently encountered in patients with multiple sclerosis who have had no history of visual impairment. A typical case was described by Halliday (1972). The patient was an intelligent man, the Managing Director of a small firm, who was quite certain that he had had no trouble with his eyes, except for having to wear glasses for reading for the past four years. This 57-year-old man had normal fields on the Goldmann perimeter and there was no pallor of the optic discs. His pattern responses were, however, grossly delayed from both eyes (Figure 6.16), with a latency for the major positivity of 166 msec for the left eye

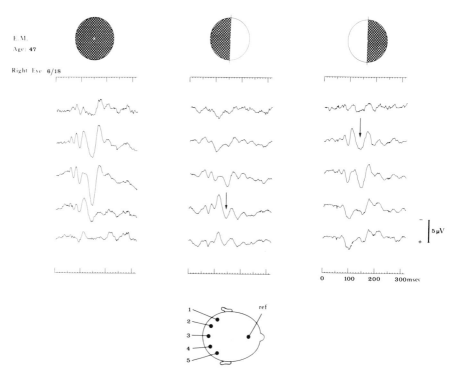

Figure 6.15 *Apparently delayed major positivity in the full-field response from the right eye of a 47-year-old patient with multiple sclerosis (left hand record). Half-field stimulation shows this positivity to be made up of the summation of 2 contralateral* $\overline{P135}$ *components. These positivities are within the normal latency range for the* $\overline{P135}$. *The appearance of a delayed response is, in fact, due to the changes characteristic of a central scotoma, and a small dense central scotoma was found on examination of the visual fields. (From Carroll and Kriss, 1981.)*

and 168 msec for the right eye. The control values for this component with the equipment in use at the time were 120.1 ± 4.0 msec. This patient presented clinically with a history of many years urgency of micturition, impotence for two years, and increasing difficulty in walking over the previous 18 months. In the past year he had noticed clumsiness of his hands, worse on the left side, slurring speech and burning paraesthesiae in the feet. On examination he had ataxia of the limbs and gait, worse on the left, increased limb jerks and bilateral extensor plantar responses. There was also a slurring dysarthria. Sensation was intact and the only abnormal eye sign was a vertical nystagmus.

The detection of clinically 'silent' plaques in the optic nerve associated with a delayed pattern response constitutes one of the most valuable clinical applications of the test. Such delayed responses can be found without any accompanying abnormal signs in the fundi, and with normal fields on perimetry and normal colour vision (Halliday et al, 1973a). Rigolet et al (1979) have compared colour vision testing, using the Hardy Rand Rittler (HRR) test and the Farnsworth 100-hue test,

Patient 33

Pattern Movement

2/sec

Left eye

Right eye

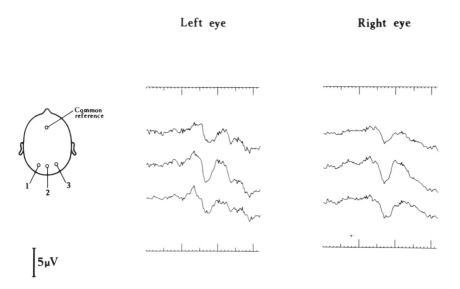

$5\mu V$

Figure 6.16 Pattern reversal responses recorded from a 57-year-old man with ataxia, dysarthria and bilateral pyramidal signs, but no history of visual impairment. He had normal fields on Goldmann perimetry and there was no pallor of the optic discs. His pupils reacted normally, but he had vertical nystagmus. (From Halliday, 1972.)

with the checkerboard reversal EP in 75 patients with possible or probable MS who had no history of optic neuritis. Only 34.7% showed a dyschromatopsia, whereas 68% showed an increased VEP latency. It appears, therefore, that the pattern evoked response is among the most sensitive tests for persisting damage to the visual pathways. Its particular value in 'silent' lesions is that it provides the clinician with information which he cannot readily get in any other way. Notwithstanding its diagnostic non-specificity, the finding of a delayed visual EP in a patient presenting with a single spinal lesion, for instance, helps to provide a firm basis for the diagnosis of disseminated sclerosis. It may thus enable the patient to avoid the inconvenience of a myelogram unless there is some other compelling reason for suspecting spinal compression.

Incidence of delayed pattern responses in multiple sclerosis

Halliday et al (1973a) found delayed pattern EPs in 52 out of 73 patients (71%) referred because of suspected multiple sclerosis. When the diagnostic criteria of McAlpine were applied to these patients (McAlpine, 1972), 34 satisfied the criteria for definite multiple sclerosis, 5 for probable multiple sclerosis and 12 for possible multiple sclerosis, whereas 22 of the patients failed to qualify even for the possible group. Three of the latter had delayed responses (14%), whereas 49 of the 51 patients making up the first three groups had delays (96%). The range of delays encountered in the multiple sclerosis groups in this study is shown in Figure 6.17 and is very similar to that encountered in the optic neuritis study (see Figure 6.6). The mean delay in the multiple sclerosis patients was 43.3 ± 20.1 msec, only 8.3 msec longer than that in the optic neuritis group. The maximum delay encountered (100 msec) and the false negative rate (2 out of 51) was also similar to that in the earlier study. The percentage incidence of delayed pattern responses in the many subsequent published studies of multiple sclerosis patients has varied a good deal and appreciably lower overall 'detection rates' have been reported (see Table 6.2).

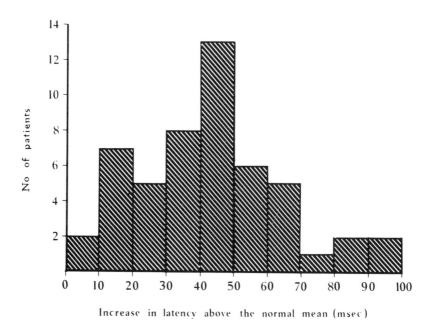

Figure 6.17 *Range of increase in latency of the major positivity of the pattern reversal EP recorded from the more affected of the 2 eyes in 51 patients with multiple sclerosis. (From Halliday et al, 1973a.)*

The lowest overall rate of abnormality in any study was 50%. All the published studies are agreed in reporting a much higher incidence of abnormal pattern EPs from the definite diagnostic group (invariably over 75%) than for the probable or possible diagnostic categories. In this context it has to be remembered that the EP test is of more diagnostic importance in the probable and possible cases, where it may serve to settle the diagnostic problem. Table 6.3 collects the comparable published data classified in terms of the presence or absence of a history of optic neuritis. Again all the studies have reported a very high rate of abnormality for those cases with definite optic neuritis (invariably over 82%) but much more

Table 6.2 PERCENTAGE OF MULTIPLE SCLEROSIS PATIENTS SHOWING ABNORMAL PATTERN REVERSAL RESPONSES

Reference	N	Overall %	'Definite' %	'Probable' %	'Possible' %
Halliday, McDonald and Mushin, 1973a					
All suspected MS cases	73	71	—	—	—
Cases satisfying diagnostic criteria	51	96	97	100	92
Asselman, Chadwick & Marsden, 1975	51	67	84	84	21
Lowitzsch et al, 1976	135	73	82	60	65
Mastaglia, Black & Collins, 1976	68	50	83	33	33
Purves & Low, 1976					
Delayed beyond normal latency	20	65	—	—	—
Including L/R eye discrepancies	20	80	—	—	—
Celesia & Daly, 1977b					
Delayed beyond normal latency	53	70	78	33	60
Including L/R discrepancies and reduced HF flicker response		77	81	50	80
Chain et al, 1977	43	77	100	100	65
Hennerici, Wenzel & Freund, 1977					
Checkerboard reversal response	57	61	81	67	43
Response to small foveal square		88	94	94	78
Matthews, Small, Small & Pountney, 1977	113	62	75	58	38
Collins, Black & Mastaglia, 1978	98	52	78	50	23
Kayed, Rosjo and Kass, 1978	60	—	92	61	39
Nilsson, 1978					
Checkerboard	38	68	79	90	30
LED display		81	84	90	70
Shahrokhi, Chiappa & Young, 1978	149	57	82	52	28
Lowitzsch, 1980	251	73	83	77	60
Bodis-Wollner et al, 1979					
Sinusoidal grating. All suspected MS cases	103	62	90	66	-(15)
Tackmann et al, 1979	54	70	96	43	45
Trojaborg & Petersen, 1979	50	74	96	58	20

variable rates for the patients with no history of visual impairment. The variability in the detection rates achieved in the different studies enumerated in Tables 6.2 and 6.3 is indicated by the range of values reported, which are summarized in Table 6.4. It is to be noted that the greatest variability between laboratories is encountered for the probable or possible categories, which represent just that part of the MS patient population where the test is of most clinical value (Halliday, 1980c).

Table 6.3 INCIDENCE OF DELAYED VEPs TO A PATTERN REVERSAL STIMULUS IN MULTIPLE SCLEROSIS PATIENTS WITH AND WITHOUT A HISTORY OF VISUAL DISTURBANCE

| Reference | Definite, probable & possible MS cases | | | | | | Definite MS cases only | | | | | |
| | Overall | | With history of optic neuritis | | Without visual history | | Overall | | With history of optic neuritis | | Without visual history | |
	N	Percent delayed	N	Percent delayed	N	Percent delayed	N	Percent delayed	N	Percent delayed	N	Percent delayed
Halliday et al (1973a)	51	96	24	100	27	93	34	97	17	100	17	94
Asselman et al (1975)	51	67	15	100	36	53	31	84	11	100	20	75
Lowitzsch et al (1976)	135	73	95	82	40	50	73	82	—	—	—	—
Hennerici et al (1977) Checkerboard reversal	57	61	—	—	—	—	16	81	—	100	—	57
Foveal square	57	88	—	—	—	—	—	94	—	100	92	86
Zeese (1977)	—	—	—	—	—	—	26	92*	10	90*	16	94*
Matthews et al (1977)	113	62	36	83	77	52	61	75	28	93	33	61
Nilsson (1978) Checkerboard	38	68	14	93	24	54	19	79	—	—	—	—
LED matrix	—	81	—	93	—	75	—	84	—	—	—	—
Shahrokhi et al (1978)	149	57	62	87	87	36	60	82	41	90	19	63
Tackmann et al (1979)	54	70	25	92	29	52	27	96	19	95	8	100
Trojaborg & Petersen (1979)	50	62	20	96	30	52	28	89	16	94	12	85

*Delayed compared with healthy control group. Comparative figures for patient control group about 20% lower

The underlying reasons for the variability in the percentage of abnormal pattern reversal responses recorded in different laboratories is obscure, but at least two sets of factors must be operating, one related to differences in the stimulating and recording technique and the other to variations in the patient populations under test. The effect of stimulus parameters on the detection rate has been discussed at length elsewhere by the author (Halliday, 1980c). The importance of this factor is illustrated by those studies in which two or more techniques of pattern stimulation have been used on the same group of patients. Examples of such studies are those by Hennerici et al (1977) and Nilsson (1978), who increased their overall percentage of abnormal pattern responses by 27% and 13% respectively by adopting a different stimulus technique (see Tables 6.2 and 6.3). Again, it is to be noted that the largest increase occurred in precisely those diagnostic groups where the test was of most value to the clinician (i.e. patients without a history of optic neuritis or falling within the probable or possible diagnostic categories). It cannot be supposed that we have yet determined the optimal stimulating technique for clinical EP testing. It can also be seen from Tables 6.2 and 6.3 that the sensitivity of the test can be improved by at least 10% by the inclusion of extra measurements, the normal limits of which have been well defined. Purves and Low (1976) increased the overall percentage of abnormalities in their study by 15% by including the measurement of interocular latency differences, while the study by Celesia and Daly (1977b) raised the percentage from 70 to 77% by identifying both interocular latency differences and reduced responses to high frequency flicker.

Table 6.4 RANGE OF VEP ABNORMALITY RATES IN DIFFERENT M.S. STUDIES

	Definite	**Probable**	**Possible**	**Overall**
Limits of Range	75-100%	33-100%	20-92%	50-96%
Difference	25%	66%	72%	46%

	With optic neuritis	**Without optic neuritis**	**Overall**	
Limits of Range	82-100%	36-93%	57-96%	
Difference	18%	57%	39%	All MS
Limits of Range	90-100%	57-100%	75-97%	
Difference	10%	43%	22%	Definite MS only

Studies of the flash EP in multiple sclerosis

As would be expected from the results in optic neuritis (Halliday et al, 1972) the flash EP has proved much less sensitive than the pattern reversal EP when the two responses have been compared in the same group of patients (Halliday et al, 1973a; Duwaer and Spekreijse, 1978; Mauguière et al, 1979; Lowitzsch et al, 1980; Harding et al, 1980; Wilson and Keyser, 1980). Nonetheless, a large number of published studies have reported abnormalities in the flash response in multiple sclerosis, which were quite marked enough to distinguish statistically between a group of patients and a group of healthy controls (Rouher et al, 1969; Richey et al,

1971; Namerow and Enns, 1972; Feinsod et al, 1973; Feinsod and Hoyt, 1975; Regan et al, 1976; Paty et al, 1976; Babel et al, 1977; Ellenberger and Ziegler, 1977; Feinsod et al, 1977; Regan et al, 1977; Paty et al, 1980).

Defects in high frequency following in demyelinating disease

Sclabassi et al (1974) established the existence of a clear defect in the ability of the somatosensory response to follow high frequencies of stimulation in patients with demyelinating disease. The severity of the defect, measured in terms of the maximum frequency at which following would occur, correlated with the severity of the disease. Thus in severely affected multiple sclerosis patients the normal response to trains of stimuli at 100 Hz was abolished and the maximum frequency at which following could occur was reduced to 40 Hz. Regan's group have reported what appears to be a very similar defect in the visual modality, manifest as a reduced ability to respond to high frequency flicker stimulation (Milner et al, 1974; Regan et al, 1976). The deficit appears to be closely related to the reduced critical flicker fusion frequency, which is characteristically found in multiple sclerosis patients (Parsons and Miller, 1957; Titcombe and Willison, 1961; Namerow, 1971). Celesia and Daly (1977b) have proposed routinely measuring the critical frequency of photic driving (CFPD) in patient testing, representing the highest frequency of flash stimulation capable of evoking a distinct train of responses in any particular individual. The characteristic reduction in this high frequency response in demyelinating disease appears to be a quite distinct defect and can occur in patients who have normal pattern reversal responses (Celesia and Daly, 1977b). It seems likely that this represents the result of the reduced ability to conduct fast trains of impulses, already mentioned, which is known to be characteristic of the demyelinated nerve fibre. Regan et al (1976) found a reduced flicker response in 5 out of 13 patients presenting with spinal multiple sclerosis. Six of the 13 also had abnormalities of the pattern reversal EP, but only 2 of the patients were abnormal on both tests. The authors suggested that the patients whose spinal syndrome was of recent onset and unaccompanied by visual signs were more likely to present with the flicker defect, whereas patients with long-standing spinal disease accompanied by visual impairment tended to have delayed pattern responses.

Cohen et al (1980) found the CFPD to yield a higher number of abnormal responses than the checkerboard reversal EP in 27 patients with definite, probable or possible multiple sclerosis, but the difference was not significant. As in the two earlier studies mentioned, there were some patients showing abnormalities on only one of the two tests, emphasizing the value of including both. The CFPD may be of particular value where lowered acuity makes it impossible to obtain a pattern response.

Other alternative stimulation procedures in multiple sclerosis: pattern onset and offset responses and low intensity pattern stimuli

There is some evidence to suggest that detection rates in multiple sclerosis may be increased by the adoption of pattern appearance stimuli rather than pattern reversal stimulation. The study by Hennerici et al (1977) already mentioned produced a 15% increase in the hit rate by recording the responses to a small foveal square subtending 45' in place of the 20° checkerboard stimulus of 70' checks (see Tables 6.2 and 6.3). By the same means Diener and Schiebler (1980) increased the rate from 57% to 73% in those patients without a history of optic neuritis, and from 43% to 67% in the possible MS group. However, Oepen et al (1982a), in comparing a 20° checkerboard reversal stimulus with central foveal stimulation in 200 patients with manifest or suspected MS, found the foveal stimulus much less effective, the response being delayed in only 25% as against 40% for the checkerboard. Moreover, the foveal EP was unobtainable in a third of the patients. These conflicting findings emphasize the importance and difficulty of accurately identifying the relevant stimulus variables. Kriss, Altrocchi and Halliday (unpublished) have compared pattern reversal and pattern onset and offset responses for the same 32° checkerboard field of 50' checks and the same mean luminance, and found the pattern onset and offset responses yielded a lower abnormality rate in a small group of patients with multiple sclerosis. Ochs and Aminoff (1981) and Riemslag et al (1982), on the other hand, have obtained higher abnormality rates for pattern onset and/or offset responses than for pattern reversal. Only further work, combined with a careful scrutiny and control of all the relevant stimulus parameters, will resolve these apparently conflicting results. The potential value of such studies is, however, of obvious importance to the ultimate improvement of EP testing techniques.

The study by Cant et al (1978) has drawn attention to the fact that lowered stimulus intensity in itself may increase the detection rate of delayed responses in demyelinating disease, since the slope of latency against stimulus intensity is apparently steeper than normal in some affected patients, especially in the diagnostically important probable and possible categories. A further study by Hennerici and Wist (1982) supports this conclusion.

Delayed pattern responses in progressive spastic paraparesis

The incidence of delayed pattern responses in patients presenting with progressive spastic paraparesis has been significantly lower in most published studies than the overall rate achieved in patients with multiple sclerosis. This is no doubt partly due to the inclusion of a proportion of cases in which the aetiology is not primary demyelinating disease. Even taking this into account, however, it appears probable that there is a significantly lower incidence of delayed pattern responses in patients with multiple sclerosis presenting in this way. This presumably represents a lower incidence of optic nerve plaques at the time of clinical presentation in this patient group.

Figures from a number of published studies are shown in Table 6.5. The diagnostic criteria employed in the different studies has varied a good deal. As might be expected, those studies which have distinguished between undiagnosed cases and patients in whom the diagnosis of multiple sclerosis could be made on other grounds have invariably shown a higher incidence of pattern EP abnormalities in the latter group. The high overall rates achieved by Bynke et al (1977) and Matthews et al (1977) reflect the high proportion of cases in these two studies where the diagnosis of multiple sclerosis was considered likely (all

Table 6.5 ABNORMALITIES OF THE PATTERN EP IN PROGRESSIVE SPASTIC PARAPARESIS

Reference	Diagnosis	N	Abnormal VEP	%
Halliday, McDonald and Mushin (1974)	Multiple sclerosis	10	8	80
	Cervical spondylosis	2	0	0
	Not diagnosed	13	5	38
	Overall	25	13	52
	Cord compression	2	0	0
Asselman, Chadwick and Marsden (1975)	Multiple sclerosis	34	23	68
	Not diagnosed	10	1	10
	Overall	44	24	55
	Cord compression	6	0	0
	Acute remitting cord lesion	8	2	25
	Spinocerebellar degeneration	5	3	60
	Tropical spastic paraparesis	2	1	50
Bynke, Olsson and Rosén (1977)	With clinical eye signs and CSF abnormalities	5	5	100
	With CSF abnormalities but no eye signs	8	8	100
	Heterogenous group of doubtful aetiology	8	6	80
	Without eye signs or CSF abnormalities	4	0	0
	Overall	25	19	76
Hennerici, Wenzel and Freund (1977)	Multiple sclerosis	20	13[1]	65[1]
			16[2]	80[2]
	Undiagnosed	14	5[1]	36[1]
			6[2]	43[2]
	Overall	34	18[1]	53[1]
			22[2]	65[2]
Matthews, Small, Small and Pountney (1977)	Undiagnosed (possible MS, alternative diagnoses excluded)	9	7[3]	78
Paty et al, 1978	Chronic progressive	72	—	44
Blumhardt, Barrett and Halliday (1982a)	Acute/subacute	31	3	10
	Chronic remitting	36	12	33
	Chronic progressive	64	23	36
	Overall	131	38	29

[1]Checkerboard stimulus with 70′ checks and 20′ diameter field   [2]Foveal square subtending 45′
[3]Including 3 with only L/R latency discrepancy

Matthews' cases fell by definition into the possible MS group and 80% of the patients studied by Bynke et al had CSF abnormalities and/or eye signs in addition to the spinal syndrome). Excluding these two studies the overall rates for checkerboard stimulation varied between 52 and 55%, except in the studies by Paty et al (1978) and Blumhardt et al (1982a), where rather lower overall hit rates of 44% and 29% were obtained. The latter study is significant in that stringent criteria were applied in selecting the patients for the trial with the aim of excluding those with any clear clinical evidence of a lesion above the foramen magnum. Included in the study were 11 patients with acute transverse myelitis, one of whom had delayed pattern responses.

The studies by Asselman et al (1975) and Blumhardt et al (1982a) also included some cases presenting with fluctuating cord lesions, which were accompanied by an incidence of delayed EPs varying between 25 and 33%. The study by Matthews et al (1977) included 39 patients with a single episode of neurological symptoms other than visual failure, three of whom had subacute paraplegia, and also seven patients with chronic undiagnosed neurological disease (e.g. progressive cerebellar ataxia). Two of the acute group and one of the chronic group had abnormal VEPs, including one paraplegic and two patients who presented with sensory symptoms, one of whom subsequently developed definite MS at follow-up.

Among the other conditions entering into the differential diagnosis of progressive spastic paraplegia, in which the VEP may be implicated, are hereditary spastic paraplegia and subacute combined degeneration secondary to pernicious anaemia. Both these conditions will be dealt with below (see pages 217 and 224).

Asymptomatic delayed responses in association with isolated brainstem lesions

Results here have been rather variable. Halliday et al (1973a) found no delayed pattern EPs in six cases and Matthews et al (1977) similarly found none in 16 such cases. Asselman et al (1975), however, found six out of 13 patients with delayed responses and Hennerici et al (1977) found two out of four with abnormal EPs to checkerboard reversal and three out of four to their foveal square stimulus.

Which modality EP test is most useful in the diagnosis of MS?

The status of an EP abnormality in MS is like that of a good clinical sign, and its significance has to be interpreted in the light of the whole clinical context in which it occurs. As has been emphasized, the EP tests are of most value when revealing clinically 'silent' lesions of one of the sensory pathways (visual, auditory or somatosensory). The value of a monocular VEP abnormality will vary with the clinical presentation of the case. A delayed VEP in the clinically unaffected eye in a patient presenting with unilateral optic neuritis is not so significant or informative as a similar subclinical abnormality occurring in a patient presenting with an isolated brainstem or spinal cord syndrome. In exactly the same way, a clearly abnormal BAEP or SEP will gain significance if it is found in the context of a patient presenting with apparently 'pure' retrobulbar neuritis.

The incidence of VEP abnormalities in the absence of a history of optic neuritis has been high in all the published studies (Table 6.3). Indeed, Halliday, McDonald and Mushin (1977) found a substantially higher incidence of *binocular* delays among those multiple sclerosis patients without a history of optic neuritis (81%) than in those with (54%). However, more significant than such overall figures are the figures obtained in the diagnostically more important probable and possible groups. Mastaglia et al (1980) found VEP evidence of optic nerve lesions in 13 out of 33 early probable or latent cases (39%), and of these 13, 11 (84%) were subclinical. Similarly, 21 out of 96 suspected patients (22%) had abnormal VEPs, and of these, 11 (52%) were subclinical. Four out of 5 progressive cases had abnormal VEPs and of these, 2 (50%) were subclinical. They found that subclinical abnormalities of the VEP were particularly helpful in patients in whom the diagnosis was not clinically definite, allowing reclassification of 10 patients from the early probable or latent to the clinically definite group, and 9 patients in the suspected group to the early probable or latent groups. A substantial number of patients can avoid myelography, angiography or pneumoencephalography, or at the very least have it deferred, on the basis of the VEP results.

A number of studies have compared the yield of the VEP with the BAEP and/or SEP on the same group of patients. Stockard et al (1979) found that pattern reversal EPs were abnormal in one-half to two-thirds of all patients with MS and revealed subclinical optic nerve lesions in a third (35 of 107) of patients who had *definite* MS but no signs or symptoms of optic neuropathy. The BAEP, by comparison, was abnormal in only one-third of all MS patients, providing evidence of subclinical lesions in about one-tenth. Chiappa (1980) recorded the pattern reversal EP, BAEP, and median nerve SEP in 70 patients with MS (combined definite, probable and possible). Clinically unsuspected lesions were revealed by 37% of the VEPs, 24% of the BAEPs and 41% of the SEPs. His yield for the BAEP appears somewhat higher than that reported by Stockard et al (1979) and that for the SEP is even higher than for the VEP. Other studies comparing SEP and VEP tests have found the VEP giving a higher overall incidence of abnormality than the SEP, but lower yields for the diagnostically important probable and possible groups. Trojaborg and Petersen (1979), for instance, recorded abnormal pattern VEPs in 36 out of 50 patients with MS (72%), while their rates for abnormalities of the SEP to median or peroneal nerve stimulation were 30/50 (60%) and 32/50 (64%) respectively. Relative rates for the definite, probable and possible cases were 96%, 58% and 20% for the VEP, 64%, 67% and 40% for the median nerve SEP and 64%, 75% and 50% for the peroneal nerve SEP. The peroneal nerve response was therefore particularly favourable for the probable and possible groups. However, it must be remembered that the possible category by definition contains those cases with an undiagnosed spinal cord syndrome in whom MS is suspected. Mastaglia et al (1976) found the median SEP superior to the pattern EP in 52 patients (63% as against 48% abnormal respectively), whereas Small et al (1978) got the opposite result (58% for the SEP, 74% for the VEP).

For the clinician the importance of an EP abnormality depends on its diagnostic significance in any particular patient. Kjaer (1982) in a recent study of the BAEP, VEP, SEP and blink reflexes found that the VEP most often led to the reclassification of patients from the suspected to possible or from possible to probable or definite groups (57% of 49 patients), while the BAEP was the next most successful (42% of 67 patients tested). The SEP results, however, led to reclassification in only

3 (13%) of the 23 cases studied by him, although 55% of those tested were abnormal. The VEP also proved the most clinically useful test in the studies by Maurer and Lowitzsch (1982), Lowitzsch and Maurer (1982) and Deltenre et al (1982). In the study by Tackmann et al (1979) the combined abnormalities in the patients with early probable or latent, progressive possible (paraplegia) and suspected MS were 17/32 (53%) for the VEP, 7/31 (23%) for the BAEP, 11/26 (42%) for the subcortical SEP to median nerve stimulation and 11/31 (35%) for the cortical SEP. Rates were also obtained for the blink reflex, 13/28 (46%), and electronystagmography, 18/32 (56%). The latter test therefore proved better than any of the EP tests in this study.

HEREDITARY OPTIC NEUROPATHIES

Hereditary spastic paraplegia

Happel et al (1980) have recorded the flash EP in both autosomal dominant and recessive forms of hereditary spastic paraplegia (HSP). Six affected members of a large kindred with autosomal recessive HSP were studied as well as 5 obligate heterozygotes (the children of patients with the recessive condition) and 5 affected members of a family with autosomal dominant HSP. There was no quantitative or qualitative difference between the flash VEPs in the two types of HSP, but all showed prolonged latencies. In 9 out of 11 patients the delay was marked, while in the two other patients, both early cases, the latencies were slightly prolonged but not beyond normal limits. The responses of the most advanced cases also showed a reduced amplitude and degradation of the normal waveform. The abnormalities were invariably binocular (a notable difference from the abnormalities of multiple sclerosis patients), and they were unaccompanied by any clinical signs of visual impairment. All the patients had normal acuity, colour vision and fundi, and none had any field defects. The obligate heterozygotes all had normal responses, so that the VEP does not apppear to be of any value in detecting the carrier state.

Pedersen and Trojaborg (1981) have recently reported a study on the pattern reversal EP, as well as the SEP and BAEP, in 13 patients from 8 families with familial spastic paraplegia, 9 autosomal dominant and 4 recessive. In contrast to the 2 families studied by Happel et al (1980) only 3 of the patients showed an increased $\overline{P100}$ latency (in 2 of them from both eyes) the other 10 having responses within the normal range. The 2 binocularly delayed cases were of the dominant type, while the uniocularly delayed case was recessive, so that again delayed VEPs were not confined to either genetic type.

Friedreich's ataxia

A number of the earlier studies (e.g. Halliday et al, 1973a; Asselman et al, 1975) reported finding delayed pattern reversal responses in cases with spinocerebellar degeneration. Carroll et al (1980c) have recently published a study of the pattern EP abnormalities in 22 patients with Friedreich's ataxia selected with stringent diagnostic criteria. The particular interest of this group of patients is that the underlying pathology of this condition is now accepted as being an axonal degeneration. The results on this group can therefore be validly compared with those obtained in primary demyelinating disease to represent the 'typical' findings to be expected in Wallerian degeneration on the one hand and segmental demyelination on the other. Although visual acuity was normal in half the patients and was only mildly impaired (up to 6/18) in the other half, 12 of the 22 patients showed delayed $\overline{P100}$ components to the standard 0-16° checkerboard reversal stimulus and a further two showed abnormalities in the responses to half-field or central-field stimuli. Many of the responses were of small amplitude and one patient

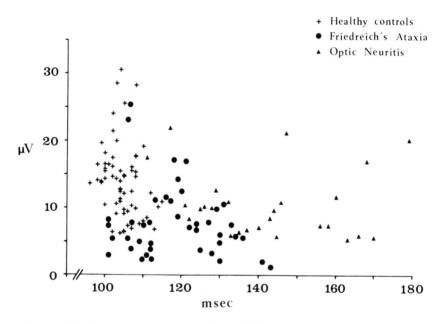

Figure 6.18 *Latency and amplitude of the $\overline{P100}$ component from each eye of 31 healthy controls (+), 21 patients with Friedreich's ataxia (●) and from the affected eyes of 24 patients who had recovered from a single typical episode of either monocular (22) or binocular (2) optic neuritis (▲). In contrast to the patients with Friedreich's ataxia the cases of optic neuritis show a clear dissociation between the $\overline{P100}$ latency increase and the amplitude changes. Mean $\overline{P100}$ latencies and amplitudes for the 3 groups were: Normals 105 msec, 14.03 μV; Friedreich's ataxia patients 118 msec, 7.6 μV; Optic neuritis 142 msec, 10.4 μV. (From Carroll et al, 1980c.)*

showed no pattern response to the standard stimulus in one eye although the acuity was still 6/18. There were some striking differences in the character of the abnormalities compared with those encountered in primary demyelinating disease (see Figure 6.18). Among these were that (1) the responses, even where abnormal, were generally very similar in the two eyes and showed none of the gross unilateral changes encountered in multiple sclerosis. As a consequence there were few additional abnormalities to be detected by examining latency, amplitude or waveform differences between the two eyes; (2) the range of delays of the $\overline{P100}$ component was much smaller than that encountered in demyelinating disease;

the maximum delay recorded was 143 msec; (3) although the amplitude of the patients' responses could not be defined individually as below the normal range, owing to the large variability of response size in the healthy population, the patients' responses were as a group significantly reduced in amplitude compared with either the healthy population or an age-matched group of patients with demyelinating disease (Figure 6.18); (4) in contrast to the situation in demyelinating optic neuritis, where amplitude and latency vary independently of each other (Figures 6.2 and 6.3), there was a highly significant inverse correlation between the latency and amplitude of the response in the group of patients with delayed $\overline{P100}$ components (Figure 6.18); (5) as in the patients with optic neuritis, there was some correlation between the reduction in the amplitude and the visual acuity level (Figure 6.19), although the slope appears steeper.

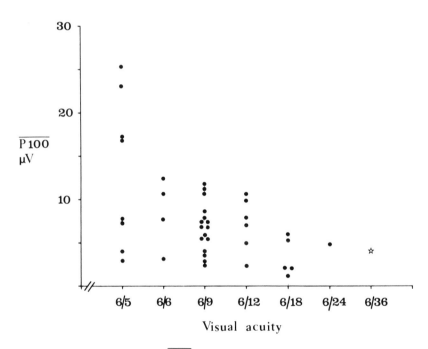

Figure 6.19 *Relation between $\overline{P100}$ amplitude and visual acuity in 22 patients with Friedreich's ataxia. The single eye with an acuity worse than 6/24 (marked with an asterisk) was from a patient who had sustained a penetrating left eye injury in the past. Amplitude and acuity was significantly correlated (p < 0.001). (From Carroll et al, 1980c.)*

As already stated, 12 out of the 22 patients (55%) had the $\overline{P100}$ component delayed more than 2.5 standard deviations above the normal mean. An example of such a delayed response is shown in Figure 6.20. In about 45% of the patients, therefore, the response latency was within the normal range. However, this group of patients also showed a highly significant reduction in the amplitude of the pattern response, even though this was not beyond normal limits in an individual case

F. S.
Case 10

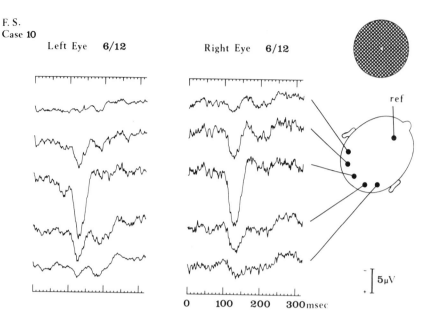

Figure 6.20 *Bilaterally delayed pattern reversal responses from a 33-year-old woman with Friedreich's ataxia. Note that the responses are very similar from each eye, with $\overline{P100}$ latencies of 131 msec and 129 msec respectively (upper limit of normal 115 msec). (From Carroll et al, 1980c.)*

I.N.
Case 14

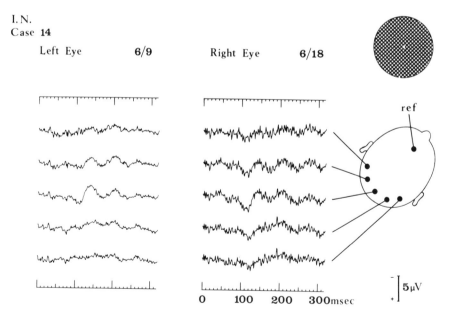

Figure 6.21 *Example of a pattern response of very low amplitude, but normal latency, from a 31-year-old man with Friedreich's ataxia. (From Carroll et al, 1980c.)*

(Figure 6.18). A typical example of such a reduced pattern EP of normal latency is shown in Figure 6.21. Neither temporal dispersion nor waveform changes were encountered in this group of patients. This feature of the responses distinguishes them from many of those encountered in compressive lesions, where waveform change is common, and from some of those seen in demyelinating disease.

The mean amplitude of the $\overline{P100}$ for the Friedreich's ataxia group was 7.6 ± 5.3 µV as compared with 14.03 ± 5.5µV for the healthy controls. The amplitude was significantly smaller than for either the normals (p < 0.001) or the age-matched optic neuritis cases (p < 0.01). Many of the Friedreich's ataxia patients had $\overline{P100}$ amplitudes less than 6 µV, the lowest amplitude recorded in the healthy control group. The abnormalities in the pattern response correlated well with the finding of temporal pallor on fundoscopy.

Wenzel et al (1982) recorded the pattern EP in 35 patients with Friedreich's ataxia using a TV stimulator, and found abnormal responses in 54% of their cases, in good agreement with the study by Carroll et al (1980c). Pedersen and Trojaborg (1981) examined the pattern EP, SEP and BAEP in 7 patients with Friedreich's ataxia and also in 11 patients with hereditary cerebellar ataxia with onset between the 3rd and 5th decade, 7 of the latter group showing autosomal dominant inheritance and 3 recessive. Five of the 7 Friedreich patients had abnormal VEPs (in 1 case uniocular) with increased $\overline{P100}$ latencies and reduced amplitudes. Four of the 11 patients with late onset hereditary cerebellar ataxia had increased $\overline{P100}$ latencies from both eyes and 6 had responses of normal latency, while no responses could be obtained in one other patient. The mean increase in latency was smaller than for the Friedreich patients.

Leber's optic atrophy

Dorfman et al (1977) studied the checkerboard reversal EP serially in two brothers with Leber's optic neuropathy during the active phase of the disease. The responses were normal until the onset of visual symptoms, but developed a progressively prolonged latency and reduced amplitude in parallel with the diminishing visual acuity. The response was eventually abolished in 2 of the 4 eyes. They also noted a change in the waveform of the response with the development of a bifid positivity. The VEPs in asymptomatic family members appeared normal.

Carroll and Mastaglia (1979) have studied the checkerboard pattern reversal response in 14 clinically affected members of a single family with Leber's optic neuropathy. Nine of these patients, all except two of whom had severe visual impairment of 6/60 or worse, had no recordable pattern responses, while four of the five others showed marked abnormalities of the major positivity, including reduced amplitude, a broadened or even bifid waveform and delayed latency. The abnormalities were generally equally marked in the responses from both eyes, but were either restricted to, or more marked in, the affected eye in two patients with only monocular involvement. In a follow-up study of six of these patients after an interval of 13-15 months, the EP findings had either remained unchanged or shown further deterioration. There was thus no evidence of the increases in amplitude with returning acuity nor of the rarely encountered return to normal latency observed in patients with primary demyelinating disease. The authors do not give detailed information about the latency changes in their patients, but comment that the responses were in general less delayed than those found in patients with demyelinating optic neuropathy, but that they had a more marked reduction in amplitude and alteration in waveform. In the absence of half-field stimulation it is not clear whether the 'delayed' positivity should be regarded as a $\overline{P100}$ of prolonged latency or an undelayed $\overline{P135}$ associated with a central scotoma, although the latter explanation seems the more likely. Central field defects were noted in all but two of the patients. The atypical bifid positivity found in six of the 14 subjects is also likely to represent the type of waveform change associated with a central scotomatous defect (Blumhardt et al, 1978; Halliday, 1976; Halliday et al, 1979; Kriss et al, 1982). However, the checkerboard stimulus used in this study was limited to the 0-3° central field and was made up of 12′ checks, so that it would not have been very favourable for detecting any such change.

Babel et al (1977) report that the flash EP was abolished in 9 out of 14 eyes from patients with Leber's optic neuropathy. The amplitude was pathologically diminished in all five of the other cases and three of them showed delayed latencies. They also report a case in which the flash EP was still present after the ERG had been abolished.

Dominant hereditary optic atrophy

Babel et al (1977) were able to record the flash EP in only one out of six patients with hereditary optic atrophy. The surviving response was an occipital VEP of reduced amplitude but normal latency. The flash ERG in both Leber's and hereditary optic atrophy is usually normal. Total optic atrophy is therefore characterized by an abolished occipital EP and a persistent ERG, while in incomplete optic atrophy the EP may still be present but of reduced amplitude. Cases of both types are found among patients with hereditary optic atrophy. The author's own experience with the pattern EP in cases of dominant hereditary optic atrophy is that these cases show a response of normal latency with an amplitude diminishing in parallel with the visual failure. Halliday et al (1977b), for instance, refer to three families with congenital optic atrophy in whom it was only possible to record a pattern EP of very small amplitude associated with severe visual impairment. Some patients may show a scotomatous defect on perimetry and this again may be associated with an apparently delayed or bifid positivity, representing an exaggerated contribution from the paramacular $\overline{P135}$ component. Such waveform changes are usually less florid and less frequently encountered in this condition than they are, for instance, in toxic amblyopia. Only 2 of 12 cases recorded in the author's laboratory (Carroll et al, unpublished) had normal pattern responses, but the responses were only completely absent in one case, and five had a recognizable $\overline{P100}$ of normal latency. An example of the apparently delayed positivity encountered in some patients in association with the scotomatous changes is shown in Figure 6.22. Half-field stimulation demonstrates that there is a reduction in the ipsilateral NPN complex combined with an enhancement of the contralateral PNP such as is seen in association with experimental central scotomata (see Figures 3.33-34). The asymmetric full-field positive component at approximately 135 msec has contributions from the paramacular $\overline{P135}$ components from each half-field.

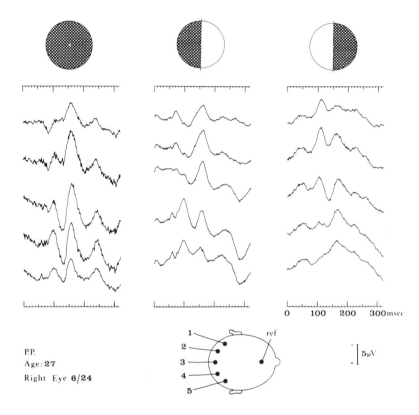

Figure 6.22 *Pattern reversal EPs from the right eye of a 27-year-old man with dominant hereditary optic atrophy. Note that the major positivity of the full-field response is made up largely of the summated contralateral paramacular P135 components from each half-field, although there is also a small contribution from the residual ipsilateral P100 component from the nasal field. The responses are therefore consistent with the centrocaecal scotoma so frequently observed in this condition. (From Carroll and Kriss, 1981.)*

Harding and Crews (1982) have reported on the flash and pattern reversal EPs in 27 members of 6 affected families with dominant optic atrophy. Relatively few of these patients showed a central scotoma on Goldmann perimetry, but they found the flash EP in most of the affected patients exhibiting a PNP-type response with a negative component at a latency of about 100 msec. Pattern stimulation also gave PNP-type responses in some cases, but more commonly the pattern EP showed a reduction in amplitude. Neither the flash nor pattern PNP complexes were found to be significantly associated with central field defects in this study.

Charcot-Marie-Tooth disease

Tackmann and Radu (1980) have recorded delayed checkerboard reversal EPs in 5 out of 9 patients with Charcot-Marie-Tooth disease (CMT), 8 of whom came from 6 families with an autosomal dominant inheritance. None of the patients had any clinical signs of optic nerve involvement. Motor nerve conduction velocities ranged from 17-29 metres/second. A checkerboard of 41' squares, subtending 12°, evoked pathologically delayed $\overline{P100}$s in 7 eyes, but the interocular differences were within normal limits. The delayed responses all fell within 5 msec of the upper end of the normal latency range. The mean amplitude of the VEP was significantly lowered to about half that in the control group. McLeod et al (1978) have reported similar findings in Charcot-Marie-Tooth disease associated with Leber's optic atrophy. Our own observations of CMT disease have confirmed the incidence of prolonged latencies in a proportion of cases. (Halliday et al, 1981).

We recorded 15 cases, all except 2 of which had a markedly reduced motor conduction velocity, putting them into the Type I CMTD group, characterized pathologically by segmental demyelination. Unequivocally delayed pattern responses to the standard 16° checkerboard were recorded in 3 patients, all of whom showed clinical evidence of CNS involvement, and a borderline delay was recorded in one other. Three further cases exhibited an abnormal response only to stimulation of the central 4°. One other patient with a central scotoma had the typical associated VEP change. Overall, therefore, 4 out of 15 patients had definitely 'abnormal' pattern EPs and another 4 had borderline changes. The group data showed only a small, but insignificant, increase of 4 msec in the mean $\overline{P100}$ latency, which was largely attributable to the 3 patients with definitely delayed responses. The findings were thus markedly different from those in Friedreich's ataxia.

SUBACUTE COMBINED DEGENERATION

Troncoso et al (1979) have recorded abnormal checkerboard reversal EPs in all three patients with pernicious anaemia and subacute combined degeneration studied by them. Two of the three patients had abnormally low serum B_{12} levels and a positive Schilling's test, and all three showed marked reticulocytosis following B_{12} treatment. The only visual abnormality detectable clinically was mildly defective colour vision in one patient who also exhibited multiple bilateral small flame-shaped retinal haemorrhages. The normal data from this study from a control group of 26 eyes gave a mean $\overline{P100}$ latency of 99.4 msec $\pm$ 5.2 msec. The authors adopted as their criterion of abnormality any response lying beyond the 95% percentile, which they took as 107.0 msec. On this index, 5 of the 6 eyes gave responses beyond the normal range. However, it is clear that if the more acceptable 2.5 s.d. had been taken as the criterion, giving an upper limit of normal of 112.4 msec, only one of the six eyes would have been classified as delayed. Fine and Hallett (1980) have recorded sensory nerve action potentials, the subcortical and cortical SEPs, the BAEP and the checkerboard reversal EP in 3 patients with subacute combined degeneration. The BAEPs were normal, but both SEPs and VEPs showed increased latencies, these being more marked for the somatosensory responses, especially from the lower limb. All 3 cases showed cortical SEPs delayed by a few msec and 2 out of 3 had delayed $\overline{P100}$s, between 114 and 134 msec. The upper limit of normal latency is given by these authors as 108 msec, although no mean or standard deviation is given for the control group and there is no indication of the criterion adopted. These results on patients with subacute combined degeneration are of great interest because of their relevance to the differential diagnosis of patients presenting with a spinal cord syndrome, and also because of the possible implication of B_{12} deficiency in nutritional amblyopia. The VEP in the latter condition is dealt with in Chapter 7 (page 262).

COMPRESSIVE LESIONS OF THE OPTIC NERVE

The pattern EP has proved particularly sensitive to the effect of compression of the optic nerve, and changes can be seen early, even before visual acuity is greatly impaired and when clinical signs are still minimal (Halliday et al, 1976). A gross distortion in the waveform of the response is the most characteristic abnormality seen. The peak latency may also be slightly delayed, but the absolute increase in latency is usually much smaller than that seen in primary demyelinating disease. For instance, none of the 19 patients with compressive lesions of the anterior visual pathways studied by Halliday et al (1976) had P100 components delayed more than 20 msec beyond the upper limit of the normal latency range for their age, and the longest latency recorded in any patient was 137 msec. By contrast, the mean delay in the 51 patients with multiple sclerosis studied in the same laboratory was 43 msec, and individual patients were encountered with delays up to 100 msec (see Figure 6.17).

A striking example of the sensitivity of the pattern response to early compression is provided by the patient whose responses are shown in Figure 6.23. A 46-year-old woman presented on 17.11.72 with a history of blurring of vision and headaches for ten months. Visual acuity was still normal (VAR 6/9, VAL 6/6), but compared with a well-formed pattern EP of normal latency from the left eye, the response from the right eye is markedly altered in waveform, with a broadening of the positivity, which, unlike that from the other eye, has no well-defined peak. The two negative peaks preceding and following the positivity have also become blunted. Formal measurement of such a response will indicate a 'delay' in the positive peak from the right eye, but it is not clear whether this is simply due to the distortion of the normal waveform, as the onset of the positivity is not appreciably delayed. At the time of this record, the patient was undiagnosed. She returned for follow-up, six months later, on 23.5.73, by which time acuity in the right eye was down to the perception of hand movements. On this occasion the pattern response from this eye is almost abolished, although there is a suggestion of a small very delayed positive inflexion at 150-160 msec. There is also a striking change in the response from the other, supposedly unaffected, eye, whose acuity was still 6/6. The positivity is reduced in amplitude and its peak is delayed by a few milliseconds, although not beyond the upper limit of the normal range. The initial negative component has been almost completely lost. It is worth emphasizing that there was no sign of any abnormality from this eye on clinical testing. On this occasion, air encephalography was carried out and a right anterior clinoid meningioma was found and removed at operation. The following record, taken a few days later, post-operatively, shows no improvement in the pattern response from the affected eye (visual acuity 6/60), but the response from the 'unaffected' eye shows a remarkable degree of recovery, with an increased amplitude of the response and a partial return

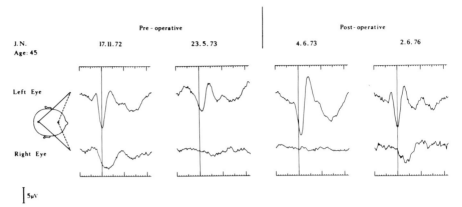

Figure 6.23 *Serial recordings of the midline pattern reversal response from each eye of a patient with a right anterior clinoid meningioma. At the time of the first record she was undiagnosed but had a 10-month history of blurring of vision in the right eye with some temporal pallor of the right optic disc. Visual acuity in this eye was 6/9 and the waveform of the response was greatly altered. Six months later acuity in this eye was reduced to the perception of hand movements and the pattern response was almost abolished. At this stage the diagnosis was made by air encephalography and the tumour was surgically removed. Ten days later the acuity in the right eye had improved to 6/60, but the pattern response had not returned. Three years later, although the acuity had remained unchanged at 6/60, the response from the right eye shows a dramatic improvement and resembles that in the initial pre-operative record. Note the subtler serial changes apparent in the response from the clinically unaffected left eye.*

of the early negative component. The peak latency is still, however, showing the few milliseconds delay which had been observed in the second record. In the last record, taken three years later, the response from the left eye has returned to its original normal form, with a well-developed initial negativity and a return to the original peak latency. The response from the right eye, in spite of an unaltered visual acuity at 6/60, has also shown remarkable improvement since the third record, although the form of the response still shows many of the abnormal features observed in the original record of 17.11.72. Both the degree of alteration of the response from the affected eye at the earliest attendance, when the visual acuity and clinical signs were minimal, and the significant changes in the response from the 'unaffected' left eye, illustrate the sensitivity of the pattern response to the early effects of compressive lesions.

Orbital lesions may cause somewhat less marked changes, particularly in the early stages, presumably because the contents of the orbit can expand forward to alleviate the effects of compression. Three of the four cases studied by Halliday et al (1976) showed only a reduction in amplitude, although the fourth, a 58-year-old man with a neurilemmoma, had a pattern response which was both reduced in amplitude and delayed in the affected eye (Figure 6.24). Where the tumour is well encapsulated at the apex of the orbit, however, the effects of compression may be more severe. Figure 6.25 shows the pattern reversal, pattern onset/offset and flash EPs recorded from a 55-year-old woman, whose CAT scan is shown in Figure 6.26.

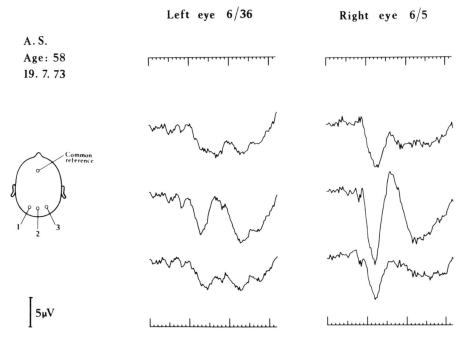

Left eye 6/36   Right eye 6/5

A. S.
Age: 58
19. 7. 73

Common reference

1   2   3

5μV

Figure 6.24 *Monocular pattern reversal EPs from a 58-year-old man with an intra-orbital neurilemmoma of the left optic nerve sheath. Note the normal response from the right eye and the delayed response of reduced amplitude from the left eye. (From Halliday and Mushin, 1980.)*

At the time of this recording visual acuity in the affected eye was reduced to the perception of light. The pattern reversal and pattern onset/offset responses are both abolished from this eye, but the flash EP is still recordable, and shows a marked delay compared with the flash response from the unaffected eye. This illustrates the usefulness of the flash EP, which is more robust than either the pattern reversal or pattern onset/offset responses, and may still be obtainable even where visual function is grossly impaired.

Intracranial tumours, particularly sphenoidal wing and suprasellar meningiomas, produce marked changes in the pattern response early in the clinical syndrome. Four of the five cases studied by Halliday et al (1976) had absent responses from the affected eye, although in one of these patients the flash response was still present at this time and could be seen to be delayed.

Babel et al (1977) recorded the flash EP in 17 cases of compression due to a tumour and found it absent in 5. Of the 12 persisting responses, 10 had a reduced amplitude and 4 a delayed latency. These authors stress the value of the flash EP in compressive lesions and emphasize the occurrence of abnormalities even from an eye showing no visual impairment. As with the pattern response, surgical decompression, if followed by rapid post-operative improvement in the flash EP, is a good prognostic sign. Even the flash response may show early changes in

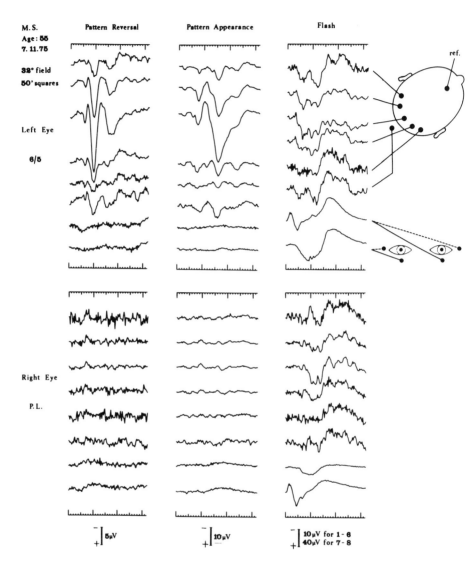

Figure 6.25 *Pattern reversal, pattern appearance and flash evoked EPs recorded in a 55-year-old woman with a space-occupying lesion of the right orbit (see Figure 6.26). Both pattern reversal and pattern appearance responses are abolished from the affected eye, but the flash response is still present, although definitely delayed in latency compared with the response from the other eye. (From Halliday and Mushin, 1980.)*

compressive lesions. Babel et al describe an 11-year-old boy with a pinealoma who had a significantly reduced flash EP at a time when the visual acuity was still good and the fields practically normal.

Rouher et al (1969), who recorded the flash response in 11 patients with compressive lesions of the optic nerve, stress that there is frequently a clear discordance between the clinical and electrophysiological findings. They found that by the use of red and blue monochromatic filters placed in front of the flash tube to stimulate selectively the central and peripheral parts of the field, they were on many occasions able to predict the post-operative loss of central vision from the abolition of the flash EP to red light. Ebe et al (1964) recorded six patients with bilateral optic atrophy secondary to a brain tumour. The flash ERG was normal in all except one of the 12 eyes, but the occipital EP was abolished in nine and was pathological in the other three eyes.

Among other studies of the checkerboard reversal EP in optic nerve compression have been those of Asselman et al (1975), who found delayed pattern EPs in each of two patients, Mastaglia et al (1976) who recorded normal pattern EPs

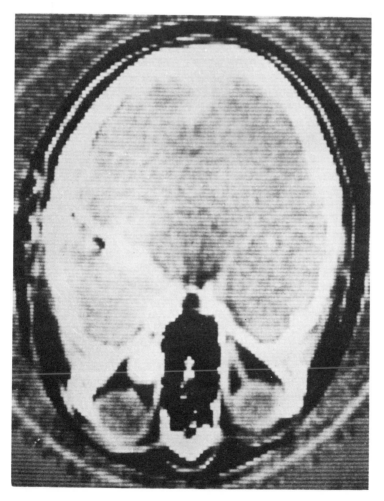

Figure 6.26 *Computerized axial tomography (CAT) scan from the patient whose VEPs are illustrated in Figure 6.25, showing the well-encapsulated mass at the apex of the right orbit. (From Halliday and Mushin, 1980.)*

in two patients 2-3 years after removal of suprasellar craniopharyngiomas, and a delayed response pre- and post-operatively in an 80-year-old woman with a pituitary adenoma, and Hennerici et al (1977) who recorded delayed pattern EPs in two patients with posterior fossa tumours.

Presellar aneurysm

Mastaglia et al (1976) report finding normal pattern responses in a patient with intermittent visual loss due to an aneurysm of the anterior communicating artery, but they also recorded grossly abnormal responses with no recognizable components in another patient with a presellar carotid aneurysm. Figure 6.27 was recorded in the author's department from a 57-year-old woman with a history of 12 months progressive, but variable, loss of vision in the left eye. Investigation revealed a giant aneurysm arising from the left internal carotid artery in the region of the left anterior choroid and extending medially over the sella. During the recording session of 30-45 minutes duration, the pattern EP and the visual acuity came and went in parallel while the left eye responses were being recorded, presumably due to changes in the size of the mass impinging on and compressing the optic nerve fibres. Figure 6.27 shows all the responses recorded serially from the affected eye during this session, some to full-field and some to half-field stimulation. The results emphasize the extreme lability of the reversible conduction block produced by some compressive lesions.

Optic nerve glioma

In the author's experience the changes in the pattern response associated with intrinsic tumours of the optic nerve are rather similar to those encountered with extrinsic compression. The waveform of the response tends to be distorted early in the disease, and the pattern response is reduced in amplitude and eventually abolished in parallel with the increasing visual impairment. The test may continue to give useful information, however, with regard to the extension of the tumour posteriorly to involve the chiasmal fibres or even the fibres on the opposite side. A good example of this is shown in Figure 6.28, which illustrates three serial recordings taken over a three year period from a girl with a right optic nerve glioma. At the time of the first record, made at the age of 11, only a vestige of the pattern response from the affected eye was still present (visual acuity was already down to perception of hand movements) and no response could be recorded on the two subsequent attendances (there is some obtrusive background alpha in the third record). The responses from the left eye, on the other hand, show a clear asymmetry of the type seen in temporal hemianopia (i.e. a right half-field response from the left eye). In the subsequent two records this asymmetry has had added to it a progressively 'scotomatous' type of change, with relative attenuation of the ipsilateral macular NPN complex and relative enhancement of the contralateral paramacular PNP complex (see pages 113-116 for an explanation). The asymmetry demonstrates that the tumour is already involving the function of the fibres crossing from the left eye in the chiasma. It must therefore, even at the age of 11, have

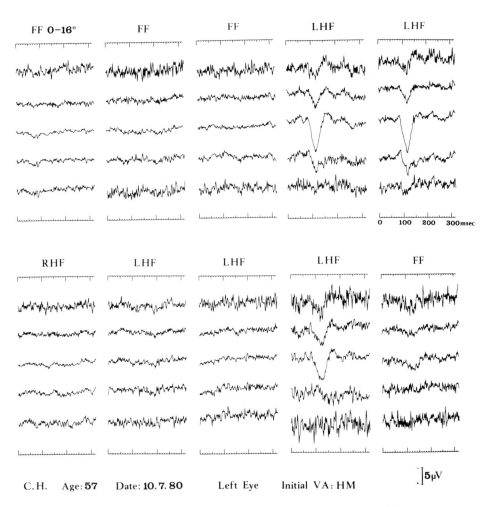

FF 0–16°   FF   FF   LHF   LHF

0   100   200   300 msec

RHF   LHF   LHF   LHF   FF

C.H.   Age: 57   Date: 10. 7. 80   Left Eye   Initial VA: HM

5 µV

Figure 6.27 *Ten consecutive average pattern reversal responses recorded during one continuous session in a 57-year-old woman with compression of the left optic nerve due to a giant aneurysm arising from the left internal carotid artery. The first 3 responses were recorded to a full-field checkerboard stimulus subtending a radius of 16° from the fixation point, and then to a left half-field stimulus (twice) a right half-field stimulus (once) the left half-field stimulus again (three times) and the full-field stimulus again. The patient, having being unable to see the stimulus, suddenly reported that she could clearly see it during the recording of the fourth and fifth responses. It then became invisible again until it reappeared during the ninth record and finally disappeared during the last record. The subjective fluctuations in vision therefore closely paralleled the appearance and disappearance of the pattern EP. (Kriss and Halliday, unpublished).*

extended back to chiasmal levels. The further changes indicate the development of a central scotoma in the surviving half-field of the good eye and must therefore involve spread of the tumour to affect the uncrossed fibres from the left side.

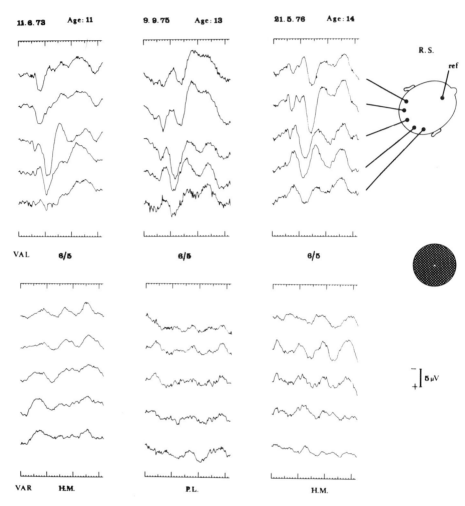

Figure 6.28 *Serial records of the pattern reversal response at the age of 11, 13 and 14 years in a patient with a right optic nerve glioma. Apart from the small residual midline positivity seen in the first record, no clear response can be identified in the records from the right eye (below), but the responses from the left eye (above) show the typical asymmetry associated with a temporal hemianopia, with the major positive component appearing in the right-sided and midline channels. (compare Figure 3.14 and 7.14-15). Note the additional changes typical of the gradual development of a central scotoma in the 'preserved' nasal field of the left eye, with the contralateral PNP complex becoming increasingly dominant over the ipsilateral NPN complex (compare Figures 3.33-34). (From Halliday, 1976.)*

Vaughan and Katzman (1964) recorded normal flash ERGs in an infant with bilateral optic nerve gliomas. The occipital flash EP was absent in the more severely affected left eye and of abnormal form and reduced in amplitude from the other eye, where only an asymmetrical wave III could be recognized. Mastaglia et al (1976) recorded a grossly abnormal pattern reversal EP with no recognizable components in one patient with optic nerve glioma.

DIAGNOSTIC SIGNIFICANCE OF DIFFERENT PATTERN EP ABNORMALITIES

A refreshingly original approach to the clinical application of pattern-evoked response recording is provided in the paper by Ikeda et al (1978), who have adopted the opposite strategy to most published studies by first attempting to classify the types of pattern reversal EP abnormality encountered in a busy clinic, and then going on to examine the type of clinical case associated with each class of VEP abnormality. They looked at the VEP and ERG abnormalities recorded in patients presenting with suspected optic nerve lesions in the Vision Research Unit at St Thomas' Hospital, London. After excluding patients with hereditary optic atrophy, systemic disorders or optic nerve lesions associated with retinal disease, they ended up with a series of records from 83 patients with suspected primary optic nerve lesions. They found that these could be divided into three categories:

1. Those with a normal ERG and a delayed pattern response of normal amplitude (including those with an abnormally large latency discrepancy between the response from the two eyes).
2. Those records with a subnormal ERG accompanying a pattern response of reduced amplitude and delayed latency.
3. Those records with a subnormal ERG accompanied by a pattern response of normal latency but often reduced amplitude.

They suggest that the significance of these three types is that they point to different pathological lesions. The delayed pattern response of normal amplitude in the first group suggests a demyelinating lesion of the optic nerve, while the additional reduction in the size of the ERG and in the amplitude of the cortical response in the second group suggests an added element of axonal involvement, leading to both orthograde and retrograde transneuronal degeneration. The reduced amplitude of both ERG and cortical response with an undelayed latency in the third group suggests a generalized cellular and axonal involvement, without demyelination.

Having classified their records, the authors then went on to look and see what were the clinical findings in the patients falling into the three groups:

1. They found that the first group included patients who were finally diagnosed as multiple sclerosis with optic neuritis, but that it comprised particularly those patients who had either no history of any visual deficit or only a sudden loss of vision from which they had recovered.
2. The second group, with a reduced amplitude of the response and some subnormality of the ERG, also included patients diagnosed as having demyelinating disease, but these were typically those in whom visual loss was the main feature, and this was often more severe and permanent. There were also included in this group, unlike category 1, a number of patients with

suspected ischaemic optic neuropathy and patients with compressive lesions affecting the optic nerve or chiasma. Most of the patients in this group had temporal pallor and pupillary defects.

3. The third group of patients, who showed reduced amplitude of both the ERG and the cortical response but no change in latency, could be divided into two distinct clinical diagnostic categories. The first of these comprised 17 patients with toxic amblyopia, either secondary to tobacco and alcohol (15 patients) or in two cases to West Indian amblyopia or quinine amblyopia. The changes in the VEP and ERG were reversible with a combination of vitamin B_{12} and abstinence. The other sub-group all came with a long history of progressive painless visual loss and bilateral optic atrophy of no known cause. There was no family history of visual loss, and none of the patients had a history of drinking or smoking. This group therefore comprises non-familial bilateral optic atrophy of unknown cause.

The results of this study are particularly interesting because they represent one of the most careful and authoritative reports of ERG changes in association with optic nerve lesions.

It has to be emphasized, as the earlier studies have repeatedly pointed out (Halliday et al, 1973a, 1977, 1976), that none of the EP abnormalities encountered is specific for any pathological lesion. Delays may be encountered, not only in primary demyelinating disease, but also in compressive lesions, spinocerebellar degenerations, ischaemic optic neuropathy and a host of other conditions mentioned elsewhere in this book. An EP abnormality has the status of a good clinical sign and must, like an upgoing toe, be interpreted in the clinical context of the case in which it presents itself. Certain features of the EP may be characteristic of a particular disease, but they are not specific for it, with the possible exception of the very much enhanced response of myoclonic epilepsy. Thus, delays of more than 30 msec or so are much commoner in multiple sclerosis than in compressive lesions, while a uniocular abnormality would be unusual in conditions like Friedreich's ataxia or Leber's optic atrophy. But exceptions do occur to these general rules, and the wise evoked potential worker will exercise caution and restraint in interpreting his findings.

7

The Visual Evoked Potential in the Investigation of Chiasmal and Retro-chiasmal Lesions and Field Defects

A.M. Halliday

INTRODUCTION

The VEP recorded in association with field defects comes from the spared field

In studying field defects with the visual evoked potential one is recording the partial absence of the normal response, rather than a positive abnormality. In hemianopia, for instance, the response which can be recorded is actually derived from stimulation of the preserved half-field and corresponds to the type of response produced by stimulation of that half-field in a healthy subject. Unless there is also some other additional lesion affecting the area of preserved vision (e.g. a partial demyelinating lesion of the afferent pathways concerned) the response will have a normal latency and waveform and will differ from the healthy response only by virtue of the loss of the contribution from the blind area of the field.

This principle, which is broadly true with only a few exceptions which will be mentioned later, implies that the recognition of abnormal responses in the presence of field defects is equivalent to distinguishing the responses produced in the healthy subject by stimulating smaller component parts of the field from the normal full-field response. This topic has already been discussed in some detail in Chapter 3 in relation to the normal VEP. It was shown there that the normal full-field response can be regarded as the sum of the responses from each half-field. In its turn the half-field response is equivalent to the algebraic summation of the responses to the upper and lower quadrants making up the half-field. In general, the response from any area of the visual field is equal to the sum of the responses from its constituent parts.

This principle seems to apply down to quite small areas of the field, although, because of the diminishing size of the response from smaller areas, there is a limit to the extent to which it can be experimentally verified. Apart from the general increase in amplitude with increasing stimulus size, the main differences between the responses from different parts of the field lie in the important changes in the topography of the VEP over the back of the head when different areas of the field are stimulated, changes which no doubt reflect the varying position and orientation of the retinotopically-organized cortical generator areas in relation to the scalp electrodes. There are also significant alterations in the waveform of the response when comparing half-field or quadrant stimulation with the composite full-field response. These are due to the asymmetric form of the half-field responses (both for left and right half-fields and for upper and lower half-fields) in which components of opposite polarity may be recorded on different parts of the head, which disappear through cancellation when both parts of the field are combined in the full-field response. A number of examples of this process are illustrated in Figures 3.31 and 3.32.

The clinical value of the VEP in the study of field defects

From what has been said it might be supposed that the use of the visual EP in field defects provided a method of carrying out an objective form of perimetry, not requiring the co-operation of the subject. This is not quite true for two complementary reasons. In the first place, the use of the pattern response to study field defects requires a certain minimum amount of subjective co-operation from the patient with regard to fixation. In a hemianopic patient good fixation is not as essential as it is, for instance, in the study of half-field responses in healthy subjects, because a large stimulus field, designed to include all the areas of preserved vision, will itself produce the characteristic asymmetry of the field defect (Figure 7.1). But the patient must be willing to co-operate to the extent of watching the stimulus field throughout the recording session. In the second place, the EP technique cannot really be regarded as competitive with traditional subjective perimetry. The latter technique can in a relatively short time yield detailed information about the shape and position of field defects, even of small scotomata, of a kind which the VEP technique could not hope to equal.

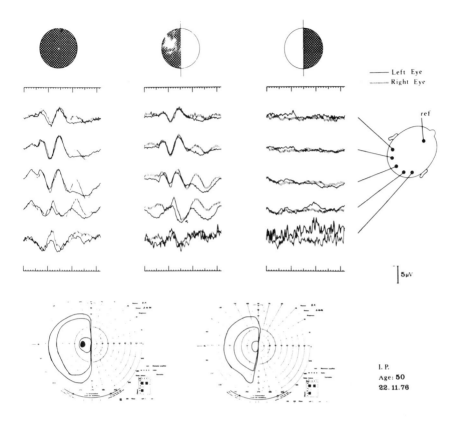

Figure 7.1 *Full-field and half-field pattern responses from a patient after left hemispherectomy. Note the macula-splitting homonymous hemianopia. No response is detectable above the background noise level on stimulation of the right half-field. The full-field and left half-field responses are virtually identical from each eye. Note that the large amplitude $\overline{P100}$ and its accompanying ipsilateral waves are maximal from the scalp overlying the excised hemisphere. Compare Figure 7.2. (From Blumhardt and Halliday, 1979.)*

There are, however, a few clinical contexts in which the visual EP can provide valuable diagnostic data which is not readily accessible by any other means. In the first place, being an objective technique it can sometimes provide decisive evidence in determining whether a particular case of visual impairment is functional or organic (Halliday, 1972). In the second place, there are at least two circumstances in which the VEP test has proved more sensitive than traditional perimetry in detecting a lesion of the visual pathways. It appears that the VEP is particularly vulnerable to the effect of an early compressive lesion and may show definite signs of an abnormal response at a time when the visual acuity is unimpaired and the fields are apparently normal. An example of this, in a patient with an early meningioma compressing the right optic nerve, has already been described (see Figure 6.23). The same sensitivity is shown to compressive lesions affecting the chiasmal and retrochiasmal fibres, where the typical defect is not in the response from one eye, but in a combination of abnormalities in the responses to monocular stimulation of either eye. These abnormalities may be homonymous or heteronymous depending on the site of the compression. In general, the pattern EP abnormality mirrors the character of the accompanying field defect (Blumhardt et al, 1977), but in early compression similar VEP abnormalities may be found before any field defect is evident on routine perimetry (Halliday et al, 1976; Gott et al, 1979).

Another type of lesion in which the VEP has shown itself more sensitive than other clinical tests, including perimetry, is, of course, in demyelinating disease. VEP abnormalities are frequently found in the presence of normal fields, fundi and colour vision and in the absence of any clinical history or signs of visual impairment (Halliday et al, 1973a). Although the optic nerve is very commonly affected, plaques may also be located further back in the chiasma or in the retrochiasmal visual pathways. Here the clinically 'silent' abnormality of the pattern EP is associated with the response to stimulation of only one or other half-field, rather than with the response from the left or right eyes (Halliday, 1978b, 1978c). In the full-field monocular responses this will usually declare itself in the form of an asymmetry of the same kind as that associated with hemianopia (Figure 7.11 below).

A further situation in which the topography of the pattern EP may be altered in a way not directly predictable from the accompanying field defect (if any) may arise where the intracranial contents are grossly disturbed or displaced so that the normal anatomical relationship of the generator areas to the overlying scalp electrodes is altered. Such altered responses may be encountered, for example, in association with a porencephalic cyst (Harding et al, 1980) or with an expanding space-occupying lesion displacing the midline structures to one side. Such cases are, however, relatively rare among the patients referred for diagnostic VEP testing.

THE VEP IN HEMIANOPIA: CROSSED AND UNCROSSED ASYMMETRIES

As one might expect, the defect of one half-field in a patient with hemianopia unmasks the asymmetry of the intact unilateral half-field response. This is then recorded ipsilaterally to the preserved half-field, i.e. contralaterally to the hemianopia. There are two major types of asymmetry encountered, which we have suggested naming 'uncrossed' and 'crossed' respectively (Halliday et al, 1976). The first is typical of a homonymous hemianopia, secondary to a lesion behind the chiasma on one side, and the second is typical of bitemporal hemianopia, secondary to a chiasmal lesion. The distinction depends on separate full-field pattern stimulation of each eye. If the asymmetry is the same for both eyes, it is 'uncrossed'; if it switches sides when the other eye is stimulated, it is 'crossed'. In either case the response from any one eye resembles the half-field response which can be recorded in a healthy subject by stimulation confined to the area corresponding to the preserved half-field (compare Figures 3.14-3.16).

Homonymous hemianopic responses following hemispherectomy

One of the most complete and uncomplicated forms of homonymous hemianopia is that seen following hemispherectomy. There is a macula-splitting field defect with the border between the blind and preserved half-field following the vertical meridian in the midline. Figure 7.1 shows the pattern reversal responses recorded in a 50-year-old woman 30 years after a left hemispherectomy for intractable epilepsy (Blumhardt and Halliday, 1979). Computerized axial tomography at the time of the recording showed some dilatation of the ventricles in the surviving right hemisphere (Figure 7.2), but the midline was not displaced and the skull contents appeared to be in normal relationship to the scalp electrodes at the occipital pole. The wide-field 0-16° checkerboard stimulus produces a response closely resembling a left half-field response in the healthy subject (cf Figure 3.14). The major positivity, forming part of a triphasic NPN complex, is recorded on the left side over the empty vault, and a normal contralateral PNP complex is seen over the right side of the head. Both the distribution and waveform of the response are entirely normal if it is thought of as a left half-field response from the surviving area of vision. Half-field stimulation confirms the origin of the response from the left half-field (Figure 7.1 middle and right hand records). The left half-field stimulus produces a record virtually identical with that of the full-field; there is no response to the right half-field stimulus.

A similar picture for a patient with a left homonymous hemianopia is shown in Figure 7.3. This 47-year-old woman had had a right hemispherectomy for epilepsy at the age of 26. The fact that both the ipsilateral triphasic NPN complex and the contralateral PNP complex of the half-field response are seen in these hemispherectomy cases is compelling evidence that all six sub-components of the normal half-field response (see page 105) are generated in the hemisphere

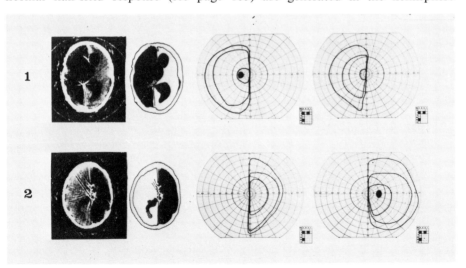

Figure 7.2 *CAT scans from (1) the patient with a left hemispherectomy, whose pattern EPs are shown in Figure 7.1; and (2) the patient with a right hemispherectomy whose pattern responses are shown in Figure 7.3.*

contralateral to the stimulated half-field. There is therefore no evidence to suggest the participation of the ipsilateral hemisphere in the normal half-field response, following transcallosal spread of activity across to the other side, as has been suggested by some authors (Beauchamp et al, 1976; Wildberger et al, 1976b).

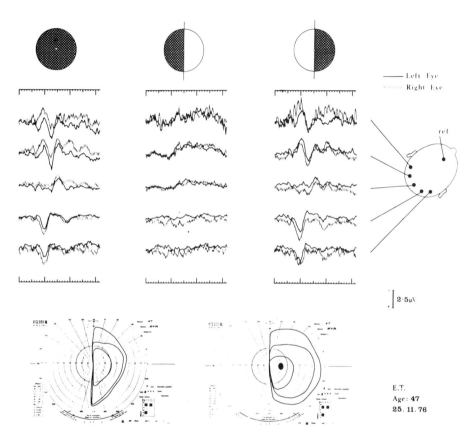

Figure 7.3 *Full- and half-field pattern responses recorded in a 47-year-old patient with a right hemispherectomy. No clearly recognizable components are detected above the background noise level on stimulation of the left half-field. This is confirmed by the virtually identical full- and right half-field responses. Note that the right half-field response has a 'transitional' midline waveform due to the dominant contralateral component, as found in 10% of healthy half-field responses. The ipsilateral complex (NPN) is recorded from the scalp overlying the excised hemisphere and all components are at normal latency. (From Blumhardt and Halliday, 1981.)*

Homonymous hemianopia following occipital lobectomy

Similar recordings can be obtained from patients following total or sub-total occipital lobectomies, provided that the hemianopic field defect includes the area of the pattern stimulus on the affected side (Blumhardt et al, 1977). Figure 7.4 shows

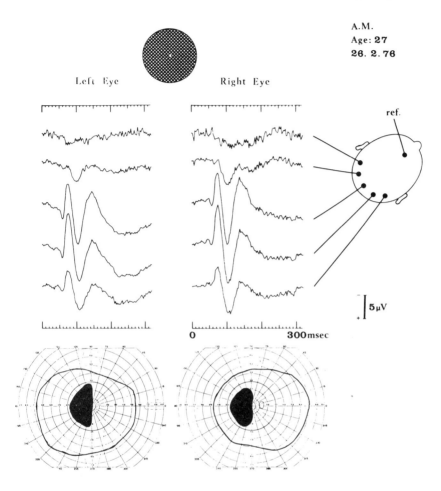

Figure 7.4 *Monocular responses to full-field stimulation of a patient after sub-total right occipital lobectomy for an arterio-venous malformation. Goldmann perimetry showed a total homonymous macula-splitting scotoma extending out to about 25° radius. Note the uncrossed asymmetry of the response, similar for stimulation of each eye. (From Blumhardt et al, 1977.)*

the wide-field pattern reversal responses from each eye of a 27-year-old woman who had presented clinically with a small left homonymous scotoma extending out some 10° from the fixation point. She was found to have a small cystic arteriovenous malformation on the medial surface of the right occipital pole. This and a small surrounding block of cortical tissue, measuring 2.5 x 1 x 1 cm, was removed surgically from the mesial surface of the occipital lobe, near the pole. Following the operation there was a dense macula-splitting homonymous scotoma extending out to 25° eccentricity. Visual acuity remained normal. The wide-field stimulus, which extended only out to 16°, well within the scotomatous area of the field on the left, produced a response with the asymmetry typical for a right half-field stimulus. When half-field stimulation was attempted (Figure 7.5), however, there was a

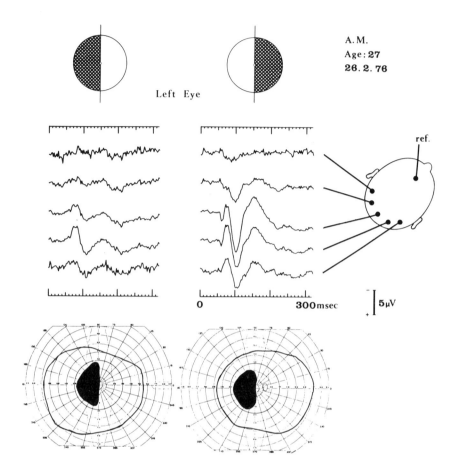

Figure 7.5 *Monocular responses to half-field pattern reversal in the patient whose full-field responses are shown in Figure 7.4. Note, however, the small response from the 'blind' left half-field, which has the same type of asymmetry as the right half-field response. This is almost certainly due to the formation of a pseudofovea leading to inaccurate fixation, with some of the stimulus falling in the preserved right half-field. Compare Figure 7.6. (From Blumhardt et al, 1977).*

similar, although much smaller, asymmetric response to the left half-field stimulus. This illustrates the problem of the development of a pseudofovea in some patients with hemianopia. The patient had fixated the central spot of light in the stimulus field at a point some way within the preserved right half-field. Consequently part of the left half-field stimulus encroaches on the preserved right half-field and produces a small VEP with the normal asymmetry typical of a right half-field response. The pattern of asymmetry serves to confirm that the response is not really coming from the blind left half-field. With eccentric fixation by shifting the fixation point 2° away from the vertical edge of the half-field checkerboard stimulus (Figure 7.6) the supposed 'left half-field response' is abolished, but the right half-field response is

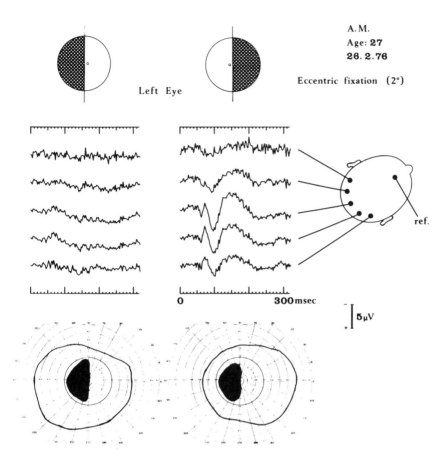

Figure 7.6 *Monocular half-field responses to pattern reversal in the same patient as in Figures 7.4 and 7.5 after the introduction of an eccentric fixation point positioned 2° into the unstimulated half-field. Note the absence of response from the left half-field. (From Blumhardt et al, 1977.)*

also reduced in amplitude because of the loss of the response from the vertical strip to the right of the new fixation point. This case illustrates well the problems of fixation in hemianopic field defects and the need to use the pattern of asymmetry of the response as a check for the possible development of a pseudofovea.

A somewhat different situation is represented by the patient whose responses are shown in Figure 7.7, who had also undergone a sub-total right occipital lobectomy for an arteriovenous malformation. He had an area of preserved peripheral vision in the left upper quadrant with a macula-splitting left homonymous field defect below it. In this case normal fixation was preserved and the half-field responses simply confirmed the fact that the full-field asymmetry was reproduced, both in amplitude and distribution, by the right half-field stimulus, while there was no response from the left half-field.

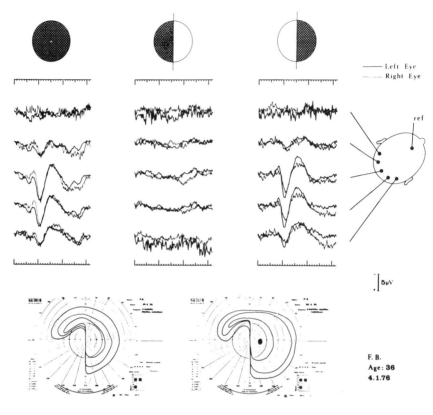

Figure 7.7 Superimposed monocular half-field responses to pattern reversal in a 36-year-old man with an incomplete left homonymous hemianopia, following a sub-total right occipital lobectomy for an arterio-venous malformation. Note the absence of any identifiable response from the left half-field and the similarity of the response from the full-field and the right half-field. (From Blumhardt et al, 1982b.)

Homonymous hemianopia secondary to posterior cerebrovascular accidents

The uncrossed asymmetries associated with hemianopic field defects do not seem to vary with differences in the underlying pathology. This is understandable if one remembers that the recorded response is coming from the preserved, and therefore presumably unaffected, half-field. The results are sometimes less clear-cut in the case of cerebrovascular lesions, because the field defect may be incongruent in the two eyes and may have spared portions of central vision. Figure 7.8 shows the wide-field pattern reversal responses recorded from each eye of a 26-year-old man with a vascular lesion of the left posterior cerebral circulation. As can be seen from the perimeter charts there is an incomplete right homonymous hemianopia and the defect is incongruent in the two eyes. Nonetheless the pattern responses show the typical asymmetry of a left half-field response, with the $\overline{P100}$ in the midline and left-sided channels, ipsilateral to the preserved half-field.

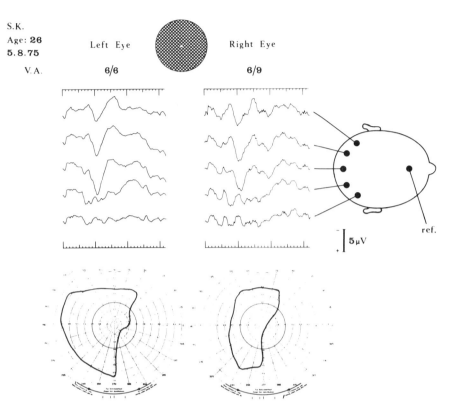

Figure 7.8 *Monocular pattern responses, showing an uncrossed asymmetry, in a 26-year-old man with right homonymous hemianopia, secondary to a cerebrovascular lesion affecting the left posterior cerebral circulation.*

In Figure 7.9 recorded from a 42-year-old man with a right occipital infarction, the left homonymous hemianopia is again associated with the type of uncrossed asymmetry characteristic of the normal right half-field response. There is also a prominent contralateral P135 component. The right half-field response is very like the full-field response, but left half-field stimulation shows a small residual pattern EP to be still present with a clear ipsilateral positivity of small amplitude from the midline and left-sided channels. For this response also there is a prominent contralateral positive wave. Half-field stimulation can be very helpful in such cases in identifying the P100 component by its ipsilateral distribution and clarifying the often obscured compound response from the full wide-field stimulus.

Homonymous hemianopia in chiasmal and retrochiasmal demyelinating lesions

Plaques are frequently found at post-mortem in the visual pathways behind the optic nerve, particularly in the chiasma, and, as in their more anterior location, they may either be associated with overt clinical impairment or be asymptomatic. Figure

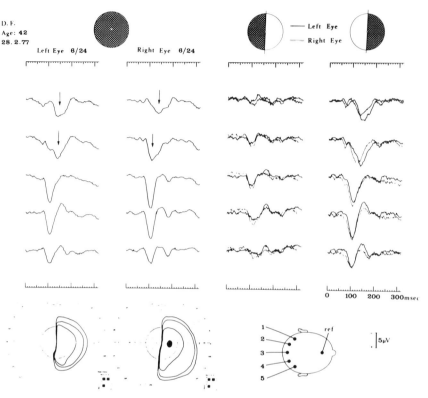

Figure 7.9 *Monocular full-field and half-field responses to pattern reversal in a 42-year-old man with a right occipital infarction and left homonymous hemianopia. Note the similarity of the full-field and right half-field responses from each eye and the small amplitude of the residual left half-field response. There is a prominent contralateral $\overline{P135}$ component (marked by the arrows), which might appear as a delayed ipsilateral $\overline{P100}$, but is identified as a contralateral $\overline{P135}$ by half-field stimulation. (From Blumhardt et al, 1982b.)*

7.10 illustrates the wide-field pattern responses from a 31-year-old woman with multiple sclerosis. At the time of the recording she had multiple opacities in both hemispheres on the CAT scan, associated clinically with a right homonymous hemianopia and hemiparesis. The field defect was incongruent, as can be seen from the perimeter chart, and there was some marked peripheral constriction of the preserved field, particularly for the right eye. The responses show the typical uncrossed asymmetric pattern characteristic of the normal left half-field response. There is a very well developed contralateral PNP complex, with particularly large P135 components. These too show some marked differences in distribution and waveform for the left and right eye.

An example of a clinically 'silent' hemianopic defect in multiple sclerosis is shown in Figures 7.11 and 7.12. This 30-year-old woman presented with an acuity of 6/5 in each eye and no field defect had been noted, but the wide-field pattern stimulus produced responses showing a typical uncrossed asymmetry, suggestive of

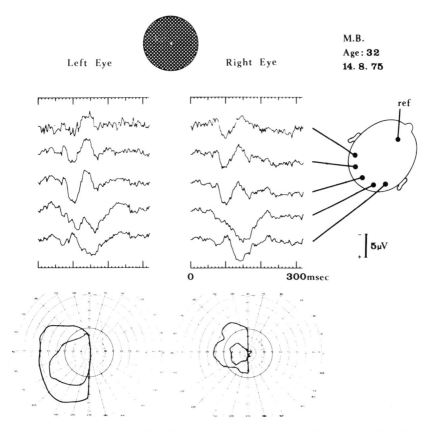

Figure 7.10 *Monocular full-field responses from a patient with multiple sclerosis, associated with a right homonymous hemianopia and a right hemiparesis. Note the typical uncrossed asymmetry. (From Halliday, 1978c.)*

a left homonymous hemianopia (see Figure 7.11). Half-field stimulation confirmed that the full-field response was duplicated by stimulation of the right half-field alone (Figure 7.12). The response to the left half-field stimulus, however, showed some striking and significant abnormalities. There was a low amplitude midline and ipsilateral positivity in the response from each eye, but this was of altered and grossly broadened waveform with no clearly defined peak but a definitely delayed mean latency. This abnormal response from the left half-field was therefore showing the typical latency change encountered in association with demyelinating lesions. Careful re-testing of the patient's fields showed a subtle defect of colour vision in the left half-fields, a red object appearing somewhat yellower and 'desaturated' if presented anywhere to the left of the fixation point.

Hemianopic field defects associated with compressive lesions

One of the commonest causes of hemianopic field defects is compression of the optic chiasm by a suprasellar mass. The typical defect is a bitemporal hemianopia, produced by compression of the fibres crossing the chiasma from the nasal retina of each eye and projecting to the contralateral hemisphere. Less commonly, where the compression has impinged mainly on the fibres leaving the chiasma posteriorly on one side, a typical homonymous field defect may be produced. Even more rarely, where this has occurred bilaterally, a binasal hemianopia may be encountered. Both 'crossed' and 'uncrossed' asymmetries of the pattern EP are therefore very commonly encountered in association with an expanding suprasellar mass, such as a pituitary adenoma or a craniopharyngioma (Halliday et al, 1976; Blumhardt et al, 1977). Unlike more anterior compressive lesions affecting one optic nerve (e.g. a sphenoidal wing meningioma), the typical abnormality involves the responses from both eyes, and half-field stimulation may be of considerable value in clarifying the situation.

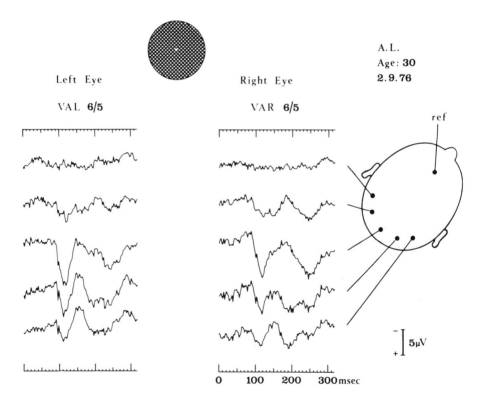

Figure 7.11 *Responses evoked by a whole-field pattern reversal stimulus from the left and right eye of a patient with suspected multiple sclerosis. Note the uncrossed asymmetry, similar for the two eyes, which would be typical for a right homonymous hemianopia. The patient, however, had no gross field defect on perimetry. Compare Figure 7.12. (From Halliday, 1978c.)*

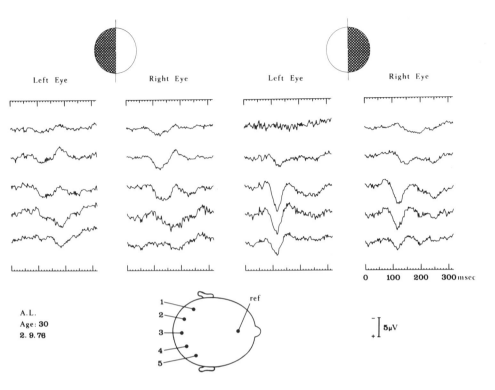

Figure 7.12 *Half-field responses to pattern reversal in the patient whose whole-field responses are shown in Figure 7.11. The right half-field responses are similar to the whole-field responses shown in Figure 7.11 and confirm that the major positivity is coming from the right half-field. The left half-field responses are abnormal, with an ipsilateral positivity of reduced amplitude, altered waveform and delayed latency. The picture is suggestive of a clinically 'silent' plaque affecting the retrochiasmal fibres on the right side. Clinical examination revealed a subtle defect in the left half-fields, a red object appearing somewhat yellower anywhere to the left of the fixation point. (From Halliday, 1978c.)*

Figure 7.13 shows the record from a 39-year-old man with a pituitary adenoma compressing the fibres crossing in the optic chiasma. The perimeter charts demonstrate the typical bitemporal hemianopia, which is incomplete, with a small area of preserved vision in the temporal fields below the fixation point. The pattern EPs show the characteristic asymmetry of the response from the preserved half-field. The $\overline{P100}$ component is seen at the midline and right-sided channels for the left eye and in the midline and left-sided channels for the right eye. This is the typical *crossed asymmetry* which reverses when the pattern stimulus is presented to the other eye. Contralateral to the relatively preserved nasal fields, a PNP complex is seen with a particularly prominent $\overline{P135}$ component.

Another example of a crossed asymmetry, from a 48-year-old man with chiasmal compression secondary to a craniopharyngioma, is shown in Figure 7.14.

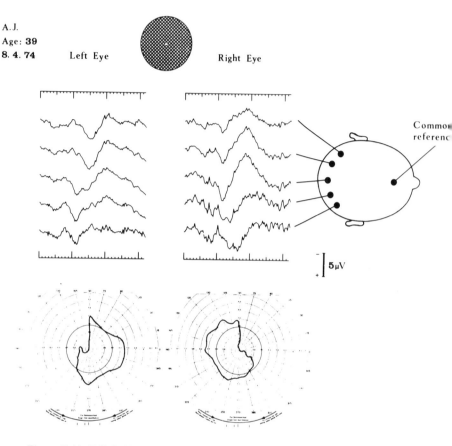

Figure 7.13 *Full-field pattern EPs from a 39-year-old man with a pituitary adenoma, associated with bitemporal hemianopia. Note the crossed asymmetry, the P100 component being seen at the midline and ipsilateral to the preserved nasal field, on the right side for the left eye response and on the left side for the right eye response. (From Halliday, 1978a.)*

There is again a bitemporal hemianopia associated with asymmetric responses in which the major positivity switches sides according to which eye is being stimulated, being seen ipsilaterally to the preserved nasal field in each case. Again there is a particularly prominent P135 component in the contralateral PNP complexes. It is only with half-field stimulation that one can confidently distinguish this P135 from a delayed P100 in the opposite hemisphere. Half-field stimulation, however, makes it perfectly clear that this positivity is, like the ipsilateral P100 component, coming from the preserved nasal fields (Figure 7.15). It is not, therefore, to be interpreted as a delayed positivity, originating in a response from the temporal half-field (Halliday et al, 1979a).

An example of an uncrossed asymmetry associated with a suprasellar compressive lesion is shown in Figure 7.16, recorded in a 50-year-old woman with a pituitary adenoma (Halliday et al, 1976). Pre-operative perimetry showed an

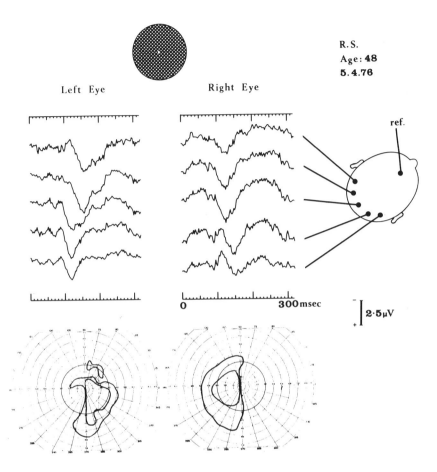

Figure 7.14 *Example of a crossed asymmetry in the pattern reversal EP of a patient with bitemporal hemianopia due to chiasmal compression by a craniopharyngioma. There is an unusually prominent contralateral positivity, particularly for the left eye, which can be identified by half-field stimulation as a P135. Compare Figure 7.15. (From Blumhardt et al, 1977.)*

incongruent right homonymous hemianopia with preserved acuity in each eye (6/5, 6/5). The pre-operative pattern EPs show the typical uncrossed asymmetry of a left half-field response. Following surgery, the field defect had disappeared and the EP asymmetry has also been abolished. However, the acuity in the left eye had deteriorated to 6/9 and, paralleling this, the amplitude of the response from the left eye is reduced.

Intra-operative monitoring of the VEP during the surgical decompression of a suprasellar mass suggests that the recovery of the normal VEP may take place very soon after the decompression. Gutin et al (1980) have recorded the return of the flash EP 3 hours after aspiration of an inoperable cystic craniopharyngioma. In an earlier study Wilson et al (1976) used an LED array, mounted in scleral shells placed

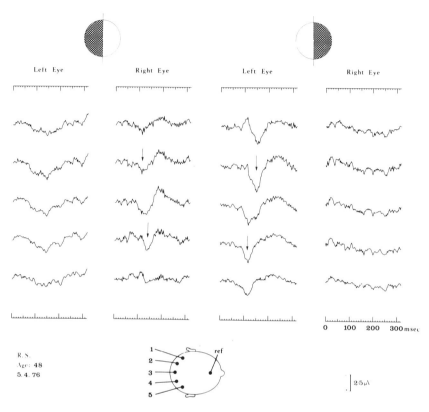

Figure 7.15 *Half-field responses from the patient whose full-field responses are shown in Figure 7.14. All the major features of the full-field response are arising from stimulation of the nasal half-field of each eye, while the responses from the temporal fields are relatively featureless. In particular, the later contralateral positive wave is seen to be the $\overline{P135}$ component of the contralateral PNP complex of the half-field response, and not a delayed $\overline{P100}$ component arising from the temporal half-field. (From Halliday et al, 1979a.)*

under the lids of each eye, to monitor the luminance EP in 4 patients undergoing parasellar surgery and noted marked depression of the response followed by recovery within 2 to 3 minutes during manipulation of the chiasm.

In general the EP changes with more posterior lesions follow the incidence of the field defect itself and disappear when the fields return to normal. However, as in the case of optic nerve lesions, the pattern EP seems particularly vulnerable and sensitive to the effects of early compression. Halliday et al (1976) found abnormal asymmetric pattern responses in two of their patients in whom the fields appeared normal, and subsequent experience has confirmed that a pattern EP asymmetry may become apparent before there is any clinically obvious change in the fields (Blumhardt et al, 1977). Since the CAT scan is often at a disadvantage in demonstrating lesions in the base of the skull, the pattern EP may therefore be particularly useful in the early monitoring of cases of suspected expanding lesions in the region of the sella turcica. The responses may be less useful in more advanced cases, particularly where the acuity is so much reduced that the pattern response is unobtainable from one eye. Figure 7.17 shows a record from a 29-year-old man with a craniopharyngioma in which pre-operative acuity was reduced to the perception of hand movements in the left eye. Acuity in the right eye was better than 6/12, and there was an incomplete temporal hemianopia in this eye. No pattern response could be obtained from the left eye, and the response from the right eye is of much reduced amplitude and shows the asymmetry typical of a right half-field defect. Post-operatively, when the acuity returned to 6/5 in each eye, the pattern EPs have also markedly improved. However, the waveform is still abnormal, with a definite suggestion of a crossed asymmetry, the $\overline{\text{P100}}$ component having a clear left-sided distribution from the right eye and a suggestion of a right-sided distribution from the left eye.

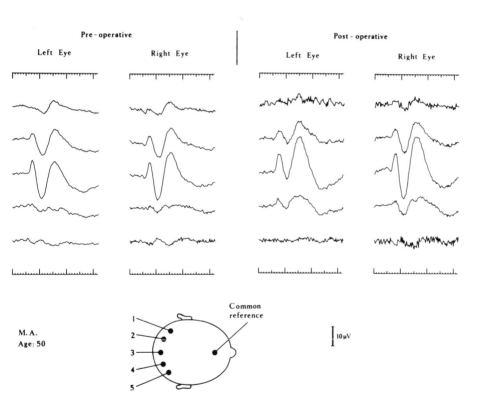

Figure 7.16 *Pre-operative and post-operative pattern EPs recorded from each eye of a patient with a pituitary adenoma. The pre-operative records show an uncrossed asymmetry, paralleling the incongruent right homonymous hemianopia revealed by perimetry at this time. Note the loss of this asymmetry following the operation. The amplitude of the response from the left eye is significantly reduced post-operatively, and the acuity in this eye was reduced from 6/5 to 6/9. (From Halliday et al, 1976.)*

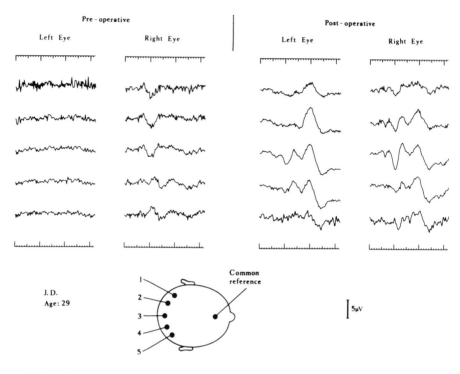

Figure 7.17 *Pre-operative and post-operative pattern reversal EPs in a patient with a craniopharyngioma. There was no response pre-operatively from the left eye, in which the visual acuity was reduced to the perception of hand movements. In the right eye the response is small and asymmetric, the reduced major positive component appearing at normal latency in the midline and left-sided channels, while the channels to the right of the midline show a slightly later negative component followed by a positivity. Acuity in the right eye was better than 6/12 and there was a temporal field defect sparing the midline. Post-operatively both responses are markedly improved, paralleling the return of normal acuity, but are still very abnormal, exhibiting a residual crossed asymmetry. (From Halliday et al, 1976.)*

Gott et al (1979) have confirmed the value of the pattern reversal EP as 'an accurate and reliable means of assessing suprasellar extension of a tumour resulting in optic nerve compression'. They recorded this response in 83 patients with pituitary tumours established by CAT scan and found VEP abnormalities in 12, correlating with radiological evidence of a suprasellar mass. Only 4 of them had accompanying visual field defects on Goldmann or tangent screen perimetry. However, with the stimulus parameters and recording montage used, they found 'hemispheric amplitude asymmetries' only in 2 of the 12 with abnormal responses, the others being reported as showing a delayed latency of the response. It seems likely that this conclusion was due to the reliance largely on electrodes near the midline (O_1, O_2, and O_z) referred to the vertex (C_z), which would be expected to be in the transitional zone between ipsilateral $\overline{P100}$ and contralateral $\overline{P135}$

components of the half-field response (see Blumhardt et al, 1978; Halliday, 1980b). The stimulus parameters also included an unusually long transition time of 20 msec for the checkerboard reversal, which was produced by the rotating mirror and projector technique. One other patient with a pituitary tumour, but with no evidence of suprasellar extension, also produced abnormal VEPs, and the authors stress the importance of evaluating all patients for visual problems unrelated to the tumour.

Compressive lesions situated more posteriorly in the visual pathways may be associated with typical uncrossed asymmetries, indistinguishable from those encountered in vascular lesions of the hemisphere or following surgical resection. However, such lesions appear to have little or no effect on the pattern EP unless they actually impinge on the visual pathways themselves. Even extensive vascular or space-occupying lesions within the hemispheres may be associated with completely normal pattern EPs, when there is no associated field defect (Blumhardt and Halliday, 1981; Blumhardt et al, 1982b).

LIMITS OF NORMAL ASYMMETRY IN THE PATTERN AND FLASH RESPONSES

Some degree of asymmetry is frequently encountered among the responses from the healthy population. (Tables 7.1-7.4). With our own standard 0-16° wide-field checkerboard stimulus of 50′ checks the amplitude of the $\overline{P100}$ component at the electrode 5 cm out on either side of the mid-occipital electrode does not exceed a difference of 3:1 for the normal population at the $+ 2.5$ s.d. level. If homologous measurements for the separate half-field amplitudes are taken, however, the upper limit of asymmetry for the normal population is reduced to approximately 2:1 (Blumhardt and Halliday, 1981). There are therefore great advantages in resorting to half-field stimulation for the detection of abnormal asymmetries in hemianopic or quadrantanopic patients. In a series of 26 patients with homonymous hemianopic field defects (16 complete and 10 incomplete) the $\overline{P100}$ for the wide-field stimulus was beyond the upper limit of the amplitude ratio for both eyes in 14 of the 26 cases (54%), but these figures were increased to 18 out of 25 (72%) if the half-field amplitude ratios were measured; one case did not have half-field recording (Blumhardt and Halliday, 1981; Blumhardt et al, 1982b). Two other cases exceeded the normal asymmetry for one of the two eyes on full-field stimulation, and three others on half-field stimulation, bringing the figures up to 62% and 81% respectively for an abnormal asymmetry present in either one or both eyes.

It must also be apparent that to adequately record and quantify the asymmetries of the pattern response, multi-channel recording is essential. It is also important to choose a suitable montage, particularly as regards the location of the occipital electrodes near the midline and the choice of reference (see Chapter 1, page 23, Figures 1.10-1.13). It seems likely that the 'normal' pattern responses reported in three cases of hemianopia by Asselman et al (1975) and in five similar patients by Celesia and Daly (1977b) are due to reliance on recording only the midline response. In this respect, the conventional electrodes of the 10-20 system O_1 and O_2 are placed too near the midline to be optimal for recording the asymmetries associated with the half-field response. It is also desirable to choose a reference, such as the mid-frontal electrode, which is both unlateralized and outside the area from which the half-field response can be picked up (see Figure 1.10 and Halliday et al, 1979; Halliday, 1980b).

Table 7.1 MEAN $\overline{P100}$ AMPLITUDE RATIOS IN 50 HEALTHY INDIVIDUALS MEASURED AT THE ELECTRODES 5 cms TO EITHER SIDE OF THE MIDOCCIPUT IN RESPONSE TO A 0-16° FULL-FIELD CHECKERBOARD REVERSAL STIMULUS

Eye	Mean ratio	Upper normal limit (+2.5 s.d)
Left	1.58 ± 0.559	2.98
Right	1.60 ± 0.553	2.93

(From Blumhardt and Halliday, 1981)

Table 7.2 MEAN $\overline{P100}$ AMPLITUDE RATIOS IN 50 HEALTHY INDIVIDUALS MEASURED AT THE IPSILATERAL ELECTRODE 5 cms OUT FROM THE MIDOCCIPUT IN RESPONSE TO A 0-16° HALF-FIELD CHECKBOARD REVERSAL STIMULUS

A. Homonymous half-field comparison
(left eye vs. right eye)

Half-field	Mean ratio	Upper normal limit (+ 2.5 s.d.)
Left	1.24 ± 0.223	1.81
Right	1.29 ± 0.250	1.92

B. Heteronymous half-field comparison
(left half-field vs. right half-field)

Eye	Mean ratio	Upper normal limit (+2.5 s.d.)
Left	1.36 ± 0.331	2.19
Right	1.34 ± 0.296	2.08

(Data from Blumhardt and Halliday, 1979, 1981)

Table 7.3 MEAN P̄100 LATENCIES IN 50 HEALTHY INDIVIDUALS MEASURED AT THE ELECTRODES 5 cm LATERAL TO THE MIDOCCIPUT IN RESPONSE TO A 0-16° FULL-FIELD CHECKERBOARD REVERSAL STIMULUS

Eye	Electrode	Mean latency	Upper normal limit (+2.5 s.d.)
Left	Left	105.5 ± 10.3	131.3
	Right	107.2 ± 7.6	126.1
Right	Left	107.6 ± 9.4	131.1
	Right	107.3 ± 8.9	129.6

(Data from Blumhardt and Halliday, 1979, 1981)

Table 7.4 MEAN P̄100 LATENCIES IN 50 HEALTHY INDIVIDUALS MEASURED AT THE IPSILATERAL ELECTRODE 5 cm OUT FROM THE MIDOCCIPUT IN RESPONSE TO A 0-16° HALF-FIELD CHECKERBOARD REVERSAL STIMULUS

Eye	Half-field	Mean latency	Upper normal limit (+2.5 s.d.)
Left	Left	105.3 ± 4.94	117.7
	Right	106.0 ± 2.88	115.7
Right	Left	106.0 ± 4.74	117.9
	Right	104.8 ± 4.02	114.9

(Data from Blumhardt and Halliday, 1979, 1981)

Flash EPs in hemianopia and quadrantanopia

Before pattern reversal stimulation was introduced, a number of studies of the flash response in hemianopia or quadrantanopia were published. These studies, which have been reviewed in detail by the author elsewhere (Halliday, 1975b), succeeded in demonstrating clear asymmetries in a number of hemianopic patients, but the results were very variable and the abnormalities seen were not as clearly distinguished from the normal response in the healthy population as they are in the case of the pattern reversal EP. This is in line with what would be expected from the comparison of the VEPs to flash and pattern stimulation of each half-field in healthy individuals (see Figures 3.17-3.18). Nonetheless, a high proportion of patients with bitemporal hemianopia associated with a chiasmal lesion have abnormal flash EPs (Müller, 1962; Vaughan and Katzman, 1964; Jacobson et al, 1968; Lehmann et al, 1969). Asymmetries of the response were also recorded from many patients with homonymous hemianopia (Cohn, 1963; Vaughan et al, 1963; Vaughan and Katzman, 1964; Kooi et al, 1965; Jacobson et al, 1968; Oosterhuis et al, 1969; Harding et al, 1970; Feinsod et al, 1975a). However, some of these studies also found asymmetries in the responses from the healthy population and there was a considerable overlap between the normal and hemianopic group. The response was particularly likely to fail to show any abnormality if there was any degree of central sparing of the visual field (Vaughan and Katzman, 1964; Oosterhuis et al, 1969), although not all studies found this to be so (Kooi et al, 1965).

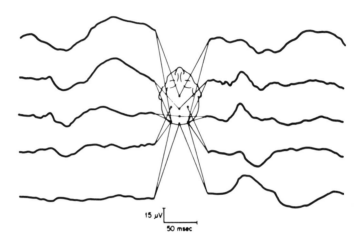

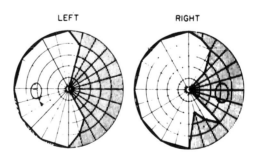

Patient Ch.; age 56 years; clinical diagnosis, left posterior cerebral artery occlusion. VER and visual fields. Evoked response was recorded with various electrode placements. Positive deflection, with peak at 52 msec is maximal on normal side, with occipital electrode referred to vertex or midparietal lead. Depression of this wave is clearly evident on abnormal side.

Figure 7.18 *Flash evoked response recorded from a 56-year-old patient with an incomplete right homonymous hemianopia secondary to a left posterior cerebral artery occlusion. (From Vaughan et al, 1963.)*

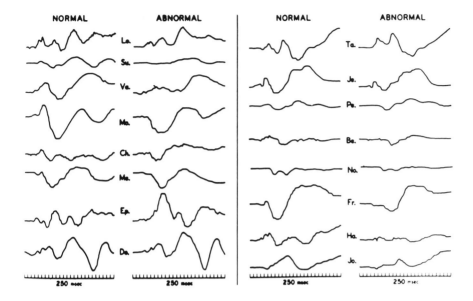

NORMAL   ABNORMAL   NORMAL   ABNORMAL

Figure 7.19 Comparison of the full-field flash evoked response recorded from electrodes on the normal and abnormal side in a series of patients with hemianopia or quadrantanopia. (From Vaughan et al, 1963.)

Figure 7.18 and Figure 7.19 from the study by Vaughan et al (1963), illustrate the type of asymmetries which may be encountered in association with hemianopic and quadrantanopic defects and the very high degree of variability in the waveform of the flash response. It is this variability which makes it unrewarding to use the flash EP in the clinical testing of patients with field defects. In the occipital-to-vertex leads in Figure 7.18 there is a clear asymmetry in the response from the two sides of the head with phase reversal of the components between 50 and 100 msec. The record is from a 56-year-old patient with a left posterior cerebral artery occlusion associated with a right homonymous hemianopia. Figure 7.19 from the same study compares the responses from the normal and abnormal sides in 11 patients with dense hemianopic defects, two with a quandrantanopia (Ep, Me) and three patients with a homonymous field defect sparing the central 10° or more of the involved field (Do, Ta, Je). As can be seen, the degree of asymmetry varies widely, even in those patients with comparable field defects.

The authors found that the best criterion for an abnormal asymmetry in the flash response appeared to be the difference between the smaller and larger amplitudes of the $\overline{P45}$ component recorded from the left and right occipital electrodes with reference to the vertex. This had a mean value of 19.5% ± 12.5% in a control group of 32 normal individuals, so that any asymmetry of more than 50% could be considered significantly abnormal at the 1% level of confidence. On this criterion, 16 of the 25 hemianopic patients in whom this peak could be identified exceeded the normal limits. Two of the other nine patients had at least 10° of the central field spared and there was some doubt about the field defect in four others. This careful study leaves little doubt that the flash response can be effectively used to detect asymmetries in some hemianopic patients, and this has been confirmed by subsequent studies. Equally, there seems little question that, because of its greater sensitivity and consistency, the pattern response is better suited to the detection of field defects than the flash response where the acuity level is high enough to permit its use.

Special stimulating techniques for the detection of asymmetries

A number of other special techniques have been tried for the detection of field defects. Regan and Cartwright (1970) have advocated the use of *simultaneous* steady state pattern reversal stimulation of different sectors of the visual field (e.g. the two half-fields or the four quadrants), each stimulus being locked to a slightly different frequency. The responses can be separately averaged, even from the same occipital electrode, by cross-correlation with the stimulus frequency, either by averaging or by the use of narrow band Fourier analysis. The same technique can be used to obtain luminance responses by employing sinusoidally modulated light panels. With this technique, Regan and Heron (1969) demonstrated marked asymmetries in the responses of a patient with right homonymous hemianopia with macula sparing, and also studied changes in the VEP associated with migraine (Regan and Heron, 1970). There have been a few other subsequent studies of field defects using the steady state response, either with averaging of pattern reversal responses (Wildberger et al, 1976b; Kuroiwa and Celesia, 1981) or Fourier analysis of the lateralized occipital response to short trains of flashes (Starr et al, 1978; Celesia et al, 1978).

Rowe (1981) has introduced a simple and practical technique for simultaneous recording of the left and right half-field responses, which speeds up routine testing and minimizes the risk of wandering fixation. The left and right half-field checkerboard stimuli are presented simultaneously on a TV display, together with a central fixation point, and reversed alternately with an interval of 250 msec between each reversal. The average, carried out over an epoch of 500 msec, provides a record of both responses on the same time base.

Pattern EPs in the detection of small field defects

It has already been pointed out that the response recorded in patients with field defects originates in the preserved areas of vision. For this reason, the smaller the defect, the less easy it is to detect any abnormality when using a fairly large stimulus field of the type suitable as a clinical screening test. The patient with a small macular hole, secondary to an embolus, whose pattern EPs are shown in Figures 5.14-16, is a good illustration of this point. Small scotomata situated near the fixation point are, in fact, especially favourably placed for EP detection, because the pattern response comes predominantly from the central areas of vision. Moreover, the relative independence of the sub-components of the macular and paramacular pattern EP means that dense central scotomata, such as are encountered in toxic amblyopia, are especially easy to record because of their characteristic waveform change with its apparent inversion of the $\overline{\text{P100}}$ component. However, even more peripheral field defects may cause significant changes in the pattern EP if they are sufficiently large.

One appproach which can be adopted if the localization of the field defect is already known, is to explore small areas of the visual fields with a localized stimulus. This method has been employed with both the luminance EP (De Haas, 1972) and the pattern reversal EP (Halliday, 1972). Figure 7.20 shows the responses from a 43-year-old woman who complained of visual impairment starting suddenly a few days after an attack of cholecystitis, treated with Ampicillin. Her visual symptoms had been diagnosed as hysterical, but on re-examination, she appeared to have a right inferior quandrantanopia. Binocular stimulation of each lower quadrant separately confirmed the diagnosis, the response from the right inferior quadrant showing a clear reduction in amplitude associated with a phase-reversal across the midline. Cappin and Nissim (1975) have used the steady-state checkerboard reversal response from homonymous quadrants in each eye to demonstrate asymmetries associated with the quadrantic field defects in glaucoma (see page 172).

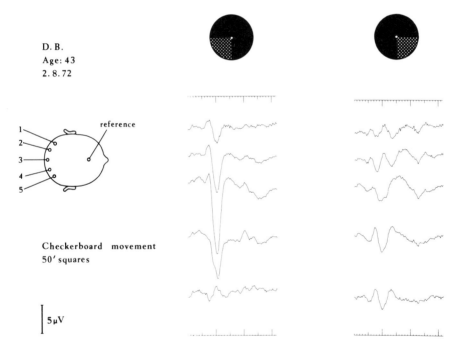

Figure 7.20 *Responses to binocular stimulation of the left and right inferior quadrants in a 43-year-old woman presenting with a complaint of visual impairment, following an attack of acute cholecystitis 5 months previously. She proved to have a right inferior quadrantanopia. See text for further details. (From Halliday, 1972.)*

Howe and Mitchell (1980) found that substantial improvement in the detection of homonymous field defects secondary to migraine or cerebrovascular disease could be achieved by resorting to quadrantic rather than half-field stimulation. The use of different check sizes (20′ and 50′) to differentiate central and peripheral responses was helpful in recording field defects in those cases with macular sparing.

The development of a scotomatous change in serial records may be of clinical significance, as in the case of the patient already described in Chapter 6 (Figure 6.28), in whom the spread of an optic nerve glioma to involve the chiasmal fibres was associated with the development of an asymmetry typical of a temporal hemianopia in the response from the 'unaffected eye', while the further spread to involve the central fibres on the other side of the head was associated with the development of the waveform changes characteristic of a central scotoma. The latter can be seen in Figure 6.28 as a progressive accentuation of the contralateral PNP components (particularly the N105) derived from the paramacular areas of the preserved nasal field response from the left eye, in the serial VEPs recorded over a 3-year period.

TOXIC AND NUTRITIONAL AMBLYOPIA

Among the clinical conditions particularly associated with a dense central scotomatous defect are the amblyopias secondary to metabolic poisons and malnutrition. Rouher et al (1969) recorded the flash EP in six cases with toxic neuropathy secondary to an excessive consumption of tobacco and/or alcohol. They found that while the response to white or blue flash stimulation was unaltered, the response to a red flash was abolished or very much diminished, paralleling the gravity of the clinical defect. Their stimulus was a flash delivered through a monochromatic red filter of wavelength 658 nm. Babel et al (1977) report flash ERG and EP recordings on much larger groups of patients with alcohol-tobacco amblyopia or intoxication by myambutol. Of the 90 eyes examined in the former group only two had normal ERGs. Oscillatory potentials were looked for in 70 of these patients and were normal in only four. The flash EP was examined in 50 eyes but could not be recorded in eight of them. Only three of the responses were of normal amplitude, whereas only ten had an abnormal latency according to these authors. In view of the changes in the pattern response waveform with central scotomata, it seems likely that at least some of these latency changes may in fact be due to the recording of a late paramacular positivity following loss of the normal major positive component. In 38 patients undergoing myambutol (ethambutol-dihydrochloride) treatment, on an average daily dose of 1 gm of the drug, there was a steady rise in the number of abnormal responses over the first three months, especially in the ERG. Of the 38 eyes recorded, a third had abnormal ERGs and flash EPs, but by the end of three months of treatment the proportion of abnormalities had risen to 100% of the ERGs and 75% of the VEPs (although only a total of ten eyes were recorded after this time).

The pattern reversal EP shows a characteristic change in association with the central scotoma of tobacco-alcohol amblyopia, as originally described by Halliday (1976). There is a relative loss of the normal NPN complex derived predominantly from stimulation of the macular area and it is replaced by the phase-reversed PNP complex characteristic of the response to paramacular stimulation in the healthy subject (Blumhardt et al, 1978). Figure 7.21 shows the typical appearance in a

58-year-old man with a long history of high alcohol intake, which was combined with being a poor eater and smoking half an ounce of tobacco a day. It is to be noted that the negativity, as seen in the response to the wide field 0-16° checkerboard stimulus, has a maximum amplitude at the electrodes 5 cm to either side of the midline and not at the mid-occipital electrode itself. This is unlike the $\overline{P100}$ component and is characteristic of the contralateral response to stimulation in each half-field, which originates particularly from stimulation of the paramacular region. The identification of the negativity as a contralateral response can be verified by resort to half-field stimulation. Figure 7.22 shows a similar wide field response in a 74-year-old man with tobacco amblyopia. Figure 7.23 records the half-field responses in the same patient. It can be seen that the full-field negativity is made up of the contralateral components from each half-field and that the normal ipsilateral positivity is missing (Halliday et al, 1979a).

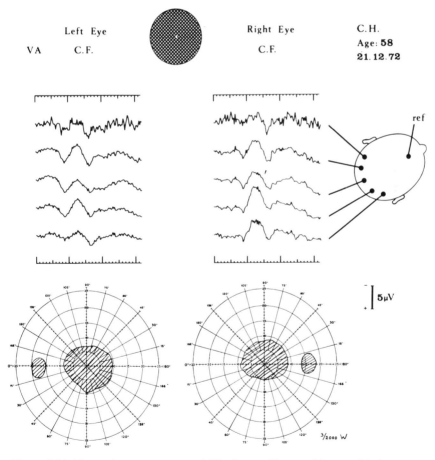

Figure 7.21 *Monocular pattern reversal EPs from a 58-year-old man with dense central scotomata, secondary to tobacco-alcohol amblyopia, showing the characteristic replacement of the normal midline NPN complex by the more lateralized PNP complexes derived from the paramacular stimulus. (From Halliday, 1976.)*

Ikeda et al (1978) have recorded the checkerboard reversal response in 15 patients with bilateral visual disturbance associated with a long history of smoking and drinking, one case of West Indian amblyopia and one patient with quinine amblyopia. The latency of the $\overline{P100}$ was generally within the normal range, but the amplitude was markedly reduced in both eyes, with a mean of 3.6 ± 2.1 µV (range 0-7.0) as compared with 15.8 ± 5.3 µV (range 8.1-32.0) in a control group of healthy volunteers. The flash ERG, measured with corneal electrodes in accordance with the routine given in Chapter 4, was also depressed, showing an increase of the threshold intensity required to produce a measurable scotopic b-wave (normally below five log units), a decreased slope of the b-wave amplitude/intensity curve (normally 100 µV per log unit increment), and a reduced amplitude of the b-wavelets to 30 Hz red flicker (normally >100 µV).

These changes were reversible with treatment, the amplitude of the flash EP increasing in parallel with the improvement in the visual acuity level. The subnormal ERG parameters also showed a return towards normality.

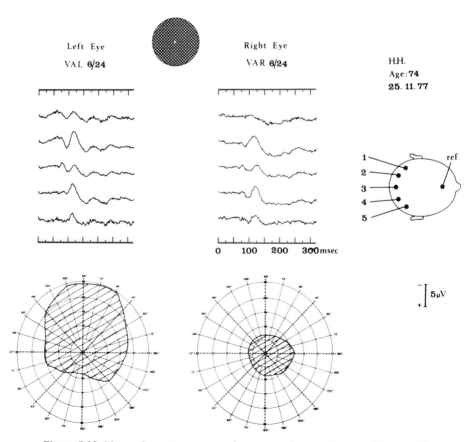

Figure 7.22 *Monocular pattern reversal responses from a 74-year-old man with dense binocular central scotomata due to toxic optic neuropathy. The responses show similar features to those of the patient illustrated in Figure 7.21. Compare 7.23. (From Halliday et al, 1979a.)*

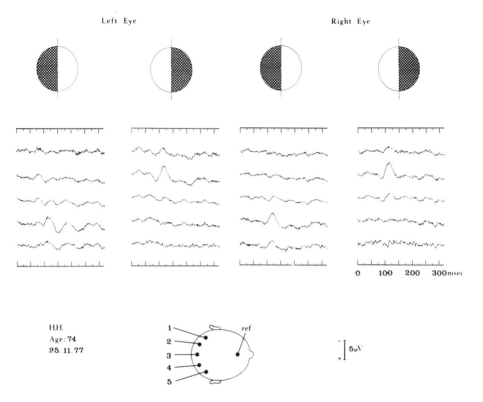

Figure 7.23 *Half-field responses from the patient whose full-field responses are shown in Figure 7.22. Note that the PNP complexes of the full-field response are shown to have a contralateral distribution for each half-field stimulus. (From Halliday et al, 1979a.)*

Figure 7.24 shows the responses recorded by the present author in a case of tobacco-alcohol amblyopia with an incomplete and asymmetric centro-caecal scotoma in each eye. In the left eye the contralateral negativity from the preserved paramacular retina to the right of the fixation point is clearly seen. Figure 7.25 shows responses recorded in the same patient six weeks later, after intensive treatment with B_{12} injections. The acuity has returned to 6/5 in each eye and the field defects had resolved. The major positive component has returned, but is still of somewhat abnormal waveform and rather small amplitude, with a peak latency near the upper limit of the normal range. These findings parallel those of Ikeda et al (1978), in which the mean latency of the $\overline{P100}$ component was significantly delayed compared with the normal (p < 0.001), but only by a few milliseconds, most of the individual values falling within the normal range.

Kriss et al (1982) have studied both full- and half-field pattern EPs in 24 patients with toxic optic neuropathy, 13 of them being recorded on more than one occasion. Fifteen of the patients also had their flash EPs recorded. The $\overline{P100}$ was much reduced in amplitude and altered in waveform, the major positivity appearing in the grand average of the full-field response as a broad midline component peaking at 130 msec. At the electrodes 5 cm to either side of the midline the response had a PNP configuration with $\overline{P80}$, $\overline{N105}$ and $\overline{P140}$ components, the latter being the largest of the three. In two-thirds of the records a small $\overline{N105}$ was also seen at the midline. The midline positivity was thus largely a $\overline{P135}$ component, the $\overline{P100}$ being identifiable in only 15% of records. Half-field stimulation confirmed these conclusions. The flash EP showed a much simplified bifid waveform with $\overline{P70}$, $\overline{N96}$ and $\overline{P130}$ components, but there was only partial agreement between the morphology of pattern and flash

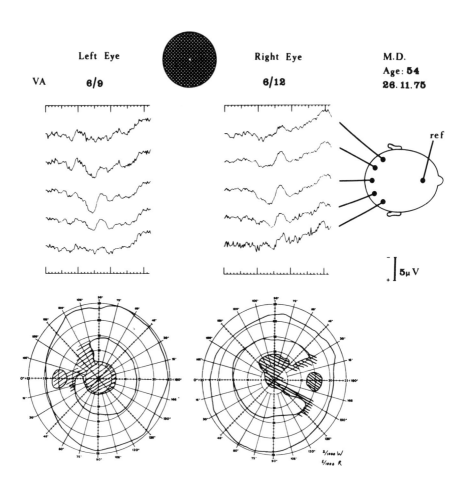

Figure 7.24 *Monocular full-field pattern responses from a 54-year-old man with toxic optic neuropathy. In the response from the left eye a PNP complex can be seen in the left-sided channels, suggesting a paramacular response from the right half-field, whereas in the response from the right eye there is a small ill-formed positivity in the left-sided and midline channels at about the same latency, suggestive of some residual macular response from the left half-field of this eye. Note the correlation of these inferences with the areas of preserved vision identified by perimetry. Compare Figure 7.25.*

waveforms when comparing individual patients. With treatment the amplitude of the responses increased. The changes in the flash EP are similar to those reported by Harding et al (1980) in West Indian amblyopia and some hereditary optic atrophies.

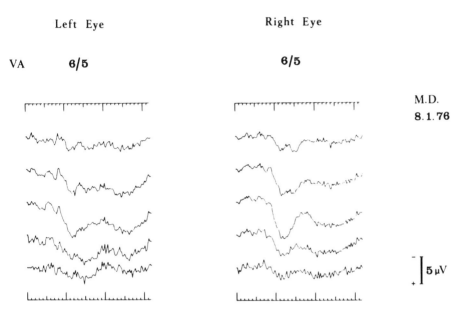

Left Eye   Right Eye

VA   6/5   6/5

M.D.
8.1.76

5 µV

Figure 7.25 *Monocular pattern EPs recorded in the same patient as in Figure 7.24 after 6 weeks treatment with vitamin B_{12}. Note the recovery of the midline positivity, which is nonetheless slightly delayed and poorly defined. Acuity in each eye has improved to 6/5.*

VEP ASYMMETRIES IN ALBINISM

An unusual form of crossed asymmetry, unaccompanied by any corresponding field defect, is encountered in albino subjects. This is a result of the peculiar anatomical anomaly characteristic of this condition, which has been extensively studied in the Siamese cat, but appears to be common to all species so far examined, including man (Guillery et al, 1975). In the normal individual each hemisphere receives a retino-cortical projection carrying visual information from the temporal half-field of the contralateral eye. This information, which arises in the nasal hemiretina, is transmitted by the fibres crossing in the optic chiasma. The corresponding information from the nasal half-field of the ipsilateral eye is carried by uncrossed fibres passing back to the cortical receiving areas on the same side. In the albino there is a misrouting of these retinocortical projections, such that, in addition to the projection from the whole of the temporal half-field, up to 20° of the nasal half-field fibres also cross in the chiasma to reach the other side. Each hemisphere therefore receives a predominantly monocular input from the contralateral eye, while the ipsilateral projection from the nasal half-field is limited to the more peripheral areas.

The misrouting of a large part of the projection from the nasal half-field to the contralateral hemisphere leads to a disorganization of the normal retinotopic cortical mapping. This appears to be dealt with in two distinct ways. In one, the so-called 'Boston' pattern, the anomalous nasal half-field representation is simply interpolated between V1 and V2 on either side of the border between areas 17 and 18 (Hubel and Wiesel, 1971). In the other variant, the so-called 'Mid-Western' pattern, the representation of the fixation point remains at the 17/18 border, as in the normal projection, and the anomalous nasal half-field projection overlies the mirror image projection of the temporal half-field. In this variant, there is some degree of suppression of the nasal half-field input, which is represented by relatively few cortical units (Kaas and Guillery, 1973). Both anomalies have been studied mainly in the Siamese cat, but it seems probable that similar abnormalities exist in albinos of other species, since the same basic anatomical misrouting is known to occur in them also.

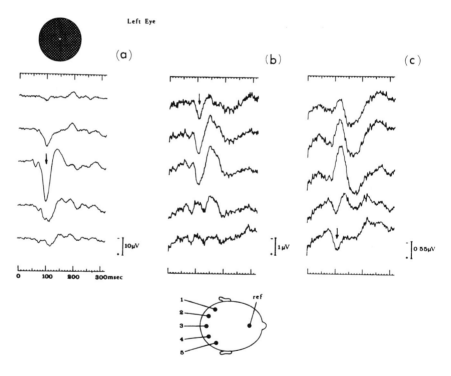

Figure 7.26 *Full-field pattern responses from the left eye of a normal subject (left hand record), as compared with the grand average of 5 albino subjects with a P100 (arrow) distribution ipsilateral to the stimulated left eye (middle records) and the grand average of 9 albino subjects with a contralateral P100 (arrow) distribution. The two distinct patterns of asymmetry found in the albino patients are illustrated in these two records. Note the much smaller amplitude of the responses from the albinos (see calibration). (From Carroll et al, 1980a.)*

Striking asymmetries in the monocular VEPs to both flash (Creel et al, 1974, 1978) and pattern stimulation (Creel, 1979; Coleman et al, 1979; Carroll et al, 1980a, 1980b) have been demonstrated. There are technical difficulties in carrying out these studies, as the responses from albino subjects are often of very low amplitude, due to the impaired acuity. There is also frequently a congenital nystagmus which necessitates special care in maintaining adequate fixation with half-field stimulation. However, in a careful study of the checkerboard pattern reversal response in 15 human albinos, Carroll et al (1980a, 1980b) have established that there is a marked asymmetry in every case, clearly distinguishing the albino responses from those of normal subjects (Figure 7.26). The asymmetry invariably resembled that produced by stimulation of the temporal half-field in the same eye. However, two quite distinct, and in some respects opposite, types of asymmetry were encountered in the albino group. In one the asymmetry resembled that produced by temporal half-field stimulation in a normal subject, in that the $\overline{P100}$ was ipsilateral to the stimulated eye or temporal half-field. In the other the opposite was the case, with the $\overline{P100}$ appearing contralateral to the stimulated eye or temporal half-field. In the latter case there was often a very prominent contralateral negative component (see Figure 7.26). Responses from the nasal half-field were in general similar to those for the temporal half-field, but were of small amplitude, particularly for the responses of the first type. Further details will be found in the paper by Carroll et al (1980b).

THE VEP ASSOCIATED WITH VARIOUS INTRACRANIAL LESIONS

The flash and pattern EP in cortical blindness

Although the occipital flash responses are frequently severely reduced or abolished in patients with cortical blindness (Kooi and Sharbrough, 1966; Brindley et al, 1969; Rouher et al, 1968; Bodis-Wollner, 1977), this is not always the case, and persistent flash responses may be found in the presence of apparently total cortical blindness, either confined to the vertex region (Kooi and Sharbrough, 1966; Paty et al, 1974) or at the occiput (Spehlmann et al, 1977). It is not clear whether these responses are mediated by extrageniculo-calcarine pathways. Many of the cases studied have been vascular in origin, where the exact extent and completeness of the lesion of the specific visual pathways is difficult to establish accurately.

Even more surprising and difficult to explain is the evidence that the pattern EP too may be apparently normal in some patients who appear to be totally blind following bilateral occipital infarction. Bodis-Wollner et al (1977) have described a 6-year-old boy with features suggestive of a disconnection syndrome of the primary visual receiving area in Area 17, following an acute febrile illness at the age of two years, which left him behaviourally blind. Although he was unable to localize a bright light or avoid obstacles, and showed no blink reflex to light or menace, he had well-preserved and essentially normal VEPs, both to diffuse flash and to 8 Hz stimulation with a reversing checkerboard or grating. The only EP abnormality appeared to be a loss of this steady-state response to fine gratings of high spatial frequency (5-6 cycles per degree or more). Computerized tomography demonstrated extensive destruction of both occipital lobes, with sparing of medial structures corresponding to part of the optic radiation and striate cortex.

A case apparently demonstrating the complementary situation of bilateral destruction of the striate area with preservation of Areas 18 and 19 has been described by Celesia et al (1980). This was a 72-year-old hypertensive woman with apparently total blindness of more than two years duration. She had no optokinetic nystagmus, and, although she still maintained that she could detect large moving objects, she was unable to detect a bright light being moved or turned on and off in front of her and performed at chance level when guessing. Nonetheless, both flash ERG and occipital flash EP were normal and pattern stimulation, with a 16° checkerboard of $\overline{27'}$ checks and a luminance of 52 foot-lamberts, produced a response with a $\overline{P100}$ of normal latency, although the initial negativity was missing. The critical frequency of photic driving (CFPD) to trains of flash stimuli was decreased from the normal value of 48/sec to 38/sec. Computerized tomography showed extensive destruction of the occipital lobes, involving Area 17 bilaterally and part of Area 18 on the left side, as well as both lingual gyri. There was bilateral sparing of all of Area 19 and part of Area 18.

In another study of a 69-year-old hypertensive woman recovering from a bilateral homonymous hemianopsia with macular sparing, Bodis-Wollner (1977) recorded the steady state EPs to sinusoidal gratings of varying spatial frequency, presented on an oscilloscope screen subtending 5° and reversed at 8 Hz. It was found that she had lost the responses to fine gratings, while the responses to coarser gratings were preserved, although at higher contrast than normal. When responses were present, they followed the simple linear relationship between contrast level and amplitude, originally demonstrated in the normal grating response by Campbell and Maffei (1970). Over the subsequent 4 weeks, her responsiveness to fine gratings improved, and this was paralleled by an improvement in her subjective ability to detect the gratings, measured in terms of the threshold contrast. On the initial examination after admission she had been unable to see gratings of more than 2.1 cycles/degree, but 2 weeks later she could detect them up to 17 cycles/degree and by 4 weeks, up to 26 cycles/degree. On the same three occasions pattern EPs could be recorded from gratings of up to 2.1 cycles/degree, 10 cycles/degree and 16 cycles/degree respectively. The finest detectable grating for the normal population is of 45 cycles/degree, corresponding to a bar width of 40 seconds and a visual acuity of 6/4.5.

The relatively close correlation between subjective visual acuity and grating EP amplitude in this recovering patient is in striking contrast to the apparently complete dissociation between the two in both the blind patients already mentioned. At present there seems no adequate explanation of these apparently conflicting findings, but it is clear that the presence of a normal pattern EP, while it may be necessary, is not sufficient to guarantee normal vision.

There is only very little evidence that cortical lesions anterior to the occipital lobes can affect the VEP. Feinsod et al (1974) have described a syndrome of 'suprastriate hemianopia' in a 52-year-old woman with a dense homonymous hemianopia accompanied by alexia, acalculia and object and colour anomia following a subarachnoid haemorrhage. The early occipital flash response was normal in waveform, but lacked a late component on the left side, which reappeared on recovery (Feinsod et al, 1975). Recovery followed surgical removal of a small superficial parieto-occipital arterio-venous malformation with an underlying haematoma. The right homonymous field defect and the associated parietal signs cleared within the first post-operative days and the flash EP recorded on the seventh day showed the late wave on the left side to have reappeared. The published record suggests the possibility that these authors may have been recording the $\overline{N150}$ component to the visual stimulus, which is known to be sensitive to attention (Hillyard et al, 1978).

The pattern EP in hysterical blindness

The author has reported elsewhere the value of the pattern EP in distinguishing between functional and organic sensory loss (Halliday, 1972). Unlike the flash EP, the pattern EP is usually very sensitive to the reduction of visual acuity and the finding of an objectively normal response in the presence of a complaint of gross visual impairment can generally provide a firm and confident basis for the diagnosis of hysterical sensory loss. This is particularly true where the loss is uniocular. However, as has already been emphasized, the situation is by no means so clear where there is any question of cortical blindness secondary to bilateral occipital lesions. Fortunately, the clinical features will usually serve to clarify or exclude this possibility.

Figure 7.27 shows the pattern reversal responses from a 15-year-old schoolgirl who was complaining of complete blindness in the right eye. She had woken up one morning four weeks previously unable to see out of the eye and said that if the left eye was closed, it was as if both eyes were closed, even if the right eye was open. Although there were no hysterical features in the previous history, she had been moody and quarrelsome and had recently had a row with her boy friend. Clinical examination revealed no abnormality, and both pupils reacted normally to light. The pattern response of normal amplitude and latency from the 'blind' right eye strongly supported a diagnosis of functional blindness.

Figure 7.28 shows the pattern responses from a 12-year-old girl with unilateral blindness of sudden onset following an injury to the eye. Nine months previously she had accidentally scratched the right eye with a cactus thorn embedded in the finger of her right hand. There was an abrasion of the eye, for which she received treatment, including an eye patch. When the patch was removed 10 days later, she complained of intermittent pain behind the eye and the visual acuity had dropped to the perception of light. Clinical examination revealed no abnormality and optokinetic nystagmus was normal from each eye, suggesting that the cortical visual function was not impaired. The pattern response from this eye was of the same waveform, latency and amplitude as that from its normal fellow.

The pattern response may be equally valuable, of course, in providing evidence of organic impairment in the presence of an hysterical overlay (Halliday, 1972). Figure 7.29 illustrates the pattern EPs from a 33-year-old woman presenting with gross hysterical symptoms, who nonetheless proved to have an underlying diagnosis of multiple sclerosis. The EP test in this patient established clearly for the first time the existence of organic disease after many years of varying clinical opinions as to the diagnosis.

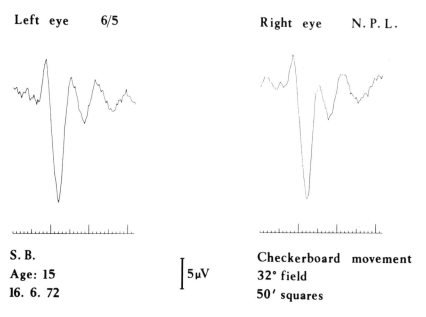

Left eye   6/5   Right eye   N. P. L.

S. B.   Checkerboard movement
Age: 15   ⎰5 µV   32° field
16. 6. 72   50′ squares

Figure 7.27 *Monocular pattern reversal EPs from a 15-year-old girl presenting with a complaint of complete loss of vision in the right eye. (From Halliday, 1972.)*

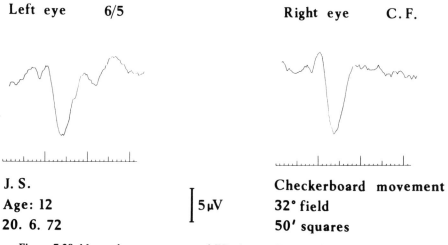

Left eye   6/5   Right eye   C. F.

J. S.   Checkerboard movement
Age: 12   ⎰5 µV   32° field
20. 6. 72   50′ squares

Figure 7.28 *Monocular pattern reversal EPs from a 15-year-old girl complaining of sudden blindness in the right eye, following a minor corneal abrasion. (From Halliday, 1972.)*

Patient 19

Pattern Movement

2/sec

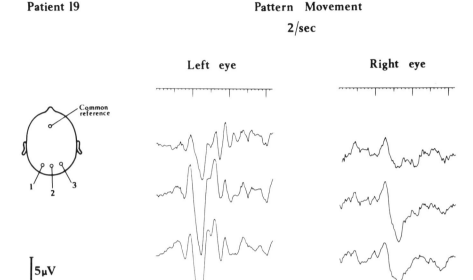

Figure 7.29 Pattern reversal responses from each eye of an undiagnosed 33-year-old patient with numerous hospital admissions for a variety of complaints over the previous 5 years (see text). (From Halliday, 1972.)

The pattern EP in migraine

Regan and Heron (1970) demonstrated lateralized amplitude asymmetries of the steady state checkerboard reversal response of more than 1.5:1 in three out of five migrainous patients recorded between attacks. They also showed a clear asymmetry in the course of the attack. Flicker responses also exhibited definite asymmetries at the time, but the ratio between the responses to nasal and temporal half-field stimulation could be quite different for the two types of EPs. The change during an attack could be as much as 500%.

Gawel et al (1979, 1980b) compared the transient checkerboard reversal response in 30 migraine patients with 30 age- and sex-matched controls, using binocular, monocular and hemifield stimulation. They found the major positivity delayed by 5-8 msec in the migraine patients ($p < 0.01$) and it was also greater in amplitude, particularly in those patients with consistently unilateral headaches. They further noted a slightly later $\overline{P100}$ in the right half-field response of the migraine patients, which was not seen in the normal group (3-4 msec, $p < 0.04$).

Papilloedema

Neither the pattern EP nor the flash EP shows any abnormality in papilloedema, so that a rise of intracranial pressure in itself is not sufficient to alter these responses. This result, which has been repeatedly confirmed in the author's experience, is in agreement with the findings of others. Rouher et al (1969) recorded normal flash responses in five patients with papilloedema and Babel et al (1977) in 12. The latter authors, however, also reported a waveform change of unknown significance in the later positive wave (their component C). The latencies were invariably normal. Asselman et al (1975) recorded normal pattern EPs in two patients with papilloedema. The author has recorded normal pattern EPs in a much larger number of similar patients.

Benign intracranial hypertension

Hume and Cant (1976) recorded pattern reversal EPs in two patients with benign intracranial hypertension. Both had delayed responses (up to 152 msec in one case) which improved after treatment.

Hydrocephalus

Jacobson et al (1968) found normal ERGs and almost abolished flash EPs in a 12-year-old patient with optic atrophy secondary to hydrocephalus and aqueduct stenosis. McInnes (1980) recorded the pattern EP and SEP in 10 patients with hydrocephalus, secondary to a variety of conditions such as aqueduct stenosis and posterior fossa tumour. The SEPs were invariably normal from both upper and lower limbs, but 2 of the VEPs were delayed and 6 had abnormal waveforms. Four of the 5 patients treated with ventriculo-peritoneal shunts showed a return to a normal configuration, but the 2 patients with delayed VEPs (both children with secondarily enlarged skulls) showed no change.

Flash evoked responses in photosensitive epilepsy

Flash stimulation, as well as eliciting an ERG and an occipital VEP, may also induce changes in the background EEG activity and evoke short-latency responses in the skeletal musculature. All four effects may be seen following flash stimulation in some photosensitive or myoclonic epileptics.

Hishikawa et al (1967) studied the EEG and flash EP in 15 photosensitive epileptics, 8 of whom had clinical attacks induced by viewing television. All had bilateral generalized spike-and-wave induced by intermittent photic stimulation of both eyes (the so-called 'photo-convulsive response'), and in about half the discharges appeared first in the occipital region and only subsequently spread almost simultaneously to involve the other areas. Photic stimulation was equally effective in REM sleep as in waking, but ineffective during slow wave sleep and drowsiness. Covering one eye also rendered the stimulation ineffective in all except one patient. Both stimulus and background intensity were important in determining the response. The flash EP showed an occipital spike which could often be recorded clearly in response to the first, second or third flash in the train, although it was frequently smaller, and a few milliseconds later, to the next 1 or 2 stimuli in the sequence. The latency of this early response varied from 35 msec to 50 msec in different patients. Meier-Ewert and Broughton (1967) studied the EMG response to flash stimulation (the so-called 'photo-myoclonic response') in 11 epileptics, including 2 patients with progressive myoclonic epilepsy (one with Lafora body disease) and 7 with petit mal, and also in 2 non-epileptic subjects.

The photo-myoclonic response consisted of a short-latency biphasic potential lasting 15-20 msec, appearing first over the frontal and temporal muscles (55 msec) and spreading caudally and peripherally to involve other muscles with an approximate speed of 30-40 m/sec. Although the amplitude of the response was very variable, the latencies for each muscle were stable in any one individual. The response could be recorded in deltoid (61 msec), biceps (64 msec), forearm flexors (65 msec), cervical trapezius-inion (78 msec), quadriceps (83 msec) and gastrocnemius (95 msec). These authors concluded that it represented an enhancement of the photo-motor response recorded at similar latencies in the healthy individual by Bickford (1964, 1966). The jerks involved both agonists and antagonists simultaneously, although the response tended to be of larger amplitude in flexors than extensors. In direct contradiction to Hishikawa et al (1967), Meier-Ewert and Broughton (1967) found both photo-convulsive and photo-myoclonic responses greatly depressed in REM sleep.

Broughton et al (1969) went on to examine the flash EP in the same 9 photosensitive epileptics together with 1 further patient with progressive myoclonic epilepsy. The SEP to median nerve stimulation at the wrist was also recorded in 8 of the patients. They noted an increased amplitude of the VEP, which was statistically significant for components N42, P58, N179 and P218. The N179 component was significantly later than in the controls (N142). Another important difference was that the VEP in the epileptics spread significantly further anteriorly to apppear at the C_3 and C_4 electrodes, particularly with respect to the early components (N42, P58 and P123). The authors were able to confirm the cortical origin of the VEP components by simultaneous cortical and scalp recordings in 2 epileptics during surgical biopsy.

The SEP in the photosensitive epileptics also showed abnormalities, including a much more widespread distribution than normal of all SEP components with significantly increased amplitudes of all the peaks from P25 on, but not for P15 or N19. N34 and the succeeding positivity (P44 in normals, P61 in the epileptics) were over 6 times larger than normal in mean amplitude and P25 over 3 times larger. The corresponding increases in the VEP were not so great as in the SEP.

This latter conclusion agrees with the findings of the present author, who compared the flash VEP and SEP in a large series of patients with progressive myoclonic epilepsy, and found both the mean increase in amplitude and the number of patients with responses beyond the upper limit of the normal amplitude range far greater for the SEP than the VEP (Halliday and Halliday, 1980). Figure 7.30 illustrates the SEP to stimulation of the index and middle fingers of each hand and the VEP to flash and pattern reversal stimuli recorded during the same session in a girl with myoclonic epilepsy. Note the very large SEPs appearing at the electrodes overlying the contralateral Rolandic area, and the waveform and topography of the flash EP which shows an early (50-60 msec) occipital spike which radiates forward to involve the central electrodes near the midline. The pattern reversal response has a slightly delayed P100 (note the monopolar montage used for the pattern response as compared with the bipolar montage for the flash response).

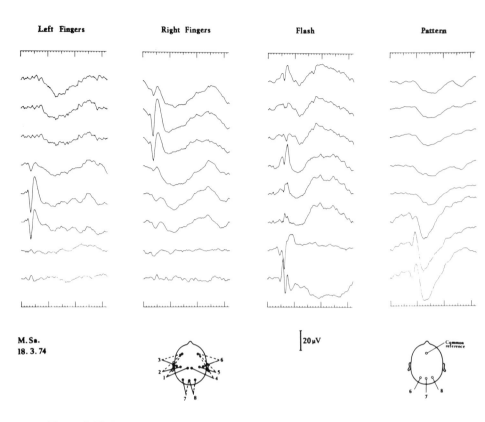

Left Fingers   **Right Fingers**   **Flash**   **Pattern**

M.Sa.
18.3.74

$20 \mu V$

Figure 7.30 *Somatosensory, flash and pattern reversal EPs from a patient with progressive myoclonic epilepsy. Note the large amplitude of the somatosensory responses, which also show an enhanced second negative component (compare Figure 7.31a), the large early components of the flash response radiating to the central channels and the large amplitude of the pattern reversal response, which in this case is also delayed, perhaps due to the associated pathology. Note the different montage used for the pattern responses.*

Figure 7.31 illustrates the amplitude distribution for the $\overline{P33}$ component of the SEP, recorded in a similar way from 22 myoclonic epileptics in (a) and from 32 healthy individuals in (b). Only half the patients have $\overline{P33}$ amplitudes within the normal range and the largest response has an amplitude 15 times greater than the normal mean. The mean amplitude in the myoclonics is 4.53 times greater than that in the controls. By comparison, the amplitudes of the $\overline{N50}$-$\overline{P100}$ components of the flash EP are shown in Figure 7.32 for 17 of the same patients, compared with those of 24 healthy individuals. Only 4 patients had values beyond the normal range, and the largest response was just over 5 times greater than the normal mean, while the mean increase in amplitude was 1.69.

The large SEPs and VEPs encountered in progressive myoclonic epilepsy are associated particularly with the incidence of the myoclonic jerking and the accompanying EEG spike discharges and are not seen in those patients recorded

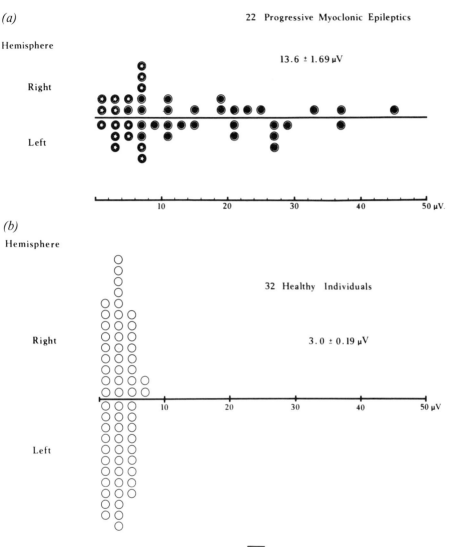

Figure 7.31 (a) Amplitude distribution of the $\overline{P32}$ of the SEP to contralateral digital nerve stimulation in 22 progressive myoclonic epileptic patients. The patients who were jerking at the time are indicated by the solid black circles, while those who were not jerking are asterisked; (b) amplitude distribution of the $\overline{P32}$ of the SEP in 32 healthy individuals. The mean and standard deviation are given in each case. (From Halliday and Halliday, 1980.)

when not jerking (Halliday, 1967b; Halliday and Halliday, 1980). This can be seen in the values for the individuals who were not jerking in Figures 7.31 and 7.32, whose responses are marked with an asterisk. In a similar way, the size of an enhanced response can be reduced to normal values by medication which controls the jerking. This was demonstrated by Ebe et al (1969) in a study of the effect of intravenous diazepam in 7 of their 10 photosensitive epileptics. Photo-convulsive and photo-myoclonic responses were very rapidly blocked by the infusion of 7.5-10 mgm of the drug, spontaneous epileptic discharges were abolished, and the early components of both SEP and flash VEP decreased in amplitude and became more localized. Figure 7.33 shows a similar change in size of SEP and VEP occurring between 2 recording sessions, 16 days apart, in an elderly familial myoclonic epileptic whose severe jerking had been controlled by clonazepam in the interim.

Flash Evoked Responses

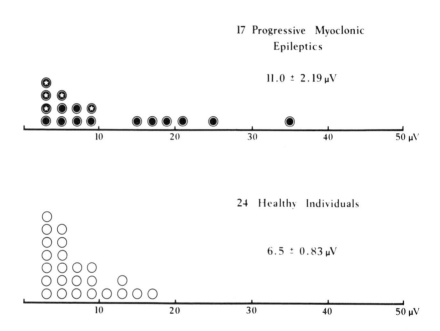

Figure 7.32 *Amplitude distribution of the* $\overline{N50}$*-*$\overline{P100}$ *component of the occipital VEP to flash stimulation in a group of progressive myoclonic epileptics and a control group of healthy subjects. The flash responses were recorded from a pair of occipital electrodes, one 3 cm above the inion in the midline and the other 3 cm to the left of this midoccipital electrode. (From Halliday and Halliday, 1980.)*

It is interesting that no similar enhancement of either SEP or VEP is found in association with the jerking of patients with benign essential myoclonus (Halliday and Halliday, 1980). In this condition, which is characteristically inherited as an autosomal dominant, the EEG is usually quite normal.

Bablouzian et al (1969) reported consistently larger amplitude occipital responses to a train of 3/sec flash stimuli in 4 'light-sensitive' individuals compared with 10 normal controls, with the components of maximum amplitude occurring later (183 msec as against 81 msec) and an increase in peak amplitude with repetitive stimulation.

Panayiotopoulos et al (1970) observed the occipital spike previously reported by Hishikawa et al (1967) in 21 out of 23 photosensitive epileptics following patterned flash stimulation (produced by a grid placed in front of the flash tube), finding it to be triphasic with a P85, a N102 and a variable later positive component. They noted that the spike was never seen after the first flash but appeared 0.2-3.0 seconds after the onset of a 5-9/sec flash train. The components of the occipital spike bore no simple relationship with the VEP components recorded at lower flash frequencies

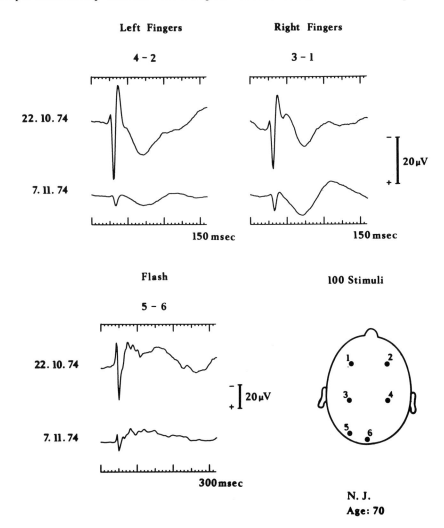

Figure 7.33 Effect of anti-myoclonic medication on the SEP and flash VEP in a severe progressive myoclonic epileptic. The first record (22.10.74) was taken while the patient was suffering from uncontrollable myoclonic jerking; the second (7.11.74) a fortnight after starting Clonazepam 0.5 mg four times daily. At the time of the second record, when the SEP amplitude had fallen to normal levels, the jerking had completely stopped. Note that the flash evoked response has also been reduced in amplitude. (From Halliday and Halliday, 1980.)

(1-4 Hz) in the same patients or in normal subjects. In a later study of 38 photosensitive epileptics, 21 of whom had attacks related to watching television, they confirmed that the occipital spikes preceded the photo-convulsive response in 87% of cases, and that there was no simple time relationship between the spikes and the components of the VEP to lower flash rates (Panayiotopoulos et al, 1972).

There have been a large number of combined clinical and electrophysiological studies of the effect of stimulation on the jerking and associated evoked EEG abnormalities in progressive myoclonic epilepsy since the pioneer study of Grinker et al (1938). Dawson's studies (1946, 1947b) were particularly fruitful as they led to his development of the method of SEP recording through the scalp in the healthy individual, first by the method of photographic superimposition (1947a) and later by averaging (1951, 1954a). Other notable studies have been those by Carels (1960) and Watson and Denny Brown (1955). The author has reviewed this literature several times elsewhere (Halliday, 1967a, 1967b, 1967c, 1967d, 1974; Halliday and Halliday, 1980). The recent application of jerk-locked averaging to this condition by Shibasaki and Kuroiwa (1975) is dealt with in Chapter 14.

The VEP in cerebromacular degeneration

Among the group of progressive myoclonic epileptics is a sub-group of patients with a variety of lipidoses, who fall within the loose diagnostic category of 'amaurotic family idiocy'. This sub-group includes several distinct pathological types, including neuronal ceroid lipofuscinosis (Batten's disease), Gaucher's disease (King, 1975) and the 'cherry-red-spot myoclonus' syndrome associated with sialidase deficiency (Thomas et al, 1979; Swallow et al, 1979). Neuronal ceroid lipofuscinosis, often called the 'late infantile form of amaurotic family idiocy' in the earlier literature (e.g. Carels, 1960), produces a very characteristic and apparently paradoxical combination of electrophysiological findings at a certain stage in its progression, to which Harden and Pampiglione have drawn attention (Harden and Pampiglione, 1972; Harden et al, 1973; Pampiglione and Harden, 1973). The flash ERG may be greatly depressed, or altogether lost, at a time when flash stimulation is still capable of evoking very greatly enlarged occipital EPs of up to 10 or 20 times those in a control group. The large amplitude occipital spikes, produced by low frequency photic stimulation (<3 Hz), reaching 50-500 µV in size, can be readily seen on the raw EEG record and produce a characteristic picture which can be diagnostically helpful. Green (1971) observed this picture in 7 out of 20 patients with Batten's disease and concluded that there was no single neurophysiological finding pathognomonic of this condition. Tackmann and Kuhlendahl (1979) have published findings on 3 further cases.

In a later publication Harden and Pampiglione (1977) discuss the differences in the ERG, VEP and EEG findings characteristic of various metabolic disorders. In Tay-Sachs disease (17 cases) they find the ERG unaffected, in keeping with the preservation of function of the outer retinal receptor elements (rods, cones and bipolar cells), the abnormal inclusions affecting particularly the ganglion cells. The flash VEP is recordable in the early stages of the disease, but the early components (before 100 msec) become poorly defined after 1 year and by 16 months of age the occipital VEP is no longer detectable. Five cases of Santavuori disease showed rapid flattening of the EEG by the age of 3-4 years, with the ERG and flash EP amplitude decreasing in parallel with it, reflecting the very rapid cell destruction in cortex and retina. Twenty-one cases of Bielschowsky-Jansky disease ('classical' neuronal ceroid lipofuscinosis or Batten's disease) showed the changes already described, the early loss of the ERG being related to the involvement of all retinal layers in the lesion. The large occipital VEP, unlike that in 'simple' photosensitive epilepsy, was not significantly reduced by resort to monocular stimulation. In 5 cases of Spielmeyer-Vogt disease, the ERG disappeared early and the occipital VEP was also eventually lost, although it persisted at small amplitude in some patients.

Parkinsonism

Bodis-Wollner and Yahr (1978) reported significant increases in the latency of the pattern reversal response in 35 patients with Parkinson's disease. The stimulus used was a somewhat unusual one, being a 2 Hz reversal of a vertical sinusoidal grating of 2.3 cycles per degree spatial frequency, displayed on a cathode ray oscilloscope screen subtending 3.8°. The mean luminance was low (4 cd/m^2) and the contrast level 0.7. The Parkinsonian patients gave major positivities with a mean latency of 143 ± 28 msec for the left eye and 139 ± 22 msec for the right eye, as against 116 ± 9 msec for either eye in a group of 26 patient controls suffering from other disorders. There was also a significant increase in the interocular latency difference from 3 ± 3.5 msec in the controls to 13 ± 17 msec in the Parkinsonians. Patients were screened for opacities or raised intraocular pressure, and the latency increase was independent of age. Twenty-four out of 30 of the Parkinsonians were classified as beyond the normal range on a discriminant function analysis. Curiously, the duration of the disease was *inversely* correlated with the latency increase, which the authors suggest may be related to the clinical subdivision of patients with Parkinson's disease into a 'malignant' and 'benign' group, on the basis of a fast or slow clinical evolution.

In a study, employing the more usual black-and-white checkerboard reversal stimulus, with a field size of 32°, checks of 50′ and a higher mean luminance (116 cd/m^2), carried out in the author's own department, no significant difference was found in the $\overline{P100}$ latency in a group of Parkinsonian patients (Kriss, Dell and Halliday, unpublished). More recently, a similar study by Gawel et al (1980a) has reported small but significant group mean increases (10 msec, p < 0.001) in the checkerboard reversal response latency in Parkinson's disease. An increased interocular latency difference was also noted (6.5 msec in the patients as against 1.7 msec in the controls, p < 0.001). However, there is some doubt about the validity of their control group, which contained a large preponderance of women. Since the difference in latency of the patient group was only a few milliseconds, and women are known to have a significantly shorter mean latency for the pattern response (see Chapter 3, page 89), it is possible that this result is fortuitous. Some past studies have included a number of Parkinsonian patients among their neurological control groups (e.g. Zeese, 1977; Celesia and Daly, 1977b). Celesia and Daly had 6 Parkinsonians in a group of neurological patients tested for both checkerboard reversal EPs and the critical frequency of photic driving. They reported them as entirely normal in every particular.

Huntington's chorea

Ellenberger et al (1978) studied the flash EP in a group of patients with Huntington's chorea and found that, while the latency of the major component was not significantly different from normal, the amplitude of the response was diminished compared with that in the control group. This agrees with the results of a study in the author's own department (Lawson et al, 1981), where exactly the same conclusions were reached in a study of the pattern reversal EP, and a similar study by Oepen et al (1982b). All three studies have found normal latencies and reduced amplitudes, a result which would be consistent with either a general axonal degeneration of the visual pathways or an impaired function of the cortical generator areas.

Effect of hypothermia and circulatory arrest on the VEP

Reilly et al (1978) recorded the flash EP in 8 infants, under 1 year of age, undergoing hypothermia (20-23°C) and total circulatory arrest for periods from 10-57 minutes in the course of open heart surgery for congenital defects. They found a progressive increase in the latency of the major positivity, P_2 (Ciganek's wave IV), during cooling and a complete loss of the VEP by the time that circulation arrest was instituted, in spite of the persistence of low voltage EEG activity. This confirms the similar results obtained in animal studies (Wolin et al, 1964). These observations indicate, without the need for further support, that the absence of the flash VEP has no useful place in the diagnosis of brain death, since the response may be absent when there is still spontaneous low-voltage EEG activity present. The presence of the flash EP may, however, be a valuable pointer to the preserved function of the cortical generator areas where this is in doubt.

8

Electrocochleography

W.P.R. Gibson

Electrocochleography is the recording of electric potentials originating from the cochlea and primary cochlear nerve fibres after acoustic stimulation. In clinical work the clearest potentials are obtained by using a transtympanic electrode. Adequate potentials may also be obtained using an electrode placed on the tympanic membrane or, provided it is placed carefully, within the external acoustic meatus. Placement of the transtympanic electrode or extratympanic electrode requires the services of an otologist. It is not surprising, given these circumstances, that the main appeal of the electrocochleogram is otological rather than neurological. The electrocochleogram provides a unique electrical picture of the cochlea both in health and disease. It is also important as it represents the initial neural process, and a clear understanding of the potentials is useful for those working with other potentials derived from higher levels of the auditory system.

HISTORICAL REVIEW

Adrian (1926) first recorded the action potentials of sensory nerves in animals. Some years later Wever and Bray (1930) demonstrated potentials from the animal cochlea; they believed initially that they had recorded a series of action potentials but Saul and Davis (1932) managed to record the true action potentials and it was subsequently shown that the earlier recordings had been of the cochlear microphonic. The summating potential was not described until many years later, when it was found almost simultaneously by Davis et al (1950) and by Békésy (1950).

Attempts to record these cochlear potentials in human subjects met with little success as the round window membrane was hidden deep within its niche and the amplifiers were not sufficiently stable to allow recordings from more distant sites (Fromm et al, 1935; Andreev et al, 1939; Perlman and Case, 1941). Lempert et al (1950) were forced to conclude that the recording of human cochlear potentials was impractical until better apparatus was available.

The better apparatus did arrive. Stable, biological amplifiers allowed Ruben and his group to obtain good recordings during middle ear surgery (Ruben et al, 1960, 1961, 1963), but it was the advent of electronic averaging techniques which really revolutionized the subject. Ronis (1966) used such a method first during middle ear surgery. At this time further development of electrocochleography within the USA halted as serious problems arose concerning possible malpractice claims.

The next event was the recording of cochlear potentials using averaging techniques from patients not undergoing middle ear surgery (so-called 'non-surgical recordings'). Yoshie et al (1967) were perhaps the first group to obtain such recordings using an electrode embedded in the external acoustic meatus. Sohmer and Feinmesser (1967) placed their electrode on the earlobe and Spreng and Keidel (1967) used the mastoid and scalp. It was the Bordeaux group (Portmann et al, 1968; Aran and Lebert, 1968) who returned to the transtympanic method suggested by Lempert et al (1950) and they encountered such clear recordings that their technique was rapidly adopted by many other workers.

Despite the fact that complications resulting from a transtympanic electrode appear to be extremely rare (Crowley et al, 1975), there has been reluctance to use the method, especially in the U.S.A., because of a fear of possible litigation. Several teams have attempted to find a non-invasive technique (among others Coats and Dickey, 1970; Cullen et al, 1972; Montandon et al, 1975a, 1975b; Humphries et al, 1977; Khechinashvili and Kevanishvili, 1974) but the drawback is that the potentials are 15 times smaller and the threshold reliability is poor compared to the transtympanic recordings.

Furthermore, recordings of the cochlear microphonic (CM) can only be obtained safely using a transtympanic electrode. If the electrode is not placed on the bony promontory but further from the ear, the intervening living tissue will produce mechano-electric artefacts which are difficult to distinguish from the CM. A clear 'microphonic' can be obtained by placing a pair of electrodes 3 cm apart on the back of the arm and then subjecting the array to a loud acoustic stimulus. The only really safe method of ensuring that the CM is true is to observe its attenuation and phase alteration when the non-test ear receives a sound of sufficient intensity to evoke the stapedius reflex. Further details are given later in this chapter.

TERMINOLOGY

The most acceptable abbreviation for electrocochleography is ECochG, as ECOG has already been used to describe the electrocorticogram. The action potential (AP) is shown by most clinical workers with its main negative peak, with respect to the active electrode, as a downward deflection. Electrophysiologists may object, but too late as the clinicians have already won the day!

THE COCHLEAR POTENTIALS

Three types of electrical activity are evoked by acoustic stimulation which can be recorded from the normal cochlea using the ECochG.

(a) The action potential (AP)

The AP recorded from near the round window membrane represents an integral of the combined activity of many individual nerve fibre action potentials firing in a manner determined by their position along the cochlear partition and by the nature of the travelling wave initiating their excitation. The fibres within the basal turn of the cochlea fire in close unison and so contribute to the major component of the click-evoked AP (Figure 8.1). The relationship between the single unit activity and the whole nerve AP has been established by Goldstein and Kiang (1958). The AP has a pattern which is quite different from that of the acoustic stimulus which elicits it, and so the response cannot be confused with electrical or mechanical artefacts. The AP has a precise threshold which indicates the threshold for neural activity leaving the cochlea. This threshold relates closely to the hearing threshold. Hence the AP can be used confidently as an objective method of assessing hearing in the higher audiometric frequencies.

(b) The cochlear microphonic (CM)

The CM is an alternating potential originating from the cuticular surface of the hair cells within the organ of Corti. The electrical waveform of the CM so closely resembles the electrical waveform of the stimulus (Figure 8.2) that care must be taken not to confuse it with any artefacts encountered by the recording system. Using a transtympanic electrode, it is only the outer hair cells lying within a few millimeters of the round window membrane that contribute to the recorded CM regardless of the frequency of the acoustic stimulus. The CM varies considerably in both amplitude and phase between different normal subjects, and varies if the electrode is placed in different positions around the round window niche in the same subject. The CM has no true threshold, as the level at which the CM can no longer be identified depends on the quality and gain of the recording amplifiers. Even if a criterion CM voltage level is used to determine a threshold, this threshold does not bear any clear relationship to the threshold of hearing. The clinical value of the CM is restricted to neuro-otological diagnosis.

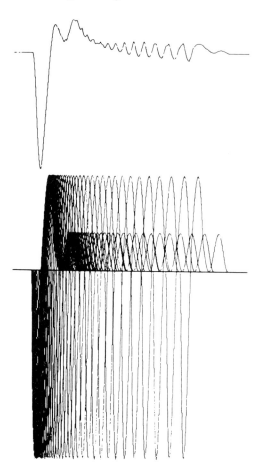

Figure 8.1 *The lower trace proportionally represents the action potentials (AP) arising from the many auditory fibres during the 12 msec immediately following a click stimulus. The APs on the left arise from the basal coil and fire first with the greatest synchrony, while those towards the right fire with progressively less synchrony. The manner of firing can be calculated from the pattern of the Békésy travelling wave. The upper trace represents the whole nerve AP composed of the algebraic summation of all the individual APs and resembles closely the click-evoked AP obtained using transtympanic electrocochleography.*

(c) The summating potential (SP)

The SP is a multi-component potential arising from any non-linear source of electrical activity within the cochlea (Dallos et al, 1972). A major source results

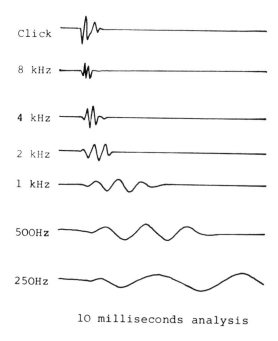

Click

8 kHz

4 kHz

2 kHz

1 kHz

500Hz

250Hz

10 milliseconds analysis

Figure 8.2 The cochlear microphonic (CM) as evoked by a click or by various different tone bursts of 2 sine waves duration. The recordings show the accuracy of the cochlea in transforming the acoustic energy into the electrical waveform of the stimulus.

from asymmetrical vibration of the basilar membrane, causing the CM to be generated unequally with a predominance towards one electrical polarity (Whitfield and Ross, 1965) (Figure 8.3). In the normal ear, the SP is only generated at high stimulus intensities; its polarity is negative with respect to the transtympanic electrode. The SP occurs simultaneously with the CM and persists for the duration of the basilar membrane vibration. At high stimulus intensities, the SP amplitude may exceed that of the CM. This is explained by remembering that the CM represents the sum of individual hair cell CMs which are generated in different phases according to their position along the basilar membrane, and the total CM is therefore a vector quantity. The SP is not phase sensitive and its amplitude is directly proportional to the amount of basilar membrane displacement. The total SP is therefore an algebraic quantity. The largest CM contributions come from the hair cells nearest the recording electrode, while the SP includes contributions from more distant sites along the basilar membrane. The SP has therefore some frequency specificity but it cannot be used for threshold estimations.

(d) Pathological cochlear potentials

In addition to the normal cochlear potentials, there are almost certainly other cochlear potentials which can be obtained from the ear when its physiology is

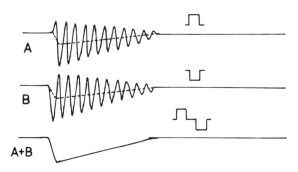

Figure 8.3 *A diagram of a possible mode of generation of the summating potential (SP). A represents the CM obtained from a high intensity tone burst. B represents the CM obtained from the same stimulus presented in the opposite phase. In each trace the baseline (dotted line) is distorted so that adding the traces (A+B), the CM is eliminated leaving the baseline shift clearly evident. The baseline shift is the SP.*

disturbed by pathological processes. Kiang and Peake (1960) identified a 'slow potential' in the denervated cat cochlea. This potential resembles the SP except that its onset latency is 0.7-1 milliseconds after the onset of the CM. Beagley and Gibson (1978) have recorded a similar potential from patients having VIII nerve tumours.

More recently Aran et al (1980) report finding a short latency (0.3 msec) diphasic response in guinea pig's ears after total destruction of the cochlea by amikacin. They speculate that the response arises from vestibular receptors.

INSTRUMENTATION

The apparatus needed for recording the ECochG is similar to that used for recording the other fast acoustically-evoked electrical potentials (brainstem responses, myogenic responses and middle latency responses). If one already possesses the equipment for these tests, then the only extra requirements for ECochG are a special electrode for placement through or onto the tympanic membrane and a co-operative otologist to place it.

The specific requirements for ECochG are now discussed.

The stimulating equipment

The stimulus is provided by a stimulus generator, which produces the electrical waveform, and it is then amplified and fed to an electromechanical transducer. The transducer may either be a loudspeaker or an earphone; it changes the electrical signal to an acoustic waveform with a degree of precision which depends on the quality of the transducer. The intensity of the stimulus is varied by an attenuator, usually providing 5 dB steps from 0 - 120 dB HL.

A loudspeaker has several disadvantages for ECochG. The main disadvantage is that unless the test chamber is anechoic, sounds bounce off walls, etc., and cause reverberations which may evoke secondary responses which can mar the recordings. Obviously a closed acoustic system would be ideal but the position of the active electrode usually prevents such a system. One method of electrode placement which does allow the use of a closed acoustic system has been described by Elberling and Salomon (1971). Clinically some compromise suffices, and an adequate system is provided by attaching an earphone to the ring support placed around the test ear (Figure 8.4). The earphone should be mu-metal screened to prevent electromagnetic artifacts.

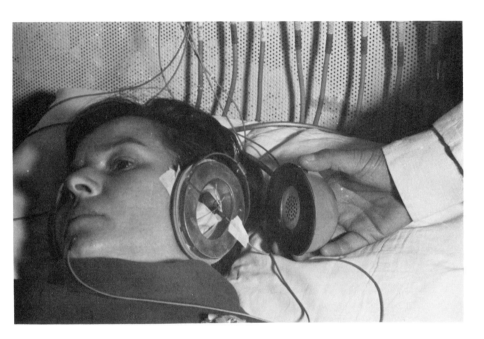

Figure 8.4 *The ring support which holds the transtympanic electrode in position. A mu-metal screened earphone is attached magnetically to this support.*

The stimulus requirements

The AP is best evoked by a brief stimulus with a rapid onset. Ideally the stimulus should fulfil three requirements; it must be exact in timing so that the latency of the response is clear, it must be frequency-specific and its intensity must be known. A click stimulus meets the first requirement but has no frequency-specificity; nevertheless it evokes an excellent 'whole-nerve' AP. A frequency-specific stimulus is a pure tone devoid of any click artefacts. Such a stimulus must have a gradual rise and fall to avoid high frequency transients. This slow rise time prevents the stimulus meeting the first requirement and does not allow for close synchrony of firing of the individual nerves within the basal turn of the cochlea. As a result the ECochG is poorly formed and there can be difficulties in identifying it using stimulus intensities which are barely greater than the subject's hearing threshold. Obviously there is a conflict of stimulus requirements for ECochG. Davis (1976) has summarized the situation crisply; 'on the one hand the stimulus must be brief to evoke a clear response, but on the other hand it should have a long rise time to be frequency-specific'. Three types of stimuli provide a compromise and allow some frequency information to be gained (Figure 8.5).

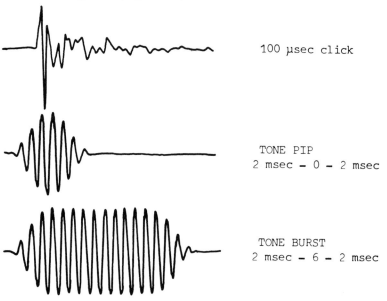

100 µsec click

TONE PIP
2 msec – 0 – 2 msec

TONE BURST
2 msec – 6 – 2 msec

Figure 8.5 *Three types of stimulus commonly used for ECochG: (a) a click with a very fast rise time and a gradually decaying fall; (b) a tone pip with a rise time and fall time of 2 msec and no plateau; (c) a tone burst with a rise and fall time of 2 msec and a plateau of 6 msec. (The author thanks H.A. Beagley for these traces which were generated using a microprocessor system.)*

(a) **Filtered clicks** are produced by filtering unwanted frequencies from a click by using high and low pass filters. The resulting waveform has a sudden onset with a gradually decaying 'tail' which oscillates at the predetermined frequency. Unfortunately, the onset of such a stimulus inevitably contains transients of higher frequency which are themselves capable of evoking an AP response.

(b) **Tone pips** are produced by passing a single sinusoidal wave, which begins and ends at zero crossing, through high and low pass filters. These stimuli have maximal energy for only the period of a single sinusoid.

(c) **Tone bursts** are periods of tone stimulation which are shaped so that they have a rise time of 1 or more milliseconds and a plateau of maximal energy lasting several milliseconds before a preset fall time. These stimuli are useful for ECochG as they enable some measurement of the CM, SP and slow component (SC)* potentials. At the lower audiometric frequencies, they do not evoke clear responses.

*See pages 288, 296 and 308.

Masking noise

A major advantage of ECochG is that it is never necessary to mask the non-test ear. Masking noise can be delivered to the test ear to improve the frequency-specificity of the AP response, and one method of using high pass masking to derive the AP from limited segments of the cochlea will be described later in this chapter.

The recording equipment

The recording equipment for ECochG is basically the same as that for other forms of evoked response audiometry. The bioelectric activity is obtained from electrodes and then amplified. The typical impedance of a transtympanic electrode is 60 kilohms. The amplifiers must have a high common mode rejection (over 120 dB) and a high input impedance (over 1 Megohm). These characteristics are available on most commercial ERA apparatus. The signal is filtered to limit unwanted bioelectric activity. The typical ECochG bandpass is 3.2 Hz to 3.2 KHz with a gradual filter slope of 6-20 dB per octave outside these limits. The use of higher settings (e.g. 250 Hz) for the high pass (or low cut) filter causes distortion of the AP, renders the SP unobtainable and limits the recording of the CM. If the ECochG is to be used purely for the purpose of determining threshold, this may be acceptable but it severely limits its neuro-otological rôle as many of the pathological low frequency changes are unobtainable. The filtered, amplified signals are averaged in the usual fashion.

The recording electrodes

The reference and earth electrodes are placed on the skin at the ipsilateral mastoid or earlobe and at the nasion or chin respectively. Any high quality EEG electrodes can be used. Commonly the silver/silver chloride dome-shaped disc electrodes, 0.6 mm diameter, are employed.

The active electrode is specialized and the type is dependent on the site used. Transtympanic electrodes are made from a thin steel wire (Figure 8.6) which is insulated except at its extreme tip and at the opposite end where it is gripped by the electrode holder. Provision can be made for varying the total length of the electrode assembly from 4 - 6 cm by arranging for the electrode to slide up and down in the holder. The extratympanic electrode usually rests upon the posterior-inferior rim of the tympanic membrane. It is made of flexible wire with a ball of silver of 1 mm diameter coated with silver chloride at the end which makes contact with the membrane. This electrode is generally fixed in position with a quick drying glue. Other workers have been trying to develop an electrode which fits on a spring loaded clip which can be placed in the meatus by non-medically qualified technicians (Durrant, 1977).

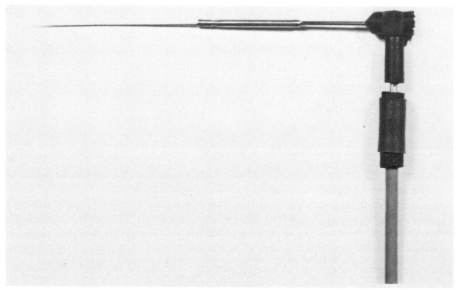

Figure 8.6 *The transtympanic electrode (total length 5 cm).*

TESTING PROCEDURES

The test procedure varies according to the age of the patient and their ability to co-operate with the test. All patients should be tested lying comfortably on a couch. A major advantage of ECochG is that a subject can be tested under full general anaesthesia. It is impossible to perform ERA on some small children while they are awake. Sedatives can act quite unpredictably, and some children are so affected that they remain deeply asleep for hours, while other children who are given the same dosage may remain wide awake and unco-operative. An expertly given general anaesthetic is probably safer, especially if the child suffers from other problems such as brain damage. It is not necessary to use general anaesthesia for co-operative adults.

Children

The subject of anaesthesia is discussed by Hutton (1976). Ketamine® is favoured by many clinics; Hutton (1976) recommends a dose of 1 mg intramuscularly for each 35 cm^2 of body surface area. The dose ensures that the child is still for 30-45 minutes, which is usually adequate for the test period. The advantage of Ketamine® is safety, as the laryngeal reflexes are not affected. The disadvantage is that it can cause unpleasant hallucinations, especially in older subjects. Ketamine® should probably not be given to subjects over 5 years of age. Another disadvantage is that it may take the child several hours to awaken fully, and nursing supervision is required.

Standard anaesthesia has the advantage that recovery is much faster and that it can be used for older subjects. Halothane ® is the agent preferred by the author. Arrangements must be made to vent the expired gases outside the close confines of the test chamber. Hutton (1976) describes the use of an Enderby valve. He vents the expired gases through a long rubber tube which leads outside the test area, and to prevent reflux he places the valve near the patient's head.

It may be argued that, whenever general anaesthesia is required, the potentials should be obtained by the transtympanic method. The insertion of the electrode is justifiable as the potentials obtained are larger and more reliable. Surely, if the child has been anaesthetized it makes sense to obtain optimal potentials, especially as the probability of any complication due to the use of a transtympanic electrode is slight.

Adults

Transtympanic electrocochleography on co-operative adults does not require any general anaesthesia or sedation; in fact, many clinics, especially in France, perform the test without any anaesthesia whatsoever. Local anaesthesia is possible and can add to the comfort of the patient. Local anaesthesia can be obtained by injection of the post-auricular branch of the vagus by piercing the skin behind the pinna immediately above the midpoint of the posterior meatal wall. In the author's experience patients found this more unpleasant than the insertion of an electrode through an unanaesthetized tympanic membrane.

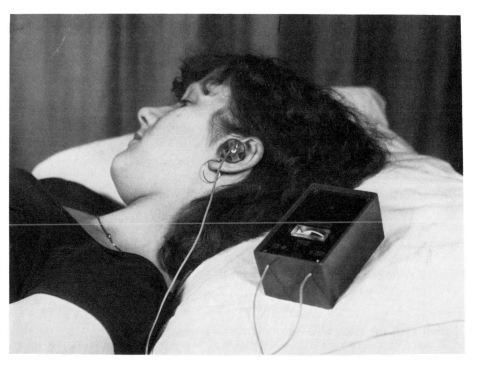

Figure 8.7 *A subject undergoing iontophoresis to anaesthetize her tympanic membrane prior to the insertion of the needle electrode.*

Spraying the tympanic membrane with local anaesthetic solution is useless as it does not penetrate squamous epithelium. The best method of local anaesthesia is iontophoresis (Ramsden et al, 1977a). This technique employs a small direct current to drive the positive ions of the anaesthetic solution into the tissues. The tympanic membrane is inspected to ensure there is no perforation and that the meatus is free of wax. The meatus is then filled with a fresh solution of 2% lignocaine and 1:2,000 adrenaline in equal quantities. A larger negative electrode is placed on the patient's forearm covering a wide area, to avoid blistering, and a positive electrode is introduced into the fluid in the ear without touching the meatus. A current of 0.5 amperes is applied for 10 minutes (Figure 8.7). The tympanic membrane is then fully anaesthetized for a period of 45 minutes. The patient will still hear the electrode being inserted if he has normal hearing and will still experience slight discomfort when the electrode touches the promontory.

The patient must be warned not to move his head while the needle is inserted. Special care must be taken when testing deaf patients. The author has not found it necessary to use sedatives or psychotropic drugs but some workers do give their patients a small dose of diazepam (Valium ®) prior to the test.

IDENTIFICATION OF THE NORMAL POTENTIALS

Several different electrical components are obtained from the cochlea by ECochG. There are some useful techniques for identifying the specific elements concerned.

Isolation of the action potential (AP)

The AP can be conveniently distinguished from the CM by alternating the phase of the stimulus during averaging. At moderate stimulus intensities (below 80 dB HL), the CM reverses its phase completely in parallel with the change of phase of the stimulus. The AP is not so phase sensitive and remains largely unaltered except when using stimulus frequencies below 1 KHz.

The responses to one phase of stimulation may be fed to one averager store (A) while the responses to the other phase of stimulation are fed to another store (B). If the responses are then added (A + B) the CM is suppressed and the AP is clearly seen (Figure 8.8).

At low frequencies (e.g. 500 Hz), this technique will blur the AP response as its latency alters considerably if the stimulus phase reverses (Elberling and Salomon, 1971).

Isolation of the cochlear microphonic (CM)

The CM may be isolated from the other electrical potentials by using alternate phases of stimulation and by subtracting the responses in one phase (A) from those obtained in the other phase (B) (Figure 8.8).

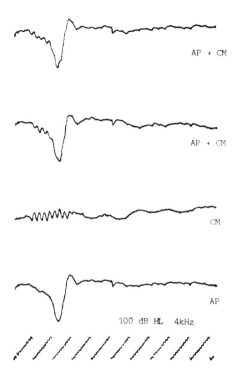

Figure 8.8 *The usual method of separating the AP and CM by combining the responses from stimuli presented in alternating phases. The top trace represents the responses to one type of stimulus; the second trace shows the response obtained when the stimulus is presented in the opposite phase. The CM faithfully follows the change of phase of the stimulus whereas the AP maintains its polarity independently of the phase. Subtracting the traces isolates the CM, and adding them isolates the AP (the amplitude of the AP is halved in the lowest figure).*

Isolation of summating potential (SP)

The technique of multiplexing the responses to alternate stimuli of opposite phases suppresses the CM, and the resulting average (A + B) reveals not only the AP but also the SP contributions. The SP can be identified by using a subtraction technique based on the adaptation of the AP at fast interstimulus intervals (ISI) (Figure 8.9). First a stimulus repetition rate of 5 per second is used which provides a long ISI and the AP and SP are obtained at their maximum values (store A); next, the responses are obtained at a short ISI (100 or 200 stimuli per second) and the AP is considerably reduced, due to neural adaptation, while the SP is unaltered (store B). Finally, subtraction of store A from B reveals that part of the AP which underwent adaptation without any SP contribution. By comparing the various traces, it is simple to obtain a fairly accurate indication of the SP contribution to the

ECochG waveform. The denervated cochlea may provide an SP-like potential called the 'slow component' which can be isolated using a similar technique.

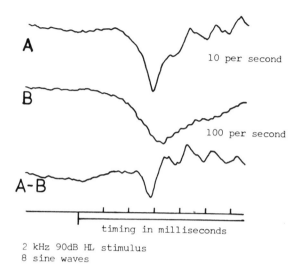

Figure 8.9 *A means of identifying the SP. The CM is suppressed in the usual way (see Figure 8.8). Using a long interstimulus interval, both the AP and SP are obtained at their maximum amplitude (A). At a short interstimulus interval (B), the amplitude of the SP is unaffected but the AP shows considerable adaptation. Subtraction of the traces (A-B) reveals AP alone without any SP contribution.*

High pass masking techniques

High pass masking (HPM) noise is noise that passes through a sharp high pass filter of 60-100 dB per octave which prevents the sound energy below the specific frequency of the filter from emerging. The resulting noise is therefore limited to the higher frequencies. This HPM noise is presented continuously to the cochlea and simultaneously a click stimulus is used to obtain the AP. This AP is produced only by the nerve fibres in the more apical (low frequency) part of cochlea as the more basal (high frequency) regions of the cochlea are masked by the noise. By using HPM with different cut-off frequencies, it is possible to derive the AP from limited cochlea segments. For example (Figure 8.10), the click AP is first obtained in the presence of 4 KHz HPM noise and stored (A), next the click AP is obtained in the presence of 2 KHz HPM noise and stored (B). Subtraction of the two stores (A – B) reveals the AP arising from the segment of the cochlea representing 2 - 4 KHz.

This technique can be used to obtain a frequency specific AP (Figure 8.11) which can be used to estimate the pure tone threshold audiogram. Unfortunately, the technique is rather time-consuming and, as tone pips also provide some frequency specificity, the latter method is more practical as a clinical procedure.

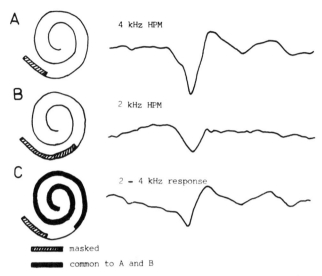

Figure 8.10 *The use of high-pass masking to isolate the AP from a distinct segment of the cochlea. (A full description of this Figure is given in the text).*

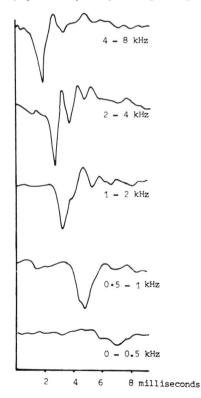

Figure 8.11 *The frequency-specific AP obtained by using a high-pass masking technique. The frequency range of each AP is indicated according to the bands of high-pass masking noise used (see Figure 8.10).*

Notched noise

Picton and his co-workers (1979) have suggested that notched noise can be used to mask the frequency spread of acoustic energy in brief tone pips. They reported that the thresholds obtained were more frequency specific and accurate to within 20 dB of the conventional audiometric thresholds. The slope of the filters producing the notched noise must be extremely sharp (45-60 dB/octave) to prevent the noise masking the responses.

THE NORMAL ELECTROCOCHLEOGRAM

The action potential

The normal ear invariably provides clear responses when a transtympanic electrode is used, but the potentials can be more difficult to identify from more distant sites. This is explained as due to the electrical activity being readily conducted through the cochlear fluids, but being rapidly attenuated as it passes through the more resistant tissues such as bone. Obviously the closer the electrode lies to the round window membrane, the larger the potentials. The average peak-to-peak amplitudes of the click-evoked or whole-nerve action potential varies considerably. In a study of normal or near normal ears the action potential at 110 dB HL varied from 1 to over 60 μV with an average amplitude of 7 μV (Figure 8.12). Those subjects who only provide a small AP may cause difficulties when an extratympanic electrode is employed.

The amplitude of the AP derived from an ear canal electrode is approximately 15 times smaller than that obtained from a transtympanic electrode. Often the AP is so

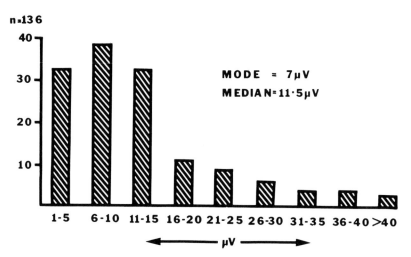

Figure 8.12 *The range of AP amplitudes encountered clinically on testing subjects with normal hearing and some patients with minor hearing impairments (from data compiled by H.A. Beagley).*

small that it cannot be distinguished from the background noise. Yoshie (1973) remarked that the AP threshold was on average 17.6 dB less sensitive when recorded directly from the ear canal as compared with the promontory.

The AP is even smaller when obtained from the ear lobe or mastoid — approximately 30 times smaller than that obtained by the transtympanic method. It is unusual to be able to identify the mastoid recorded AP within 40 dB of the cochlear threshold.

The input/output functions

The change in the amplitude and latency of the response with changes in stimulus intensity are known as the input/output functions. The most obvious feature is that the amplitude decreases and the latency lengthens as the stimulus intensity becomes less (Figure 8.13). The AP is usually measured in microvolts from its main negative peak to the following positive peak, and its latency is determined by measuring the time elapsed in milliseconds between the onset of the stimulus (at the tympanic membrane) to the main negative peak.

The amplitude/intensity graph shows two main areas known as the 'H curve' and the 'L curve' (see Figure 8.13). The 'H' curve, or high intensity area, was thought to correspond to the output of the inner hair cells, while the 'L' curve or low intensity portion was thought to correspond to the output of the outer hair cells. This is likely to be an over-simplification and the true explanation may relate to the tuning curves of individual nerve fibres (Evans, 1975).

The latency/intensity graph often shows a marked change corresponding to the

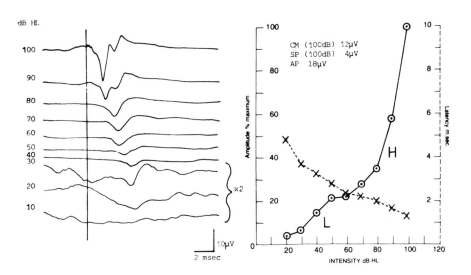

Figure 8.13 *The normal electrocochleogram. The click-evoked AP at varying intensities is shown on the left side. The amplitude/intensity graph is expressed as a percentage of the largest response. The latency/intensity graph is shown in dotted lines. Note the two distinct segments of the amplitude/intensity graph: the H (high level) portion and the L (low level) portion.*

transition between the 'H' and 'L' areas of the amplitude/intensity graph. The click-evoked AP also shows changes in the waveform corresponding to the amplitude changes. At high intensities it has a monophasic character and the first negative deflection is the largest, followed by a smaller N_2 and perhaps an N_3 peak. At lower intensities it is the second negative deflection (N_2) which appears to become dominant and can be detected down to the cochlear threshold. At the point of transition between the 'H' and 'L' areas, the AP often has a double peaked waveform (see Figure 8.13).

The frequency-specificity of the AP

The AP can only be clearly identified when a number of individual nerve fibres fire in synchrony to provide a recognizable net electrical change. A click stimulates the entire length of the basilar membrane but the fibres in the basal turn provide the major component of the AP, as the individual fibres placed higher along the cochlear turns do not fire with sufficient synchrony to produce a clear response. This is partly because the travelling wave responsible for activating the nerve endings becomes progressively damped as it travels towards the apex (Zwicker and Fastl, 1972), and partly because the velocity of the travelling wave slows as it approaches the apex, so that there is a decrease in the number of hair cells firing per unit time (Zerlin, 1969).

Pure tone bursts of short duration can be used to evoke a frequency specific AP

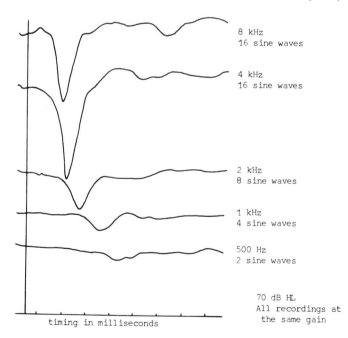

8 kHz
16 sine waves

4 kHz
16 sine waves

2 kHz
8 sine waves

1 kHz
4 sine waves

500 Hz
2 sine waves

70 dB HL
All recordings at
the same gain

timing in milliseconds

Figure 8.14 *The frequency specific AP obtained using short tone bursts from a normal ear. The amplifier gain was kept constant to illustrate the difficulty of obtaining clear responses using low frequency stimuli.*

(Figure 8.14). The latency of these APs directly reflect the speed of the travelling wave. At high stimulus intensities the frequency specificity is poor, as these stimuli activate a considerable length of basilar membrane, but at intensities below 60 dB the frequency specificity is good (Eggermont and Odenthal, 1974a). The frequency specific AP can be clearly identified using stimuli between 2 - 8 KHz, but at lower frequencies the synchrony of the AP is poor, making threshold estimation hazardous. It is not practically possible to evoke an AP using frequencies below 500 Hz. This finding limits the use of ECochG to the higher audiometric frequencies.

It is possible to identify the responses to low frequency stimulation using the high-pass masking technique but the procedure is too time-consuming for routine clinical application. Tone pips provide a reasonable clinical estimation of hearing at 500 Hz and 1 KHz and the use of notched noise (Picton et al, 1979) may further aid the frequency specificity.

Test/retest reliability

The repeatability of ECochG responses is better than for any other method of evoked response audiometry (ERA). For frequencies above 2 KHz, the AP threshold accurately identifies the cochlear threshold within ± 10 dB. The correlation between the psycho-acoustic threshold and the ECochG threshold deteriorates as the stimulus frequency becomes progressively lower, and Gibson (1978) reported a gap of up to 60 dB on average at 500 Hz.

The normal cochlear microphonic (CM)

The normal CM has an amplitude between 5 - 25 µV for 110 dB HL click stimulation (Gibson, 1978). The amplitude of the CM increases as the stimulus frequency is lowered. The amplitude increase relates to the larger number of hair cells within the basal turn providing electrical responses which are essentially in phase, and in no way relates to any true frequency specificity.

The normal CM has a characteristic amplitude/intensity function which reaches a maximum at 100 - 110 dB HL. This finding does not ensure freedom from electrical artifacts which may exhibit identical amplitude/intensity characteristics. The wisest method of investigating the validity of the CM responses is by using the stapedius muscle reflex (Elberling and Salomon, 1973). A click stimulus delivered with a long interstimulus interval does not evoke a stapedius muscle contraction at the instant that the CM is recorded (the latency of the CM is approximately 0.3 msec, while that of the stapedius muscle is 15 msec). If noise is introduced into the contralateral ear with sufficient intensity to cause a bilateral stapedius muscle contraction, the amplitude of the CM should be reduced by an amount corresponding to a stimulus reduction of approximately 10 dB and the phase of the CM shifts by nearly 90 degrees. The CM recorded by transtympanic ECochG at moderate intensities (60 - 90 dB HL) exhibits these characteristics clearly, but the CM recorded by extratympanic electrodes does not show any such alteration in the author's experience.

The normal summating potential (SP)

The normal summating potential can be identified using stimulus intensities over 70 dB HL. There is a wide variation in the amplitudes obtained from normal ears. In a series of 33 normal ears tested by the author, the SP amplitudes varied from 0.5 to 10 μV using a 100 dB HL click stimulus. It was noticeable that the larger amplitudes were related to the recordings which gave the larger AP amplitudes. As the clinical significance of the SP rests on whether it is relatively enlarged as compared with the AP and causes a distortion of the SP/AP complex, the width of the SP/AP complex has been used as a measure (Gibson, 1980). Normal ears never yield a width of over 3 msec using a click stimulus, whereas ears affected by endolymphatic hydrops often have a SP/AP complex of over 3 msec width. There are nevertheless several pitfalls to this approach which stem from the fact that the SP duration is related to the duration of the stimulus. The acoustic duration of a click stimulus depends on the amount of acoustic 'ringing' and hence on the quality of the transducer, etc.

Recently the author has changed his approach and now expresses the SP amplitude as a percentage ratio of the AP amplitude. In a series of 33 normal ears, the SP/AP ratio ranged from 10 to 63 per cent (mean 25.03%, s.d. 13.7) using a 100 dB HL click stimulus. Although the range of normal is large, the difference in the SP/AP ratio between ears with a hearing loss due to pure hair cell damage and those with endolymphatic hydrops is marked and will be discussed later in this Chapter.

THE ELECTROCOCHLEOGRAM IN PATHOLOGICAL CONDITIONS

The ECochG shows changes which may be directly related to pathological conditions which occur within the cochlea. These changes have considerable diagnostic significance for the otologist. In general, the ECochG remains unaltered in most conditions affecting the CNS, so that ECochG data has limited value to the neurologist, except in some cases where the disparity between the ECochG potentials and the potentials obtained from higher levels of the auditory tract clearly indicate an interrupting lesion. The various changes which have been noted will be described separately, although it is possible for an ear to be affected by more than one pathological process, making interpretation of the ECochG more complex.

Conductive hearing loss

The ECochG in conductive hearing loss is similar to that obtained from a normal ear except that a greater stimulus intensity is required, as the input/output functions are shifted to the right in a manner analogous to the speech audiogram. A 40 dB conductive hearing loss provides an ECochG using a 110 dB HL stimulus identical with that obtained from the normal ear at 70 dB HL. The AP may have a double peak similar to that seen in the transition between the 'H' and 'L' regions on the normal input/output graph. The CM and the SP are reduced. At lower intensities, the latency of the AP is much longer than that of the normal ear for corresponding intensities. A conductive loss of 70 dB yields a small AP with a latency of 3 msec or more, compared with the normal latency of 1.4-1.8 msec.

Cochlear (recruiting) hearing loss

Many different pathological conditions can damage the hair cells within the cochlea (sensory damage). One phenomenon which is very characteristic of a sensory hearing loss is loudness recruitment and the sensation of an abnormally rapid increase in loudness when sounds of increasing intensity are presented to the affected ear. Loudness recruitment has been explained by the selective vulnerability of the outer hair cells and by a deterioration in the tuning characteristics of the afferent nerve fibres (Evans, 1975).

The input/output characteristics of the AP obtained from an ear with sensory damage provide a clear indication of recruitment (Figure 8.15). The amplitude/intensity functions are steep and resemble the 'H' part of the normal graph. The latency/intensity functions are flat. Inspection of the actual recordings often reveals a diphasic AP, as the positive peak which follows the main negative peak (N_1) is relatively enhanced. The main negative peak is present down to the cochlear threshold and, unlike the situation in the normal ear, no significant N_2 low frequency contribution appears. This finding tempted Teas et al (1962) to postulate that the 'H' part of the amplitude/intensity graph was derived mainly from inner

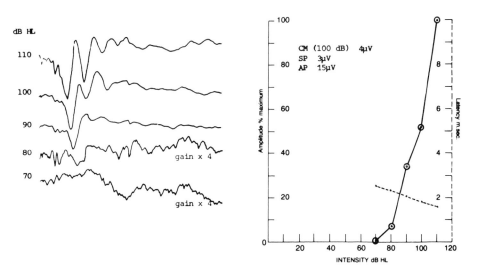

Figure 8.15 *The electrocochleogram from an ear with a recruiting (sensory, hair cell) hearing loss. Note the diphasic pattern of the AP. The amplitude/intensity graph resembles the H portion of the normal graph (see Figure 8.13) and the latency remains relatively constant.*

hair cells and the 'L' part was derived mainly from outer hair cells. It seems likely that this hypothesis is essentially true although the actual mechanisms involved are likely complex (Evans, 1975).

The CM may vary considerably in amplitude between different patients. It is theoretically possible for a patchy hair cell loss within the basal cochlear turn to provide a larger CM than normal, as the remaining clumps of hair cells could act together in the same phase. In practice, the CM is almost always small and it is rarely visible (<0.1 µV) at stimulus intensities less than 90 dB HL when the loss exceeds 50 dB. The SP/AP ratio in 50 ears affected by hair cell damage varied from 0 - 29% (mean 10.94%, s.d. 9.35). Usually the SP makes an insignificant contribution to the SP/AP waveform which has a diphasic pattern.

Acoustic trauma and noise-induced hearing loss

The characteristic feature of an early noise-induced hearing loss is an area of damaged hair cells within the basal turn of the cochlea, causing a dip in the pure tone audiogram at a particular frequency, e.g. 4 KHz. As the hearing loss progresses, the hair cell damage becomes more widespread within the basal turn, so that hearing for all the higher frequencies becomes affected. Whenever there is a selective loss of hair cells within the basal turn, the AP shows a characteristic 'W' shape (Figure 8.16). This is caused by a relative enhancement of the N_2. The

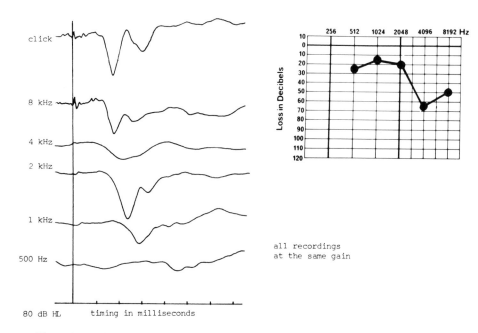

Figure 8.16 *The electrocochleogram obtained using tone bursts at different frequencies from an ear affected by a high frequency sensory loss. The pure tone audiogram is shown and resembles that seen after noise exposure. Note the W-shaped pattern of the click evoked AP and the distortion of the high frequency (4 KHz) evoked AP.*

explanation is that the N_1 component which is derived from the basal turn is greatly reduced while the N_2 retains its normal amplitude. Usually the N_2 is swamped by the greater N_1.

The CM in these cases is usually minute (<0.1 µV at 90 dB HL). The SP can rarely be identified using click or high frequency (over 2 KHz) stimuli.

Ototoxicity causing hearing loss

The aminoglycoside group of antibiotics are the best known of the ototoxic drugs but there are several other drugs which also cause either a temporary or permanent hearing loss. Originally it was assumed that aminoglycosides, such as streptomycin, affected the eighth nerve but it has now been shown that the primary lesion is a loss of hair cells (Hawkins and Engstrom, 1964).

Gentamicin is more vestibulo-toxic than cochleo-toxic in man. Moffat and Ramsden (1977) reported one case of profound hearing loss and noted ECochG characteristics which resembled a severe sensory hearing loss. Tobramycin causes a localized loss of outer hair cells within the basal cochlea turn, and the ECochG resembles that encountered on testing acoustic trauma cases. Wilson and Ramsden (1977) have reported a similar change affecting the AP as soon as 5 minutes after the infusion of tobramycin. It may be that the ECochG can be used to assess the vulnerability of an ear to an ototoxic agent before a prolonged course of treatment.

Hearing loss due to labyrinthine window rupture

The author has knowledge of only 4 patients tested using ECochG who were later found to have a labyrinthine window rupture. In each case the potentials were minute. The AP had a diphasic pattern with a slightly enhanced negative SP. In 2 cases there was a fairly pronounced positive SP preceding the AP. The CM was minute in every case. It has been suggested that the ECochG changes in form when the patient is tilted and the author noted an increase in amplitude of the AP in one patient when the head was turned so that the electrode lay vertically. The patient was later at surgery found to have a round window rupture.

Sudden hearing loss

Sudden hearing loss should be considered an otological emergency. If left untreated, approximately 50 per cent of patients exhibit some recovery and a further 33 per cent gain full recovery (Siegel, 1975). Because of this, many authorities feel that treatment of any sort is difficult to justify. Nevertheless, 17 per cent of untreated patients do not regain hearing and identification of these patients and early treatment with steroids or vasodilators may lead to recovery in a few cases.

Graham et al (1978) reported the results of electrocochleography in 70 patients and found that the ECochG helped considerably in localizing the underlying pathology to either the cochlea or the eighth nerve. Some evidence was obtained that the presence of a large CM favoured spontaneous recovery. Patients with a relatively large SP, indicating endolymphatic hydrops, are also more likely to recover.

More recently Hirasugi et al (1979) have studied 20 patients with sudden hearing loss. Interestingly, they reported the prognosis in respect of the SP/AP ratio. In their series, the normal SP was 25% of the amplitude of the AP. In cases of sudden hearing loss, all the ears with an SP/AP ratio of over 27% recovered, whereas recovery was unusual when the SP/AP ratio was below 27%.

Ménière's disorder

Ménière's disorder is an idiopathic condition characterized by episodes of rotational vertigo associated with tinnitus and hearing loss. ECochG can be of great value not only in excluding other known causes of this symptom triad, such as vertebro-basilar ischaemia and congenital syphilis, but in reaching the correct diagnosis with certainty. The striking feature of the ECochG is the presence of a SP which is so large in relation to the AP that the waveform becomes widened (Figure 8.17). Gibson et al (1977) found that the more clinically certain the diagnosis of Ménière's disorder, the more likely the presence of the abnormal SP.

The author has examined a series of 25 patients tested consecutively that had clinically definite Ménière's disorder. The SP amplitude varied from 1.25 µV to 18 µV. It was interesting that a few Ménière's patients had larger SP amplitudes than

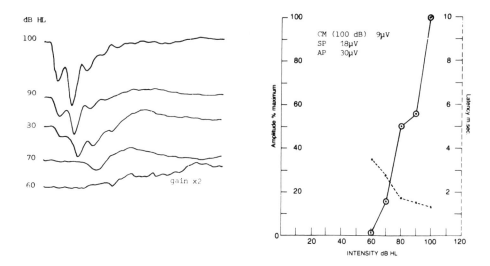

Figure 8.17 *The electrocochleogram from an ear affected by Ménière's disorder. The striking feature is the large SP contribution which causes an apparent widening of the SP/AP complex.*

any of the normal patients evaluated. The SP/AP ratio in the Ménière's affected ears varied from 29.4% to 88.8% (mean 50.2%, s.d. 14.23). Although there is some overlap in these values with normal hearing ears, there is virtually no overlap with ears affected by purely sensory lesions. If the patient has a hearing loss of over 40 dB at 2 - 4 KHz, then the ECochG does appear to provide a very useful means of distinguishing between those ears affected by hair cell damage and those affected by endolymphatic hydrops. Coats (1981) has recently supported the clinical value of the SP/AP ratio for the diagnosis of Ménière's disease. He defines the normal limits of the SP amplitude as a function of the AP amplitude. Sixty-eight percent of Ménière's ears gave SP amplitudes that exceeded the upper limit of normal, while only 7 percent of ears with hair cell damage and no endolymphatic hydrops exceeded this limit.

Moffat et al (1978) found that glycerol dehydration reduced the size of the abnormal SP in patients with endolymphatic hydrops and postulated that the SP could be directly related to the presence of endolymphatic hydrops.

The CM in Ménière's disorder tends to be small and distorted. Gibson et al (1977) reported that the CM to a 110 dB HL click stimulus was less than 2 μV in 58 per cent of their patients.

The author has tested 2 patients during a severe attack of vertigo and was unable to detect the abnormal SP in either case. In fact, the potentials were difficult to obtain and the AP threshold was far worse than the subjective threshold. These cases were thought to have ruptured their cochlear duct, but whether this mixing of cochlear fluids can explain the milder episodes of vertigo is unknown.

The ECochG changes in the presence of endolymphatic hydrops are so characteristic that some optimism can be voiced that the ECochG will provide interesting data on the subject.

Syphilitic hearing loss

This condition causes endolymphatic hydrops and produces symptoms similar to Ménière's disorder. There is, in addition, extensive hair cell loss, especially in the basal turn of the cochlea, with retrograde degeneration of the eighth nerve and spiral ganglion. Ramsden et al (1977b) investigated 30 cases. The most characteristic ECochG waveform was an early 'W' shape comprising an early negative SP followed by a small diphasic AP (Figure 8.18). The CM was minute. The interesting feature was that in none of the cases did the SP affect the positive-going limb of the AP, the common finding in Ménière's disorder. Perhaps this finding is related to the difference in the degree of hair cell damage in the two conditions.

Eighth nerve tumours

The commonest tumour affecting the VIII cranial nerve is a Schwannoma arising from the myelin sheath of the vestibular nerve (acoustic neuroma). This tumour can affect the hearing either by interfering with the cochlear blood supply or by directly damaging the afferent nerve fibres.

The ECochG findings reflect the different mechanisms involved. In 70 per cent of subjects, there is a widened waveform resembling the waveform seen in Ménière's disorder (Figure 8.19) (Gibson and Beagley, 1976). In 20 per cent of these cases further analysis reveals that there is a relative enhancement of the SP and it seems likely that these tumours are associated with endolymphatic hydrops. In many cases the widening is probably due to a slow component (SC) contribution similar to that encountered in the denervated animal cochlea (Kiang and Peake, 1960). This component is similar to the SP, as it does not exhibit adaptation and the subtraction technique provides a residual AP. The SC differs from the SP as its onset latency is 0.7 - 0.9 msec after the onset of the CM. The SC is more prominent at high frequencies (4 and 8 KHz), whereas the SP is maximal at 2 KHz.

The CM is large in over 90 per cent of ears affected by VIII nerve tumours and it is often larger than the CM obtained from the unaffected ear. This enhancement could be explained by a loss of efferent control, as the efferent fibres pass down the vestibular nerve before crossing to the acoustic nerve.

The more medially the tumour affects the nerve, the less likely there is to be a widened waveform and the more likely it is that the AP threshold will be more sensitive, or lower, than the psycho-acoustic threshold. Gibson and Beagley (1976) found that the ECochG threshold was 20 dB lower than the subjective hearing threshold in nearly one third of the patients they tested. These patients are likely to exhibit abnormalities of the brainstem potentials and the diagnosis may be more certain if both ECochG and BAEP (see Chapter 9) are undertaken.

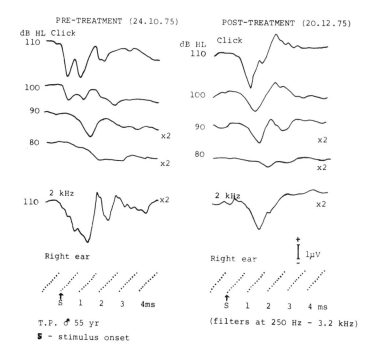

Figure 8.18 *The electrocochleogram of a patient suffering from congenital syphilis (tarda). Pre-treatment, the ECochG showed an early SP contribution which gave a 'W' configuration. After treatment with steroids and penicillin, the ECochG assumed a more normal shape. (From Ramsden et al, 1977, by permission of Annals of Otology, Rhinology and Laryngology.)*

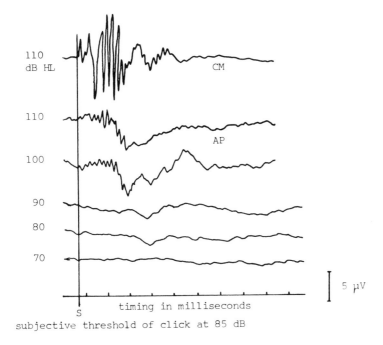

110
dB HL

CM

110

AP

100

90

80

70

5 μV

S
timing in milliseconds

subjective threshold of click at 85 dB

Figure 8.19 *The electrocochleogram from an ear with an acoustic neuroma. The CM is relatively large compared with the AP. The AP is widened and distorted and has a threshold which is more sensitive than the psycho-acoustic threshold.*

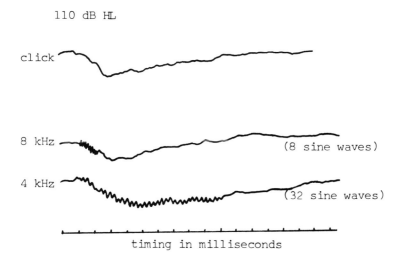

110 dB HL

click

8 kHz

(8 sine waves)

4 kHz

(32 sine waves)

timing in milliseconds

Figure 8.20 *Neurofibromatosis. The ECochG is extremely wide and this widening is not clearly dependent on the stimulus duration.*

Neurofibromatosis

The neuroma in neurofibromatosis acts differently to the acoustic neuroma in that it actually infiltrates the nerve itself. The lesion usually lies very laterally, often within the modiolus of the cochlea. The ECochG usually reveals a markedly widened waveform which is totally dominated by a SC contribution (Figure 8.20). The CM is usually very large.

Other posterior fossa tumours

The ECochG has been reported in a variety of lesions (Beagley and Gibson, 1976). In general, the ECochG resembles that described for the acoustic neuroma. Basilar artery ectasia (Gibson and Wallace, 1975) does not cause much widening, but the AP threshold may be lower than the psycho-acoustic threshold. Meningiomata do not generally affect the ECochG waveform, although again the subjective threshold is higher than the ECochG threshold (Figure 8.21). Children

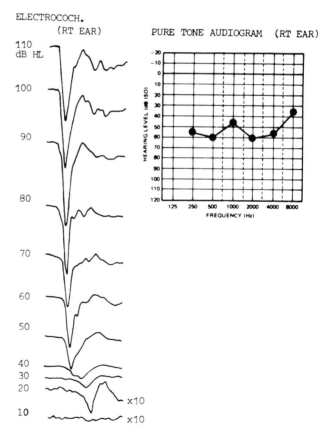

Figure 8.21 *The electrocochleogram and audiogram of a patient with a posterior fossa meningioma. Note that the electrocochleogram is normal despite the marked audiometric hearing loss.*

with hearing loss due to kernicterus often exhibit a wide distorted ECochG waveform with a large CM. A similar finding was noted in a patient with a brainstem astrocytoma (Beagley and Gibson, 1976). The use of ECochG in detecting brainstem lesions is limited, as the test only records the retrograde affect these tumours exert on the cochlea and primary VIII nerve fibres.

Final conclusions

This brief description of ECochG has left several fields unmentioned. Further information can be obtained elsewhere (Gibson, 1978). The ECochG has its chief use at present as a hearing test in young children under general anaesthesia. This rôle may become less important as the use of brainstem evoked response audiometry is developed. It is likely that the main value of ECochG will then lie in the differential diagnosis and management of pathological conditions affecting the cochlea.

9

The Use of Auditory Evoked Potentials for the Estimation of Hearing

W.P.R. Gibson

INTRODUCTION

Although auditory evoked potentials (AEPs) were recognized in the human electroencephalogram in 1939 (P. Davis, 1939; H. Davis et al, 1939), it was not until after the introduction of electronic methods of averaging and summing the responses (Geisler, Frishkopf and Rosenblith, 1958) that the clinical use of the AEP was appreciated. Over 20 years of extensive investigation have followed and it is now possible to record many different AEPs in man arising from the cochlea, brainstem, auditory cortex and from muscles which react to acoustic stimulation. These AEPs have several important diagnostic uses in both otology and neurology but, without doubt, their most important clinical use is as an 'objective' means of assessing the auditory threshold.

The term threshold requires some explanation. In the audiometric field, the threshold refers to the limit of stimulus intensity below which the stimulus ceases to be audible. The auditory threshold is therefore a psycho-acoustic measure which involves not just neural transmission to the auditory cortex but the ability of the subject to associate the information meaningfully so that he actually perceives the sound. Auditory evoked potentials, with the possible exception of the very late AEPs such as the contingent negative variation, do not measure the entire perceptual process but merely indicate the function of the auditory system at a certain level. The AEP threshold is the limit of stimulus intensity below which the potential ceases to be recognizable. The AEP threshold can be used to assess the auditory threshold only by making the assumption that the higher functions of the auditory system are intact. In clinical work, this assumption is rarely unacceptable.

There are two main groups of patients in which electrophysiological methods of assessing the auditory threshold are of special value. The first and most obvious is young children suspected of having impaired hearing. An 'objective' test is particularly useful for children suffering from multiple handicaps such as blindness and dementia as such children can be very difficult to assess using behavioural tests alone. The second group is made up of adults who may not give reliable responses during conventional audiometry. This latter group includes patients with disorders, such as senile dementia, which impair their ability to give voluntary responses and those with a possible non-organic hearing loss.

The value of electric response audiometry (ERA) requires careful appraisal. It is true that ERA provides an accurate means of assessing hearing, especially in the higher audiometric frequencies, and can be used on any subject, including young children. The danger is that the availability of such tests may polarize audiologists into two extreme groups: those who consider that electrophysiological tests have the most important rôle in auditory assessment, rendering behavioural tests outdated; and those who regard electrical tests with the utmost suspicion, feeling that the properly conducted behavioural test is the only test of any real value, that electrophysiological tests may undermine their status as clinicians and that these tests are an expensive waste of personnel and money. Both these groups hold views that are bigotted and unhealthy.

In the first case it must be remembered that ERA often fails to detect important islands of preserved hearing at low frequencies. Complete reliance on a machine is unwise as the machine or operator may be faulty and either fail to record a response, or worse, misinterpret some artifact as a true potential. Often considerable 'subjective' judgement is required in determining the threshold of the response (Rapin and Schimmel, 1977).

In the second case equally strong arguments exist. No matter how expert the clinician is in performing behavioural tests there is always a risk of error. Some clinicians avoid the possibility of error by failing to provide a definite answer until they have retested the child several times. Such management can lead to the loss of many vital months before correct auditory rehabilitation is instituted.

It should be obvious that the correct use of ERA is as an adjunct to behavioural testing when dealing with the 'difficult to test' patient. Final diagnosis should be reached after careful consideration of the results of both behavioural and electrophysiological testing.

There are several different AEPs which can be used to assess the auditory threshold and each has its own advocates. This chapter will attempt to review the relative advantages and disadvantages of each method as a hearing test. The picture that will emerge is that there is not a single optimal test but that the choice depends on the particular clinical requirements. Apart from assessment of the auditory theshold, the AEP can provide valuable diagnostic information regarding the actual cause of the hearing dysfunction. This matter is discussed only briefly in this chapter as it is dealt with extensively elsewhere (see Chapters 8 and 10).

ELECTROCOCHLEOGRAPHY

Electrocochleography (ECochG) is concerned with the electrical potentials of the cochlea and VIII nerve. The cochlear potentials, cochlear microphonic (CM) and summating potential (SP) have no direct value in the assessment of hearing although they may help in reaching the diagnosis of the underlying pathological condition. The VIII nerve action potential (AP) provides a reliable measure of the cochlear threshold and can be used with confidence to estimate hearing.

Methodological considerations

Electrocochleography involves the placement of the active electrode either through the tympanic membrane (transtympanic) or within the external auditory meatus (extratympanic electrocochleography). The AP or NI wave recorded from the mastoid has a threshold at 40-60 dB SL and has limited use as a threshold test, especially as the later NV (brainstem electrical potential) provides a much better means of assessing the auditory threshold (see later in this chapter). Extratympanic ECochG also has several disadvantages as a threshold measure; the potential is much smaller and may be difficult to identify in partially-hearing ears; the AP threshold lies at 20-40 dB SL, and background noise may obscure the responses unless the electrode is actually embedded into the meatus. Both extra- and transtympanic ECochG can be performed in adults without any anaesthesia or sedation but has to be performed using general anaesthesia in young children.

The AP threshold can be estimated using two different methods. The simplest method is to record the response using decreasing stimulus intensities and then to judge (i) the intensity at which the response first becomes absent and (ii) the intensity at which it is just visible after increasing the stimulus intensity again. The determination of these end points should be repeated on at least two independent trials. The AP threshold is then taken as the mean of these two intensity levels. A more precise method of judging the threshold relies on the input/output (I/O) functions. The AP decreases in amplitude, and its latency increases, as the stimulus intensity diminishes. Near to threshold the amplitude/intensity function is reasonably linear and the AP threshold can be estimated from this I/O function by interpolation or extrapolation to a criterion voltage level (e.g. 0.2 or 0.1 µV). The I/O functions also have value in determining whether the hearing loss is conductive or sensory, while the AP pattern and CM and SP provide further diagnostic information (See Chapter 8).

Advantages of ECochG

No masking of the non-test ear is needed. In conventional audiometry, it can be difficult to determine whether one ear is completely functionless ('dead') if the other ear hears normally, as it can be impossible to prevent the sound delivered to the bad ear being heard through the good ear. ECochG can be extremely useful in resolving such dilemmas.

General anaesthesia does not affect the AP threshold. This is useful when dealing with hyperactive children who react to sedatives in an unpredictable manner. The clinician soon appreciates the advantage of general anaesthesia as the test can be completed within a known period allowing him to organize his own daily timetable, whereas the other tests under sedatives can take hours to complete, as the child may either fail to quieten under the first dose or become alarmingly comatose requiring anxious supervision until he awakens. Another advantage from the ENT surgeon's viewpoint is that the test can be performed after aspirating the fluid of serous otitis media, or it can be combined with other surgical procedures.

The reliability of the test is excellent. At frequencies between 1 and 8 KHz this is the most robust method of ERA.

Disadvantages of ECochG

The need for general anaesthesia and for a minor surgical procedure is viewed as a disadvantage by non-otologists. Unless they can procure the services of a co-operative surgeon, the test cannot be carried out.

Transtympanic placement may theoretically lead to complications and even exacerbate the hearing loss. Patients with non-organic hearing loss may accuse the surgeon of having caused some symptoms, such as vertigo or tinnitus. In reality, the incidence of serious complications is minimal (Crowley et al, 1975) but, nevertheless, ECochG is not recommended for the evaluation of non-organic hearing loss.

Low frequency information (below 500 Hz) is unobtainable and important islands of residual hearing can be overlooked.

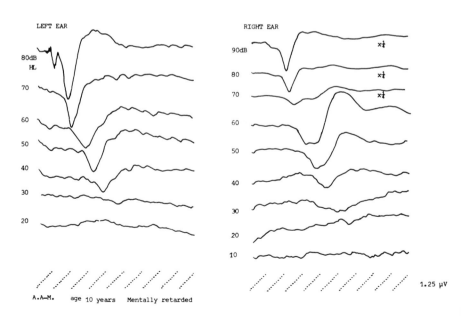

Figure 9.1 *The electrocochleogram obtained from a mentally-retarded girl with normal hearing.*

Bone conduction thresholds are for practical purposes impossible. Several workers have tried to obtain bone conduction thresholds but the procedure is fraught with problems of acoustic control and artifact generation (Berlin et al, 1978).

Central hearing disorders will not affect the ECochG potentials. Centrally placed tumours can cause hearing loss in the presence of a normal ECochG threshold (Morrison et al, 1976).

The reliability and accuracy of ECochG

The test/retest reliability of the ECochG is better than that of other AEPs. The difference between the ECochG threshold and the audiometric threshold at 2 - 8 KHz is within –5 to +10 dB in 85% of subjects and within 25 dB in the remainder who have not given such large amplitude potentials. If the suprathreshold response is over 10 μV, then one can be certain that the ECochG will accurately indicate the audiometric threshold for the same stimulus. At 1 KHz the discrepancy between the ECochG threshold and the audiometric threshold is larger, reaching 40 dB, and at 500 Hz the gap may reach 60 dB (Gibson, 1978).

Examples of clinical use of transtympanic ECochG

Aran (1971) provides many excellent examples of ECochG used for hearing estimation. Beagley et al (1974) reviewed 106 clinical cases and following this publication over 2,000 children have been successfully tested at The Nuffield Speech and Hearing Centre in London without a single known serious complication. Two examples from the author's experience will be described.

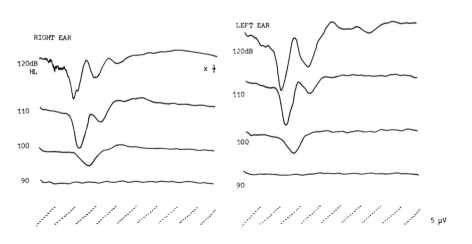

F.A.B.   age 4 years Mentally retarded ?not hearing

Figure 9.2 *The electrocochleogram from a child with severe bilateral sensory hearing loss.*

1. A.A-M age 10 years. This young girl from Saudi Arabia was extremely retarded and was referred as doubt still existed as to whether she had a hearing loss contributing to her retardation. Despite several attempts at behavioural testing, a conclusive answer was not reached and at least two paediatric audiologists were offering conflicting opinions. The transtympanic ECochG was obtained without difficulty (Figure 9.1) and revealed normal peripheral auditory function.

2. F.A.B. age 4 years. A young boy from Iraq who was mentally retarded and epileptic. The ECochG revealed a 90 dB hearing loss in both ears (Figure 9.2) and the amplitude and latency functions suggest a cochlear (sensory) hearing loss with recruitment.

THE ACOUSTIC BRAINSTEM ELECTRIC POTENTIALS

There are several types of acoustic brainstem potentials: the short-latency brainstem auditory evoked potential (BAEP), as described by Jewett and Williston (1971), which comprises a series of 6 or 7 mastoid negative potentials occurring in response to the onset of a transient stimulus; the frequency following response (FFR) which is a sustained response elicited by the continuance of a more prolonged sinusoidal acoustic stimulus. The FFR resembles the cochlear microphonic as it follows the electrical waveform of the stimulus but the onset latency of the first wave of the response is approximately 6 msec. A third auditory brainstem potential is perhaps the sonomotor (myogenic) response as this response has a neural pathway traversing the brainstem.

The brainstem auditory evoked potential (BAEP)

The BAEP occurs within 10 msec of the stimulus onset, and each of the seven constituent components can be labelled NI, NII, etc., according to Jewett's classification. The neural origin of each potential is discussed in Chapter 10. It is the fifth mastoid negative potential or NV and the following positive-going deflection (FFP7) that provides the best means of estimating the auditory threshold. Following Hallowell Davis' nomenclature, FFP7 is an abbreviation for 'far field potential at approximately 7 msec'. Both the NV and the FFP7 are thought to arise from the region of the inferior colliculus.

Methodological considerations

The BAEP can be obtained using 3 standard EEG electrodes attached to the skin surface over each mastoid and the vertex respectively. Some workers have suggested placing the central electrode in the midline immediately below the hairline on the forehead, but this position does not provide such a large or clear NV potential as the vertex. The potentials are very small, measuring less than 1 μV, and, unless the subject remains still and relaxed, it is not possible to distinguish the potentials from the background noise. Adults can be tested lying comfortably with their heads supported by a pillow to prevent muscle artifact. Children are best tested while they are asleep; young children need careful sedation but neonates can sometimes be tested during natural sleep after feeds. It may take some time for a child to settle as the effect of sedatives is unpredictable. It is not wise to test children in a harried atmosphere.

In addition to the estimation of threshold using the NV or FFP7, the BAEP can provide important information concerning the cause of a hearing disorder. The NV has a latency which alters in parallel with the N_1 (or the AP of the ECochG) as the stimulus intensity changes. The NV latency/intensity functions can be used to distinguish between conductive and sensory (recruiting) hearing loss. The NV amplitude tends to be too variable, especially in children, for proper interpretation of the amplitude/intensity functions, but a sudden collapse of response amplitude as the stimulus intensity nears the threshold is suggestive of recruitment. The NV latency, amplitude and reproducibility also alters significantly in the presence of some retrocochlear conditions (Chapter 10).

Advantages of the BAEP

Non-invasive technique. Any sensible person can soon learn to attach the electrodes correctly and medical qualifications are not needed.

Sedatives do not affect the responses which can be identified just as easily as when the subject is awake. This is a considerable advantage for testing young children.

Abnormal EEG activity does not affect the response.

The BAEP is recognizable even in premature babies (Schulman-Galambos and Galambos, 1975). The BAEP can be used for the auditory screening of babies before they leave the premature baby unit.

The reliability of the test is excellent, especially using stimulus frequencies between 500 Hz and 8 KHz.

Changes in the individual components of the BAEP have important neurological implications which can be as significant for the clinical management as the assessment of the auditory threshold (see Chapter 10).

Disadvantages of the BAEP

The potentials are minute, making identification difficult without careful averaging of many hundreds of individual responses. At near threshold levels in infants it may be necessary to average as many as 8,000 responses. It is fortunate that averaging can proceed at a stimulus repetition rate of 20 - 40 per second, for, otherwise, the time taken to identify each BAEP would be excessive. Despite the large number of averages, the responses can be easily obscured by muscle potentials; hence the necessity to test young children while they are asleep.

Masking of the non-test ear is necessary whenever the possibility of cross-over exists. Basically masking is required whenever the difference between test ear and non-test ear with better hearing exceeds 40 dB.

The assessment of low frequency hearing is poor and, like the ECochG, residual islands of low frequency hearing (below 500 Hz) may not be detected.

A pathological condition which affects the auditory mechanism above the level of the inferior colliculus would not alter the BAEP threshold. In practice this situation is extremely rare.

The reliability and accuracy of the BAEP

The brainstem EPs have high reliability in younger subjects. The optimum age is 10 to 30 years as the waveform becomes less consistent as the subject's age increases beyond 30 years (Beagley and Sheldrake, 1978). Hecox and Galambos (1974) described the maturation of the BAEP during the first few months of life. At birth the latencies of the later waves are longer, the amplitudes are small and the NIII and NV are most prominent. As the child gets older the latencies decrease until by the age of 2 years the typical adult waveform is obtained (Schulman-Galambos and Galambos, 1975). The latencies are much more constant than the amplitudes when the same subject is retested on different occasions (Kendall and Lawes, 1978).

The difference between the NV or FFP7 threshold and the auditory threshold is generally less than 10 dB (Davis, 1976). Antonelli (1976) found that 75 per cent of subjects had a BAEP threshold of 10 - 30 dB SL at 1 KHz. Ryerson and Beagley (1981) compared the BAEP and ECochG thresholds at 1 KHz and found that the BAEP was marginally more accurate for assessing the auditory threshold. At 500 Hz, the BAEP appears to be definitely more accurate than the ECochG, but at

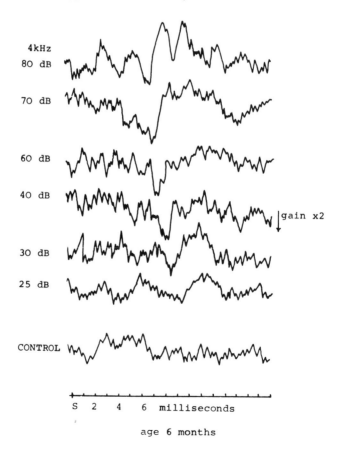

Figure 9.3 *Brainstem auditory potentials from a normal child, aged six months.*

this frequency the NV is a slow, flattish potential with an onset latency of at least 10 msec and, unless the bandpass of the recording system admits low frequencies (e.g. the high pass filter must be around 1 - 5 Hz and not 100 Hz or more) the NV cannot be recorded (Davis and Hirsh, 1976).

Examples of clinical use of the BAEP

1. T.B., aged six months. This small boy has a father, uncle and paternal grandfather with hereditary, sensory hearing loss. Screening tests suggested normal hearing but an electrophysiological test was required to confirm these clinical impressions. The BAEP is an ideal non-invasive technique for this age group and the recordings showed normal brainstem auditory function (Figure 9.3).

2. J.S., aged 18 months. This child suffered from meningitis at the age of 14 months. Following the meningitis there was no further speech development. The BAEP shows a click threshold of 65 dB (Figure 9.4). After being given a hearing aid and with auditory training, his speech returned and is now quite normal.

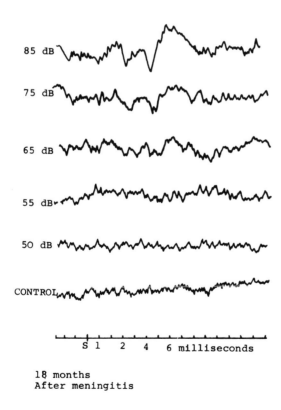

Figure 9.4 Brainstem auditory potentials from a child, aged 18 months, with partial hearing loss.

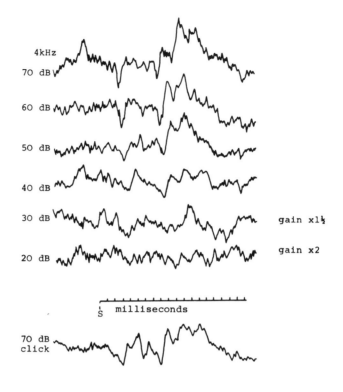

Figure 9.5 *Brainstem auditory potentials from a neonate of only 37 weeks gestational age.*

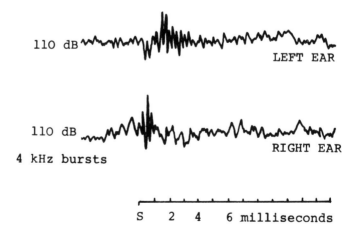

Figure 9.6 *Brainstem auditory potentials from a deaf child, aged 6 months.*

3. R.O'S, aged 37 weeks gestational age. A tiny baby born at 32 weeks who survived after intensive nursing. The BAEP waveform had a small amplitude but could be identified (Figure 9.5) although the NIII and NV were not especially prominent.

4. P.B., aged 6 months. A baby born with multiple handicaps, including blindness. The nurses had noticed that he did not respond to sound. The BAEP showed total absence of any potential except for an artefactual microphonic which is visible at the maximum stimulus intensity (Figure 9.6). Subsequent behavioural testing appeared to confirm the deafness, but the child died within one year.

The frequency following response (FFR)

The FFR is a frequency specific response which is similar in shape to a microphonic but has an onset latency of approximately 6 msec. The latency increases with decreasing stimulus intensity. The FFR is thought to arise by slow dendritic activity within the brainstem, possibly from the region of the inferior colliculus (Smith et al, 1975). Gardi et al (1979a), however, found that aspirating the inferior colliculus did not alter the FFR, so it may be that it is generated elsewhere or possibly that there is more than one generator site (Worden and Marsh, 1968).

Methodological considerations

The FFR has maximum amplitude using stimulus frequencies below 1 KHz and it is difficult to identify at higher frequencies. The bandpass of the recording system should be approximately 10 - 10,000 Hz. The electrodes and the electrode positions are the same as those used for the BAEP, although a systematic investigation of the optimal electrode positions has not yet been published. The stimuli are presented at a rate of 5 - 25 per second and comprise 4 - 6 sine waves. About 2000 stimulus trials are needed to elicit an identifiable FFR.

Advantages of the FFR

The recording procedure is non-invasive.

The FFR does not appear to be altered by sleep.

The response offers a measure of low frequency hearing unlike any of the other short latency AEPs.

Disadvantages of the FFR

The waveform can easily be confused with electrical and mechanical artifacts and care must be taken to avoid these.

The higher audiometric frequencies are not measurable.

Little work has yet been accomplished regarding its use in young children and babies.

The FFR threshold does not relate very exactly to the auditory threshold.

The reliability and accuracy of the FFR

The FFR threshold varies from 20 dB SL (Stillman et al, 1976) to 50 dB (Davis, 1976). Most investigators agree that an identifiable response can be recorded at 45 dB SL. The amplitude of the FFR is larger if binaural, rather than monaural, stimuli are used, but even so the response is minute and has a peak-to-peak amplitude of less than 0.1 µV. Davis and Hirsh (1976) report that click stimuli and tone pip stimuli (500 Hz, 2 - 4 msec duration, 1 - 2 msec rise and fall time) elicit complicated FFR waveforms as low as 10 dB SL while longer duration stimuli (500 Hz, 15 - 20 msec duration, 2 - 4 msec rise and fall time) have a somewhat higher threshold (40 - 50 dB SL) but evoke a clear following phenomenon.

To date little work has been accomplished in adults and no studies on children have been published.

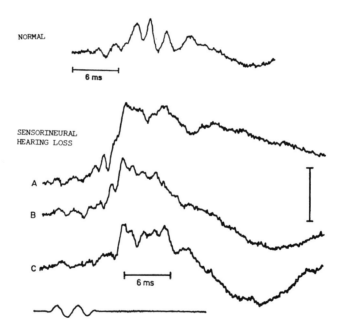

Figure 9.7 *The frequency following response obtained from a normal hearing subject and from 3 hearing-impaired subjects. (Adapted from Stillman et al, 1976.)*

The clinical use of the FFR

After its discovery, it was hoped that the FFR would complement the use of the BAEP by providing the missing low frequency information. Some promising studies have been published. Stillman et al (1976) studied populations of normal subjects, deaf-blind subjects and subjects exhibiting learning disorders and mild speech discrimination deficits. Figure 9.7 shows examples of their findings and illustrates the difference between the FFR of a normal subject and 3 subjects with mildly impaired hearing. Gardi et al (1979b) were able to record the FFR from full-term healthy neonates. Figure 9.8 shows the FFR recorded at different intensity levels in a normal subject (Picton et al, 1977).

Despite these promising reports, there are major problems regarding the clinical use of the FFR. The FFR has a higher threshold than the BAEP and is more artifact prone. More disturbingly there is a strong suspicion that a significant part of the response arises from low frequency firing of nerve fibres within the basal turn of the cochlea (Davis and Hirsh, 1976). This can be predicted on considering the phenomenon of periodicity pitch. There is also a dispute concerning the origins of the FFR. Hou and Lipscomb (1979) compared the decline of the cochlear microphonic and FFR in chinchillas after death and found they were directly related. This finding suggests that the FFR originates mostly within the cochlea rather than in the brainstem. Gardi et al (1979a), however, in a study of the cat found that only 25% of the FFR was generated within the cochlea, while 50% came from the cochlear nucleus and 25% from other brainstem structures.

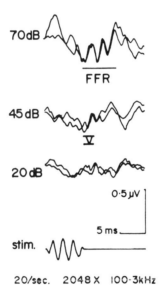

Figure 9.8 *The frequency following responses resulting from stimulation at different intensity levels. (Reproduced from Picton et al, 1977, by permission of The Journal of Otolaryngology.)*

The sonomotor potentials

The sonomotor potentials (Davis, 1965) are acoustically-evoked muscle reflexes. The neural pathway involves the brainstem but not higher cortical levels.

Although all the muscles of the body react to very loud sounds, it is the muscles of the scalp which react most consistently. There are two main sonomotor potentials, the inion response and the post-auricular muscle response (PAM). Sonomotor potentials can also be recorded from the jaw muscles (Meier-Ewert et al, 1974).

Historically the sonomotor potentials were the first auditory EPs to be recorded using electronic averaging techniques (Geisler et al, 1958). The potentials were thought originally to be neural in origin, but Bickford et al (1963a, 1963b) showed clearly by a number of different experiments that the true source was myogenic. The earliest recordings were of the inion response which is recorded maximally from an active electrode placed over the inion (a small bony protuberance at the back of the skull in the midline immediately above the nape of the neck). The inion response is very dependent on the muscle tension in the neck muscles and cannot usually be recorded within 40 dB of the auditory threshold. The inion response has been abandoned as a hearing test because it was found that intense sound could stimulate the vestibular receptors and lead to a response even in a deaf subject (Cody et al, 1964; Gibson, 1974).

The post-auricular sonomotor response was first reported by Kiang et al (1963). This response is also very dependent on muscle tone and it can be absent in normally-hearing subjects. Nevertheless, the PAM response can only be elicited through cochlear, and not vestibular, stimulation, so it has some rôle as a hearing test (Yoshie and Okudaira, 1969; Gibson, 1978). The PAM response has also been called 'the crossed acoustic response' (Douek et al, 1973), a name chosen in order to stress the importance of obtaining the response from behind both ears simultaneously. The author now regrets this term as it may give the erroneous impression that the response can only be obtained on the contralateral side of the head.

Some methodological considerations (PAM response)

The optimum active electrode position is immediately over the main bulk of the muscle as close to the attachment of the pinna as possible. The response amplitude is reduced by 90 per cent if the active electrode is moved 2 cm from the optimal position. The reference electrode can be placed at several convenient sites, but Gibson (1974) favoured the neck immediately below the muscle, as this avoided contamination by other muscle potentials. The reliability of the response is considerably enhanced by recording simultaneously from both sides, as the side which will provide the larger potential is difficult to predict.

The PAM response can only be recorded with reasonable reliability using stimuli with a fast rise time such as acoustic clicks. Attempts to record it with 1,000 Hz tone bursts were unsuccessful (Cody and Bickford, 1969). The recording amplifier bandpass should be approximately 1 - 200 Hz. Although the high cut causes some response distortion, it is worth-while as it removes an appreciable amount of background noise. Artifact rejection facilities are essential if young active children are to be tested. Usually 150 stimulus trials are sufficient to evoke a response at a rate of 10 stimuli per second, but it is wise to continue averaging until 2,000 trials are completed before declaring a 'no response' situation.

The identification of the PAM from an active child requires either good subjective judgement or can be achieved by machine scoring. The subjective judgement depends on seeing the response at around 15 msec build up slowly on the averager screen. The slow build-up is a measure of consistency and distinguishes it from the occasional random artefact of larger amplitude. If recordings are taken from both sides of the head, then there should be a response with the same latency in both averager channels. Machine scoring holds several advantages for this particular auditory EP and Fraser et al (1978) have developed a simple machine which appears to work well under clinical conditions.

Advantages of the PAM response

The only real advantage of the PAM response is that it can be used as a quick 'objective' screening method for young active children. Gibson (1974) tested 166 young children, many of whom were deemed untestable on behavioural measures, and, without sedation, failed to get meaningful information in only 2 children. The test time is under 15 minutes and the electrodes can be simply pressed into position without trying to reduce the skin/electrode impedance by scratching the underlying skin.

Disadvantages of the PAM response

There are many disadvantages. The chief drawback is the poor reliability of the test. The stimulus requirements limit the test to the higher audiometric frequencies and masking of the non-test ear is required when unilateral hearing loss exists.

The test does not provide a means of assessing the auditory threshold, but merely shows whether or not a child can hear a click at 80 dB HL or at 50 dB HL.

The reliability and accuracy of the PAM response

The reliability of the PAM is worse than any other auditory EP mentioned in this Chapter. The response is absent at 70 dB in as many as 20% of adult subjects if recordings are taken only from one side. Gibson (1974) managed to identify a response at 30 dB SL in 92% of subjects by recording from both sides simultaneously and by asking the non-responders to perform various tasks such as gritting their teeth or putting their chin onto their chest. He found that, providing a response was obtained that was over 2 µV at high stimulus intensities, then the response lay within 30 dB of the auditory threshold.

The clinical use of the PAM response

The response has been used as an auditory test for neonates (Douek, 1981) and for children and adults (Gibson, 1974). Whenever consistent responses are obtained, the input/output functions show a nearly exponential rise in amplitude and a 3 msec decrease in latency as the stimulus intensity increases (Figure 9.9). A recruiting hearing loss is revealed by an abrupt change in latency with increasing intensity, similar to the BAEP, unlike the almost static response latency in the ECochG in such cases.

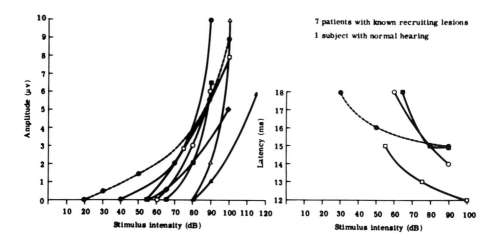

Figure 9.9 *The amplitude and latency versus stimulus intensity functions for the post-auricular sonomotor potential. The dotted line shows a typical subject with normal hearing, the solid lines show 7 subjects with sensory (recruiting) hearing loss.*

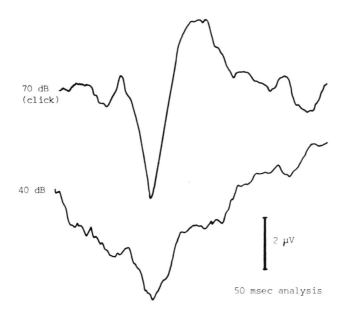

Figure 9.10 *The post-auricular sonomotor responses obtained from a severely autistic child*

1. A severely autistic child, aged 6, was found to be almost untestable using conventional behavioural means and as a screening test the PAM was helpful in confirming that the child had normal hearing. The PAM was recorded within 10 minutes without sedation (Figure 9.10).

2. A subject, totally deaf in the right ear, was tested, who had normal caloric responses in both ears. It can be seen (Figure 9.11) that no PAM response was obtained from either side of the head on stimulating the deaf ear. The inion response, however, could still be clearly obtained on stimulating each ear. Gibson (1974) tested 6 other totally deaf subjects who had normal vestibular function, and did not obtain the PAM response in any of them.

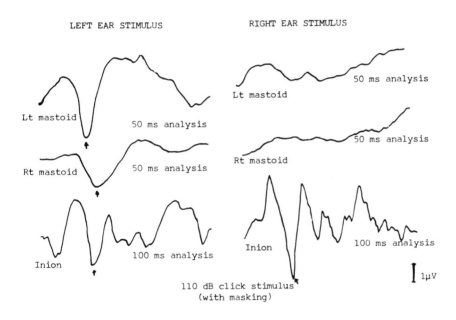

Figure 9.11 *The sonomotor responses obtained from a subject with a total right hearing loss. Note that although the post-auricular response is absent on the affected side, the inion response is still present.*

THE CORTICAL POTENTIALS

The cortical auditory evoked potentials can be classified according to their onset latencies. The fast cortical potentials fall into the group of medium latency auditory responses as they occur at a time between the short-latency responses, such as the ECochG, BAEP and FFR, and the long-latency cortical responses. These intermediate potentials have latencies from 8 - 80 msec. The slow cortical potentials to transient stimuli have latencies between 50 - 250 msec. The late positive cortical potential or P300 has a latency of approximately 300 msec and its behaviour is different to the 50 - 250 msec cortical potentials. There are also slower cortical potentials such as the contingent negative variation (CNV). The sustained potential or DC cortical potential has an onset latency of 150 msec but its duration may last several seconds. The discussion of the cortical potentials begins with the slow (vertex) potential which historically preceded the other potentials and which has been extensively investigated as a hearing test.

The slow cortical potential or vertex potential

The slow cortical potential or vertex potential was first described by P. Davis (1939) and by Hallowell Davis and his colleagues (1939) from an analysis of the raw electroencephalogram. It took considerable skill to identify the evoked auditory potentials buried amongst the EEG noise, particularly at faster stimulus repetition rates. Much of the earlier work involved photographic superimposition, but it was the application of electronic averaging and summating techniques that allowed the potential to be seen clearly (Davis and Yoshie, 1963). Soon afterwards the slow potential was developed into a useful audiometric test, but the optimistic view that it would provide a definitive means of assessing the hearing of young children was later proved to be misplaced.

The slow cortical potential has also been called the 'vertex potential' (Bancaud et al, 1953; Gastaut, 1953) but this is not a very suitable title as virtually all the AEPs except for the ECochG are recorded using a vertex active electrode.

The typical adult response has a small inconsistent positive peak (P_1) (with respect to the vertex electrode) at 50 - 75 msec followed by a much larger negative peak (N_1) at 100 - 150 msec and a large positive peak (P_2) at 175 - 200 msec. A later negative peak (N_2) at 200 - 250 msec is usually small in the adult but may be the largest potential in a young child.

The exact origin of the slow cortical potentials is still uncertain. Vaughan and Ritter (1970) suggested that the potentials arose from the primary auditory cortex and the temporo-parietal association cortex, but Kooi et al (1971) were unable to confirm their work. Now most workers believe that the N_1, P_2 and N_2 components represent a widespread activation of the frontal cortex (Picton et al, 1974).

Methodological considerations

The slow potential is recorded using standard EEG electrodes which are attached to the skin surface at the vertex and over either mastoid. The response waveform is little altered by recording from the side ipsilateral or contralateral to the stimulated ear. The stimuli are tone bursts presented at a rate of one each second or every two seconds; faster rates cause marked attenuation of the potentials. Between 30 and 64 stimulus trials are needed to obtain a clear averaged response. Each average response takes 1 - 2 minutes to accumulate, during which time movements must be avoided, as the response can easily be obscured by spurious muscle potentials. The optimal test frequencies are 250, 500 and 1,000 Hz (Antinoro and Skinner, 1968).

Advantages of the slow potential

The test procedure is non-invasive

The stimulus is a pure tone burst. Such a stimulus is easy to calibrate and the responses can be compared directly with the familiar pure tone audiogram.

The frequency range of the test corresponds to the most important hearing frequencies.

Disadvantages of the slow potential

The response waveform alters drastically at different sleep stages and sedation can make the response unidentifiable.

Young children have a poorly developed response waveform which may vary considerably on retesting. The adult waveform is not reached until the age of 7 years.

Abnormally large EEG potentials obscure the averaged response.

Muscle artifacts can also easily obscure the response.

Masking of the non-test ear has to be used whenever there is a wide difference between the threshold of the two ears.

The slow cortical response to tactile stimuli closely resembles the auditory response and, whenever low frequency stimuli at high intensities are used, the possibility that one is recording a tactile response to mechanical stimulation should not be overlooked.

The reliability and accuracy of the slow potential

Excellent recordings with accurate threshold determination can invariably be obtained on testing healthy young adults, but the responses from patients can be disappointing. The slow potential threshold accurately indicates the audiometric threshold in young adults. Jones, Harding and Smith (1980) found the thresholds to be identical in 81% of 23 young normal adults, and all the subjects had a difference between the slow potential and audiometric thresholds of less than 10 dB. The estimations were less accurate in 46 adults with hearing disorders; at 250 Hz the threshold difference was –50 to +20 dB, at 1 KHz from –30 to +20 dB, and at 4 KHz from –35 to +45 dB. The difference between the slow potential threshold and the audiometric threshold in children aged 7 - 14 years was –10 to +25 dB at 250 Hz, –30 to +25 dB at 1 KHz and –10 to +30 dB at 4 KHz. The slow potential threshold and audiometric threshold discrepancies are more marked in children under 7 years of age and this problem is exacerbated whenever sedation is required.

The clinical use of the slow potential

At present the slow potential is of limited use for the testing of young children. Contraindications include epilepsy, muscle tics and spasms, abnormal EEG activity and the need for sedation. The chief clinical use of the slow potential is for the detection of possible non-organic hearing loss in older children and adults.

The cortical potentials of a normal hearing adult are shown in Figure 9.12. The N_1/P_2 complex is prominent. In contrast the potentials from a 31-year-old female child (Figure 9.13) are much more difficult to identify. This child was sedated and this figure represents one of the better recordings.

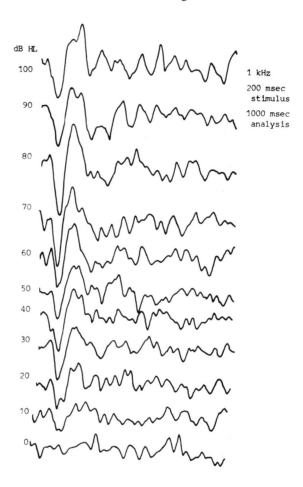

Figure 9.12 *The slow cortical potentials obtained from a normal hearing adult.*

The middle latency responses (MLR)

The MLR share a common time domain with the sonomotor (myogenic) responses and, following the first descriptions (Mast, 1963; Goldstein, 1967) of the MLR, many years passed until sceptical investigators were finally convinced that they were truly neurogenic. The individual components of the MLR have been labelled N_0, P_0, N_a, P_a and P_b to avoid confusion with the N_1, P_2, etc. of the slow cortical potential. The latency of each peak is as follows: N_0, 8 - 10 msec; P_0, 10 - 13

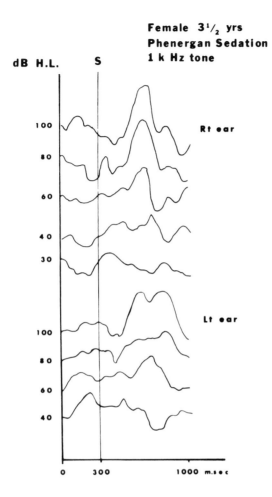

Female 3¹/₂ yrs
Phenergan Sedation
1 k Hz tone

dB H.L.   S

100   Rt ear
80
60
40
30

                       Lt ear
100
80
60
40

0   300   1000 m.sec

Figure 9.13 *The slow cortical potentials obtained from a young child using sedation. Note the dominance of the N₂ component which can be traced to a threshold of 35 dB for the upper traces (right ear) and to 50 dB for the lower traces (left ear). (Reproduced from Beagley et al, 1972, by permission of Sound.)*

msec; N$_a$, 16 - 30 msec; P$_a$, 30 - 45 msec; N$_b$, 40 - 60 msec and P$_b$, 55 - 80 msec. The P$_b$ component is probably the P$_1$ component of the slow cortical response. The N$_0$, P$_0$ and N$_a$ components overlap in latency with known myogenic responses arising from the post-auricular and inion regions of the scalp. It appears that the N$_a$/P$_a$ complex provides the most stable waveform which can be used to estimate the response threshold.

The precise origin of the MLR is unknown but it has been suggested that the earliest components arise from the medial geniculate body and the later components arise from the primary auditory cortex (Picton et al, 1974).

Methodological considerations

The MLRs are recorded maximally at the vertex with a reference on the ipsilateral mastoid or earlobe. Mendel (1974) recommends that the bandpass of the recording system is 25 to 175 Hz with a roll-off of 6 dB per octave. The optimal stimulus is a click or a tone burst with a fast rise time, but, to provide some frequency specificity, Mendel (1974) suggests using a stimulus with a rise and fall time of 2 msec and a plateau of 2 msec. The usual stimulus repetition rate is 10 per sec.

The MLRs have peak amplitudes of approximately 1 - 2 μV at 60 dB SL. Trials of 1,000 or more stimuli are needed to elicit a clear response especially at near threshold intensities. The subject should be relaxed, preferably lying down comfortably, because the MLR can easily be swamped by myogenic potentials.

The input/output functions of the MLRs have limited use, as the response waveform is too variable. The threshold is usually judged subjectively by several observers who have to decide whether or not a response is present in a particular recording. The latency is the most stable measure and could have a possible use in determining brainstem function (Robinson and Rudge, 1977b).

Advantages of the MLR

The test procedure is non-invasive.

The responses are fairly stable in sleep and can be identified with the same degree of certainty as when the subject is awake.

The MLRs are recognizable in young infants.

The frequency range of the test is excellent, as clear responses can be obtained at 500 Hz.

Disadvantages of the MLR

The chief disadvantage of the MLRs is their poor reliability.

The need to mask the non-test ear whenever the test ear is 50 dB deafer has to be remembered.

The reliability and accuracy of the MLR

Goldstein and Rodman (1967) compared the MLR and the subjective auditory threshold, using clicks, and reported that the MLR could be identified at 30 dB SL in 80% of normal subjects and in about half the subjects at ±5 dB SL. The relationship is not so favourable using tone pips, and Horowitz et al (1966) reported more difficulty in identifying responses at near behavioural threshold intensities in patients with partial hearing losses. Engel (1971) reported the presence of MLR in only 8 out of 24 babies that he tested.

Mendel et al (1977) found the MLR more reliable than other investigators and detected the responses in all 18 infants tested in one series. Nevertheless, the present author has not had a great deal of success, and Davis (1976) reported difficulties using the MLR to assess the hearing of young children. Similar disappointing results are reported by Skinner and Glattke (1977).

The clinical use of the MLR

The clinical use of the MLR as a hearing test remains uncertain because most workers find the responses inconsistent. It would appear that their only advantage was their stability during sleep, and since the BAEP shares this advantage, most workers have turned to this more reliable response.

There are few examples of clinical recordings available in the literature. Figure 9.14 shows the composite MLR from groups of six infants at different ages. Figure 9.15 shows the responses obtained from a normal hearing adult.

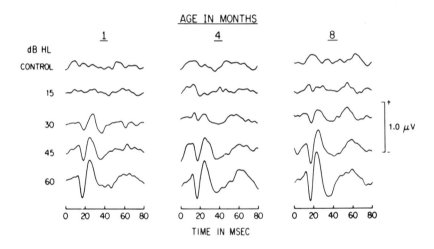

Figure 9.14 *The middle latency responses recorded at different ages in the first year of life. Each set of responses represents the average from 6 infants. (Reproduced from Mendel et al, 1977, by permission Annals of Otology, Rhinology and Laryngology.)*

The $\overline{P300}$ potential

The $\overline{P300}$ potential is the late positive component of the slow vertex potential with an onset latency of approximately 300 msec. The $\overline{P300}$ can be grouped with the late sustained (DC) potential and the CNV as 'perceptual responses'. The earlier AEPs (ECochG, BAEP, FFR and MLR) are not altered by the subject's psychological state, attention, intentions, etc. The perceptual responses are not fully investigated as audiometric tests, but should provide a means of assessing higher hearing functions, such as the subject's ability to comprehend speech and to associate sound meaningfully.

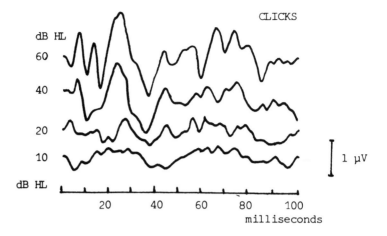

Figure 9.15 *The middle latency responses recorded from a normal hearing adult.*

The $\overline{P300}$ can be distinguished from the earlier AEP components and from the CNV. Unlike the earlier potentials, the $\overline{P300}$ relates to the amount of task-relevant information in the stimulus. Sutton et al (1967) showed that the amplitude varied considerably according to whether or not the subject felt he had guessed correctly the significance of the stimulus, relating it to the resolution of the subject's uncertainty about the stimulus. The main factors that increase P300 amplitude are the improbability of the stimulus, and the fact that the subject is attending to it. Its designation as a target (task-related) stimulus is also important. In fact, the $\overline{P300}$ can be obtained when the subject detects an absent stimulus within a train of regularly presented stimuli, provided this is unexpected (Simson et al, 1976). Donald and Goff (1971) distinguished the CNV from the $\overline{P300}$ by a simple experiment. They presented subjects with a click which was followed two seconds later by a tone to which the subject was asked to respond by pressing a button. During 75 per cent of the trials an unpleasant electric shock was given and, if the electric shocks were made to correspond with pressing the button, a large increase in the $\overline{P300}$ occurred, although there was no change in the CNV.

The available evidence suggests that the $\overline{P300}$ arises from a wider area of the cortex than the N_2 and that it involves the parietal association areas (Picton et al, 1977).

Methodological considerations

The recording parameters are similar to those used for recording the other components of the slow vertex potential. The electrodes are usually positioned on the vertex and over the mastoid on either side. The bandpass of the recording system must include the low frequencies. The stimulus is usually a tone burst of 100 - 200 msec duration.

The advantages and disadvantages of the $\overline{P300}$

The advantages and disadvantages of using the $\overline{P300}$ as a clinical test are not known yet, as the test is still confined to the research laboratory. The obvious advantage is that the potential provides a measure of higher auditory functions. Theoretically, at least, its amplitude does not decrease with decreasing stimulus intensity, and the threshold may be simpler to judge. The response can also be used to assess the subject's ability to discriminate and could provide a means of 'objective' speech audiometry. Furthermore, the test could provide interesting data concerning autism, dyslexia and learning and speech disorders.

The obvious disadvantage concerning its use as a threshold audiometric test is the requirement that the subject pays attention to the stimulus, although there is a $\overline{P300}$ component which has been identified which does not require attention (Squires et al, 1975).

The clinical use of the $\overline{P300}$

A simple illustration of the potential clinical use of the $\overline{P300}$ is provided by Picton et al (1977). In this example, a 1.1 KHz tone was presented randomly among a train of 1 KHz tones with a probability of 0.2. The evoked potential resulting from the 1.1 KHz tones was averaged. The subject either ignored the tones and read a book or was asked to pay particular attention to the 1.1 KHz tones. It can be seen (Figure 9.16) that the $\overline{P300}$ can only be identified when the subject is paying attention. This useful test of the subject's ability to discriminate may possibly have implications for speech audiometry, as the subject could be asked to ignore or pay attention to certain words or words with particular meanings. At present the clinical possibilities of the $\overline{P300}$ are unexplored.

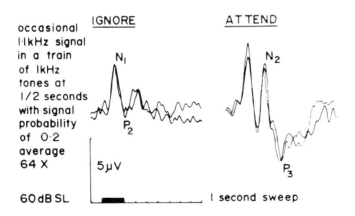

Figure 9.16 *The $\overline{P300}$ as a function of attention. The traces show the averaged responses to an occasional stimulus when a subject is ignoring the stimulus and reading a book, and when she is actively attending and keeping count of the signals. Note that the $\overline{P300}$ is only present during attention. (Reproduced from Picton et al, 1977, by permission of The Journal of Otolaryngology.)*

The sustained or DC potential

This DC potential has also been called the 'steady' or 'sustained' potential. It was initially recognized as a change in the raw EEG recordings (Kohler and Wegener, 1955), but it can be identified more easily using averaging techniques (Keidel, 1971). The DC potential consists of a negative baseline shift in the EEG which persists between the slow cortical responses that mark the onset and offset of a long duration pure tone stimulus (Picton et al, 1978a, 1978b). The exact origin of the potential is unknown, but studies reveal that it is derived maximally over the vertex and frontal regions and that its origin probably extends less posteriorly than the N_1 and P_2 components of the slow cortical response. The DC potential decreases in amplitude as the stimulus intensities fall. The amplitude is, however, somewhat diminished whenever the subject fails to pay attention to the stimulus. A small DC potential can even be identified during sleep.

Some methodological considerations

The electrode positions are similar to those used to record other cortical potentials (active-vertex, mastoid-reference). The bandpass of the recording amplifiers must accept DC activity. This requirement can lead to problems with electrode stability and these problems will be discussed when dealing with the CNV response. The stimulus is usually a tone burst of 600 msec or more. At a stimulus repetition rate of one per 2 sec, the DC potential has an amplitude of approximately one third of the slow cortical response occurring at onset; at higher stimulus repetition rates, the DC potential adapts less than the slow cortical response. The DC potential decreases in amplitude at stimulus frequencies over 2 KHz. Normally about 32 stimulus trials are needed to obtain a clear averaged response.

The advantages and disadvantages of the sustained DC potential

This potential has not yet been used clinically, so the advantages and disadvantages are not known with certainty. The most obvious advantage is that the response can be evoked using speech stimuli. Attempts to use the onset responses, such as the slow cortical response, for speech testing have been thwarted by the fact that the slow cortical response is only evoked by the onset of the word and the potential is completed before the word has finished. The DC potential may also have some value in demonstrating that the subject is paying attention to the stimulus.

There are several disadvantages. The subject must remain very still and the response is less easily identified whenever the subject is sedated. It is unlikely that the potential has any use for testing young children. The exact relationship between the response threshold and the psycho-acoustic threshold is not known and may depend on the amount of attention paid to each stimulus by the subject.

The clinical use of the DC potential

At present the clinical use of the DC potential is uncertain. Picton et al (1977) provide an example of using the DC potential to determine the auditory threshold for a pure tone stimulus (Figure 9.17). It would be interesting to show the response using speech stimuli, but no published work is available.

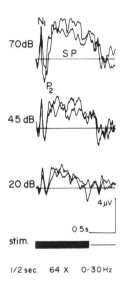

Figure 9.17 *The sustained evoked DC potential in threshold determination. The subject was a young adult and the stimulus tone 500 Hz. (Reproduced from Picton et al, 1977, by permission of The Journal of Otolaryngology.)*

The contingent negative variation (CNV)

The contingent negative variation (CNV) is a slow DC baseline shift of the EEG record which occurs when the subject is expecting to have to perform some perceptual or behavioural task. The CNV was first described by Walter et al (1964). In CNV audiometry, the subject is first given an audible stimulus and told that soon after this sound, a light will come on and continue to flash rapidly. He is asked to prevent the light from flashing by pressing a button as quickly as possible after it comes on. After several trials, the paradigm is established. The subject learns to expect the light to flash on about one second after he hears the warning sound, and a slow negative potential (CNV) develops between the auditory potential resulting from the warning sound and the visual potential resulting from the flashing light. Once the paradigm is established, the stimulus intensity of the warning sound can be reduced until the subject does not produce a CNV potential because he does not hear the warning sound. The great advantage is that the CNV amplitude is not dependent on the intensity of the stimulus but on the subject expecting the light to flash. It is therefore equally large when the sound stimulus is at near threshold .evels.

The CNV potential must be distinguished from the *Bereitschafts potential* (BP) or readiness potential, which is a similar DC EEG shift preceding voluntary movements. The CNV can be obtained without a voluntary movement but with the subject merely thinking 'press the button' when the light flashes. The BP probably has a different scalp distribution to the CNV (Cohen, 1969).

The CNV must also be distinguished from the potentials resulting from eye movements. Hillyard (1974) has tackled the problem of separating the eye potential artifacts from the 'true' CNV (Hillyard and Galambos, 1970). He found that 23% of the CNV recordings in normal subjects were composed of eye potential artefacts as the subjects had a tendency to roll their eyes downwards when they were awaiting the flashing light (or any other 'imperative stimulus'). To avoid this, CNV recordings should be obtained with the eyes open and fixated upon a target.

Some methodological considerations

The apparatus used for CNV audiometry differs from that used for other AEPs as provision has to be made for the imperative stimulus (flashing light) to occur one or two seconds after each sound stimulus and for a switch that can be used by the subject to extinguish the light. The recording electrodes are placed at the vertex and over the mastoid area. Reliable, non-polarizing electrodes are essential or a slow baseline drift appears on the recordings. The skin-to-electrode impedance should be better than 3 kilohms at 1 KHz and the leads should be kept close together to avoid sway.

The amplifiers must either be DC coupled or have a time constant of 10 sec or more. The high cut is usually between 12 and 16 Hz. The CNV is best observed after only a few stimulus trials and usually 10 - 30 are sufficient. A typical analysis period is 4 sec and consists of a 1.2 sec pre-analysis period, 300 msec during which the pure tone stimulus is delivered and then a 1 sec period until the imperative stimulus with a 1.5 sec post-analysis period. The interstimulus interval is between 2 and 5 sec.

Advantages of the CNV

The CNV is recorded using non-invasive electrodes.

The CNV amplitude does not diminish with decreasing stimulus intensity and the threshold is consequently much easier to determine.

The CNV can be used with speech stimuli.

The CNV has an important use for measuring perceptual processes. The amplitude alters, using the same stimulus intensity, when the subject is given meaningful or meaningless words. The CNV almost certainly demonstrates that the subject has truly heard, unlike the other AEPs (except perhaps the P300 and sustained DC potential) which merely show that auditory impulses have reached a certain level within the nervous system.

Disadvantages of the CNV

An operant response is required to develop a CNV and sceptics may say that the auditory threshold is better measured by observing whether or not the subject presses the button rather than by observing the EEG!

There are several difficulties in testing young children. Many young children do not appear to develop a CNV (Walter, 1966) and the need for some co-operation throughout the session, an operant response and the avoidance of sedatives make the testing of young disturbed children impracticable. Psychopathic subjects have great difficulty in establishing a CNV response and conflicting reports on whether or not anxious patients develop a CNV have been published. Knott and Irwin (1968) found small CNV amplitudes, while Low et al (1967) found no such correlation. The CNV may fade unless reinforcement of the paradigm is accomplished, as many subjects will fail to develop a CNV after a number of negative trials.

The reliability and accuracy of the CNV

The CNV cannot be obtained in 10% of normal subjects (Burian et al, 1969) so the possibility of encountering a non-responsive subject must be considered. This possibility is greater in young children, psychopaths and possibly anxious and neurotic subjects. Prevec et al (1974) tested 8 normal adults and obtained the CNV threshold at 5 - 10 dB SL in every case. The test-retest reliability is fair, as subjects

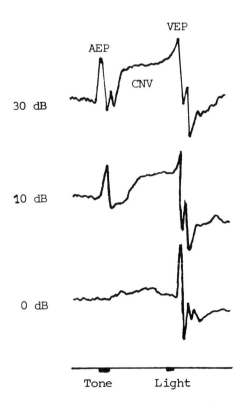

Figure 9.18 *The contingent negative variation as a measure of the hearing threshold. (Adapted from Picton et al, 1977.)*

with clear responses tend to give good responses on subsequent testing, but the amplitude of the CNV is variable as it does depend on the subject's attentiveness. Repeated testing reduces the number of non-responders to 3% (Prevec et al, 1974). Butinar et al (1978) tested 12 patients with audiological problems and obtained a mean difference between CNV and behavioural audiometry of 0.9 ± 7.8 dB with a range of –20 to +25 dB. The same authors have tested pre-school children with some success using a cartoon as the imperative stimulus.

The clinical use of the CNV

The clinical use of the CNV is scant, but there are a few interesting reports. An example of using the CNV to determine the pure tone audiometric threshold is published by Picton et al (1977) (Figure 9.18).

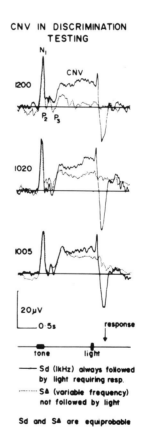

Figure 9.19 *The contingent negative variation as a test of frequency discrimination. The subject is required to respond to the light stimulus as quickly as possible. The light is preceded by a 1 KHz tone (Sd). Another tone (SΔ) is not followed by the light. When the subject can no longer distinguish Sd and SΔ an equal CNV follows both stimuli. Both tones were presented at 75 dB SL.*

Burian and his co-workers (1969, 1972) have used the CNV for objective speech audiometry. They tested two subjects with aphasia and showed that no CNV difference was observed following meaningless or meaningful words. One subject later recovered and retesting showed a clearly enhanced CNV amplitude when the meaningful words were presented.

The CNV can also be used to show that a subject can discriminate between a stimulus occurring at a slightly different frequency to other stimuli (Figure 9.19). The use of CNV as a test of discrimination could prove most interesting in the study of perceptual disorders.

FINAL CONCLUSIONS

From this brief review of the AEPs and their application as tests of hearing, it is hoped that certain characteristics will have emerged. The shorter the latency of the AEP, the less it is influenced by age, sedation and by factors such as the subject's attention and co-operation. The earliest potentials (ECochG, BAEP and FFR) provide the most suitable means of determining the hearing status of young uncooperative children but the frequency range of these tests is limited. More frequency information can be gained by using the cortical responses, but as the latency increases, the cortical responses become increasingly susceptible to external influences such as abnormal EEG patterns, age of the subject, effects of sedatives, attentiveness, etc. The middle latency responses would be useful if they could be obtained with greater reliability, while the slow cortical responses have almost been abandoned for testing young children because the waveforms are so variable. The sonomotor response (PAM) has poor reliability, but has the one advantage that it can be obtained readily from the young active (unsedated) child and may have a rôle as a simple screening test. The later response ($\overline{P300}$, DC potential and CNV) have not yet been fully investigated as clinical tests but do show promise, not merely as methods of determining pure tone audiometric thresholds, but as a means of carrying out objective speech audiometry and as tests of perception.

10

Centrally Generated Auditory Potentials

K. Robinson and P. Rudge

INTRODUCTION

Evoked potential studies of the auditory system have proved to be a significant advance both in understanding physiological mechanisms of hearing in man and particularly as a useful addition to the diagnostic armamentarium of the clinician. It is now possible to examine electrophysiologically the output of the cochlea and the VIII nerve through the techniques of electrocochleography, pioneered by Portmann and co-workers in the late 1960s. These techniques are discussed by W.P.R. Gibson in Chapters 8 and 9 and have proved most valuable to the audiologist. This chapter is concerned primarily with more central connections of the VIII nerve system and the potentials generated by them. The emphasis will inevitably be on those potentials generated by the brainstem pathways since they have been most extensively explored in both animals and man and have proved to be of use to, not only the audiologist, but also the neurologist. However, some of the later potentials probably arising from other parts of the nervous system are also discussed at length, since in preliminary studies they have shown considerable promise as a clinical tool. There will be some overlap between this chapter and those by W.P.R. Gibson, which are intended to be complementary, so it is desirable that all the chapters on the auditory evoked potentials be read to obtain a full picture of evoked potentials in this modality.

It is fortunate that all the potentials generated by the central connections of the auditory system can be optimally recorded between surface electrodes at the vertex and the ipsilateral mastoid and that latency can be usefully employed to classify these components. All the auditory evoked potentials (AEPs) so far described in the literature are tabulated in Table 10.1, together with their salient characteristics. The galvanic skin response (GSR) to an auditory stimulus is an exception to the principles outlined above, but is included for completeness.

The auditory evoked potentials recorded with a latency of 0 - 10 msec comprise the early components, or brainstem evoked potentials (BAEPs) and the frequency following response (FFR). The BAEP is best obtained with a high intensity click stimulus and consists of up to seven components, commonly called components

Table 10.1 CHARACTERISTICS OF THE AUDITORY EVOKED POTENTIALS

Classification	Latency	Evoked response	Abbreviations	DC Potential	Waveform Nomenclature	Unaffected by level of arousal
Early	< 10 msec	Electrocochleogram	E.Coch.G. E.Co.G.	Yes (SP)	Cochlear microphonic (CM) Summating potential (SP) Component I or N_1 and N_2	+ +
		Brainstem evoked potential	BSEP BAEP		Components or waves I-VII	+
		Frequency following response	FFR			
Middle	10-60 msec	Myogenic Sonomotor Post-auricular muscle response	— — PAM			
		Central nervous system responses			N_0, $P_\emptyset$, N_a, P_a, N_b, P_1	+
Late	> 60 sec	Vertex K Complex P300			$N_1 - P_2 - N_2$ P_3	
	< 1.5 sec	Contingent negative variation	CNV	Yes		
		Sustained potential		Yes		
	1.5-4.5 sec	Galvanic skin response	GSR			

I-VII respectively (Figure 10.1). The FFR is a response of about 6 msec latency with a fundamental frequency and duration equal to that of the stimulus eliciting it (Figure 10.2). Since there is considerable evidence that at least the first five components of the BAEP are generated in or near to successive nuclei on the classical auditory pathway, many laboratories have shown interest in these components. A review of the evidence for their origin would therefore seem to be an appropriate starting point.

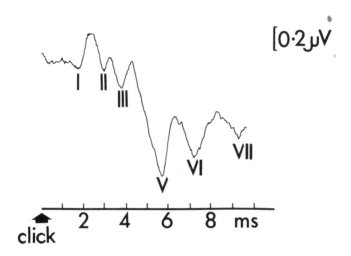

Figure 10.1 *BAEP of a normal subject. Component IV is not present as the stimulus was given at short interstimulus interval (50 msec). Stimulus onset indicated. C_z-A_2. Vertex positivity upwards.*

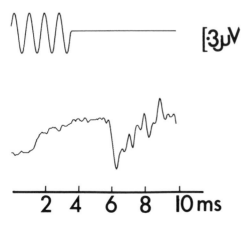

Figure 10.2 *FFR from a normal subject. Stimulus shown above (1 KHz), record below. Note FFR₁ and FFR₂ (see page 367 of text for explanation).*

BRAINSTEM EVOKED POTENTIALS

ORIGIN OF THE COMPONENTS OF THE BRAINSTEM EVOKED POTENTIALS

There is considerable evidence that the brainstem evoked potential (BAEP) arises from structures in the classical auditory pathways, which include the VIII nerve, cochlear nuclei, superior olivary complex, the lateral lemnisci and associated nuclei, and the inferior colliculi. Furthermore, the generators of some of the components are anatomically discrete. Thus an analysis of the spatio-temporal distribution of the potentials clearly indicates that components I and II in rats and cats (Plantz et al, 1974) and I, II and III in monkeys (Allen and Starr, 1978) are asymmetrically disposed over the surface of the scalp, while later components, particularly IV and V, are symmetrically arranged. A more direct approach has been applied to this problem using intracerebral recording techniques, or inducing lesions on the auditory pathways in animals, concurrently with surface recordings. In assessing these data it is important to realize that different groups of workers have used varying techniques. Thus the lesions induced by Achor and Starr (1980b) were in general small, while those of most other workers were large. On the other hand, Achor and Starr (1980a) have done much more extensive exploration with recording electrodes than other workers, in an attempt to build up a composite picture of the electrical events. These data indicate, with one exception (Berry et al, 1976), that the different components do have independent, albeit complex, generators.

Component I is dependent upon the auditory nerve. This component occurs simultaneously with the compound action potential of the nerve (N_1) recorded at the round window (Sohmer and Feinmesser, 1967; Jewett, 1970b; Jewett and Romano, 1972) and is of maximal amplitude and reverses its polarity when the recording electrode is adjacent to the nerve (Lev and Sohmer, 1972). Isolation of the VIII nerve from the brainstem abolishes all but the first component, and destruction of the nerve abolishes it (Buchwald and Huang, 1975). The cochlear microphonic may make a small contribution to this component (Achor and Starr, 1980a).

Component II depends, at least partly, upon the cochlear nuclei, especially the ventral parts, since its appearance coincides with activity in that nucleus (Jewett, 1970b; Lev and Sohmer, 1972; Achor and Starr, 1980a). Although component II disappears when the connections of the VIII nerve to the brainstem are destroyed ipsilaterally, but not contralaterally (Buchwald and Huang, 1975), this component is complex. It seems to have a small contribution from wave N_2 recorded at the round window, which probably arises from the auditory nerve and, in addition, Achor and Starr (1980b) have shown that there is a contribution from the trapezoid body.

Component III arises from generators in the region of the superior olivary complex, being maximal when recorded in this area, and the phase changes when the electrode penetrates the nucleus (Jewett, 1970; Lev and Sohmer, 1972). A midline section in the brainstem at the level of the trapezoid body abolishes component III implying a total dependence upon decussating fibres (Buchwald and Huang, 1975), although more recent work by Achor and Starr (1980a) shows that there is activity in both superior olivary nuclei after unilateral stimulation.

Publications from different laboratories reveal marked variation of the morphology of components occurring after component III. This is important in assessing the origin of these components and in particular in extrapolating the animal work to man. Earlier experiments suggested a dependence of component IV upon the inferior colliculi, the wave being of maximal amplitude when recorded from this structure, and its polarity reversed when the electrode passed through the inferior colliculus (Jewett, 1970b). Destruction of the colliculi greatly diminished, but did not abolish, either component IV or V (Lev and Sohmer, 1972). More recent work demonstrated the loss of component IV with lesions in the ventral nucleus of the lateral lemniscus (Buchwald and Huang, 1975). Furthermore, component IV depends upon both crossed and uncrossed fibres, midline lesions reducing the amplitude of the component but not abolishing it. Huang and Buchwald (1978) have recently shown that, unlike earlier components, the amplitude of component IV to binaural stimulation is smaller than anticipated from the sum of that component obtained by stimulation of each ear separately. Such a result is explicable in terms of convergence upon the generator of component IV of a crossed and uncrossed input and is consistent with their earlier experiments. Jones et al (1976), using a cryogenic technique to slow conduction in fibres and block synaptic transmission, claimed that unilateral cooling of the pons abolishes component IV and suggest this is due to the consequent asymmetric activation of a bilateral structure upon which component IV depends. This results in dispersion of the electrical activity that would normally have been seen as component IV. Such an argument is again consistent with a bilateral input to the generator and the authors thought the effect they observed was obtained from near the inferior colliculus.

There is now some controversy over the origins of component V. Until recently most workers agreed that this component depended upon the inferior colliculus or a structure just anterior to it (Jewett, 1970; Lev and Sohmer, 1972; Buchwald and Huang, 1975). Destruction of the inferior colliculi or undercutting them abolished component V (Jewett, 1970; Buchwald and Huang, 1975). In contrast Achor and Starr (1980a, 1980b) found no evidence that activity of the inferior colliculi had any effect upon the surface recorded BAEP, both from work with depth electrodes and lesions in the area. It is of interest that component V probably depends on a crossed pathway, since midline section at a lower level abolished the response (Buchwald and Huang, 1975), while unilateral cooling merely delayed, but did not abolish, the component to contralateral stimulation (Jones et al, 1976). These experiments illustrate the important point that a lesion cannot in fact define anatomically the region of generation of a component; it merely defines the structures upon which a function is necessarily dependent.

It is unknown if the so-called brainstem responses reflect activity of groups of neurones or the action potentials in fibre tracts or a combination of both. Furthermore, it should be emphasized that all the surface recorded components are the summation of electrical activity of many thousands of neurones and their processes, dispersed in anatomically discrete nuclei and tracts between which there is extensive interaction. Indeed, further work with depth electrodes and small lesions placed at various sites within the brainstem auditory pathways indicates that neuronal activity is quite widespread at any particular instant after the administration of a click stimulus (Achor and Starr, 1980a, 1980b). This work implies that events recorded at the surface are the sum of the activity of many neuronal populations and that a discrete lesion can cause considerable disruption of more than one component. Finally, it should be noted that some of these observations of the effects of lesions upon the various components of the BAEP and their supposed origins are not compatible with the generally accepted anatomical connections of the auditory pathways (e.g. see Whitfield, 1967).

Thus far we have considered the animal work. In man direct evidence on the source of these various components is, of course, more difficult to obtain; lesions within the auditory pathways cannot be produced deliberately and one must therefore use data from disease studies. Unfortunately, many pathological processes within the central nervous system cause widespread effects, since they are either inherently multifocal, as in multiple sclerosis and anoxic damage, or are associated with oedema and pressure effects, as with tumours. This greatly limits, but does not negate, the value of such cases, as one can never be sure of the exact site of damage causing alteration of the BAEP. On the other hand, the effects of discrete vascular lesions can be better localized, especially if they are long-standing, and enable useful clinico-pathological correlations to be made. Data from patients with a large variety of conditions have been obtained and these do suggest similar generators to those determined from animal work.

Component I is the only component depending upon a structure outside the brainstem, viz., the VIII cranial nerve. This component is altered by cochlear damage and surgical section of the nerve, but is often preserved in acoustic neuromata and in some of these cases (but certainly not all) the later components are absent (Sohmer et al, 1974; Starr and Hamilton, 1976; Stockard and Rossiter, 1977; Selters and Brackman, 1977). One interpretation of the acoustic neuroma observations, in which the components after wave I are absent, is that activity originating in that part of the VIII nerve adjacent to the cochlea passes centrally in the nerve until the tumour is reached, at which point there is a failure of transmission of the nerve impulses and consequent failure to activate the brainstem auditory pathways. It is usually possible to record the activity of the peripheral part of the VIII nerve as component I, but the generators of subsequent components are not necessarily activated. Further support for the auditory nerve as the generator of component I comes from the temporal coincidence of it with N_1 of the electrocochleogram and the relative resistance of this component, compared with later ones, to anoxia, a feature typical of peripheral, as against central, nervous system, fibres (Starr, 1976).

All the other components of the BAEP are thought to come from central nervous system structures. Again we must emphasize that patient data can only be used to complement the animal work except in those rare cases where discrete vascular lesions have occurred. Vascular lesions of the cochlear nuclei alter or abolish component II, while midline lesions sparing these nuclei cause abnormality of component III without change in component II (Stockard and Rossiter, 1977). This is consistent with the generators of the second component being in the region of the cochlear nuclei. Interestingly, in some patients with asymmetrical involvement of the brainstem, the delay of component III is greater when the contralateral ear is stimulated, implying that this component is more dependent upon a structure on the opposite side of the brainstem as in animal studies. Vascular lesions at a higher level such as the mid- or rostral pons, sparing structures such as the superior olivary nucleus, cause a relative increase in latency of components IV and V, the earlier components being normal.

Recently Hashimoto et al (1981) have attempted to elucidate the origins of the components of the BAEP in man at operation by placing electrodes directly upon the VIII nerve, brainstem, mesencephalon and in the ventricular system. The results obtained confirm the animal data. Component I seems to arise from the most peripheral part of the VIII nerve, i.e., that portion enveloped by peripheral myelin. Component II is more complex and seems to comprise activity from the more central part of the VIII nerve and adjacent pontine structures. Components III and IV appear to come from the pons, while component V coincides with activity in the inferior colliculus conforming with earlier animal work. Hashimoto et al (1981) also adduce evidence for activity in the medial geniculate ganglia of the thalamus resulting in component VI. This is the most direct evidence so far obtained in man on the origin of components.

From all these data one may tentatively conclude that the generators of the BAEP in man are similar to those in animals. It is hoped that when further cases of vascular disease have been studied, or an approach combining the methods of stereotaxic surgery and the computerised tomogram has been used, more precise origins may be delineated.

RECORDING THE BAEP

Electrode placement

Most workers are agreed that the BAEP recorded with electrodes on the scalp are volume-conducted potentials that reflect the activity of generators that are located deep within the brainstem.

Component I

Component I reflects activity of the VIII nerve (Sohmer and Feinmesser, 1970). Jewett and Williston (1971), using engineering concepts, described component I as a near field potential (a potential which shows significant differences in wave shape for electrodes a short distance apart) which is volume conducted. It is frequently reported that component I cannot be discerned when the BAEP is recorded between the vertex and the contralateral mastoid (Thornton, 1975a; Stockard et al, 1978), but this observation is not dependent on the concept of component I as a near field potential. With a non-cephalic reference electrode it has been confirmed that component I appears as a negative deflection at the ipsilateral mastoid. In addition, however, a positive deflection with the same latency as component I is recorded at the vertex and, with smaller amplitude, at the contralateral mastoid (Terkildsen et al, 1974; Streletz et al, 1977). The important point from this evidence is that when recordings are made between vertex and ipsilateral mastoid the contributions to component I will be out-of-phase and therefore enhance the response, whereas with vertex-contralateral mastoid recordings the contributions to component I will be in-phase and thus cancel.

Components II - V

With binaural stimulation and vertex-mastoid recordings it has been established that waves II - VI are distributed widely over the scalp. There is little attenuation, although the response is maximal at the vertex. Jewett and Williston (1971) used the concept of a far field response to distinguish these components from component I, since change in the position of the vertex electrode over a few centimetres is not critical.

Using a non-cephalic electrode as a reference it is apparent that a potential difference can be recorded with electrodes both at the vertex and at the mastoid (Terkildsen et al, 1974), which, of course, gives a cancellation effect when the potential difference is recorded between vertex and mastoid. With a non-cephalic electrode as reference to a vertex electrode the amplitude of the BAEP (apart from component I) is enhanced. The identification of an inactive non-cephalic site is even more difficult than with conventional electroencephalography. Terkildsen et al (1974) showed that the tip of the nose was not indifferent and chose as reference the left 3rd sternocostal joint. Martin and Moore (1977) chose the chin as the inactive site and tested the assumption by showing that there was no potential difference between it and the thorax. Streletz et al (1977) used a sternovertebral electrode as the indifferent site and showed that, when connected to the wrist, there was no potential difference. Most authors are, of course, aware of the perennial problem of the search for a truly indifferent site for electroencephalographic recordings and recognize that all these sites may well be isoelectric rather than indifferent.

Ipsilateral and contralateral recordings

With monaural stimulation and recording between vertex and mastoid the response recorded from the ipsilateral channel (C_z-A_{ipsi}) is consistently different to that recorded from the contralateral channel (C_z-A_{contra}). Using a series of 6 normal subjects, it has been claimed that components I - V were present in the ipsilateral channel, whereas only waves II - V were present on the contralateral channel, and that waves II and III showed phase reversal between channels whilst components IV and V were in phase. With the exception of wave II, which tended to be larger on the contralateral channel, the components on the ipsilateral channel were of larger amplitude (Thornton, 1975a). In a subsequent paper, using these normal data and a single illustrative case of a patient with a suspected 'midbrain' lesion as evidence, it was argued that those neural pathways that traverse the brainstem act as generators for the responses recorded on the contralateral channel. This concept is being used as the basis for the interpretation of records from monaural stimulation which are recorded on a contralateral as well as an ipsilateral channel (Thornton, 1976).

Stockard et al (1978) reported that in normal subjects components II and III fuse completely in the contralateral channel in some cases, whilst in others the two components move closer together.

It is the authors' opinion that attempts to label the components of the contralateral channel to conform with those of the ipsilateral channel are misguided. With mastoid-mastoid recordings and monaural stimulation it has been shown that there are components which do not coincide exactly in peak latency with those components identified in the ipsilateral channel (Picton et al, 1974; Robinson and Rudge, 1981). Figure 10.3 shows the results from a personal series. When the waveform recorded for the contralateral channel is summed algebraically with the waveform recorded independently between the two mastoid electrodes, the result is identical to the waveform recorded for the ipsilateral channel. A further pitfall which awaits those of us who take too simplistic a view of the composition of the BAEP is the post-aural sonomotor potential (post-auricular muscle potential) which has a pathway that is closely linked with the classical auditory system. It is probable that the central pathway of the post-aural sonomotor response involves at least six synapses (Gibson, 1978), and potentials from this system could be contributing to the BAEP waveform.

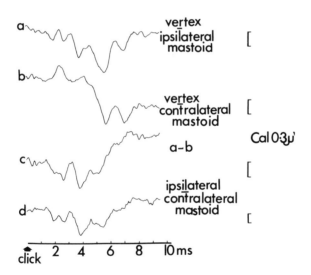

Figure 10.3 BAEP recorded from vertex-ipsilateral mastoid (a), vertex-contralateral mastoid (b) and between mastoids (d) to unilateral stimulation. Record c is the algebraic difference between records a and b. Note the similarity of traces c and d.

Choice of electrode placement

There is an element of choice regarding electrode placement, although there is compelling evidence that component I is best recorded in a vertex-ipsilateral mastoid derivation. Component I may be identified and distinguished from the cochlear microphonic by giving an auditory stimulus which reverses polarity on alternate presentations, this procedure cancelling the cochlear microphonic, whilst component I remains unchanged. At the same time stimulus artifacts will also be cancelled. Component I can be distinguished from components II onwards by its absence from the recordings between the vertex and the contralateral mastoid. In the case of the subsequent waveform there is some cancellation if vertex-mastoid differential recordings are used. Although this effect can be avoided with vertex-non-cephalic recording there are disadvantages to this. First, there is the major problem of identifying a site which is truly electrically indifferent. Secondly, it is known that the signal-to-noise ratio deteriorates considerably when the active and reference electrodes are placed far apart on the body. Thirdly, there is contamination by the ECG. The electrocardiogram can overload the amplifiers of the recording apparatus for a proportion of the stimulus presentations. As a result some of the BAEP responses are excluded from the average buffer causing slight reduction in the BAEP waveform amplitude. These electrocardiogram potentials can be excluded by restricting the presentation of the clicks to the T-P interval, although the pulse rate will then dictate, to some extent, the repetition rate of the stimulus. In spite of these limitations there is an indication for using a vertex-non-cephalic recording in those patients in whom particularly large post-auricular muscle potentials are present. These responses are picked up by the mastoid electrodes and may well overload the amplifiers of the recording apparatus on all or most of the stimulus presentations.

The stimulus

Frequency components

The most effective stimulus to evoke the BAEP is a click or high frequency tone burst. For investigation of the commoner retro-cochlear disorders, e.g. cerebello-pontine angle tumours, a click is an adequate stimulus, since it is unlikely that the lesion will be confined to a structure associated with a narrow range of frequencies. In contrast, in order to use the BAEP as a clinical tool to evaluate peripheral hearing disorders, a stimulus which tests specific frequency ranges might be of value, as the hearing deficit is often confined to a narrow frequency band, e.g. noise induced hearing loss.

There are some important technical aspects of producing a pure tone stimulus. A sinusoidal waveform can readily be produced electrically, but the resulting mechanical signal may be considerably distorted. For this reason, a pure tone stimulus should be monitored, by leading off the signal from earphones or loudspeaker with a microphone and displaying the result on an oscilloscope. Transients containing high frequency components will usually be apparent at the onset of the stimulus; these can be partially damped by increasing the rise time of the signal (shaping the onset), the steeper the rise time the greater will be the contribution of these transients to the overall signal.

At the physiological level more snags exist for those proposing to practise BAEP audiometry. First, there is an impressive amount of evidence to suggest that the BAEP is only elicited by stimuli with a significant high frequency content. Figure 10.4 shows the results of recording BAEP and middle latency components in a patient with a symmetrical high frequency cochlear hearing loss due to quinine administration for myotonia. Although middle latency components were easily elicited, BAEPs were absent on repeated testing. Secondly, the rise time of the stimulus is important; in a study using noise bursts as the stimuli it was clearly demonstrated that the latency of the BAEP was determined exclusively by the onset of the stimulus (Hecox et al, 1976) and that the sharper the onset, the shorter the latency of component V, whilst its amplitude remained unaffected. Recent animal work has emphasized further the importance of the onset of the stimulus. In the cat a sub-population of units exists within cochlear nucleus, superior olivary nucleus and, to a lesser extent, inferior colliculus, which have the shortest response latency

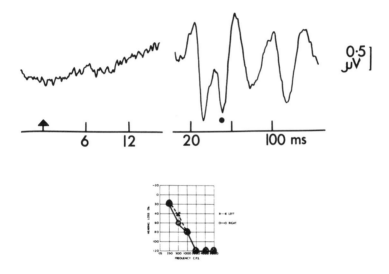

Figure 10.4 *BAEP (left) and middle latency (right) components from a patient with symmetrical high tone hearing loss due to quinine administration. P_1 indicated . Pure tone audiograms below (x---x left, o---o right, in this and subsequent figures).*

of any component. They also have the least variability of latency and have been described as 'precision units'. When surface recorded BAEPs were obtained, the latencies of the successive components corresponded most closely with this sub-population of precision units (Huang and Buchwald, 1977). These short-latency units are similar to those units described as responding to the stimulus onset with great precision in the cochlear nucleus (Radinova, 1971) and superior olivary complex (Galambos et al, 1959). These observations could be relevant to those of Hecox et al (1976) cited above. Since the frequency of a stimulus and the rapidity of its onset are inter-related there is obviously a major problem in recording the BAEP to a specific frequency. This applies in particular to those frequencies in the speech range, although there is at least one report describing the BAEP with low frequency stimuli (Suzuki et al, 1977).

An alternative method of demonstrating the physiological response to various frequency ranges is to mask the click or high frequency tone with sounds of pre-selected frequencies (Terkildsen et al, 1975). Other workers have expanded these procedures using a masking strategy where the high and low pass maskers are extended in a step-wise fashion and algebraic subtraction procedures are then used to derive response waveforms thought to represent activity initiated at specific frequency regions along the cochlea (Parker and Thornton, 1978a). No systematic difference between these derived waveforms and response waveforms recorded to specific frequencies could be detected. Thus a patient suffering from a hearing loss in a particular frequency band should give a modified derived response to that band (Parker and Thornton, 1978b).

The question of whether or not BAEPs which are truly frequency specific can be recorded over the human auditory frequency range needs to be resolved. Few aspects from the various approaches to this problem seem to knit together at present.

Interstimulus interval (ISI)

As BAEPs are of small amplitude ($<2\,\mu V$) it is necessary to average at least 512 responses to obtain a satisfactory signal-to-noise ratio. In most human evoked potential work the optimum interstimulus interval is 0.5 - 1 sec, so that averaging more than 512 responses requires long recording sessions. On the other hand, with an interstimulus interval of less than 0.5 sec there is a possibility that the slower cortical evoked potentials will overlap the period of the BAEP to the subsequent stimuli. Jewett and Williston (1971) demonstrated that it was possible to record the BAEPs at an interstimulus interval of 20 msec, although components I - IV were much less distinct. In a group of 19 controls, given clicks at interstimulus intervals of 420 msec and 50 msec presented randomly, we have shown that only component V was consistently distinct at the shorter intervals and that the parameters of this component alone remained stable (Robinson and Rudge, 1977a). Two aspects of this effect of interstimulus interval need discussing: firstly, the problem of adaptation to trains of stimuli both at the periphery and, perhaps, centrally; secondly, the effect of pathological processes, in particular demyelination, upon the ability of the auditory system to cope with short interstimulus intervals.

In an elegant experiment (Don et al, 1977), in which trains of 20 clicks were presented to one ear at an interstimulus interval of 10 msec with a 0.5 sec period between trains, it was shown that component V to the first click of the train had a latency equivalent to that recorded with an interstimulus interval of 100 msec, whilst this same component V to the twentieth click of the train had a latency equivalent to that recorded with an interstimulus interval of 10 msec. When clicks 2 - 19 were presented to the other ear the latency of component V to click 1 and click 20 was the same and equivalent to an interstimulus interval of 100 msec. These workers concluded that the effect causing an increase in latency was monaural and that it is probably due to adaptation in the peripheral part of the auditory pathway.

However, since they were unable to identify the intervening components at these interstimulus intervals, they could not prove that the changes in latency were independent of central adaptation. Similarly, in the cat, interstimulus intervals shorter than 20 msec result in large decrements in the amplitude of BAEPs recorded from implanted electrodes; however, potentials generated more centrally in the brainstem showed the same order of decrement as those originating from the peripheral structures, which suggests that the adaptation occurs only at the peripheral part of the pathway. Increases in latency also occurred, and they were of a similar order at all levels of the brainstem (Huang and Buchwald, 1977). In contrast, when a train of four pulses is presented with interstimulus intervals of 32.5, 24 and 15 msec and an intertrain interval of 90 msec, it is claimed that waves I - IV can be identified and that the change of amplitudes provides evidence that adaptation occurs at all levels of the auditory system (Thornton and Coleman, 1975).

These studies confirm that the interstimulus interval modifies the BAEP, but the site of adaptation remains uncertain. There is no doubt from electrocochleographic studies that peripheral adaptation does occur. Thus the VIII nerve action potential is unchanged with intervals between clicks of more than 50 msec but with shorter intervals this action potential is modified (Yoshie et al, 1967). A further complicating factor is that the nature of the stimulus seems to be important. Using tone bursts it has been shown that adaptation effects may persist for up to 256 msec (Eggermont and Odenthal, 1974b). In conclusion, controversy exists regarding the precise interstimulus interval for which adaptation modifies responses, as to whether central as well as peripheral processes are implicated, and also as to whether the intensity and type of the stimulus modifies the adaptation process.

Another important factor in respect of interstimulus interval is the fact that demyelination of central pathways affects the ability of the nerve fibres to conduct impulses. In animals with experimentally induced demyelination it has been shown that, as the interstimulus interval is decreased, the abnormality of nerve conduction is enhanced (McDonald and Sears, 1970; Rasminsky and Sears, 1972), a phenomenon that has been gainfully employed in the detection of demyelination occurring in multiple sclerosis. Thus in a series of 30 patients with multiple sclerosis subjected to clicks at interstimulus intervals of 420 and 50 msec, two patients had abnormal BAEPs only for the shorter interval. This indicates that abnormalities can be highlighted by stressing the auditory pathways with short interstimulus intervals.

The choice of an appropriate interstimulus interval is important and should to a certain extent be dictated by the clinical context. In multiple sclerosis a shorter interval (faster rate) that will highlight the demyelinating process is preferred. Since at very short interstimulus intervals adaptation effects are present even in normal subjects, and patients with peripheral hearing loss adapt abnormally, it must be appreciated that it may be subclinical hearing loss which is causing the abnormality rather than central pathology. A useful technique to overcome these difficulties is to present a pair of clicks 5 msec apart with an interpair interval of 45 msec. With this arrangement component I remains stable, whilst the latency of component V to the *first* click of the pair shows an increase in normal subjects which is markedly enhanced in a proportion of patients with multiple sclerosis. This is a particularly useful technique when the response to a single click at an interstimulus interval of 50 msec is borderline (Robinson and Rudge, 1977b). If, on the other hand, the aim is to demonstrate the individual components as clearly and consistently as possible, as in the investigation of cerebello-pontine angle lesions, then a long interstimulus interval rather than an increased number of sweeps should be the method of choice. The initial appeal of the BAEP to the neurologist was the possibility it presented of localizing brainstem lesions precisely, e.g. brainstem infarcts and tumours, by demonstrating the absence of components generated beyond a particular brainstem level. The results have been disappointing, although in the individual case it may still be a useful approach.

Intensity

In a previous section we have outlined some limitations of BAEP audiometry (see frequency components of the stimulus). However, there is one factor which might enhance its value as an audiometric tool, namely, the highly reproducible input-output latency and amplitude functions with changes in stimulus intensity. In an excellent review of the literature the striking latency sensitivity of component V to changes in stimulus intensity was noted (Picton et al, 1977). Furthermore, at any given intensity there was only a 0.4 msec range of latency between various laboratories and in any one laboratory the inter-subject variation was even less.

The components of the BAEP depend upon the input to the auditory system via the VIII nerve and will reflect, at least in part, the activity of the VIII nerve action potential. In experiments with electrodes implanted at various levels of the brainstem auditory pathways of the cat, latency and amplitude-intensity functions similar to those recorded with surface electrodes in humans have been obtained; the interval between components (inter-peak interval) did not change with alterations in the intensity of the stimulus, and absolute changes in the amplitude of the VIII nerve action potential were passively reflected by subsequent peaks. This suggests that, once signals have been initiated at the level of the acoustic nerve, there is little additional modification within the brainstem (Huang and Buchwald, 1978). If this is also the case in man, the BAEP should faithfully reflect VIII nerve function.

The data from electrocochleographic studies of the VIII nerve action potential in man suggest that the input-output functions are composed of two distinct parts. The first, a slowly incrementing part (L-curve), is followed by a rapidly incrementing part (H-curve) and these curves are considered to represent the output of two independent hair cell populations (Yoshie, 1968). Furthermore, it is thought that in each frequency-specific part of the cochlea the overall population of neural units may be divided into two sub-populations, since the VIII nerve action potential is bimodal, the two components being 0.8 msec apart in man. The input-output functions of the electrocochleogram reflect this bimodal waveform with an abrupt change in latency and amplitude when the stimulus level falls below 65 dB HL, at which point the first negativity is no longer predominant. The function remains relatively flat in the range of 60 - 40 dB HL, while below this level only the second negativity is present, the incrementing function changing to one of lesser slope (Eggermont and Odenthal, 1974b).

Abnormally rapid loudness growth, i.e. recruitment, is characteristic of a cochlear hearing deficit, and can be tested objectively with electrocochleography. In these cases the L part of the input-output function is absent, since the VIII nerve action potential is unimodal in waveform and the second negativity seen in the normal electrocochleogram does not occur. In contrast to this, although the BAEP does show an abnormal slope in these cases, the unimodal nature of the response has not been verified. Thus surface BAEP measures of recruitment add little information to routine audiometric testing using subjective methods in co-operative adults.

On the other hand in patients with neurological disorders there is rarely the need to monitor input-output functions and a single stimulus intensity is adequate. In our own laboratory we commonly use a high intensity of 84 dB HL in all subjects. Since the input-output function for both latency and amplitude reaches an asymptote at about 75 dB HL, any minor hearing losses will not be reflected in the BAEP, as the stimulus will be sufficiently above the patient's threshold to remain on this asymptote. In some laboratories correction for hearing loss is made by determining the patient's sensory threshold to the click for both ears separately, and a standard intensity above this level used.

In summary, recording input-output function of the BAEP is of limited value. Apart from the rare case the BAEP adds no further information to conventional audiometry and is less satisfactory than electrocochleographic techniques for the study of recruitment. For neurological problems this information is redundant.

Monaural versus binaural

In patients where there is a significant hearing loss, or a lesion involving the cerebello-pontine angle is suspected clinically, monaural stimulation is mandatory. In contrast, where multiple sclerosis is suspected we routinely use binaural stimulation. Other workers have been critical of our approach preferring unilateral stimulation for all patients. There are, however, good reasons for using binaural stimulation in patients with MS.

First, the anatomy of the auditory pathways differs from the other major sensory systems in ways that are relevant to recording and interpreting its evoked potential in demyelination. Visual and somatosensory pathways within the CNS remain unilateral for a substantial part of their course and damage to them can cause abnormalities that are confined to one side. In contrast, the central myelinated part of the auditory nerve is relatively short before it synapses within the cochlear nucleus and partially decussates. Furthermore, because of the multiple decussations at higher levels, cortical representation of auditory data is more nearly bilateral than is the case for the other sensory systems. Thus there is no *a priori* reason to use unilateral stimulation in patients with demyelination, where the chance of damage to a strictly unilateral part of the pathway is slight.*

---

* Editorial Note: In fairness to the reader it should be pointed out that many workers in the field would dispute this point. A strong argument for monaural stimulation in MS can be advanced on the grounds that, with binaural stimulation, a normal response from one ear tends to mask an abnormal one from the other ear and thus leads to an unduly high false negative rate, especially as the limits of normal variability can be more accurately defined for the ipsilateral and contralateral components of the monaural response (Prasher and Gibson, 1980a, 1980b). A further discussion of this topic by the authors of the present Chapter will be found in Chapter 11 on pages 376 and 384.

Secondly, the majority of workers agree that component V provides the most useful landmark for the interpretation of the BAEP waveform. It is relatively stable at faster inter-stimulus intervals and can be identified nearer to subjective threshold than any other component. With current recording techniques using monaural stimulation this component rarely exceeds an amplitude of 1 μV, so that any technique which enhances the amplitude of this component will be of value. Although the latency of all the components is unaltered whether stimulation is monaural or binaural, it has been shown that binaural stimulation consistently increases the amplitude of component V compared with monaural stimulation. For example, in 14 normal subjects the amplitude increases varied from less than 10% to greater than 100% (Blegvad, 1975). Figure 10.5 shows some results from a personal series of 14 normal subjects. All components, apart from component I, show an increase in amplitude with binaural stimulation and component V was always recorded with an amplitude of at least 0.7 μV. As a result normal limits can be

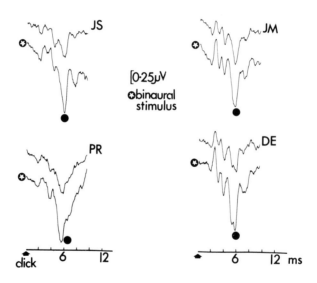

Figure 10.5 *BAEP from 4 normal subjects to monaural (above) and binaural (below) stimulation. Note the marked increase in component V (●) in each case to binaural stimulation.*

defined for the absolute amplitude of component V with binaural stimulation, a situation that does not pertain in unilateral stimulation. This is important, particularly since Achor and Starr (1980b) have shown that with experimental lesions (not specifically demyelination) alteration of amplitude, not latency, occurs.

Finally, few published results are available on the effect on the BAEP of masking the unstimulated ear. It has been claimed that the absence of component I on the contralateral channel means that masking is unnecessary. However, there is some evidence that the absence of component I is due to the particular electrode placement (see section on electrode placement). The literature on when and how to mask in conventional audiometry is vast and complicated, and there is no reason to expect the problem to be simpler in BAEP audiometry. Although masking is unnecessary when the abnormality is central, a central disorder of the auditory pathway does not preclude there also being disorders of the peripheral organ which are sufficient to alter the BAEP in a misleading way. With binaural stimulation these problems are pre-empted.

There are, however, two disadvantages to using binaural stimulation in the investigation of MS. First, data on the crossed acoustic muscle response (CAR) are not obtained. There is evidence that this response can be abnormal in demyelination and affords an opportunity of detecting damage to brainstem structures not involved in the generation of the BAEP (Clifford-Jones et al, 1979). Secondly, patients referred with a provisional diagnosis of MS may have another condition, including lesions of the cerebello-pontine angle. With binaural stimulation in these cases, although individual BAEPs are within normal limits, there is often a marked asymmetry between the two channels, a phenomenon rarely seen in multiple sclerosis and never encountered in the records from normal subjects. If, therefore, a grossly asymmetrical BAEP is obtained from the two channels in a routine investigation with binaural stimulation, the recordist should proceed to give monaural stimulation.

In the clinical section (see page 376) the results obtained by various workers using the two modes of stimulation are reviewed.

Binaural interaction

Recently four independent publications have appeared describing components which can be ascribed to binaural interaction (Ainslie and Boston (1980), Dobie and Norton (1980), Levine (1981), Robinson and Rudge (1981)). Apart from the first of these, accounts and illustrated records are similar. Thus the components of binaural interaction are visualised by subtracting the sum of the monaural (right ear plus left ear) records from that obtained by binaural stimulation. The major component occurs at a latency of 4 msec in the guinea pig (Dobie and Berlin, 1979) and 6 msec in man, so that the peak latency is similar to that of component V obtained with a vertex-ipsilateral mastoid electrode pair and either monaural or binaural stimulation. The binaural interaction components are of small amplitude and they are best demonstrated in group average records, although comparison of the individual record with the group average shows that the binaural interaction components are present in all normal subjects studied. Within defined stimulus intensities and repetition rates, Levine (1981) has excluded the effects of a middle ear reflex and acoustic cross-talk on the BAEP which might produce apparent binaural interaction components. In our own laboratory (Robinson and Rudge, 1981) we have shown that unlike the components seen with a vertex-mastoid electrode pair and monaural or binaural stimulation, the components from binaural interaction are unaffected by the sex of the subject. In addition we have shown that the components appear to be 'seen' by the vertex electrode. In this paper we drew attention to the confounding effects of components recorded maximally with an intermastoid montage on any study of binaural interaction where a mastoid electrode is used. Ainslie and Boston (1980) compared records from vertex-mastoid electrode pairs, and this may explain the disparity between their results and those of all other reports. The fact that they did not obtain a group average may be another factor here.

Thus it does appear that there are components which are best described as binaural interaction components. To date little more has been done than to record and describe them. Although it is tempting to speculate on a possible rôle for these components in studies of the functioning of the auditory pathway in man their small size and susceptibility to artifact (acoustic cross-talk) may limit this aim.

Polarity

It is a routine procedure in many laboratories to reverse the polarity of the stimulus on successive presentations, so that the contribution of both cochlear microphonic and stimulus artifact cancel and are thus removed from the BAEP waveform. The stimulus artifact is particularly obtrusive when close-fitting earphones are used, since they are directly over one of the recording electrodes. The cochlear microphonics are electrical potentials which can easily be recorded at the round window, have identical frequency characteristics to the applied stimulus, and increase with the intensity of the latter. They can also be recognized in the waveform of the surface recorded BAEP.

In our series of control subjects with normal audiometric function component V was the same for condensation (downgoing), rarefaction (upgoing) and alternating condensation and rarefaction clicks. There is compelling evidence, however, that the results from condensation clicks should be different to those for rarefaction clicks. In single fibre studies of the auditory nerve of the cat the activity of the unit is probably increased above the level of spontaneous activity with the rarefaction phase of the stimulus but not the condensation phase (Kiang, 1965). It was shown that the waveform of the VIII nerve action potential (AP) could be separated into an early (1.5 - 2 msec) component, which was in-phase for both condensation and rarefaction clicks (C-R in phase), and a late (2.5 - 4.5 msec) component, where phase depended upon the polarity of the click (C-R out of phase) (Coats and Martin, 1977). In most cases the responses to rarefaction clicks were of shorter latency, although in 15% of normal ears the action potentials of the condensation clicks were shorter. Furthermore, these authors produced evidence that differences in response to rarefaction and condensation clicks were particularly susceptible to high frequency hearing loss. When the hearing loss was in the 4 - 8 KHz range, the late component of the action potential waveform (the C-R out of phase component) became dominant, giving an increased latency of N_1 no matter where the lesion was, and, in addition, the differences between waveforms collected with condensation and rarefaction clicks were increased. In this same study the VIII nerve action potential and BAEP were monitored concurrently and it was shown that component V could also be prolonged in latency with selective high frequency hearing loss, although not to the extent of the action potential. Hence the component I-V interval shortened. These features were not present in the records of all patients with high frequency hearing loss, but were thought sufficiently common to constitute a valid objection to adding together condensation and rarefaction responses.

Other workers have shown that action potential latency and waveform are influenced by audiogram shape (Elberling, 1974; Eggermont, 1976), so that caution in the choice of polarity of the click is required. This is discussed further in the following section.

INTERPRETATION OF THE BAEP WAVEFORM

It is often claimed that the advantages of physiological testing lie in the fact that the functioning of a particular system rather than its structure can be monitored. While evoked potential recording may eventually develop this capacity, it has not yet been realised in the auditory system, where the responses to simple and unnatural stimuli are studied. Furthermore, the analysis of the waveform produced by these stimuli is, to say the least, somewhat crude. Pattern recognition techniques available in other unrelated areas of technology have not been successfully applied to the analysis of evoked potentials. In general only amplitude and latency are used to measure the BAEP waveform and to describe the functioning of a highly complicated nervous system. Nevertheless these parameters do provide useful information and hopefully the analysis techniques will mature with time.

Amplitude

In all evoked potential work amplitude has the longest history as a useful measure and it was quickly realised that amplitude was an objective assessment of threshold in any one sensory system. The amplitude of the BAEP is dependent on several variables.

1. Intensity

Intensity of the stimulus is a major determinant of amplitude. From threshold the amplitude of the BAEP is linearly related to the intensity of the stimulus over a wide range. At high intensity levels (more than 80 dB) the curve flattens out and some workers claim that beyond this the BAEP amplitude declines with increasing intensity.

Conductive hearing loss due to abnormalities of the middle ear raises the threshold to the stimulus, but thereafter a normal intensity-amplitude function is recorded. Recruitment (abnormal loudness growth), which occurs with cochlear and, less commonly, certain retrocochlear lesions, alters the amplitude-intensity curve to one with an abnormally steep slope and usually elevates the threshold. With lesions in the brainstem the amplitude of the BAEP is commonly reduced irrespective of the intensity of the stimulus.

2. Time constant (TC) of the amplifiers

The time-constant of the amplifiers can have a substantial effect, the amplitude of component V being degraded considerably between 0.8 Hz and 250 Hz (slope -6 dB octave^{-1}), whilst the earlier components remain relatively unaltered by this manipulation (Robinson and Rudge, 1977b).

3. Interstimulus interval

With interstimulus intervals of less than about 50 msec the amplitude of the BAEP can be reduced, as discussed in the section on interstimulus interval.

Measurement of amplitude

Amplitude is traditionally measured between two consecutive turning points in a wave (peak-to-peak) or between an arbitrary baseline and the peak of a particular component. Component I is normally measured from the pre-stimulus base-line and it is therefore necessary to present the stimulus at some interval after the averager is triggered. Apart from component V all the other waves are measured from the preceding peak. Since component IV is less well formed than the other

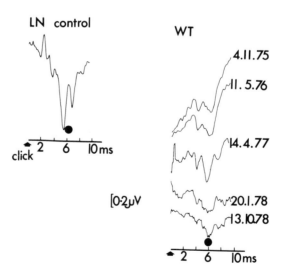

Figure 10.6 *Five consecutive BAEPs (dates indicated) from a patient with stable multiple sclerosis, showing the reproducibility of the records, in which component V is of reduced amplitude. Component V indicated (●). Note well formed component III. Last two records obtained at a faster sampling rate (12.5 as against 6.25 per msec). Normal control shown at left for comparison.*

components and is particularly vulnerable to decreasing interstimulus interval, the amplitude of component V is measured to the preceding turning point of component III.

Many workers are critical of the use of reduced amplitude as an indication of abnormality and most neurophysiologists would be reasonably sceptical about the consistency with which amplitude can be measured in the same individual on repeated testing. We have shown that an abnormality of amplitude can be reliably recorded on consecutive occasions and this is illustrated in Figure 10.6, where five records, obtained over a period of 3 years in a patient with definite but stable multiple sclerosis, are shown. We also stress that with the results of binaural stimulation in normal subjects, the statistical confidence which can be applied to amplitude is *equal* to that which can be applied to measures of latency.

In some laboratories the relative amplitude between components has been used to derive normal ranges. Since the time-constant significantly alters component V, but not other components, it is important to keep it at a pre-set value if this method is used. In our own laboratory we do not consider that components I-III can be recorded with sufficient reliability in normal subjects to be able to define statistical limits for abnormality of their relative amplitude, although a reduced component V in the presence of a large component III would be clear evidence of an abnormality.

Latency

The stimulus determinants of the latency of the BAEP components include intensity, rise time and interstimulus interval. Their effects are described in other sections. There are also other physiological factors which can alter the latency of the BAEP and these will be discussed.

1. Sex

It has been reported that the inter-peak latency (component I-V) is 0.27 msec less in females than in males (Beagley and Sheldrake, 1978; McClelland and McCrea, 1979; McClelland et al, 1980). Using a similar intensity level in our own laboratory we reviewed the results of 100 patients (males and females matched in age) referred for auditory evoked potential testing and who had normal auditory evoked potentials. The absolute latency of component V in females was on average 0.3 msec shorter than in males.

2. Age

The latency of wave I decreases with age until about six months (Galambos and Hecox, 1978), and there is a progressive shortening of the latency of component V in the first year (Hecox, 1975). Children of both sexes under the age of 14 years have the same latency of component V and, interestingly, this is similar to adult females (McClelland and McCrea, 1979; McClelland et al, 1980). At the other end of the age-scale there is a slight increase in latency of component V after the fifth decade. This may be due to the minor peripheral hearing deficits which develop later in life.

3. Temperature

In neurologically normal patients without hearing deficits, subjected to hypothermia during cardiopulmonary bypass, a change of temperature from 37°C to 27°C caused on average an increase of 1.4 msec in inter-peak (I-V) interval (Stockard et al, 1978). Taking account of such effects is important in BAEP recordings obtained from patients in coma, especially in the elderly or in cases of drug intoxication.

Since component I is dependent on the cochlear end-organ it is an attractive proposition to use the inter-peak interval between components I and V as a measure of central conduction time. While analogous measurements in the spinal sensory system, where the peripheral component (N9) is large, have proven of great value, there is a major problem in the auditory system, as component I is so small in surface recordings; indeed it cannot always be recognized with confidence. Furthermore, it has been shown that the inter-peak interval (I-V) shortens when there is significant high frequency hearing loss (Coats and Martin, 1977), although other authors have claimed that there are no significant interaural differences in inter-peak intervals in patients with normal hearing in one ear and mild to moderate high frequency hearing loss in the other ear (Stockard et al, 1978). For both these reasons we prefer to use the absolute latency of component V rather than inter-peak measurement and to use a high intensity stimulus to compensate for mild peripheral hearing loss.

FREQUENCY FOLLOWING RESPONSE (FFR)

Worden and Marsh (1968) described electrical events, recorded directly from the brainstem nuclei of the cat, which had a fundamental frequency equal to that of the sinusoidal stimulus which elicited them. They termed this the frequency-following response (FFR). With depth recordings, although without signal averaging, an FFR has been recorded in the cat directly from the cochlear nucleus, superior olivary nucleus and inferior colliculus, but from no structure at a higher level (Smith et al, 1975). When averaging techniques are used, recording from non-primary areas of the reticular formation, an FFR can be recorded (Faingold and Caspary, 1979). Frequencies of up to 5 KHz can be recorded in the cochlear nucleus, but at the inferior colliculus the highest frequency FFR obtained is 2 KHz.

In both the cat and in man a similar FFR, which faithfully follows the stimulus throughout its duration, can be recorded using surface electrodes (vertex-ipsilateral mastoid) (Figure 10.2). This FFR has a latency of 5.5 ± 1 msec and is superimposed on a slower, pedestal-like component, the latency of which is approximately 10 msec (Marsh et al, 1975). When tone bursts are used to generate this FFR, the latency of onset of the response decreases as the intensity rises, while the phase of the FFR remains the same (Smith et al, 1975). This observation implies that the initial, but not subsequent, cycle of the response is independent of subsequent components, a view confirmed by the fact that the early part of the waveform is usually of a higher frequency than the tone burst. It would appear that there is an 'on' response followed by the FFR. The FFR can be recorded with surface electrodes to frequencies of up to 2 KHz, although the amplitude of the response decreases with increase in frequency. The threshold is higher than that for any other auditory evoked potential, commonly being unobtainable with intensity levels below 50 dB SL. The subsequent amplitude-intensity function is steeper than for other auditory evoked potentials. The FFR can be recorded from infants, but is more difficult to elicit in subjects older than 40 years. It has been demonstrated that the two ears generate independent FFRs and it is postulated that each ear has a distinct population of neurons capable of subserving this (Gerken et al, 1975). Thus, there is little evidence of binaural interaction, the responses obtained by binaural stimulation being similar to the summed monaural responses, both with stimuli given in-phase and 180° out-of-phase to each ear.

There is a great deal of debate whether the FFR obtained with surface recordings represents a summation of activity originating from cochlear nucleus, superior olivary nucleus and inferior colliculus. Since there is no one frequency at which the responses at the different nuclei would be in-phase, the fact that the sinusoidal nature of the stimulus is always preserved in the FFR is against this hypothesis. However, using vertex-ipsilateal mastoid (V derivation) and ipsilateral mastoid-contralateral mastoid (H derivation) montages, it has been shown that monaural stimulation with frequencies of less than 0.5 KHz results in an FFR which contains two components, an FFR_1 and an FFR_2. These are on average 1.7 msec apart. This interval, which varies between 1.4 and 1.8 msec in different subjects, is independent of the frequency and intensity of the stimulus, and for each subject the difference is correlated with the interval separating components III and V of the BAEP to a click (Stillman et al, 1978). The two FFR components behave differently. Thus the FFR_1 is of larger amplitude than FFR_2 in the H montage, whilst in the V montage the relative amplitude of FFR_1 and FFR_2 depends on the intensity of the stimulus. Furthermore, the slower pedestal-like component of 10 msec latency is only present in the V montage. The authors have suggested that these results are evidence that there are at least two generators contributing to the FFR and that they correspond to the generators of the BAEP to click stimuli. Thus FFR_1 and component III are recorded best in the H montage, while FFR_2 and component V are recorded best in the V montage. However, against this is the fact that components III and V exhibit parallel growth in amplitude with intensity increments, whilst this is not the case for FFR_1 and FFR_2. There is also evidence from destructive lesions in animals that the FFR recorded with surface electrodes is not the summed activity from superior olivary nucleus and inferior colliculus, but is dependent on the activity from inferior colliculus alone. Simultaneous surface and depth recordings in the cat, in which the inferior colliculus was repeatedly cooled, showed that the surface FFR and depth FFR from inferior colliculus disappeared when the inferior colliculus was cooled, and reappeared with temperature reversal, whilst the potential recorded from depth electrodes in the superior olivary complex remained the same throughout (Smith et al, 1975). If the superior olivary complex was contributing to the surface recording, this should still be seen in the surface record when the inferior colliculus is cooled.

Compared with the literature on the BAEP to click stimuli the work on the FFR is sparse. We suspect that this may be due to the seemingly greater technical difficulties in recording an FFR response. There is always a great danger that the FFR is, in fact, a cochlear microphonic or a stimulus artifact, although there are tricks to dissociate these from the FFR. For example, masking the other ear with noise should decrease the amplitude of the recorded FFR. Whether the surface FFR is produced from a single generator, or is a composite response from multiple generators, has clearly to be resolved before the FFR can be used to probe the physiology of the auditory pathway. However, this need not detract from its value as a clinical tool. When an FFR to a particular tone is present, this is strong evidence for a neural response to a particular frequency at the level of the brainstem. On the other hand, with the BAEP to tonal stimuli the experimenter is never certain whether the response is to the tone, or to any sharp transients which may be present at its onset. Although the threshold to FFR is much higher than the subjective threshold in the normal, this is not of great import, since normal ranges of threshold for FFR can be defined.

MIDDLE LATENCY COMPONENTS

As mentioned previously, a useful classification of the components of the auditory evoked potential evoked by a click stimulus is on the basis of latency (Picton et al, 1974). Components occurring within the first 8 msec were called the early components by these authors, although BAEP is the more usual terminology in the literature. Components occurring between 8 - 60 msec were termed middle latency components and comprised waves N_0, P_0, N_a, P_a, and N_b. Since the frequency content of the auditory evoked potential at the latency of P_1 (the first of the late components as classified by Picton et al, 1974) is similar to that of the middle components we have included it in the middle latency group. Before 1974, these middle latency components were commonly called early components. The confusion in the literature is not confined to the nomenclature. The actual identification of the middle latency components can be difficult, since there is some risk that they will be contaminated by myogenic reflexes. Indeed there has been much debate regarding their central nervous system, as against muscular, generation, and for this reason we will review the evidence for the former before embarking on a description of the normal middle latency components.

In 1964 widespread myogenic responses to auditory stimuli were described and were called sonomotor responses (Bickford et al, 1964). These sonomotor responses had latencies ranging from 6 msec at the inion to 50 msec in the leg. One of these responses, the inion response, was shown to be increased in amplitude with increased activity of the neck muscles. As Bickford et al (1964) were able to record these sonomotor responses in three patients with sensori-neural deafness, all with normal vestibular function, they concluded that the responses to the click were initiated via the vestibular system. Other myogenic reponses were recorded from the frontalis and temporalis muscles and again the amplitude of the responses increased with increase in muscle activity. Picton et al (1974) have reviewed these various muscle-generated evoked potentials.

The threshold for these large amplitude myogenic responses tends to be at least 40 dB. Since it could be argued that the middle latency components seen below this threshold are, in fact, myogenic responses whose waveform alters abruptly at a certain stimulus intensity, it became necessary to prove that the middle latency components were indeed generated by the central nervous system, before they could be used clinically. Many workers have commented that the amplitudes of the myogenic components are radically affected by local muscle tension (Bickford et al, 1964; Cody and Bickford, 1969), yet an increase in amplitude of a cerebral evoked response with increased muscle tension would not be expected and has never been reported. Mast (1965) described a component of 30 msec latency, recorded from electrodes P_1-C_z, which seemed to require a longer recovery cycle than the response recorded from the inion. This component also had a different amplitude-intensity function to the myogenic responses and was perhaps originating from a central nervous system structure.

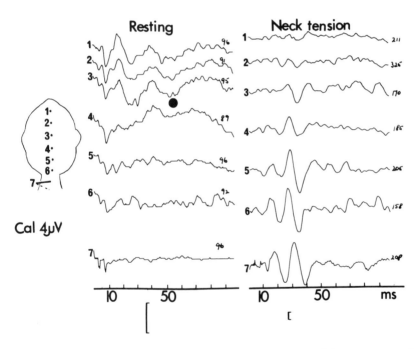

Figure 10.7 *Middle latency and myogenic components obtained from an array of sagittal electrodes (3 = C_z) with and without neck tension. As each record was obtained on different occasions an index of tension from the electromyogram is given on right of each trace. P_1 indicated. Note different gain in two conditions. See text for explanation.*

In an attempt to clarify the situation we have recorded the middle latency components from the electrodes shown in Figure 10.7 referred to the mastoid, simultaneously with the myogenic responses from electrodes between inion and neck. The electromyographic activity from the inion was rectified so that an index of the muscle activity could be derived. The amount of tension in the neck muscles was varied by altering the position of the head (forward and backward neck flexion), and by hanging weights around the neck. Six subjects were studied. With the neck muscles relaxed the middle components were seen most clearly at the C_z electrode and were progressively reduced in amplitude as the recording site was moved further away; in fact, no responses could be recognized in the inion-neck channel. With the neck muscles activated, the middle components were modified on the C_z channel, the amount of contamination was linearly related to the distance from the inion electrode and was recorded maximally by the inion-neck pair of electrodes. Thus, although both the myogenic and middle latency components can be recorded widely over the scalp, they have a very different distribution; in particular the middle components are best recorded in the C_z-mastoid pair of electrodes. We conclude that in the middle latency range there are both muscle and central nervous system generated potentials and that they can be distinguished.

Table 10.2 SOME MYOGENIC RESPONSES

Reflex	Description
P.A.M.	Diphasic negative/positive wave
	Latency of positivity 16 msec
	Great variability between and within subjects
	Can be bilateral or unilateral
	Unrelated to muscle tension
	Recorded on the ipsilateral mastoid
Temporalis	Diphasic negative/positive wave
	Latency of positivity 23 msec
	Increase with muscle tension
	Recorded from temporal area
Neck muscles	Multiple components
	Negative waves at 11 and 25 msec
	Positive waves at 17 and 34 msec
	Sensitive to muscle tension
	Recorded from inion
Frontalis	Highly variable
	Mean positive component 30 msec
	Sensitive to muscle tension

Another myogenic component in the latency range 8 - 50 msec has been reported from the post-auricular muscle (Kiang et al, 1963). In contrast to the myogenic component recorded from the inion, this component is mediated via the VII nerve and can be elicited at thresholds as low as 10 - 20 dB. The account by Kiang et al has remained the most complete documentation of the post-auricular muscle response in the normal subject, and in our own laboratory we have obtained no further information to complement it. In man the post-auricular muscle is vestigial and its development varies between individuals. In contrast to the inion respone, which can be obtained in all controls, there are at least 30% of normals in whom the post-auricular muscle response cannot be elicited, and in others it is only present on one side. We have noted that in those controls in whom a bilateral response is obtained, it is usually present bilaterally on repeated testing. Similarly, controls with a unilateral or absent post-auricular muscle response are usually consistent on subsequent testing. Whilst this muscle response does contaminate the middle latency components and is a considerable nuisance when identifying the various components, particularly in the abnormal record, we feel that this is not sufficient to invalidate the usefulness of the middle latency components. Furthermore, when the post-auricular muscle response is recorded through a coaxial needle electrode and the auditory evoked potential between the shaft of the same needle and the vertex, components P_a, N_b and P_1 occur after the reflex activity of the muscle has ceased, so that these components can be used to evaluate the central nervous system. A summary of the various myogenic responses in the range of the middle latency components is given in Table 10.2.

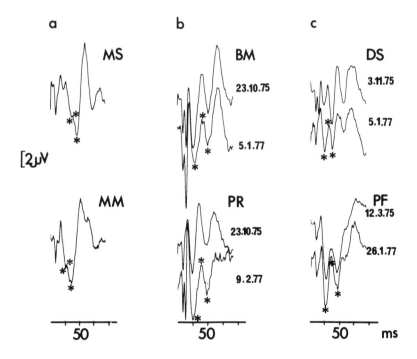

Figure 10.8 *Variations of middle latency components between 6 individuals (columns a, b, c) and consistency within an individual (columns b and c). Note variable presence of post-auricular muscle response in some records. Components* P_a, N_a, P_1 *indicated (*).*

In 1951, Dawson published his now familiar W shaped average evoked potential recorded from the sensory cortex with surface electrodes in response to stimulation of the median nerve at the wrist (Dawson, 1951; Dawson, 1954a). It is interesting that the middle latency components of the auditory evoked potential to a click stimulus have a similar W shape (Figure 10.8b). There are some common variants of this W shape in the normal. For example, in some subjects component N_b is poorly formed despite a well formed P_a and P_b component of normal latency (Figure 10.8a). Another frequently occurring variant is one with extra components at any point on the waveform between P_1 and P_2 (Figure 10.8c), although these extra components are usually easily recognized as such and do not distort the W shape of the waveform. The middle components are of variable amplitude between subjects, they are unaffected by the level of arousal, or by sedation, and can be elicited by pure tone, in addition to click, stimuli. The latency of the components remains stable on repeated testing over a period of years, presumably partly due to the fact that they are independent of the level of arousal. Another striking feature of the middle components is that each individual seems to have a particular 'signature'. Thus Figure 10.8 (b,c) shows some of the variants of the waveform seen in control subjects and also demonstrates that similar waveforms can be recorded from the same individual after a period of 1 - 2 years. Indeed if this signature could be quantified it might be possible to demonstrate in patients an abnormality on repeated testing which does not manifest itself as an increase in latency.

Compared to the early components, the middle latency ones have received little attention in the literature, presumably because of the debate over their central nervous system, versus myogenic, origin. Our experience of the use of these components in clinical practice is briefly discussed in other sections (e.g. multiple sclerosis, acoustic neuromata and other tumours) and we hope that this review will encourage more laboratories to enter into research in this area, since it could be equally fruitful as the BAEP.

11

The Use of Auditory Potentials in Neurology

K. Robinson and P. Rudge

MULTIPLE SCLEROSIS

Introduction

Since experimental demyelination of both peripheral and central nerve fibres causes abnormalities of conduction, including decrease in conduction velocity, inability to faithfully transmit trains of impulses and ultimately failure to conduct an impulse through the damaged nerve (McDonald and Sears, 1970; Rasminsky and Sears, 1972), it would seem reasonable to study latency changes of the EP in patients with demyelination. Initial human evoked potential work concentrated on the visual sensory system (see Chapters 3 to 7), where a single large potential, with a latency of about 100 msec, could be recorded in normal subjects using a checkerboard pattern as the stimulus. There is rarely any difficulty in identifying an abnormality of this component in patients with multiple sclerosis. In contrast the BAEP waveform is of complex morphology, no one component having a duration longer than 2 msec, and does not lend itself to such an easy interpretation. However, in spite of this, component V is sufficiently stable in latency and amplitude in normal subjects for abnormalities of it to be readily identified in patients with multiple sclerosis. In general one might expect the latency of an abnormal component to be greater, and the amplitude to be less, than normal, although, in such a complex system, it would be unjustified to interpret these latency findings in terms of alteration of conduction velocities of individual fibres. Whether evoked potentials recorded from scalp electrodes represent activity of nerve fibres, their synapses or cell bodies is irrelevant, provided the potential generator is beyond the damaged area and the stimulus is proximal to it. In this case the envelope of the total activity of a group of cells or their processes will be altered, such that the peak of a particular component may occur at a different time, and the total area and peak amplitude will be different to that found in the normal subjects.

The auditory system in multiple sclerosis

At first sight it is surprising that the auditory evoked potential is abnormal in patients with multiple sclerosis, a disease in which symptomatic deafness is rare. Occasionally a patient with multiple sclerosis does become deaf in one ear and in these cases it is assumed that an area of demyelination occurs in that part of the VIII nerve enveloped by central myelin, or within the cochlear nuclei on that side of the brainstem, since the auditory pathways begin to decussate after this. The VIII nerve is peculiar amongst the cranial nerves, with the exception of II, in having an envelope of central myelin for a short distance outside the brainstem, in addition to that part within the central nervous system. In spite of this the total amount of tissue vulnerable to demyelination sufficient to cause unilateral deafness is small, and this is presumably part of the reason for the rarity of unilateral deafness in multiple sclerosis. When deafness occurs, it has the characteristics of a retrocochlear or nerve fibre type (Dix, 1965). Almost invariably the deafness recovers, the pure tone audiogram being the first parameter to improve, followed by loudness function and speech (Citron et al, 1963). In four of our patients who had a symptomatic plaque within the VIII nerve or cochlear nucleus at the time of BAEP recording, the records obtained from monaural stimulation were asymmetrical. The record obtained with stimulation of the affected ear was grossly abnormal, and components I and II could not be identified on any of the records, even after using long interstimulus intervals, a procedure that would normally accentuate these components.

It is known that the VEP detects clinically silent demyelination in the visual pathways in a considerable proportion of patients with multiple sclerosis, a finding that is not surprising as the clinical symptoms of demyelination in the visual system are known to remit. However, since significant deafness is so rare in multiple sclerosis, there is little reason to believe that there will be many patients in whom there is a silent lesion of the VIII nerve and cochlear nucleus. It was thus an unexpected finding that so many patients with multiple sclerosis proved to have abnormalities in the auditory pathways.

Abnormalities of auditory evoked potentials in multiple sclerosis

In the first large series of brainstem evoked responses to be published (Robinson and Rudge, 1975) and two subsequent papers (Robinson and Rudge, 1977b; Stockard et al, 1977) abnormalities were found in a high proportion of patients with definite multiple sclerosis. These results, which implied that some involvement of the brainstem auditory pathways was common, although clinically silent, will now be discussed.

(a) Patients with clinical evidence of a brainstem lesion

We know that the brainstem is usually a clinically eloquent area, no doubt partly due to the numerous fibre systems traversing it and the fact that most of the cranial nerves are connected with it. Damage to this structure results in abnormalities of cranial nerve function, as well as motor and sensory disorders of the limbs, eye movement abnormalities being particularly prominent. Thus involvement of the medial longitudinal fasciculus frequently occurs causing an internuclear ophthalmoplegia and V and VII nerve plaques result in abnormalities of sensation and motor function of the face in multiple sclerosis. Since these structures are closely associated with those concerned with the auditory evoked potential, including the BAEP and post-auricular muscle reflex, it might be expected that patients with clinical evidence of brainstem dysfunction would have a greater chance of abnormalities of these auditory evoked potentials, especially as plaques of demyelination do not respect anatomically defined fibre tracts. This proved to be the case.

Subdivision of the patients with definite multiple sclerosis on clinical criteria into those with and those without brainstem involvement revealed that (with binaural stimulation) the former group had abnormalities of component V in 79% while the figure was 51% in the latter (Robinson and Rudge, 1977b). In the series of 30 patients with definite multiple sclerosis studied by Stockard et al (1977), all of whom had clinical evidence of brainstem involvement, a rather higher proportion (93%) of abnormalities was found (with unilateral stimulation). Unfortunately there were no patients with definite multiple sclerosis in this series in whom the brainstem was clinically normal.

In a recent paper, where we have extended our studies to patients in whom the diagnosis of multiple sclerosis is less certain (Robinson and Rudge, 1980), the striking feature has again been the correlation between a clinically detectable brainstem lesion and an abnormality of the BAEP. Approximately 80% of patients have an abnormality of the BAEP if there are clinical signs of brainstem dysfunction at the time of assessment, while those with no such signs have a much lower incidence of abnormalities. This is independent of the clinical classification of the patients.

A recent paper by Chiappa et al (1980b) using monaural stimulation is in marked contrast to these results. They found a much lower proportion of abnormalities of the BAEP in all categories of MS they studied and claimed that there was no correlation with evidence of brainstem involvement on other criteria. These results, at least as far as those patients with brainstem involvement are concerned, are probably due to the authors' idiosyncratic determination of the presence of a brainstem lesion and the fact that many were deemed to have such involvement on history alone.

(b) Patients without clinical evidence of a brainstem lesion

In our own laboratory we have studied two separate series of patients with definite multiple sclerosis in whom there was no clinical evidence of a brainstem lesion, and the BAEP was abnormal in 51% and 57% respectively (Robinson and Rudge, 1977b, 1980). The only other comparable large series is that of Chiappa et al (1980b), in which a much lower incidence (19%) of abnormalities of the BAEP was found.

In the less definite clinical categories the results of Stockard et al (1977), Robinson and Rudge (1980) and Chiappa et al (1980b) are in broad agreement as far as patients with possible multiple sclerosis and no clinical evidence of a brainstem lesion are concerned, all series having a low proportion of abnormalities (35%, 25%, 24%) respectively. In contrast, Stockard et al (1977) found a much higher proportion (77%) of abnormalities of the BAEP in patients with probable multiple sclerosis, and no clinical evidence of a brainstem lesion, than either Robinson and Rudge (20%) or Chiappa et al (21%). The reason for the discrepancy probably lies in differences in clinical classification rather than the methods of obtaining the BAEP, a similar wide variation of the proportion of abnormalities in less definite categories being found for the VEP in the literature (Halliday, 1978a).

(c) Progressive spastic paraparesis

One group of patients of considerable interest is that of progressive paraparesis in middle life, a proportion of whom are known to have MS at autopsy. These patients are classified as having clinically possible MS if no other cause is found for their disability. In a small series (18) of such patients we have found that half had an abnormal AEP, and in two thirds of these the abnormality was confined to the BAEP (Robinson and Rudge, 1980). It is of interest that this is a similar proportion of abnormalities to those who were also classified as having possible MS but who did not have the progressive spastic paraparetic form of the disease. Similar results have been obtained in the visual system.

Monaural versus binaural stimulation

In contrast to our own work (Robinson and Rudge, 1975, 1977a, 1977b, 1980) most reports in the literature of the BAEP in patients with MS are based on results of monaural stimulation (Stockard et al, 1977; Chiappa et al, 1980b; Prasher and Gibson, 1980b), the assumption being that a higher proportion of abnormalities will be detected. In published studies where bilateral and unilateral stimulation have been compared in the same patients it has been shown that the percentage of abnormalities detected is increased with monaural stimulation, particularly in the less definite categories of demyelination (Prasher and Gibson, 1980b). Thus an increase in the proportion of abnormalities detected of 20% in the definite and 10% in the probable clinical category was obtained in one series (Chiappa et al, 1980b) and 20% in the definite, 67% in the probable, and 59% in the possible categories in another (Prasher and Gibson, 1980b). These figures should not, however, be accepted uncritically. For example, Chiappa et al (1980b) do not report the results for their possible clinical category, where 12/54 of the patients had abnormalities, and the marked increase obtained in the probable category in the study of Prasher and Gibson (1980b) is based on three patients only. Furthermore Prasher and Gibson (1980b) have included abnormalities recorded between electrodes on the vertex and contralateral mastoid and have attributed these to a lesion of the contralateral pathway. Recent studies in controls and patients show that the waveform morphology of the BAEP for any electrode pair is complex and that the record from vertex-contralateral mastoid electrodes probably does not represent the contralateral pathway. The most likely candidate for components of the contralateral pathway are those recorded maximally between electrodes on each mastoid with monaural stimulation. (Robinson and Rudge, 1981).

One might expect that if the proportion of abnormalities detected was significantly increased by monaural stimulation, this would be most apparent in the clinically definite group, unless the proportion was already high with binaural stimulation. To this end we have compared monaural and binaural stimulation in 40 young patients with definite MS who were having at least one relapse per year, all of whom were ambulant at the time of testing. Twenty of these patients had a normal BAEP with binaural stimulation. With monaural stimulation, and results from records between vertex and both ipsilateral and contralateral mastoids, only four of these 20 records had additional abnormalities (3 of these had abnormal middle latency components). Thus in this study the abnormalities were increased by only 10% with monaural stimulation. The percentage increase in abnormalities with monaural stimulation in this study was not high and is rather different to the results of Chiappa et al (1980b) and Prasher and Gibson (1980b).

From the above it is clear that unilateral abnormalities of the BAEP do occur in patients with demyelination. Although this result is not predicted from the anatomy of the auditory system, a recent study of deafness in brainstem demyelinating disease has indicated that unilateral dysfunction is rather more frequent than previously supposed (Luxon, 1980). This study was not of a random sample, in that it came from a unit specifically dealing with problems of deafness in neurological disease and the degree of hearing loss was slight, but it does suggest that unilateral involvement of the auditory pathways in MS is not infrequent.

It remains to be seen which of the methods stands the test of time. For our own part we are satisfied with the results of a retrospective study of unselected patients in the differentiation of MS from other conditions (Robinson and Rudge, 1980); specificity is a necessary requirement often overlooked by those striving for higher hit rates in a particular condition.

The post-auricular muscle response

Another brainstem potential that can be evoked by auditory stimuli is the post-auricular muscle response (PAM). Since contraction of the posterior auricular muscle group occurs bilaterally to a unilateral stimulus, the reflex is sometimes called the 'crossed acoustic' response. Normal limits can be calculated for the latency difference between ipsilateral and contralateral responses and used to detect abnormalities in MS. Unfortunately the response may be absent at one or both mastoids in controls, thus limiting its usefulness.

Humphries et al (1976) tested 18 patients with MS, using this technique, and in 7 the latency difference between ipsilateral and contralateral was abnormal. These authors made no reference to clinical signs of brainstem dysfunction in their patients, but stated that the results implied a lesion in the brainstem at the level of the facial nucleus, damaging decussating fibres involved in the reflex pathways. A subsequent study from the same laboratory extended these observations (Clifford-Jones et al, 1979). They found an abnormal ipsilateral-contralateral latency difference in 75% of their patients. The proportion of abnormalities was largely independent of the McAlpine classification. They also reported a higher proportion of abnormalities in those patients with other evidence of a brainstem lesion (87%) than without (69%), this latter figure being as high as most reports for the VEP in patients with clinically silent optic nerve lesions. Neither study compared the PAM with the BAEP results in the same series of patients. In our own laboratory we collected the PAM in some 40 patients in whom we compared monaural and binaural stimulation. In this series if the PAM was abnormal, an abnormality was also found in the BAEP with one exception. The converse was not true. Thus in many cases in which the BAEP, or middle latency components, or both, were abnormal, the PAM was absent on one or both sides. There is unfortunately no way of knowing whether the absence of a response is due to a brainstem lesion or not, since the response is not always present in controls.

To conclude, although we believe that the PAM is a useful adjunct to the BAEP, the response is too unstable to use alone for the detection of brainstem lesions in MS.

Middle latency components

So far we have discussed the use of the auditory evoked potentials recorded from the brainstem in multiple sclerosis. In the literature little attention has been paid to the middle latency responses, no doubt partly due to the unknown origin of these components, particularly their central nervous system, as against muscular, generation.

We have examined a number of patients with clinically definite multiple sclerosis and shown that the middle latency components are often abnormal (Robinson and Rudge, 1977b). Thus in 66 patients with clinically definite MS 45% had abnormalities of latency of one or more component (P_a, N_b, P_1). Amplitude could not be used, as the variation in normal subjects is too great for the normal range to be calculated. As with the BAEP there was a higher proportion of abnormalities in those patients with a clinically apparent lesion in the brainstem (70%) than in those with no evidence of such involvement. Interestingly the two systems were sometimes dissociated; an abnormal BAEP could be associated with a normal middle response, this occurring in about one-third of the patients, while the converse occurred in 12%. This latter figure indicates that it is worth recording middle components, and the data as a whole show that any concept of these various components being a simple serial system is incorrect. Indeed one wonders whether the two groups of potentials are evoked from the same system at all. In two cases of proven multiple sclerosis there was a total absence of any middle latency components despite normal BAEP and PAM.

Not only is the percentage of abnormalities detected enhanced, but the inclusion of the middle latency components adds specificity to the test in the diagnosis of MS. In the authors' experience one striking feature of the middle latency components in multiple sclerosis is the relative preservation of the waveform in spite of a considerable increase in latency, a situation that does not always apply to other brainstem lesions, e.g. tumours. Thus of 8 patients studied with extrinsic or intrinsic tumours of the brainstem (excluding CP angle lesions) four could be considered unusual and perhaps abnormal (Robinson and Rudge, 1980). In particular the waveform was distorted, so that there was some difficulty in identifying the specific components. It is possible that with further refinement, recording of middle latency components would be a useful additional test in the diagnosis of this group of patients. Furthermore, although abnormalities of latency of the middle components are seen in conditions other than MS, e.g. tonsilar herniation, an abnormality of both the BAEP and the middle latency component was essentially confined to MS, with the exception of two patients with extensive vascular disease (Robinson and Rudge, 1980).

The waveform abnormalities of the BAEP in multiple sclerosis

In the investigation of multiple sclerosis, we routinely use binaural stimulation and record two channels of BAEP, viz. vertex-right mastoid and vertex-left mastoid. With adequate recordings abnormalities are usually symmetrical in the two channels, and if they are asymmetrical, monaural stimulation is indicated. Since component V is the only component which can be recorded in all normal subjects, we try to identify it in the records and indeed, if the BAEP is abnormal, this component is fortunately always involved. It is easily distinguished from other components in the normal record but can be more difficult to identify in an abnormal one; we arbitrarily define it as the most negative-going potential in the latency range of 5.5-10 msec.

There are three types of abnormalities of the BAEP waveform which typically occur in multiple sclerosis. Firstly, when there is an increase in latency of component V this component is usually easily identified and the earlier components may have a latency within normal limits. Secondly, there are the cases in which the waveform is so degraded that it is difficult to say which is component V, and in these there may be little evidence of any BAEP waveform, despite clear post-auricular muscle reflex and middle components. Thirdly, component III may be well formed and of normal latency, but component V is of greatly reduced amplitude, and indeed would be difficult to identify were it not for the presence of the normal component III.

When assessing any record it is convenient to use normal ranges based on a population comprised of both sexes and all ages. However, there are differences of latency between the sexes and with age, so that a borderline increase of latency in a young female is more likely to represent an abnormality than a similar change in an older male. In an earlier section we have discussed the importance of the interstimulus interval and have pointed out that delivering two clicks 5 msec apart at a rate of 20 pairs per sec stresses the auditory system in normal subjects. This also increased the yield of abnormality in patients by a small amount (Robinson and Rudge, 1977b). It is, however, of particular importance in the doubtful case in which there is an equivocal abnormality to single click stimulus, and in confirming that a component V of reduced amplitude is abnormal. Thus in some patients where the amplitude of component V was small but its latency normal there was an abnormal increase of latency to the paired clicks, implying that there is a similar mechanism underlying both latency increase and amplitude decrease.

The waveform abnormalities of the middle latency components in patients with MS

In assessing the abnormality of the middle latency components it is important to avoid contamination of the responses by myogenic reflexes. While in some patients the PAM can be exceptionally large, the problem can be overcome by using an alternative electrode placement, viz. vertex-inion, which gives a similar response to the vertex-mastoid record in control subjects in whom the PAM is bilaterally absent. Only those responses P_a, N_b, P_1, which occur after the PAM, are used in the analysis.

There are a variety of abnormalities of the middle latency components which have been recorded in patients with multiple sclerosis. For example, while amplitude reduction of the middle components is not sufficient evidence of CNS abnormality, complete absence of these components in the presence of normal BAEP is, and this sometimes occurs. In other cases there may be increases in latency of all the middle components. In our experience this is most often associated with clear abnormalities of the early components or with long established cases showing evidence of many lesions. Another fairly common abnormality is to have an increase in latency of P_1 in the presence of an otherwise normal auditory evoked potential in patients without clinical evidence of brainstem involvement. This occurred in 6 out of 35 patients with definite multiple sclerosis. Occasionally components P_a and N_b will be abnormal when P_1 is normal, but in our experience this is rare. Difficulty can sometimes be experienced in identification of the various middle latency components. In some normal records additional components occur between P_1 and P_2 (Figure 10.8c), but are easily identified as such. However, in abnormal records these may become exaggerated, rendering identification of individual waves difficult (Figure 11.1). A useful trick in these cases is to identify the onset of the later component complex N_1-P_2-N_2, the latency of which is too variable in normal populations to be used in isolation, but delay of which in those cases with difficulty in middle component identification can be helpful in determining the presence of an abnormality. Figure 11.2 shows the serial records in one patient with definite multiple sclerosis. These demonstrate some of the varieties of abnormalities of the BAEP. Furthermore, although the middle components were never increased in latency, there were considerable changes in waveform on different occasions which did not necessarily coincide with changes in the BAEP.

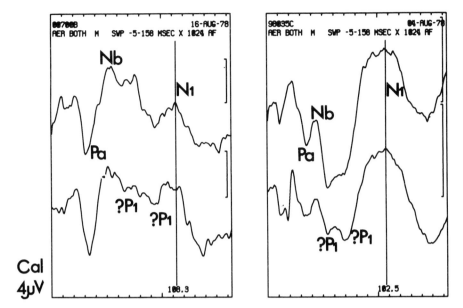

Figure 11.1 *Examples of middle components from 2 patients in whom identification of P₁ was difficult. Component N₁ of increased latency indicated. Vertex-right mastoid above, vertex-left mastoid below.*

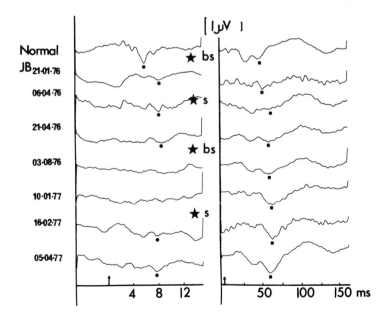

Figure 11.2 *Serial BAEP (left) and middle latency (right) records from a patient with multiple sclerosis compared with those from a normal control (top trace). Components V (●) and P₁ (■) indicated where possible. Relapses occurring between records shown (*) and site indicated (bs = brain stem, s = spinal cord).*

The BAEP and the differential diagnosis of MS

The ideal test is specific to a given disease. This is certainly not the case with the BAEP which may be abnormal in a variety of conditions other than MS, where hearing is preserved (Stockard et al, 1977; Hashimoto et al, 1980; Robinson and Rudge, 1980; Chiappa et al, 1980b). At first sight this appears to be a serious deficiency of the test, but, in fact, is not so. In the majority of patients there is no great difficulty in making the diagnosis of MS and, conversely, in those patients where the BAEP is abnormal due to another cause, the clinical features exclude multiple sclerosis, e.g. intrinsic brainstem tumours, Friedreich's ataxia. There are exceptions to this, however, which we will now briefly discuss.

(a) Patients presenting with a single acute neurological episode

A common clinical problem is the young patient who presents with a single episode indicative of an isolated lesion in the CNS. In some of these patients the disturbance might reasonably be expected to be due to the first episode of demyelination, and Small et al (1978), introduced the term 'acute undiagnosed neurological episode (AN)' to describe them. In 27 such patients we found that, if the brainstem was clinically involved, 67% had an abnormal BAEP, while in those where the lesion was remote from the brainstem, in only one was the BAEP abnormal (Robinson and Rudge, 1980). Thus if the brainstem is clinically involved in these patients, the proportion of abnormalities of the BAEP is similar to those of the definite, probable and possible MS categories of McAlpine's classification. It was therefore of great interest that patients with a known vascular disturbance involving the brainstem clinically, and who were ambulant at the time of testing, had a low proportion of abnormalities of the BAEP, indicating that the BAEP could possibly be of value in the differential diagnosis between MS and a vascular cause. However it is not yet possible to say if those with an abnormality of the AEP in fact had MS although two developed clinically definite MS in a 2 year follow-up period.

The only other report of patients with an isolated neurological episode is that of Chiappa et al (1980b), where no patients with transverse myelitis (14 cases), or optic neuritis (18 cases), had an abnormal BAEP. When evaluating these results it is important to remember that these authors obtained considerably lower proportions of abnormalities than most workers in patients with MS. Chiappa et al (1980b) also studied an ill-defined group of patients with 'cerebellar' disorders and found that 40% had an abnormal BAEP, a percentage as high as any of the MS groups studied by these workers. The significance of this latter work must await further elucidation of the clinical diagnosis.

(b) Cerebellar tonsillar herniation

Cerebellar tonsillar herniation can mimic multiple sclerosis both in clinical signs and fluctuation of the symptoms. It has been stated that an abnormal BAEP is incompatible with cerebellar ectopia (Stockard et al, 1977), but in a series of 8 patients studied by us, 5 had an abnormal AEP; in 4 of these the abnormality was of the BAEP (Robinson and Rudge, 1980). Two of these patients have been studied post-operatively and improvements in the evoked potential observed. It is of interest that in the Mayo Clinic approximately 10% of patients with Arnold Chiari malformation are reported to have deafness (Saez et al, 1976).

(c) Vascular disease

It is our impression that in order to obtain significantly abnormal records, vascular disease has to be gross. Thus Hashimoto et al (1980) reviewed a series of patients with vascular brainstem lesions, all of whom were severely disabled, and found that all had abnormal BAEPs to unilateral stimulation. Similarly, all of the smaller number of patients studied by Starr and Hamilton (1976) with an abnormal BAEP, died. In contrast, we recorded AEPs from a series of 28 patients with vascular disease, the majority of whom had clinical evidence of a brainstem lesion, and only 21% (6 patients) had an abnormal AEP, in 5 of whom the BAEP alone was abnormal. Only 3 of these patients were not ambulant and all of these had abnormal BAEPs. The abnormalities were of distorted waveform in which no single component could be recognized. This is in marked contrast to the findings in patients with a plaque of demyelination in the brainstem, where the preservation of some components is the rule. In a few younger patients who developed brainstem symptoms and, on occasion, persisting signs due to migraine, the BAEP has been normal. Even a patient with a bilateral internuclear ophthalmoplegia due to Takayashu's disease had a normal BAEP. We would, however, stress that in our series the BAEP was recorded with a binaural stimulus.

(d) Axial and extra-axial tumours

Both axial and extra-axial tumours might be confused with MS, especially in the early stages. Tumours within the brainstem, or compressing it (excluding cerebello-pontine angle masses), do cause abnormalities of the BAEP in many cases, in spite of normal routine audiometry. We have studied 8 ambulant, normally hearing patients with tumours of the brainstem or tectal plate. The BAEP was abnormal in only 2 of these, using binaural stimulation, although in some of the other cases the middle latency components of the BAEP were distorted (Robinson and Rudge, 1980).

Concluding remarks on the use of auditory evoked potentials in multiple sclerosis

There are four necessary requirements for evoked potential studies to be useful in the diagnosis of a patient suspected of having multiple sclerosis. Firstly, that the demonstration of an abnormality does indeed indicate the presence of a demyelinating lesion. This has not so far been proved, but it is reasonable to assume that it is true. Secondly, that a patient suspected of having multiple sclerosis, in whom the evoked potential is abnormal when no lesion is anticipated, subsequently is proved to have the disease. It does look as if at least some of those who have less than definite multiple sclerosis on clinical criteria, with abnormalities of the evoked potential, do pass on to the clinically definite group, at least for the visual evoked potential and probably also for the auditory evoked potential. If this is the case, the value of evoked potentials would be greatly enhanced. Thirdly, it is a necessary requirement that the abnormality of an evoked potential should be stable once established, if the techniques are to be of maximal value. In the visual system initial work suggested that this was the case, on rather indirect grounds (Halliday et al, 1973), but this is certainly not true of auditory evoked potentials. Robinson and Rudge (1978) serially followed a number of patients over three years and showed that the auditory evoked potential fluctuated quite markedly. In normal subjects the latency measures of the brainstem and middle latency responses remained remarkably stable. A similar situation exists in patients with definite multiple sclerosis, but in whom clinical relapses were not occurring. However, in patients with 'active disease', i.e. those having clinical relapses, the auditory evoked potential varies. It might be argued that this is not surprising, as the auditory system is silent clinically, so that new plaques might be expected to cause variation of the auditory evoked potential. However, it appears that this is not the correct explanation. We showed that in a group of 'active' patients, if the auditory evoked potential was normal at the onset, it remained so until a clinical brainstem episode occurred. Conversely, if the auditory evoked potential was abnormal, the waveform fluctuated with further relapses, *no matter where* the clinical sites of the new lesions were. For example, a patient might develop a change in auditory evoked potential at the time of an episode of optic neuritis. In some patients the auditory evoked potential might return to normal, having previously been abnormal for a prolonged period. A similar situation has subsequently been shown to occur in the spinal sensory system and also to a lesser extent in the visual pathways (Matthews and Small, 1979). These workers rightly comment that the basis of the use of evoked potentials in the diagnosis of multiple sclerosis lies in the 'persistence of abnormalities in the absence of relevant clinical signs (and that) this property (is) incompatible with the use of these techniques as an effective means of monitoring the course of the disease'. Robinson and Rudge (1978) proposed a general systemic effect of activity upon conduction in demyelinated fibres as a cause of this phenomenon, and one wonders whether this is a much more physiological demonstration of the finding in tissue culture that multiple sclerosis serum causes alteration of conduction (Bornstein and Crain, 1965).

Finally, the ideal test is specific to a given disease. As discussed previously, this is not the case with the AEP, which can be abnormal in a variety of conditions. There is obviously a dichotomy of interest here between the clinician requiring a test that is specific to a disease process, even if it is positive in only a small proportion of cases, and the research worker who may wish to maximize the proportion of abnormalities at the expense of specificity in a controlled group of patients. Our own experience is with a busy EP service in which the 'false positive' rate must be kept to a minimum. For this reason we use binaural stimulation in the investigation of MS. We record the BAEP with two stimulation procedures, a single click, and a pair of clicks. We then record the middle latency and later cortical potentials. In the case where the middle latency components are abnormal in the presence of a normal BAEP to binaural stimulation, we go on to record the BAEP with monaural stimulation. We also do this if there is a marked asymmetry of the BAEPs in the two mastoid-vertex channels. Thus the chances of correctly identifying component V are enhanced and any abnormality confirmed with paired stimulation. In addition this method provides information about various levels of the CNS. It also adds specificity to the test, since an abnormality of both the BAEP and middle latency components in a patient suspected of having MS supports that diagnosis (Robinson and Rudge, 1980). Although the proportions of BAEP abnormalities detected is less than with unilateral stimulation, the overall proportion of abnormalities of the AEP is similar and the investigation now has specificity.

We confirmed this approach in a recent study in which we reviewed the results from 227 patients passing through a routine laboratory, who had not been pre-selected. One hundred and thirteen (50%) of these patients did not have MS, and only 2 had abnormalities of both BAEP and middle components. Both of these had extensive vascular disease. If only the BAEP results, using binaural stimulation, are assessed, 16 of 100 patients who definitely did not have MS had abnormal BAEP, and this proportion might have been higher with monaural stimulation. Chiappa et al (1980b) analysed the data on 614 patients referred to a routine laboratory, and used monaural stimulation to record the BAEP. Only 200 of these patients had MS. Of the remainder Chiappa et al. did not report either the clinical diagnosis or the BAEP results in 342. Thus in both studies at least 50% of the patients referred to a routine clinic did not have MS. It is therefore particularly unfortunate that Chiappa et al did not give an exhaustive analysis of the BAEP in these other patients and its use in the differential diagnosis.

SPACE OCCUPYING LESIONS OF THE CEREBELLO-PONTINE ANGLE

It is logical to assume that a mass arising in, or adjacent to, the VIII nerve will affect the function of that nerve and alter information passing to the brainstem through the auditory pathways. Furthermore, a mass of any size will distort the adjacent brainstem and may also alter the passage of information within it. The detection of a space-occupying lesion in the cerebello-pontine angle (CP angle) is of considerable importance since the tumours are usually benign and can often be removed with little morbidity, provided they are detected at an early stage. Of the space-occupying lesions arising in the cerebello-pontine angle acoustic neuromas are the most common and it is to this group that we will first direct our attention.

Acoustic neuromas

Acoustic neuromas arise on the VIII nerve and usually, although not invariably, cause deafness. The problem is to differentiate this deafness from that due to disorders affecting the middle ear and cochlea. Routine audiometry will detect those patients with conductive loss due to middle ear disease. Separation of cochlear (peripheral end organ) loss from deafness due to involvement of the VIII nerve (retrocochlear, nerve fibre deafness) is more complex, although tests of tone decay, recruitment and speech audiometry will be of value in a considerable proportion of cases. In the 1970s two important non-invasive tests became available for the investigation of these patients, namely the computerized tomogram (CT scan) and the BAEP. Thus any account of the use of the BAEP in the diagnosis of acoustic neuroma would be incomplete without reference to the CT scan.

Sohmer et al (1974) studied the BAEP in 8 patients with a space-occupying lesion in the CP angle, 6 of which were proven to be acoustic neuromas. In all patients components III-V were absent, in response to unilateral stimulation of the affected ear, as was component II in some cases. These authors concluded that the presence of the tumour caused blocking of conduction in the VIII nerve at or near its junction with the brainstem. Other isolated reports have been in agreement with these results (Stockard and Rossiter, 1977; Thornton, 1975b). In our own series of acoustic neuromas we have confirmed that components III onwards may be absent, but this was not always the case. In a large proportion component V was present, albeit of increase latency. In the first published systematic study of the BAEP in a series of 36 acoustic neuromas, component V could be identified in 18 although abnormalities of latency were common (Selters and Brackmann, 1977). Similar results were obtained experimentally in animals, showing that compressive tumours can result in an increase in latency of the evoked potential (Chinn and Miller, 1975).

To date it has been the small tumours, particularly those arising in the porus, that are missed by CT scanning. It is of particular importance that the diagnostic efficiency is improved for these, since a surgical approach can be made through the ear with minimal operative morbidity. On the other hand, if diagnosis has to wait until the tumour has grown larger, the operative procedure is more hazardous, since a formal posterior fossa approach has to be made. The VII nerve is rarely spared and the other cranial nerves are at considerable risk in these cases, to say nothing of the brainstem itself. In the series of Selters and Brackmann, not only could component V be present, but it could be of normal latency, usually in those cases where the tumour was small. Thus, like the CT scan, the BAEP was in danger of reporting a false negative in these cases. It was for this reason that Selters and Brackmann extended their analysis of the waveform to look at the interaural difference calculated from the records obtained with stimulation of each ear separately. They called the interaural difference in latency of component V the IT_5. They found that this measurement was abnormal in those patients with small tumours even if the latency from each ear was in the normal range. These results have been extended with further cases (House and Brackmann, 1979) and confirmed in other independent studies (Clemis and Mitchell, 1977; Eggermont et al, 1980), although a small proportion (5-10%) are not detected.

Selters and Brackmann claimed that not only are the brainstem responses of great value in detecting acoustic neuromas, but that they can be used to separate peripheral hearing disorders, e.g. Ménière's disease, from tumours, i.e. they have added specificity to the test, a necessary requirement if it is going to be of value in clinical practice. On subjective testing most patients with Ménière's disease show abnormal growth of loudness perception (recruitment) in the affected ear. However, 10% of patients with acoustic neuromas also show this phenomenon, presumably because of the effects of the tumours on the vascular supply of the cochlea. This gives rise to a diagnostic problem. Selters and Brackmann used a high intensity stimulus, so that at least some of the patients with Ménière's disease would have a similar subjective perception of loudness to a normally hearing person at this level. They recorded the BAEP in 54 patients with no evidence of either a cerebello-pontine angle tumour or a conductive hearing loss, who were matched with the proven tumour groups for the amount of hearing deficit. Only 13 of these patients had an IT_5 greater than 0.2 msec, and when the IT_5 index was plotted against hearing loss at 4 KHz it was clear that patients with peripheral deficits and a prolonged IT_5 tended to have a loss at 4 KHz which was greater than 50 dB. By defining the IT_5 as less than 0.2 msec with hearing loss of up to 50 dB at this frequency, less than 0.3 msec with losses of 50 - 60 dB, and less than 0.4 msec with losses greater than this, only 5 peripheral lesions were falsely placed in the tumour category, whilst all the tumour cases remained abnormal. Clemis and Mitchell (1977) repeated this work but were unable to confirm the results entirely. In this study of 54 patients with a unilateral hearing deficit thought to be peripheral in origin, 19 had an IT_5 that would have put them in the tumour category by Selters and Brackmann's criteria. The lowest false positive rate was in that group of patients with unequivocal cochlear loss (Ménière's disease), but even here 20% gave a result indicative of a retrocochlear lesion. Subsequently, House and Brackmann (1979) have stated that if the hearing loss is greater than 75 dB, the IT_5 does not differentiate peripheral from acoustic tumour patients.

To date the published series of the BAEP in acoustic neuroma are from otological centres where the tumours tend to be small, as 21/35 in the series of Selters and Brackmann (1977) and 20/23 in that of Clemis and Mitchell (1977) were 2 cm or less in diameter. Our own experience is of a neurological centre where the tumours tend to be large. Apart from one unusual case of a small tumour, all our cases had unequivocal abnormalities of the BAEP from the affected ear, and we have not had to use the interaural difference to interpret these results. Indeed, since it is common in our experience for the response from the 'good' ear to be abnormal, the interaural latency may be a misleading measure in this type of patient. Selters and Brackmann also reported that the response from the 'good' ear could be abnormal. This was usually associated with a large tumour, and displacement of the brainstem determined by CT scanning. The IT_5 index is also misleading in patients with bilateral acoustic neuroma. Although these are rare, all series, including our own, have reported such occurrences.

To summarize, the BAEP is abnormal in a high proportion (at least 95%) of patients with acoustic neuromata, in all reported series. This is true for both large and small tumours, although comparison of the interaural difference is necessary to detect the latter. Conversely, there is sometimes difficulty in separating a cochlear loss due to another cause, especially if the deafness is profound. In comparison, the non-invasive use of the CT scan with present-day machines fails to detect the majority of acoustic neuroma which are confined to the porus, and a proportion of those extruding from it if they are small. More surprisingly, large tumours are also missed in some cases, especially if enhancement is not used, the IV ventricle is not visualized, or insufficiently low cuts obtained. Finally, the occurrence of a false positive result is not confined to the BAEP. In 70 consecutive patients thought to have CP angle lesions studied by us, 2 had false positive scans.

Other space-occupying lesions of the CP angle

Other space-occupying lesions of the CP angle include both intrinsic and extrinsic tumours. Like acoustic neuromas the extrinsic tumours, e.g. meningiomas and neurofibromas on other cranial nerves, are usually operable. The intrinsic lesions include brainstem tumours and secondaries, and in this group it is more important to know both the site and nature of the tumour before deciding to embark upon surgery. Of 166 cases of CP angle tumour reviewed by House and Brackmann (1979), only 20 did not have an acoustic neuroma. These authors reported that the proportion of abnormalities of the BAEP in this group was 75% compared with 98% in acoustic neuromas. In our own series we have obtained rather different results. Firstly, the proportion of patients with CP angle tumours other than acoustic neuromas is at least 30%, much higher than that reported by House and Brackmann, and again probably represents the difference of clinical material seen in a neurological, as compared to an otological centre. Secondly, the proportion of abnormalities of the BAEP was as high in this (95%) as in the acoustic

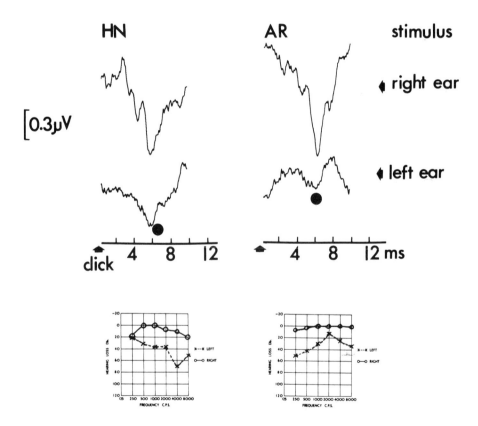

Figure 11.3 BAEP to unilateral stimulation from two patients with cerebello-pontine angle tumours. Subject H.N., left meningioma; subject A.R., left IX nerve neurofibroma. Component V indicated (●). Pure tone audiograms shown below.

neuroma group, even though the involvement of the VIII nerve, as measured by conventional audiometry, was less severe in this group. It is important to emphasize that, like those patients with small acoustic neuromas, absolute amplitude and latency may be normal, the only abnormality being asymmetry between records from the unaffected and the affected side. In addition the abnormality may mimic a peripheral hearing loss. Two such records are illustrated in Figure 11.3. In these patients, both of whom had an extrinsic space-occupying lesion of the CP angle, the only abnormality was a reduction in amplitude of all the components including component V, without a latency increase, and with a normal IT_5 index. These records make us take a conservative approach to the claim that cochlear and retrocochlear causes of hearing loss can always be differentiated by the BAEP if records from a single montage only are used. We have confirmed that borderline records were abnormal by demonstrating a latency increase of the major component in the vertex-chest record and abnormalities of the intermastoid components.

It is not uncommon in this group of patients for the abnormality of the BAEP to be unrelated to the amount of hearing loss. The two patients illustrated in Figure 11.3 had a significant hearing loss on the affected side. On the other hand, Figure 11.4 shows the BAEP of a patient of ours who had a large cerebello-pontine angle meningioma and a markedly abnormal BAEP, yet little hearing loss as measured by the pure tone audiogram.

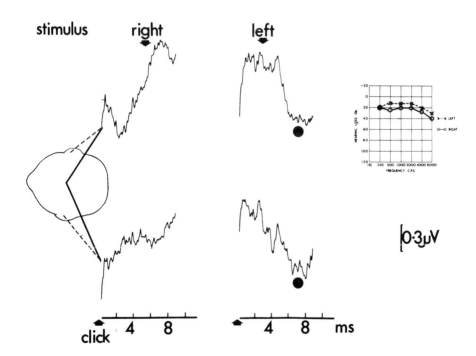

Figure 11.4 *BAEP to unilateral stimulation from a patient with a huge right cerebello-pontine angle meningioma, with minimal deafness (see audiogram). Note absence of recognizable components from either side to right ear stimulation and increased latency of component V (●) on either side to left ear stimulation.*

In conclusion, there is sufficient evidence to be excited about the rôle of the BAEP in the diagnosis of patients with space-occupying lesions of the cerebello-pontine angle, but the exploration of this technique is in its infancy. At present there is no method of predicting from the BAEP whether the tumour is intrinsic or extrinsic, whether it is a meningioma or a neurofibroma, and, if the latter, on which cranial nerve it has arisen. In addition there are some lesions that simulate CP angle tumours, and these are difficult to differentiate with the conventional BAEP, as is illustrated by the following case report.

Vascular disease of brainstem mimicking an acoustic neuroma

A 58-year-old musical instrument maker had a severe vertiginous episode preceded by a number of minor attacks. Two weeks later he rapidly became deaf in the left ear. Examination soon after this revealed a severe sensorineural deafness in the left ear, with marked tone decay, inverse recruitment and absence of speech perception. There were no other signs. The BAEP was recorded at this time and was not only grossly abnormal with stimulation of the left ear, the records were also abnormal with stimulation of the right ear. There were no features of this BAEP to distinguish it from the BAEP of patients with acoustic neuroma. There was no evidence of a cerebello-pontine angle tumour on air encephalography or computerized tomography. A vertebral angiogram revealed extensive atheroma with occlusion of several of the major vessels of the posterior circulation.

COMA AND BRAIN DEATH

The brainstem auditory evoked potentials have been shown to be of value in assessing the irreversibility of brain damage resulting in coma, particularly for that difficult group of patients in whom drug ingestion or metabolic abnormalities make assessment so problematical. Starr (1976) studied a series of patients, all of whom fulfilled the usually accepted criteria of brain death (Medical Royal Colleges, 1976). These criteria rest heavily upon clinical evidence of brainstem dysfunction, including absence of the vestibulo-ocular reflex, pupillary reactions and spontaneous respiration. A variety of conditions had led to the coma, including anoxia and hepatic failure. All the patients studied had absence of any auditory evoked potential originating from brainstem structures (component II-V) at the time that they fulfilled the clinical criteria of brain death. Furthermore, in one patient who suffered anoxia, in whom the brainstem reflexes were initially present but were slowly lost, the BAEP abnormalities paralleled the clinical decline. Ultimately all responses except component I were lost, this occurring at the time when the patient fulfilled the criteria of brain death. Starr pointed out that components became abnormal in a rostro-caudal sequence, familiar enough to the clinician with only his eyes and a torch to assist him, but of interest in that yet another physiological variable follows the same course. This has been confirmed by Uziel and Benezech (1978). Component I from the VIII nerve was particularly resistant to change and was often present, albeit with prolonged latency, after other components were lost and the patient was clinically dead.

Perhaps of more use to the clinician is the BAEP in patients who have taken an excessive dose of drugs. Starr and Achor (1975) studied a number of such patients (9), who had taken a variety of drugs including barbiturates, benzodiazepines, tricyclic antidepressants, phenothiazines and propoxyphene. The BAEPs are remarkably resilient in the face of such drug insults and can be normal in the absence of all the conventional brainstem reflexes used to ascertain death. This observation may well prove useful in one of the common causes of coma in a general hospital where neurologists, at least, are reluctant to apply conventional clinical testing of brainstem function to ascertain whether death has occurred. The converse of this, namely the absence of the BAEP must only be used as a criterion of death in the presence of all other clinical criteria.

Finally, we think that the use of auditory evoked potentials in assessing death due to trauma has not yet been fully evaluated. Greenberg et al (1977a, 1977b) studied AEPs in a series of patients subjected to head trauma. They found no correlation between the BAEP and duration of coma, neither were they able to predict a fatal outcome using the BAEP obtained during the first week after trauma, although there was a better correlation later than this. A worrying feature was the association between BAEP abnormalities and audiometric assessment obtained from those who survived. The degree of abnormality of the BAEP correlated with the degree of deafness assessed at routine audiometry. A necessary requirement in any sensory study is that the stimulus does excite the end organ and has the potential to generate nerve impulses. If the end organ is shattered, as sometimes occurs with fractures of the skull, this requirement is not fulfilled. Greenberg et al (1977a, 1977b) attempted to overcome this problem by recording the VIII nerve action potential using the ECochG, the presence of an action potential implying an intact cochlea. More recently Tsubokawa et al (1980) have studied a number of patients subjected to head injury and found that the BAEP is a reasonable guide to the likely outcome provided that it is obtained more than 12 hours after the insult. Absence of components III-V at this time indicates a poor prognosis and none of their patients with this finding did better than obtain a persistent vegetative state. There was no difference between adults and children in this respect. Other abnormalities, e.g. delay of component V, were often associated with a better outcome. Obviously further work is needed here to enable the clinician to put confidence limits upon the significance of the abnormalities seen in the BAEP after head injury, but the technique looks a promising addition to our assessment of the patient.

OTHER CONDITIONS

So far we have discussed three areas, viz. multiple sclerosis, coma and angle tumours, where the auditory evoked potential is of considerable clinical value, and have highlighted some of the limitations of this test. There are, of course, many other disorders that involve the auditory pathways and could therefore alter the auditory evoked potential. Some of these cause symptomatic deafness, especially those in which the cochlea is damaged, e.g. by ototoxic drugs, and they are the province of the audiologist. They are discussed in Chapter 8. Others involve more central structures and are the province of the neurologist. They may cause symptomatic deafness, but more commonly do not; they will now be discussed.

Lesions involving the cochlear nuclei, e.g. tumours and vascular disease, do have a profound effect upon the BAEP providing they cause symptomatic deafness. So far there are only isolated reports showing that the destruction of one cochlear nucleus grossly distorts the BAEP on unilateral stimulation (e.g. Starr and Achor, 1975). It should be pointed out that cases such as this are rare in the extreme and certainly would not alone be a justification for setting up an evoked potential laboratory. Of more importance however is the fact that such a case cannot be differentiated from an acoustic neuroma on the BAEP record, although the cluster of other neurological signs usually make it abundantly clear that this is not the diagnosis.

Progressive degenerative disorders have not been extensively studied. Markand et al (1980) in a preliminatry report examined 10 children with leucodystrophies of various types (7 had Pelizaeus-Merzbacher disease, 1 metachromatic leucodystrophy and 2 adreno-leucodystrophy) and noted that all had abnormal BAEPs, with absence of component III-V in 9 of them. Component I was normal in all except the case of metachromatic leucodystrophy. They also examined 10 patients with 'grey matter' disease, a term the authors used to describe SSPE, Batten's disease and Leigh's encephalopathy. In all except one case of Leigh's encephalopathy, the BAEPs were normal. Component VI has been reported as abnormal in a single case of adrenoleucodystrophy (Black et al, 1979).

The present authors have examined 3 adults from one family with metachromatic leucodystrophy, none of whom had a peripheral neuropathy, and the BAEP was normal in all. We have also studied 9 patients with Steele-Richardson-Olzewski's syndrome, including one with an internuclear ophthalmoplegia, and all have had remarkably normal BAEP and middle latency components. The hereditary ataxias have not been studied systematically, but can be abnormal, and abnormalities have been described in Charcot-Marie-Tooth disease (Satya-Murti et al, 1978). Chronic alcoholism has been associated with an abnormal BAEP, both in cases with cerebral pontine myelinolysis (Stockard et al, 1976) and in a small series in whom a slow tremor of the limbs, thought to imply brainstem rather than pure cerebellar involvement, was present (Rosenhamer and Silfverskiold, 1980).

One interesting area where the BAEP might prove useful is in monitoring man during hazardous procedures. Thus Sem-Jacobson (1979) has suggested that deep sea divers might have their BAEPs recorded prior to descent, so that brainstem involvement in cases of decompression sickness can be detected, and he has set up a programme to do this in one area of intensive diving activity in Europe. Another hazardous procedure is that of posterior fossa surgery, especially on the arterial tree, where one group has claimed that BAEP monitoring is useful (Hashimoto et al, 1980, 1981). Certainly it seems reasonable that the BAEP, which is so resistant in the face of anaesthesia, could be useful in such work.

Acknowledgements
We are grateful to Dr R.M. Sherratt and Dr J.D. Hood for their invaluable comments on the original manuscript of Chapters 10 and 11.

12

Somatosensory Evoked Potentials: The Normal Waveform

S.J. Jones

In the field of human evoked potentials the somatosensory modality is unique, since the opportunity exists to by-pass the peripheral receptor organs by the delivery of an electrical impulse directly (usually transcutaneously) to the nerve trunk. Although a case can be made in favour of more natural forms of stimulation (mechanical tap, pinprick, temperature change, etc.) an electrical stimulus possesses the advantage that a substantial proportion of the large diameter fibres may be activated simultaneously, resulting in a stronger and more coherent volley arriving at the central nervous system. On the other hand, however, a tolerable electrical impulse is capable of depolarizing only the fibres of largest diameter and fastest conduction velocity. These are responsible, in the main, for the sensory modalities of light touch and proprioception, although there is evidence that fibres of much smaller diameter may respond to light touch and other modalities, in addition to thermal and noxious stimuli (Iggo, 1966).

Since only large fibre input (Groups I and II) need normally be considered, the interpretation of the SEP waveform is rendered more straightforward than might have been the case were it possible to activate the entire sensory fibre population, but at the same time the potential clinical usefulness of the SEP is considerably restricted. Nevertheless it is found that SEPs are affected by a wide variety of disorders involving the peripheral and central nervous system, and have their place as an aid to clinical medicine provided the inherent limitations are borne in mind.

The first SEPs to be recorded from the scalp of a human subject were the pathologically enhanced responses of a patient with progressive myoclonic epilepsy (Dawson, 1947a, 1947b). With the adoption and development of signal averaging techniques (Dawson, 1954a) it became possible to study the individual components of the normal waveform, and this capability has recently been extended to the sequence of short latency potentials generated in the brachial plexus, spinal cord and subcortical cerebral structures. In this chapter it is intended to bring together the significant published observations, experimental and clinical, which have contributed to our understanding of the early components of the SEP waveform, and to provide a somewhat less comprehensive survey of the distribution and properties of later components. First, however, it may be useful to raise some questions of technique, which are commented on largely from the author's own experience.

SUGGESTED PROCEDURE FOR CLINICAL SEP RECORDINGS

1. Reassure the patient.

2. Mark the electrode locations (e.g. with a wax pencil). Detailed suggestions concerning location of recording electrodes are to be found later in this Chapter.

3. Attach disc electrodes using collodion, or double-sided adhesive annuli for non-hairy skin.

4. Reassure the patient. Scarify the skin under each electrode by mild pressure and rotation of a sterile, blunt (serrated tip) needle inserted through the central hole of the cup. Inject electrode jelly into the cup until a little emerges from the hole. Check that the electrode/skin impedance is less than 5 kilohms. If not, scarify the skin further. It is not necessary (or desirable) to draw blood.

5. Secure vulnerable electrodes with adhesive tape.

6. Clean the skin over the stimulation and earthing points using an alcohol-soaked swab. The earthing electrode should be located proximal to the stimulating electrode on the same limb.

7. Apply a little electrode jelly to the earthing electrode (usually an ECG plate) and attach using an appropriate strap (elastic, velcro etc).

8. Apply electrode jelly to the feet of the stimulating electrodes which should be separated by 3 - 5 cm and should each terminate in a moist felt pad ('stick-on' electrodes similar to those used for recording are suitable but less easily adjusted). Locate the electrodes longitudinally over the appropriate nerve trunk and secure with an elastic or velcro strap. For median nerve stimulation at the wrist the optimal location for the stimulating cathode (blue or black lead) is usually about 3 cm proximal to the crease of the wrist and 1 or 2 cm from the midline toward the radial side. There are theoretical reasons why the stimulating cathode should be located proximal to the anode, but at the wrist the opposite configuration seems to be equally effective and perhaps more comfortable.

9. Connect the recording and earthing leads to the head box. Switch on the amplifiers to allow them time to settle. The recording equipment (amplifiers, averager etc) should be accurately calibrated for each patient, using a signal of known amplitude and duration.

10. Connect the stimulating leads and determine the sensory threshold current or voltage by raising and lowering the stimulus intensity at least twice. Further remarks on stimulation technique are to be found later in this Chapter.

11. Reassure the patient and slowly increase the stimulus intensity to the operational level (sufficient to produce a moderate flexion of the thenar muscles in most subjects, 3 to 4 times the sensory threshold if there is no twitch and no sensory impairment).

12. Ask the patient to settle comfortably, to relax as much as possible and to open the mouth slightly to ensure relaxation of the jaw muscles. Swallowing, yawning and talking should be discouraged and the patient should remain perfectly still throughout the recording run.

13. Commence averaging. The patient should be capable of tolerating a run of 400 stimuli delivered at a rate of 2 per second. A higher stimulation rate of up to 10/sec may be employed if only short latency potentials are to be studied, but may be less well tolerated. The suggested averager epoch is 30 or 50 msec, assuming at least 256 ordinate points per channel. The epoch may need to be increased if cortical SEPs are severely delayed, and the number of sweeps increased if the signal/noise ratio is very poor. It may be found useful to eliminate the stimulus artifact by triggering the averager 1 - 4 msec after the stimulus pulse.

14. Record at least two runs from each limb to establish which peaks are consistent and which are due to variable 'noise'. If the noise obscures the consistent signal one can: (1) try to secure better relaxation, particularly of neck, jaw and scalp muscles; (2) average more sweeps in each run; (3) record more runs; (4) make use of an input monitor and a 'pause' facility, if available, to exclude the worst bursts of muscle artifact.

15. Switch off the amplifiers and remove the electrodes (collodion is soluble in acetone).

16. Measure the amplitude and latency of the consistent peaks and compare with normative values. Norms are generally derived from a large group of healthy subjects in which identical procedures have been observed, but it may be necessary to make additional allowance for the age and general stature of the patient (see below). If there is good reason to suppose that only one side of the body is involved then the other can be adopted as the control, provided the permissible range of left/right variation has been established in healthy subjects.

FURTHER HINTS ON RECORDING TECHNIQUE

Stimulation

In the vast majority of cases the whole range of SEP components can be obtained with transcutaneous stimulation of the median nerve at the wrist or the elbow. The ulnar nerve may also be stimulated at the wrist or the elbow, and the responses complement the median nerve potentials since they rely on input to the eighth cervical and first thoracic spinal cord segments, whereas the majority of median nerve input is to the sixth and seventh cervical segments. The radial nerve is less easily located in the forearm and gives rise to smaller evoked responses in spite of the preponderance of sensory fibres.

In the lower limb the posterior tibial nerve is usually accessible in the popliteal fossa, the common peroneal nerve at the neck of the fibula, and the sural, anterior tibial and posterior tibial nerves at the ankle. All of the latter can give rise to well-defined cortical potentials, but the posterior tibial nerve is the most effective for evoking spinal responses, and even this may be unsuccessful in some cases.

Stimulus parameters are not usually critical provided the nerve is accurately located and the motor threshold slightly exceeded. The stimulus pulse will usually be a square wave with a fast rise-time and a duration of less than 0.5 msec. In the author's experience there seems to be little advantage to be obtained by using a 'constant current' stimulator in preference to the 'constant voltage' type, and likewise in practice it seems to matter little whether the anode is distal or proximal to the stimulating cathode. If only short latency (up to about 25 msec) components are to be studied then the stimuli can be delivered regularly at between 2 and 10/sec, but for optimal recording of later waves the interstimulus interval should be at least 2 sec and preferably randomised.

A value can be derived for sensory conduction velocity in the arm from the change in the latency of early cortical and subcortical SEP components when the stimulus is delivered to different sites along the same nerve (see Figure 12.1). This may be of particular usefulness in severe cases of peripheral neuropathy where no sensory nerve action potentials (SNAPs) can be recorded (Desmedt et al, 1966). In such cases the cortical SEP is frequently better preserved than the SNAP, thanks possibly to trans-synaptic amplification. A broadening of the SEP waveform when the stimulus is delivered more distally (not seen to any marked degree in normal subjects) may be suggestive of increased temporal dispersion in the peripheral fibres concerned — perhaps due to diffuse segmental demyelination. In addition to the wrist and the elbow it is possible to stimulate median nerve fibres at the axilla and the tips of the thumb and the first and second fingers (Desmedt et al, 1966).

There has been considerable discussion concerning the desirability of ensuring a relatively 'pure' afferent volley by applying the stimulus to the digital nerves (containing sensory fibres only) rather than to a mixed trunk which may contain fast-conducting muscle spindle afferents and motor fibres as well as cutaneous sensory axons (see, for example, Desmedt and Brunko, 1980). However, although the response to stimulation of the median nerve is possibly more complex than that to digital nerve stimulation, there is no evidence that any components are mediated by fibres conducting faster than approximately 75 m/sec, and likewise there is no suggestion that any components are entirely due to antidromic activation of motor fibres. The larger amplitude of median nerve SEPs probably outweighs the theoretical disadvantages when considering which technique should be applied to routine clinical referrals. The same consideration has also discouraged the use of mechanical evoking stimuli (tap, vibration, etc.), although a number of studies are described later in which just such techniques have been employed to evoke cortical

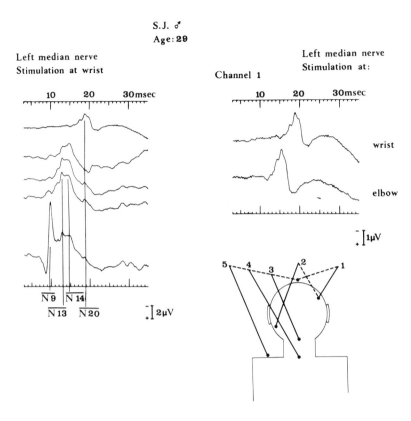

S.J. ♂
Age: 29

Left median nerve
Stimulation at wrist

Channel 1

Left median nerve
Stimulation at:

10   20   30msec

10   20   30msec

wrist

elbow

$\bar{}$|1µV

N̄9 N̄14
N̄13 N̄20

$\bar{}$|2µV

5   4   3   2   1

Figure 12.1 *Normal subcortical and early cortical SEP components showing* $\overline{N9}$ *at the clavicle,* $\overline{N11}$ *(not labelled) and* $\overline{N13}$ *at C7 and C2,* $\overline{N14}$ *relatively enhanced at the left mastoid process and* $\overline{N20}$ *over the somatosensory cortical hand area. On the right* $\overline{N20}$ *is shown following wrist and elbow stimulation, with a latency shift of 3.5 msec. (From Jones et al, 1980.)*

(for example Nakanishi et al, 1974; Salamy, 1978) and subcortical (Pratt et al, 1979) potentials. This matter is discussed by Allison et al (1979), who concluded that the advantages of median nerve stimulation considerably outweigh the disadvantages, which have yet to be convincingly demonstrated. SEPs have also variously been recorded in response to electrical stimulation of the tooth pulp (innervated by unmyelinated fibres only), painful stimulation of the skin by laser-beam and electrical impulses, and local warming or cooling of the skin (Chatrian et al, 1975; Stowell, 1977; Carmon et al, 1976; Frühstorfer et al, 1976). Other techniques increasingly employed include segmental electrical stimulation of the limbs and trunk (for example Blair, 1971), trigeminal nerve stimulation (Stöhr and Petruch, 1979) and the delivery of pairs or chains of electrical impulses to a nerve trunk (Shagass and Schwartz, 1961; Namerow et al, 1974). All of these are briefly described in this and the following Chapter.

Recording

Silver/silver chloride disc electrodes are most commonly used, with skin impedance reduced to 5 kilohms or less by scarification. Opinions will inevitably differ as to the optimum siting of recording and reference electrodes, although for median and ulnar nerve stimulation a site overlying the contralateral somatosensory cortical hand area (approximately 2 cm posterior to the vertex and 7 cm towards the tragus of the ear) is near-optimal for the majority of cortically-generated SEP components. Other parts of the body are represented along the same line connecting a point 2 cm posterior to the vertex with the external auditory

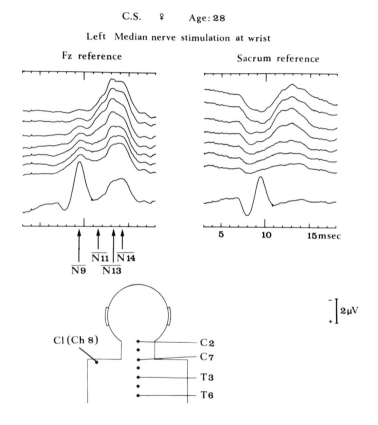

Figure 12.2 Cervical and clavicular SEP waveform in scalp (F_z) and sacrum referential recordings, illustrating the 4 major components and the much more restricted distribution with the latter reference.

meatus, the lower limbs approximately 1 cm and the facial area 9 cm from the midline. For routine recordings the 'reference' electrode is usually located on the earlobes or the midline of the frontal scalp, but it should not be assumed that these sites are indifferent. At latencies of less than 16 msec following stimulation at the wrist a sequence of negative-going potentials can be recorded from the ipsilateral shoulder, the dorsal surface of the neck between the seventh and second cervical vertebrae and the mastoid processes, while a sequence of positive-going waves at similar latencies is widely distributed over the scalp. As a purely practical procedure, therefore, one can record a larger amplitude waveform with the 'reference' electrode on the scalp rather than on the earlobe or a noncephalic site (see Figure 12.2), since the negative neck potentials will be summated with the positive-going potentials from the scalp. For topographic studies, however, a totally inactive reference site is essential, and only the lower part of the body and the contralateral arm can be considered effectively indifferent to median nerve stimulation.

It has been noted that an insufficiently extended high frequency response will cause distortion of brief EP components and artificially prolong their latency (Desmedt et al, 1974). The majority of EEG amplifiers are therefore unsuited to the recording of short latency SEPs, for which a high-frequency response flat to at least 3 KHz is recommended. The detection of slow potential shifts is limited by the time constant of the amplifier; for most purposes a value of 0.1 to 1 sec is sufficient, although a longer value is desirable for the recording of potentials above 200 msec latency. The sampling rate of the averager should ideally exceed the high-frequency response of the amplifier by a factor of 2.5 or more (at least 8 sample points/msec recommended).

Since the short-latency SEP components may be smaller than 2 μV and of similar frequency spectrum to spontaneously-occurring muscle artifacts it may be necessary to average more than 1000 responses to obtain adequate definition in some cases. As a further precaution against the misinterpretation of contaminated records repeat recordings should always be made. Automatic rejection of sweeps contaminated by high amplitude noise is a desirable luxury, although the provision of a 'pause' facility on the averager can serve to prevent the worst effects of sporadic muscle tension (caused, for example, by swallowing) if the raw input can be monitored by eye. When recording from the lumbar region a reference electrode to one side of the spine adjacent to the active site may serve to reduce the distortion of small spinal potentials by muscle and ECG interference, and the latter can also be avoided by triggering the stimulator cycle from the QRS complex, with a suitable delay such that the evoked potentials will occur when ECG activity is at a minimum.

Range of normality

A number of authors have published more or less detailed statistical criteria of SEP normality which may be useful to a newcomer in the field. It is a matter for debate whether the norms obtained by one group should ever be adopted by another, inevitably using slightly different techniques, but since there are few ways of influencing the SEP waveform by varying the parameters of an electrical nerve trunk stimulus, this argument probably applies less to the somatosensory than to the visual or auditory modalities, provided the electrode locations and amplification characteristics are similar.

A selective reference list of papers providing useful normative data is given in Table 12.1. SEP latency norms are likely to vary according to the race and sex ratio

Table 12.1 PAPERS PROVIDING USEFUL NORMATIVE DATA

Contribution	Range of components covered	Particular attention to
Goff et al (1962)	All cortical	Waveform, distribution
Giblin (1964)	Early-middle latency cortical	Latency, waveform, stimulation sites and parameters
Lueders (1970)	All cortical	Amplitude, latency, effect of ageing
Tamura (1972)	Early-middle latency cortical	Amplitude, latency, contralateral vs. ipsilateral
Tsumoto et al (1972)	All cortical	Amplitude, latency, lower limb stimulation
Matthews et al (1974)	Subcortical	Latency (corr. with arm length), waveform, distribution
Fukushima & Mayanagi (1975)	Early-middle latency cortical	Latency; upper limb, lower limb and digital stimulation
Desmedt et al (1976)	Early cortical	Amplitude, latency, maturation (digital stimulation)
Goff et al (1977)	All cortical	Amplitude, latency, distribution
Jones (1977)	Subcortical	Amplitude, latency, waveform, distribution
Shibasaki et al (1977)	All cortical	Amplitude, latency, left/right differences
Delbeke et al (1978)	Subcortical (lumbar)	Waveform, latency, lower limb stimulation
Hume & Cant (1978)	Subcortical-mid. lat. cortical	Amplitude, latency, waveform, 'central conduction time'
Jones & Small (1978)	Subcortical-early cortical	Amplitude, latency, distribution, lower limb stimulation
Kritchevsky & Wiederholt (1978)	Subcortical-early cortical	Amplitude, latency, scalp distribution
Dorfman & Bosley (1979)	Early cortical	Latency, effect of ageing
Chiappa et al (1980a)	Subcortical-early cortical	Amplitude, latency, left/right differences

of subjects comprising the normal group, simply through variation in arm length (Matthews et al, 1974). It is also well known that subdermal temperature has a marked influence on peripheral nerve conduction velocity. These factors should always be borne in mind when comparing an individual record, possibly abnormal, with normative data obtained in another laboratory.

Short latency potentials following median nerve stimulation at the wrist (recorded with a mid-frontal reference) are described with means and standard deviations of normal amplitude and latency by Jones (1977) and Chiappa et al (1980a). Kritchevsky and Wiederholt (1978) describe the positive-going complex of subcortical 'far-field' potentials which can be recorded from the scalp using a remote non-cephalic reference (technically a more difficult procedure). The potentials generated in the lower thoracic and lumbar region following posterior tibial nerve stimulation at the knee are described in detail by Delbeke et al (1978), while Jones and Small (1978) quote amplitude and latency figures for spinal, subcortical and cortical potentials following stimulation at the ankle.

The latency and distribution of cortical SEP components following median nerve stimulation is described by Goff et al (1962, 1977), with some indication of the range of normality. These authors indicate which are the most consistent peaks and which are likely to become fused in some subjects, but the labelling of components according to mean latency values is based on a fairly small number of subjects. Giblin (1964) divided his 25 normal subjects into two groups in which the initial cortical positivity (occurring at 22-31 msec) was a single peak (V-group) or bifid (W-group), and quoted latency ranges for each. Thanks to the improved resolution of amplification and averaging equipment, however, a bifid wave can now be seen in a much larger proportion of subjects. Tamura (1972) measured the amplitude and latency of cortical potentials recorded contralateral and ipsilateral to the stimulated arm. Other notable accounts with regard to tabulation of normative data include those of Lueders (1970), who studied the effects of ageing on a great many parameters of the SEP waveform, Tsumoto et al (1972) who examined the cortical responses to common peroneal nerve stimulation, and Fukushima and Mayanagi (1975) who recorded SEPs in response to stimulation of the fingers and toes in addition to the major nerve trunks in the arm and leg.

Most authors are inclined to regard the 'normal' range of amplitude and latency as lying within 2 or 2.5 standard deviations of the normal mean. This may be statistically legitimate for latency values, which approximate fairly well to a normal (Gaussian) distribution, but seems less appropriate for amplitude measures which may be scattered much more widely above the mean than below. This often results in a situation where the ± 2.5 standard deviation range encompasses amplitudes approaching or below zero. There is a case, therefore, for adopting a non-parametric criterion such that, for example, an amplitude measure could be regarded as abnormal with probability of error less than 5% if it were smaller than the corresponding measure in all subjects out of a normal group of 20, or all save one out of a group of 40 (a special case of the 'Randomization test for two independent samples', see Siegel, 1956). It should also be realised that the adoption of more than one independent criterion (for example, latency in addition to amplitude) increases the probability that a normal individual will be outside one 'normal' range by chance variation, and each criterion should therefore be made statistically more stringent.

A considerable amount of the inter-subject variation in SEP latency is attributable to variation in arm length. This factor can be virtually eliminated in an individual record by; (1) standardizing latency values according to arm length, assuming a linear relationship, or (2) measuring latencies from the peak of the $\overline{N9}$ component, which is generated in the brachial plexus and is maximally recorded over the clavicle of the stimulated arm. The adoption of one or other of these procedures is strongly recommended as a means of increasing the sensitivity and reducing the inherent error factor of the test.

The patient

A practical consideration perhaps not sufficiently appreciated is that a patient may deviate from 'normality' (as defined by the relevant physiological and psychological characteristics of the particular subjects comprising the normal group) in ways which affect the recording of EPs but are unrelated to the disease process under investigation, or are related to it only in a trivial manner. A patient may be less co-operative than a volunteer, or physically more tense and therefore less able to tolerate unfamiliar stimuli or a protracted recording session. If there is increased muscle tone as a consequence of an upper motor neurone lesion the evoked potentials may be distorted by muscular artifacts, and possibly misinterpreted if insufficient sweeps are averaged or repeat recordings are not made. Where there is sensory impairment or peripheral neuropathy involving motor fibres one's guidelines as to the effective intensity of the stimulus (a multiple of the sensory threshold current, or the presence of a direct motor response) may need to be revised or abandoned. Obesity in a patient may make transcutaneous nerve trunk stimulation more difficult owing to the thickness of interposed tissue. When these factors are borne in mind it is easy to see how records of abnormally low amplitude may sometimes be obtained for trivial reasons, and that a clinical recording should never be interpreted by blind adherence to normative data. If possible an experienced electrophysiologist should be on hand during the session to make sure all necessary steps are taken to obtain the optimum record, and the final report should be written by someone with a thorough comprehension of the limitations and pitfalls, as well as the power, of the SEP technique.

ORIGIN OF SUBCORTICALLY-GENERATED SEP COMPONENTS

Peripheral nerve

The conduction velocity of the sensory nerve action potential (SNAP) recorded from the median nerve at the wrist or the elbow following digital nerve stimulation is such that the volley must arrive at the spinal cord after less than 15 msec, or less than 12 msec following stimulation at the wrist. The earliest potential recorded over the neck and scalp following stimulation at the wrist occurs with a peak latency of 9-10 msec in most subjects, and is therefore likely to originate in the periphery. Over the clavicle ipsilateral to the stimulated arm a large positive/negative biphasic wave is recorded with latency increasing towards proximal sites (Jones, 1977; see Figure 12.3), but a positive peak alone is recorded over the scalp and neck (Cracco and Cracco, 1976; Jones, 1977; Kritchevsky and Wiederholt, 1978). These potentials appear to have a common generator, and will subsequently be referred to as 'N9' according to the polarity and approximate latency of the largest (supraclavicular) phase.

Our understanding of the electrical currents associated with the propagation of a nerve action potential, allied with the theory of the distribution of potentials in a volume conductor (for example see Woodbury, 1960), predicts that the depolarisa-

S. J.

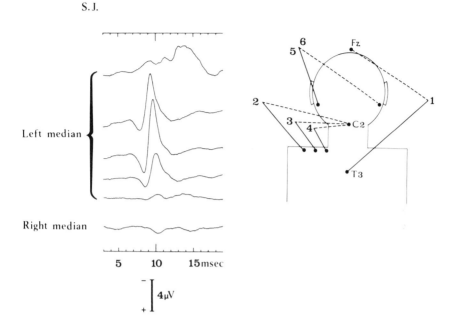

Figure 12.3 *The* $\overline{N9}$ *potential recorded from the clavicle (latency increasing from lateral to medial sites), the thoracic spine with reference to* F_z*, and the left mastoid with reference to the right (showing inversion of polarity on stimulating the contralateral arm). (From Jones, 1977.)*

tion of axonal membranes will be manifested as a positive potential field in advance of the direction of propagation, with the recorded amplitude inversely proportional to the square of the distance from the generator and directly proportional to the solid angle subtended by a cross section through the nerve trunk. A more intense but less directional negative potential is recorded by electrodes in a plane perpendicular to the depolarized region of the nerve. The distribution and latency of the positive and negative constituents of $\overline{N9}$ are therefore consistent with the field of an afferent volley passing through the brachial plexus. This hypothesis is supported by clinical evidence, since both the negative and positive components of $\overline{N9}$ may be preserved (with all succeeding potentials absent) in patients with traction lesions of the brachial plexus, when there is a rupture of the rootlets adjacent to the spinal cord and proximal to the dorsal root ganglia (Jones, 1979 and unpublished observations). In spinal recordings with a scalp reference $\overline{N9}$ is seen as a negative deflection which is greatly diminished or absent when the 'active' electrode is above the mid-cervical region (Jones, 1977; also seen in the records of Hume and Cant, 1978 and El-Negamy and Sedgwick, 1978). The use of a remote noncephalic reference site, however, reveals that this is likely to be due to a gradual reduction in the amplitude of the scalp positivity below the second cervical vertebra, presumably reflecting a gradual divergence from the axis of the approaching peripheral nerve volley. No animal analogue of $\overline{N9}$ has yet been reported, but the potential now seems to be well understood in man.

Spinal cord and brainstem

The second component occurs 2-3 msec after $\overline{N9}$, with positive polarity at scalp locations ($\overline{P12}$ according to Cracco and Cracco, 1976, and Kritchevsky and Wiederholt, 1978) but negative in the lower cervical region ($\overline{N11}$ or $\overline{N12}$, see Figure 12.2 and Matthews et al, 1974; Jones, 1977; El-Negamy and Sedgwick, 1978; Hume and Cant, 1978). Both positive and negative constituents can frequently be seen in the same individual by use of a remote noncephalic reference on the hand, foot or sacrum. The interval between $\overline{N9}$ and $\overline{N11}$ remains the same when the stimulus is delivered to the elbow instead of the wrist, indicating that the two potentials are mediated by the same group of large diameter afferent fibres (Group II, conduction velocity 60-75 m/sec). This inevitably leads one to conclude that the generator of the later potential can be no further rostral than the spinal cord, since an interval of 2 msec is insufficient time for propagated activity from the brachial plexus to reach the brainstem or higher structures.

Several authors (including Cracco and Cracco, 1976 and Kritchevsky and Wiederholt, 1978) have suggested that $\overline{P12}$ might be generated in the cuneate nucleus or medial lemniscus of the brainstem, but for the reason given above this hypothesis now seems unlikely. El-Negamy and Sedgwick (1978) reported that the N11 component evoked by the second of a pair of median nerve impulses showed signs of attenuation when the interstimulus interval (ISI) was less than 60 msec, suggesting a post-synaptic origin since the peripheral nerve potential was unattenuated even at an ISI of 10 msec. This finding is contrary to the present author's experience, however, which is that both $\overline{N9}$ and $\overline{N11}$ appear to be virtually unattenuated with an interstimulus interval as short as 4 msec (Jones, unpublished observations). In the author's opinion the majority of evidence now suggests that N11 is likely to reflect the activity of presynaptic sensory axons in the most proximal segments of the dorsal roots, and/or the spinal cord. As with $\overline{N9}$ there is a local negative field adjacent to the proposed generator area (the lower cervical region) and a positive potential more widely distributed in advance of the direction of propagation. $\overline{N11}$ is sometimes of longer latency at C2 than at C7 (Jones, 1977), although this was shown to be due to the existence of distinct subcomponents with different spatial distributions, and may not be apparent when a noncephalic reference is used.

In animals the earliest potential recorded from the dorsum of the spinal cord following dorsal root or nerve trunk stimulation is a brief 'spike' of negative polarity and less than 1 msec duration (Gasser and Graham, 1933; Bernhard, 1953). The spike was not easily occluded by repetitive stimulation and its latency was increased at more rostral recording sites, consistent with propagation in the dorsal columns of the spinal cord (Gasser and Graham, 1933). An apparently analogous positive/negative 'spike' potential has been recorded from the lower cervical region in man, using epidural (Shimoji et al, 1971, 1972, 1976, 1977, 1978) and intrathecal (Ertekin, 1973, 1976a) electrodes. With the latter technique the mean peak latency for the negative phase of this 'cord dorsum' (CD) potential was 8.3 msec following median nerve stimulation at the elbow (Ertekin, 1976a), equivalent to 11.5 or 12 msec following wrist stimulation. At the same locus it was possible to record a triphasic 'tractus' potential in response to stimulation of the posterior tibial nerve (Ertekin, 1976b). The evidence suggests, therefore, that $\overline{\text{N11}}$ may be an analogue of the CD potential, perhaps generated in the dorsal columns of the spinal cord.

The largest potential recorded from the cervical region with the reference electrode on the earlobe or scalp occurs with a mean peak latency of 13 or 14 msec from the wrist (Liberson and Kim, 1963; Schwartz and Shagass, 1964; Cracco, 1973; Matthews et al, 1974, etc.). When a noncephalic reference is used the potential is seen to be of negative polarity between C7 and C2 but undergoes phase reversal above the level of the inion (see Fig 12.4), and a positive potential of the same latency is widely recorded at scalp locations including Fz (Cracco and Cracco, 1976; Jones, 1977; Kritchevsky and Wiederholt, 1978). The cervical potential ($\overline{\text{N13}}$ in the majority of recent accounts) is apparently recorded as low as the thoracic and lumbar region when a scalp reference is used, but this is certainly due to the

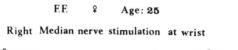

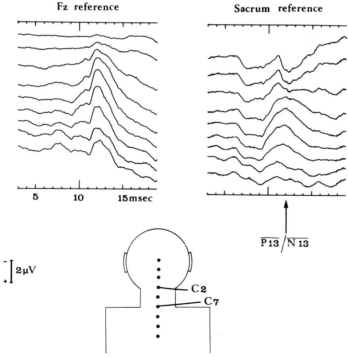

Figure 12.4 *Short latency cervical SEP components, illustrating the polarity reversal of $\overline{\text{N13}}/\overline{\text{P13}}$ across the inion, seen using a noncephalic (sacrum) reference.*

contribution from the reference. Since positive and negative constituents of $\overline{\text{N13}}$ are in synchrony whether the stimulus is delivered to the wrist or to the elbow, with latencies shorter by approximately 3.5 msec from the proximal site, it can be concluded that both rely on the same group of fast afferent fibres as is responsible for $\overline{\text{N9}}$ and $\overline{\text{N11}}$. This suggests that the generator is likely to be situated in the spinal cord or brainstem, since an interval of 4-5 msec after $\overline{\text{N9}}$ is probably insufficient time for propagated activity from the brachial plexus to reach higher cerebral structures or the cerebellum. An analogue of $\overline{\text{N13}}$ (and of other short latency SEP components) has been recorded following mechanical stimulation of the digits (Pratt et al, 1979), suggesting that a major proportion of the wave is likely to originate through activation of low threshold cutaneous afferents.

The evidence from epidural and intrathecal recordings in man is inconclusive, although with both techniques negative waves have been recorded with suitable latency to account for $\overline{\text{N13}}$. The 'N_1' potential recorded epidurally by Shimoji et al (1972) had a mean peak latency of 10.6 msec following ulnar nerve stimulation at the elbow, equivalent to about 14 msec from the wrist, and was refractory at longer interstimulus intervals than was the preceding 'spike' potential (Shimoji et al, 1978). Ertekin (1976a) recorded a large segmental 'dorsal root' (DR) potential with a mean negative peak latency of 10.2 msec following median nerve stimulation at the elbow. It was postulated that this might reflect 'the mixture of the recordable total activity passing through the spinal roots', and the relatively long latency compared with the CD potential was explained by the possibility of a contribution from smaller diameter fibres. Since the stimuli used were many times more intense than those routinely employed to elicit $\overline{\text{N13}}$ there may indeed have been significant activation of smaller diameter fibres, and Ertekin's hypothesis could be tested by comparing DR potential latencies following wrist and elbow stimulation. If, however, the DR potential is in fact the intrathecal analogue of $\overline{\text{N13}}$ (mediated by the same fibres as are responsible for $\overline{\text{N11}}$ and the CD potential), the 2 msec latency separation between CD and DR peaks recorded at the same segmental level is perhaps best accounted for by the possibility that the latter is generated postsynaptically, probably in the grey matter of the spinal cord.

In the animal experiments of Gasser and Graham (1933) and Bernhard and colleagues (1953) the 'spike' potential recorded over the dorsum of the spinal cord was followed after approximately 2 msec by a broader negative wave ('N_1') with restricted distribution and no evidence of a change in latency rostrally or caudally. N_1 was refractory at longer interstimulus intervals than the spike, and was abolished by asphyxia at an earlier stage. This and other evidence led Gasser and Graham (1933) to attribute the wave to depolarization of internuncial neurones in the dorsal horn, adjacent to the root entry zone. The potential was evoked by activation of low threshold (hence large diameter and fast conducting) sensory afferent fibres, similar to those responsible for $\overline{\text{N13}}$. The properties of N_1 were further investigated by Bernhard and Widén (1953), who found the wave to be occluded when the evoking volley was preceded by electrical stimulation of the spinal cord at a more rostral level, although reflex activity recorded from the ventral roots was unaffected. This implied a function for N_1 other than (or at least in addition to) the mediation of spinal cord reflexes — possibly the trans-synaptic activation of pathways such as the spinothalamic, spinocerebellar and spinoreticular systems. The location of the

N_1 generator in the dorsal horns was confirmed by the effect of small experimental lesions (Lindblom and Ottosson, 1953).

There are marked similarities between N_1 and the negative-going potential which is recorded from the lower thoracic and lumbar region in man following stimulation of the lower limb (best described by Delbeke et al, 1978). The lumbar wave is reportedly bifid in some subjects (as is $\overline{N13}$, Jones 1977), while N_1 has been resolved into pre- and postsynaptic constituents by the effect of a closely preceding 'conditioning' stimulus (Austin and McCouch, 1955). It seems highly plausible, therefore, that the lumbar wave, $\overline{N13}$, N_1 and the 'DR' potential are all manifestations of pre- and postsynaptic events in the dorsal horn, generated within a few centimetres of the appropriate root entry zone.

It is possible that the scalp-recorded positive wave at the same latency as $\overline{N13}$ ($\overline{P13}$, see Figure 12.4) may be the positive field in advance of a postsynaptic volley ascending from the spinal grey matter, but an alternative proposal has been put forward by Arezzo et al (1979). In the monkey it was found that the rising phase of the second of three positive potentials recorded from the scalp surface coincided with multiple unit activity in brainstem lemniscal structures (see Figure 12.5). The

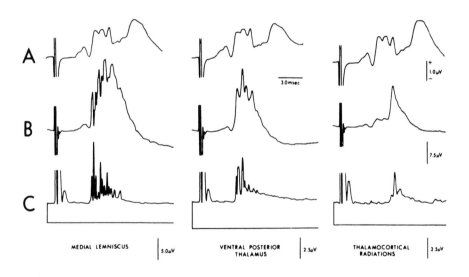

Figure 12.5 *Scalp recorded subcortical somatosensory evoked potentials in the monkey. (A) contralateral sensorimotor cortex referred to wrist in comparison with: (B) depth recordings of SEP, and (C) multiple unit activity in various structures. (From Arezzo et al, 1979.)*

first scalp positivity was believed to originate in the dorsal columns and to correspond with the $\overline{P12}$ potential in man. If it is the case that the second positive wave is analogous to $\overline{P13}$, and reflects postsynaptic activity in the medial lemniscus, then there is no justification for summating $\overline{P13}$ with $\overline{N13}$ by recording with the 'active' electrode over the cervical spine and the 'reference' on the scalp. In clinical practice, however, the large negative-going potential recorded with just such a montage can be profoundly attenuated by lesions which leave the cortical SEP (and therefore presumably the dorsal columns and medial lemniscus, see Halliday and Wakefield, 1963; Noël and Desmedt, 1975) intact. This phenomenon has been reported in cases of multiple sclerosis (Small et al, 1978; see also Figure 13.8, next chapter) and syringomyelia (Mastaglia et al, 1978). One must therefore conclude that the origin of $\overline{P13}$ remains obscure, although $\overline{N13}$ is very likely to be generated in the spinal grey matter.

In numerous published accounts, including those by Nakanishi et al (1978) and Sances et al (1978), no distinction is made between $\overline{P13}$, approximately symmetrically distributed across the scalp, and an overlapping potential ($\overline{P15}$) which is slightly lateralized over the parietal cortex contralateral to the stimulated arm and can be distinguished in many subjects by the use of a mid-frontal reference which effectively cancels $\overline{P13}$ (see Figure 12.6). $\overline{P15}$ may also be associated with a negative potential ($\overline{N14}$) of maximal amplitude in the upper neck region. $\overline{N14}$ is difficult to record in isolation from $\overline{P15}$ but is sometimes clearly seen with a non-cephalic reference (Jones, 1977, see Figure 12.2). Although $\overline{P15}$ may occur slightly later than $\overline{N14}$ in some subjects the amplitudes can be summated by recording from the mastoid process with reference to the parietal scalp contralateral to the stimulated arm (Matthews et al, 1974).

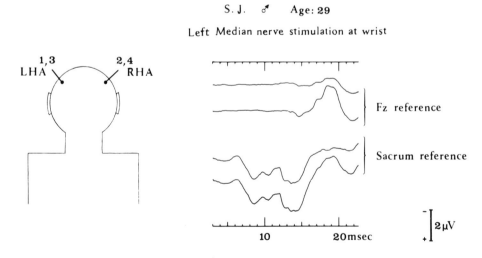

S. J. ♂ Age: 29

Left Median nerve stimulation at wrist

1,3 LHA   2,4 RHA

Fz reference

Sacrum reference

2 μV

10   20 msec

Figure 12.6 Subcortical and early cortical SEP components, recorded over the left and right somatosensory cortical hand area with reference to F_z (cancelling all subcortical potentials preceding $\overline{P15}$) and the sacrum.

In the scalp recordings obtained from monkeys by Arezzo et al (1979) both of the two positive potentials thought to originate in the brainstem lemniscal pathway had a slightly asymmetrical (contralateral) distribution, and were attenuated by frequencies of repetitive stimulation which had little effect on the initial positive wave (thought to arise presynaptically in the dorsal columns). The third positivity was coincident with unit activity in the medial lemniscus and ventral thalamus. It seems reasonable to propose, therefore, that $\overline{N14}$ may reflect postsynaptic events in the brainstem cuneate nucleus, while $\overline{P15}$ is due to the associated positive field, maximally recorded in advance of propagated activity in the medial lemniscus. This is consistent with the clinical observations of Nakanishi et al (1978), who found that a '$\overline{P15}$' potential recorded from the scalp referred to the earlobe (actually an amalgam of $\overline{P13}$ and $\overline{P15}$) was reduced or abolished by lesions involving the brainstem but not by thalamic or suprathalamic lesions. An animal analogue of the combined $\overline{P13}/\overline{P15}$ potential, recorded with the same montage in the monkey by Sances et al (1978), was abolished by section of the cervical cord but not by a cut at mid-pontine level, consistent with a generator in the lower brainstem. There have been at least two accounts describing evoked potentials recorded intracerebrally from the region of the medial lemniscus in man, but the latencies are somewhat vaguely quoted as 12-18 msec (Larson and Sances, 1968) or 10-16 msec (Liberson et al, 1970) following median nerve stimulation at the wrist.

Thalamus

Since it now seems probable that all the recently identified subcortical SEP components ($\overline{N9}$ to $\overline{P15}$) are in fact of subthalamic origin it appears necessary to examine the scalp 'cortical' waveform in more detail than has often been attempted in order to identify potentials originating in the thalamus and thalamocortical radiation. When the early components are largely cancelled by the use of a reference also on the scalp the sequence of waves recorded over the post-Rolandic somatosensory cortex commences with a negative peak at 18-21 msec latency ($\overline{N20}$), although there is frequently a shoulder on the rising edge 1-2 msec earlier. In respect of latency, therefore, the most likely candidate for a potential arising in the thalamus would seem to be the shoulder on the rising edge of $\overline{N20}$. Such a suggestion was made by Abbruzzese et al (1978), who found that two small negativities preceding $\overline{N20}$ ($\overline{N16}$ and $\overline{N17}$) were more widely distributed than the main peak, and were therefore unlikely to be simply due to the arrival of a slightly faster projection to the sensory cortex.

During the course of stereotaxic surgery for the relief of dyskinesia or intractable pain, Ervin and Mark (1964) placed electrodes in the medial and lateral nuclei of the ventro-posterior thalamus, recording a positive-going potential in response to various forms of stimulation which had a latency of 17 msec from the contralateral hand. It is not clear, however, whether the latency quoted was for onset or for peak. The initial wave was followed by a large negative/positive diphasic potential with a duration of approximately 50 msec. From the same nuclei Pagni (1967) was able to record an initially positive wave with latency (probably of onset) 13-16 msec after median nerve stimulation at the wrist, preceding the first (positive) potential recorded directly from the surface of the cortex by approximately 2 msec. A second positive thalamic deflection occurring 8 msec later was present only with strong stimuli of long duration, and was abolished under pentothal anaesthesia. Larson and Sances (1968) obtained a positive/negative biphasic response from the VPL nucleus 12-18 msec (again the values quoted are probably for onset latency) after a stimulus delivered to the wrist, although in this case the negative peak was said to coincide with $\overline{\text{N20}}$ recorded from the scalp. Similar latencies were obtained by McComas et al (1970) for unit activity in nucleus ventralis oralis posterior, in response to light touch and joint movement as well as median nerve stimulation at the wrist. Mathews et al (1970) obtained responses from the VPM nucleus which consisted of a positive peak at 16.5 msec followed by a small negativity at 20.5 msec and a second positivity at 25.0 msec. The initial positive peak latency in the VPL nucleus was 20.5 msec.

The most extensive published study to date is that of Fukushima et al (1976), who recorded positive-going potentials with mean peak latencies of 15.6 and 17.5 msec from two thalamic nuclei (nuc. ventro-caudalis and nuc. ventro-caudalis parvocellularis) following median nerve stimulation at the wrist. Responses of much longer latency were recorded from various thalamic nuclei, some of which responded to stimulation of the ipsilateral as well as the contralateral hand (see also Larson and Sances, 1968). Latencies of potentials recorded from nuc. ventro-caudalis were closely related to $\overline{\text{N20}}$ latency but were consistently shorter by 1-2 msec.

Hume and Cant (1978) reported one case in whom the potentials recorded from the ventroposterior thalamus in response to stimulation at the wrist consisted of a positive peak at 16.3 msec followed by a negativity at 19.8 msec, both preceding the scalp $\overline{\text{N20}}$ which occurred at 21.6 msec. Celesia (1979), however, concurred with earlier accounts in describing a monophasic positive-going thalamic potential with a peak latency of 17-18.7 msec, preceding $\overline{\text{N20}}$ by 1-2 msec.

Although in two of these studies (Larson and Sances, 1968; Mathews et al, 1970) negative-going thalamic potentials were recorded at a latency similar to that of $\overline{\text{N20}}$, in a third (Hume and Cant, 1978) the thalamic negativity preceded $\overline{\text{N20}}$ by approximately 2 msec. In all the other accounts described above the initial thalamic activity (at less than 20 msec latency) was positive in polarity and preceded the initial cortical potential by 1-2 msec. It is sometimes not clear whether latency values quoted were for onset or for peak but in the majority of cases the initial thalamic response must have occurred between 15.5 and 19 msec following stimulation at the wrist. This is slightly later than $\overline{\text{P15}}$ but appropriate, perhaps, for the shoulder on the rising edge of $\overline{\text{N20}}$. The apparent failure to agree on the polarity of early thalamic activity may be due to minor differences in the placement of intracerebral electrodes, compounded by source/sink effects within the thalamus and the thalamocortical radiation.

WAVEFORM AND ORIGIN OF CORTICAL SEP COMPONENTS

The most detailed description of the scalp topography of SEP components from $\overline{\text{P15}}$ onwards is that of Goff et al (1977), although some earlier accounts are not entirely superceded. Succeeding $\overline{\text{P15}}$ a total of 19 components were identified, of which 2 or 3 were thought to be myogenic artifacts generated in the muscles of the scalp, face and neck. The first negative wave ($\overline{\text{N20}}$) was fairly widely distributed over

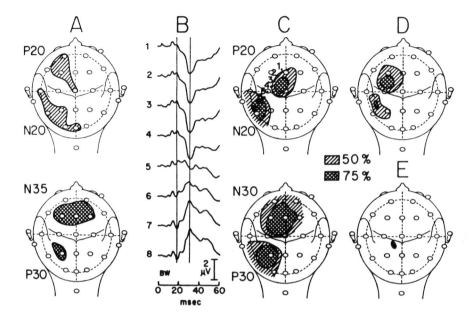

Figure 12.7 *Scalp topography of early SEP components. A: Distribution of $\overline{N20}$, $\overline{P20}$, $\overline{P30}$ and $\overline{N35}$. Pooled data from 12 subjects. B: Scalp recording from a selected subject who shows polarity inversion of the postcentral $\overline{N20}$–$\overline{P30}$ complex anterior to the central sulcus; responses are from an anterior-posterior array orthogonal to the central sulcus as shown in C. Iso-latency lines at 19 and 31 msec. C: 75% and 50% iso-potential maps, based on responses in B plus data from electrode arrays parallel to the one shown. D: predicted scalp topography for potentials generated by hypothetical dipole source located in the posterior bank of the central sulcus 7 cm from the midline. E: Calculated location of generators producing the evoked activity in B in the latency range from 20 to 40 msec. (From Allison et al, 1980.)*

the posterior quadrant of the scalp contralateral to the stimulated arm, while a potential of similar latency but opposite polarity ($\overline{P20}$) could sometimes be recorded from the anterior quadrant (see Figure 12.7). Broughton (1967) was the first to notice this apparent reversal of polarity, which is better seen at operation with electrodes on the exposed cortical surface, and may be noticed in the records of Hirsch et al (1961) and Kelly et al (1965). In infants the initial negativity is more prominent, and the antero-posterior phase reversal may be clearly seen in scalp surface recordings (see Figure 12.8). It was Broughton's hypothesis that $\overline{N20}$/$\overline{P20}$ and a later component ($\overline{P30}$/$\overline{N30}$), which also exhibits its reversal of polarity between posterior and anterior quadrants, constitute the 'primary' response of the somatosensory cortex. In animals cortical evoked potentials usually assume a positive/negative biphasic configuration when the active area is on the superficial surface, close to the recording electrode (Bartley and Bishop, 1933), but Broughton

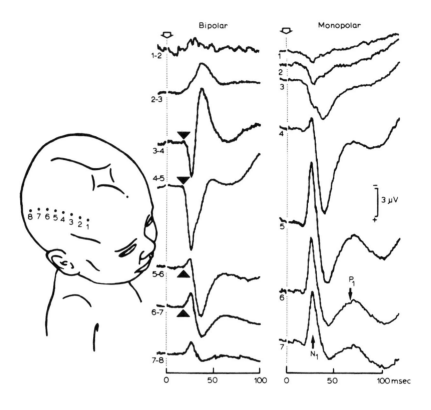

Figure 12.8 *Somatosensory evoked potentials recorded in a normal baby, aged 5 days. Electrode separation 15 mm, mid-frontal reference on right, bipolar derivation on left. (From Manil et al, 1967.)*

(1967) suggested that in man the primary cortical SEP generator may be located deep in the posterior wall of the central sulcus. If the neuronal columns are thereby oriented horizontally, then an electrode situated over the postcentral gyrus will be closer to the deep end of the columns and record the primary response with inverted polarity. This theory was examined by Allison et al (1980, see also Goff et al, 1978) and found to be consistent with recordings obtained from the pial surface in human neurosurgical patients. The observed (scalp) distribution of $\overline{P30}/\overline{N30}$ was also shown to be consistent with the computed electrical field of a point dipole source, horizontally oriented and located in the region of the central sulcus, assuming the brain to be a uniform conducting medium surrounded by two concentric spheres (representing bone and skin) of different conductivities (Goff et al, 1978). There are other authors, however, who dispute Broughton's theory on the grounds that the frontal $\overline{P20}$ is in fact of slightly longer latency than $\overline{N20}$ and more widely distributed, contralateral and ipsilateral to the stimulated arm (for example Kritchevsky and Wiederholt, 1978, Papakostopoulos and Crow, 1980). It has also been observed by Noël and Desmedt (1980) that $\overline{N30}$ may be affected by lesions of the precentral cortex which leave $\overline{P30}$ apparently intact. This suggests there may be a second generator area situated in the precentral cortex, receiving its input either from a second thalamocortical radiation or via transcortical projection from the postcentral gyrus.

In a substantial proportion of the subjects studied by Giblin (1964) the $\overline{P30}$ potential was preceded by another positivity ($\overline{P25}$) with a slightly different distribution over the post-central gyrus. It has been suggested by Allison et al (1980) that $\overline{P25}$ and a succeeding negativity ($\overline{N35}$) may represent the response of a further 'primary' receiving area, situated on the crown of the post-central gyrus and giving rise to a biphasic response of conventional polarity (positive/negative) on the scalp surface. The longer latency of this response may be explained by the possibility of a group of smaller diameter fibres projecting to the cortex from the ventro-postero-lateral nuclei of the thalamus (Jones and Powell, 1970). Even with the likelihood of at least 3 generator areas this model does not explain all the known properties of the $\overline{N20}/\overline{P25}/\overline{P30}$ sequence (for example in the recordings of Giblin (1964) $\overline{P25}$ was evoked by less intense stimuli than were required to elicit $\overline{P30}$), but it is now widely accepted that the potentials occurring between 20 and 30 msec after an electrical stimulus to the median nerve at the wrist are likely to originate in a restricted area of cortex which may be regarded as the primary sensory receiving area of the hand.

By stimulating at the wrist and the elbow it can be demonstrated that the $\overline{N20}/\overline{P25}/\overline{P30}$ complex is mediated (as are all subcortical potentials) by large diameter peripheral axons conducting at approximately 60-75 m/sec in the forearm (Desmedt and Noël, 1973; Allison et al, 1980). Fibres of this conduction velocity are mainly concerned with tactile sensibility, although many convey proprioceptive information from joint receptors and secondary sensory endings in the muscle spindles. On entry to the CNS collaterals are sent off which synapse in the spinal grey matter, but a large proportion of axons are continued centrally in the dorsal columns before synapsing in the cuneate nucleus of the brainstem. Halliday and Wakefield (1963) found that patients with spinal cord lesions causing impairment of joint-position sense (and therefore presumed to have involvement of the dorsal columns) had SEPs which were delayed, attenuated or absent, whereas no SEP abnormalities were found in patients where there was impairment of pain and temperature sensation alone. Giblin (1964) and Fukushima and Mayanagi (1975) have since confirmed these findings, and Namerow (1969) reported that the SEP waveform was unchanged following surgical section of the spinothalamic tracts. Noël and Desmedt (1975) studied patients with vascular lesions of the lateral medulla or ventrolateral thalamus (causing loss of pain and temperature sensation) and found the SEP waveform to be unaltered, whereas other brainstem and thalamic lesions causing impairment of joint-position sense did result in delayed or attenuated SEPs. Cryogenic ablation of the VPL region of the thalamus (which receives input from the dorsal columns via the cuneate nucleus) was found to abolish all cortically generated SEP components of up to 125 msec latency (Domino et al, 1965), while there was no effect of lesions involving other thalamic nuclei. Finally, in support of what may be termed the 'one-track' model of SEP generation, Stohr and Goldring (1969) reported that all potentials recorded from the cortical surface during surgery were abolished by surgical excision of the hand area of the primary sensorimotor cortex. This is compatible with an observation by Williamson et al (1970), that in patients with vascular lesions involving the cerebral hemispheres at or above thalamic level all the scalp-recorded SEP components were affected to an equal degree or not at all. This suggested, not only that the primary hand area is essential for the mediation of all cortically generated SEP components, but also that all components are likely to originate within a small area of cortex, since none were selectively abolished by lesions involving other areas.

With regard to the last observation, however, there is now conflicting evidence from at least three groups of Japanese workers studying the effects of cerebrovascular disease. Miyoshi et al (1971) used the data of Lueders (1970) to define normal limits in several age ranges, and was able to demonstrate cortical SEP abnormalities in a large proportion of cerebrovascular patients. In the majority of cases, however, the early components (particularly $\overline{N20}$) remained within normal limits, particularly when sensory loss was confined to the modalities of temperature and pain. Shibasaki et al (1977) reported that early SEP components were affected only when there was evidence that the internal capsule was involved, whereas later components were abnormal even with lesions confined to the frontal cortex. Tsumoto et al (1973) found specific abnormalities of the $\overline{N35}$ and $\overline{P45}$ components in 5 out 6 cases with diminished pain and temperature sensibility alone, caused by cerebrovascular lesions at or above thalamic level. The same authors described one case in whom late potentials were absent over the affected hemisphere following stimulation of either arm, while early potentials were bilaterally normal. This conflicts with the earlier findings of Giblin (1964), Larson et al (1966a) and Williamson et al (1970), all of whom failed to demonstrate a dissociation between early and late SEP components as a result of cerebrovascular lesions. Giblin (1964), however, noted the presence of 'extra' components at 35-65 msec latency for some cases in whom the lesion caused no sensory loss.

The possibility that a functional relationship might exist between late components of the cortical SEP waveform and the sensory modalities of temperature and pain has been investigated more directly by the use of thermal and noxious evoking stimuli. Duclaux et al (1974) were able to record scalp potentials in response to rapid cooling of the hand, although not to warming. A positive potential of about 325 msec latency and 200-325 msec duration was maximal over the cortical hand area contralateral to the stimulated arm. A negative-going potential evoked by skin cooling was recorded by Frühstorfer et al (1976), with a mean peak latency of about 400 msec from the hand and 230 msec from the lip, suggesting a peripheral conduction velocity in the order of 4-5 m/sec. Less consistently it was possible to record a response to warming the same area of skin, with an even longer latency suggesting a conduction velocity of about 2.5 m/sec. A skin-warming response was obtained with slightly shorter latency by Chatt and Kenshalo (1977), who also recorded a smaller, later wave from the hemisphere ipsilateral to the stimulated hand. Using a stimulus consisting of the rapid transfer of hot and cold water in a closed tank, with the hand in contact with the external surface, these authors appear to have overcome the main practical difficulty of obtaining an evoked response to thermal stimulation, which is the production of an abrupt but essentially 'pure' stimulus without any likelihood of mechanical deformation of the skin.

There is now considerable evidence that pain may be regarded as a true sensory modality, mediated (at least in part) by small myelinated and unmyelinated fibres sensitive to stimuli which damage or threaten to damage the bodily tissue. It has been reported that electrical stimulation of the tooth pulp gives rise to an impression of pure pain (that is, without any element of touch, thermal sensation, etc.), and using this technique Chatrian et al (1975) were able to record a sequence of potentials from the midline of the scalp at 43 to 250 msec latency (Figure 12.9).

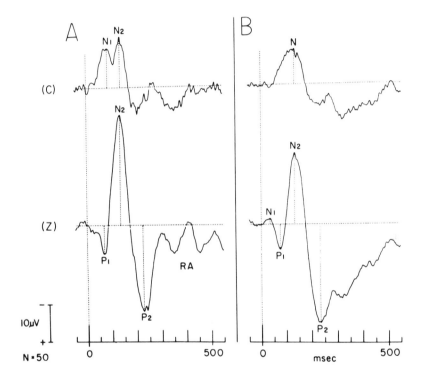

Figure 12.9 *Somatosensory evoked potentials recorded over low contralateral postcentral (C) and midline (Z) areas in response to stimulation of the tooth pulp (inion reference). Examples of waveform in 2 normal subjects (A and B). (From Chatrian et al, 1975.)*

These waves were topographically distinct from a negativity (occasionally bifid) at 80 to 150 msec latency which was bilaterally distributed in the low postcentral region but of slightly longer latency on the ipsilateral side. All the potentials were abolished by local anaesthesia, and none were present in a subject who was congenitally indifferent to pain. A similar technique was used by Chen et al (1979), who showed that the amplitude of the earlier midline potentials ($\overline{N65}$, $\overline{P120}$ and $\overline{N175}$) was related to the objective intensity of the stimulus, whereas that of two later peaks ($\overline{P260}$ and $\overline{N340}$) was correlated with the subjective intensity of the pain.

More controversially Carmon et al (1976) and Stowell (1977) studied the responses to noxious thermal (laser beam) and electrical stimulation of the forearm and hand. Carmon et al (1976) recorded a negative/positive wave of about 160 and 270 msec latency which was maximal at the vertex and was correlated in amplitude with the subjective intensity of pain (although the objective stimulus intensity remained constant). It is not possible to decide, however, whether this was a primary 'pain' response due to activation of specific cortical areas, a non-specific 'arousal' response mediated by the brainstem reticular formation, or an 'attentional' response analogous to the vertex potentials discussed by Hillyard and Picton (1978). Similar uncertainty surrounds the 'dominant positive complex' of Stowell (1977) which had a latency of 170 to 290 msec and an amplitude which was related to the subjective intensity of pain rather than to the objective intensity of a cutaneous electric shock. A major disadvantage of both these studies was that the stimuli were likely to have activated all manner of cutaneous receptors in addition to specific nociceptors. The findings may yet be of interest in the context of pain research, but at this time it is difficult to conceive of any likely clinical applications.

Other relevant studies of long latency SEP components in normal individuals include that of Yamada et al (1977), who found that ischaemia of the arm (induced by inflation of a pressure cuff and causing a progressive loss of vibration and joint-position sense in the hand) produced a gradual change in the waveform of the cortical SEP following median nerve stimulation at the wrist. The initial effect was attenuation of 'N_1' (20 msec latency) and 'N_4' (135 msec) but relative preservation of 'N_2' (30 msec) and 'N_3' (64 msec) components. After a further period of ischaemia, during which there was a gradual impairment of all sensory modalities, barring long latency pain perception, only a slow negative potential was evoked by high intensity median nerve shocks.

Nakanishi et al (1974) followed the example of, among others, Halliday and Mason (1964), Franzen and Offenloch (1965), Posthumus Meyjes (1969) and Larsson and Prevec (1970) in stimulating the fingers with a mechanical tap in an attempt to produce SEPs by specific activation of mechano-receptive fibres. It was found that the responses to skin tapping were very similar to those produced by a pinprick on the same area of skin, each having a major positive component at 32-36 msec latency. The responses to both stimuli were reported to be abnormal in 7 out of 8 patients with spinal cord and brainstem lesions causing impairment of pain and temperature perception but no loss of joint-position sense. Although the study did not achieve a dissociation between tap- and pinprick-evoked responses, the results did suggest that cutaneous afferents might contribute to the SEP waveform via pathways other than the dorsal column/medial lemniscal system, which was presumably unaffected in these patients. An alternative explanation might be, however, that abnormality of the mechanically-evoked SEP is simply a more sensitive sign of a dorsal column lesion than is the clinical impairment of joint-position sense. Many years earlier it had been observed by Alajouanine et al (1958) that cortical SEPs following low intensity electrical stimuli were of abnormal waveform in 2 out of 4 patients with loss of 'spinothalamic' type sensation caused by a unilateral brainstem lesion (Wallenberg syndrome), but of normal configuration following high intensity shocks. Once again, however, the most likely explanation would appear to be that low intensity stimulation was effective in revealing minimal involvement of the lemniscal pathway.

Other properties of the middle latency ($\overline{\text{P45}}$ on) and late cortical SEP components provide few clues as to whether all depend on prior activation of the primary sensory cortex via the dorsal columns and the medial lemniscus, or whether some are mediated by slower conducting multisynaptic pathways. It was reported by Giblin (1964) that the component with the lowest stimulus intensity threshold was $\overline{\text{P45}}$, and this component has also been found particularly sensitive to surgical anaesthesia (Clark and Rosner, 1973; see below). The scalp distribution of $\overline{\text{P45}}$ is wider than that of $\overline{\text{P30}}$, mainly in the medial and anterior directions (Goff et al, 1977). It is possible, therefore, (as suggested by Giblin, 1964), that $\overline{\text{P45}}$ may represent an early 'association' response generated outside the primary somatosensory receiving area but dependent on the integrity of the latter. After $\overline{\text{P45}}$ the potentials become more widespread with even less certainty as to their origin. A 'somatic late response' ($\overline{\text{P100}}$ and $\overline{\text{N200}}$, Goff et al, 1978) has a distribution similar to that of the earliest cortical potentials when recorded from the pial surface and, like them, shows an inversion of polarity anterior and posterior to the central sulcus. Although the origin and significance of this wave remain obscure, it is likely to be a separate entity from the specific potentials of similar latency evoked by thermal stimuli, and from the vertex potential ($\overline{\text{N140}}/\overline{\text{P190}}$, Goff et al, 1977) which is non-specific in so far as similar waves can be recorded following visual and auditory stimulation (see Hillyard and Picton, 1978; Hillyard et al, 1978). The latter and other 'cognitive' EP components are described elsewhere in this volume.

SEP COMPONENTS RECORDED FROM THE IPSILATERAL HEMISPHERE

Although the sequence of subcortically-generated potentials at 9-15 msec latency is recorded by electrodes on the ipsilateral as well as the contralateral side of the scalp, there is a divergence of opinion as to whether 'specific' cortically-generated potentials can be recorded by ipsilateral electrodes. Tamura (1972) and Salamy (1978) both reported the existence of ipsilateral responses which were delayed by 4-8 msec (in adults) compared with the contralateral waveform. Tamura (1972) found no interhemispheric latency difference for 'P$_1$' ($\overline{\text{P15}}$), but succeeding components ($\overline{\text{N20}}$, $\overline{\text{P30}}$, $\overline{\text{N35}}$ and $\overline{\text{P45}}$ contralaterally) were of longer latency by 4.5-6.7 msec on the ipsilateral side in a group of subjects aged 9-18 years, and by 5.5-7.9 msec in a group aged 19-20 years. The ipsilateral components were less consistently recorded than their contralateral counterparts, but were quantifiable in terms of amplitude and latency in 50-70% of recordings. Other authors have been unable to replicate these findings (for example, see Tsumoto et al, 1973; Goff et al, 1977), and it is conceivable that in Tamura's study activity at the reference location (the ear, although whether ipsilateral or contralateral to the stimulated arm was not stated) may have contributed to the 'ipsilateral' waveform.

Salamy (1978) recorded potentials from the ipsilateral and contralateral scalp (with the reference electrode on the midline) in response to an unusual vibratory stimulus of 50 msec duration, delivered to the index finger. The initial positive potential (occurring at approximately 40 msec) and succeeding negativity and positivity were present on either side of the scalp, but the ipsilateral latencies were longer by 20-28 msec in a group of children aged 4-5 years. In adults the latency difference was only 4-8 msec — comparable with values obtained by Tamura (1972). Both authors suggested the latency difference might be a manifestation of interhemispheric conduction time through the corpus callosum.

Further evidence concerning the origin of potentials possibly generated in the ipsilateral hemisphere comes from the effect of unilateral cerebrovascular lesions. Larson et al (1966a) found that all components were absent when the recording electrode was located over the damaged hemisphere and the unaffected (ipsilateral) arm was stimulated. In a similar investigation performed by Liberson (1966) the potentials recorded over the intact hemisphere following stimulation of the ipsilateral (affected) arm were abolished when the responses of the involved hemisphere to the same stimulus were severely abnormal. Tamura (1972) found that with stimulation of the affected arm all ipsilateral and contralateral potentials were abolished while, in contrast to the findings of Larson et al (1966), those produced by stimulation of the intact arm were fully preserved. Although these studies are not in complete agreement (and do not resolve the main issue as to whether ipsilateral responses normally exist at all) they are all compatible with the existence of a transcallosal projection from the contralateral hemisphere, rather than a separate ipsilateral ascending pathway.

Contrary to the above conclusion, however, there is evidence that in some cases of hemispherectomy long latency potentials may be recorded over the intact hemisphere following stimulation of the ipsilateral (affected) arm (Hazemann et al, 1969; Matsumita et al, 1971, although not supported by Stohr and Goldring, 1969 or Noël and Desmedt, 1980). This seems to imply the existence of a direct projection to the ipsilateral hemisphere. It might be argued that abnormal development takes place in patients with a hemispherectomy performed relatively early in life, and that such ipsilateral projections may be undeveloped in normal adults, but Fukushima et al (1976) have demonstrated that evoked potentials can be recorded from certain nuclei of the human thalamus (nuc. centrum medianum, dorso-medialis, ventro-lateralis and pulvinar) following stimulation of the ipsilateral as well as the contralateral arm. The ipsilateral responses were of longer latency, suggesting that they may first rely on a projection to the contralateral thalamus followed by interhemispheric transfer at subcortical level.

EFFECTS OF REPETITIVE STIMULATION

By delivering pairs of electrical stimuli to a nerve trunk and varying the inter-stimulus interval (ISI), Allison (1962) found that the generator of the initial negative potential (N20) appeared to be fully recovered 200 msec after the first stimulus, while long latency potentials required an ISI of at least 2 sec. Additionally, however, both Allison (1962) and Shagass and Schwartz (1961) found that the 'recovery

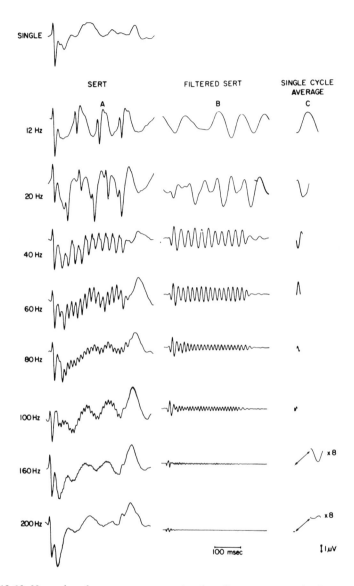

Figure 12.10 *Normal scalp response to a train of median nerve stimuli, duration 250 msec, frequency 12-200 Hz. The response was filtered to exclude all frequencies but a narrow band centred on the stimulation frequency, and the oscillatory response so obtained was reduced to a single cycle by averaging. (From Namerow et al, 1974.)*

function' of the amplitude of the second response against ISI was 'U' shaped. The amplitude of $\overline{P27}$ measured from the peak of $\overline{N20}$ following ulnar nerve stimulation at the wrist was fully recovered or even slightly enhanced when the 'test' impulse was delivered as little as 17.5 msec after the 'conditioning' stimulus, but was depressed at longer intervals between 20 and approximately 110 msec (Shagass and Schwartz, 1961). At short ISIs, however, it was apparent that the response to the second stimulus was contaminated by longer latency potentials evoked by the first, and therefore a waveform subtraction technique was employed, whereby the response to a single stimulus alternately presented with the doublets could be subtracted from the doublet response waveform (Schwartz and Shagass, 1964). At the neuronal level, however, it is possible that the later activity evoked by the first stimulus of the doublet may be influenced in some way by the arrival of the second volley, and may therefore not be identical to the corresponding activity evoked by an isolated stimulus, even allowing for the fact that the recorded waveform is distorted by the algebraic summation of two responses. Under such circumstances the waveform subtraction technique may not reveal the potentials attributable to the second stimulus without residual contamination.

Namerow et al (1974) studied the cortical response to trains of stimuli delivered to the median nerve at the wrist. A waveform was obtained in which an oscillatory potential at the intra-train frequency was apparently superimposed on a sequence of slower potentials evoked by the initial stimulus (see Figure 12.10). By filtering the waveform to exclude all frequencies but those within a narrow bandwidth centred on the intra-train stimulus frequency, and condensing the resultant oscillatory waveform to a single cycle by an averaging technique, it was possible to derive a function for oscillatory potential amplitude against intra-train stimulus frequency. This function was found to be a sensitive index of somatosensory system involvement in multiple sclerosis (Sclabassi et al, 1974). The scalp distribution of the oscillatory potential was similar to that of the early cortical SEP components ($\overline{N20}$ to $\overline{P45}$). Measurement of the phase angle of the oscillatory response with respect to the stimuli revealed a difference between responses recorded pre- and postcentrally, suggesting to the authors that more than one area of cortex might be active. However, this phenomenon might simply be analogous to the phase reversal of early components reported by Broughton (1967), and attributed to a single dipolar source.

MYOGENIC SEP COMPONENTS

The possibility that neurogenic evoked potentials might be distorted by stimulus-related activity in the scalp and neck musculature has received considerable attention, following the work of Bickford et al (1964) who established that the $\overline{N15}$ and $\overline{P20}$ components evoked by auditory click stimuli were enhanced by voluntary tension in the neck muscles, and were in fact due to a fast reflex loop involving the post-auricular muscle. In the somatosensory modality Cracco and Bickford (1968) found that stimulus-bound myogenic artifacts were present even in relaxed subjects, with a latency and scalp distribution similar to some neurogenic potentials. In the topographic study of Goff et al (1977), however, although 2 or 3 of the 21 components identified were thought to be of myogenic origin, only a positive wave at a latency of approximately 65 msec was of similar distribution to cortically generated potentials, and there was thought to be little contamination of the more important short latency components. Spontaneous EMG activity can, of course, cause distortion of any component, but this is in theory surmountable by achieving sufficient relaxation and averaging sufficiently large numbers of sweeps.

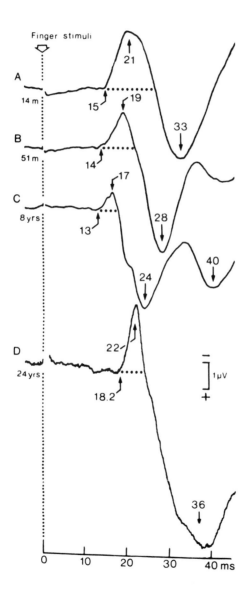

Figure 12.11 *Comparison of scalp SEPs to stimulation of the contralateral hand (forehead reference) in normal humans aged 14 months, 51 months, 8 years and 24 years. (From Desmedt et al, 1976.)*

MATURATIONAL CHANGES

The SEP waveform recorded from the scalp of the human neonate is considerably different from that of the adult, with a later and more prominent initial negative potential (onset at approximately 23 msec and duration 15 msec following stimulation of the fingers), sometimes exhibiting a clear inversion of polarity between the contralateral posterior and anterior quadrants (Manil et al, 1967). The initial negativity (probably equivalent to $\overline{N20}$) undergoes a progressive reduction of amplitude and duration throughout infancy and childhood (Desmedt et al, 1976). Onset latency, however, shows an initial rapid reduction during the first few months, followed by a period of relative constancy up to at least 8 years (Hrbek et al, 1968; Desmedt et al, 1976; see Figure 12.11). There is then a gradual increase to adult latency values in the mid to late teens. Allowing for increasing body size, the maturation of afferent sensory pathway conduction velocity (peripheral and central) measured to the onset of $\overline{N20}$ is apparently complete at age 7-8 years, although the amplitude and duration of $\overline{N20}$ undergo further maturational changes independent of bodily growth.

At the other end of the age spectrum Lueders (1970) found no significant effect of ageing on the first and fourth positive-going SEP components studied (mean peak latencies 33 and 300 msec), but a significant latency increase for two intervening positive peaks at approximately 45 and 100 msec. This was, however, with a fairly short inter-stimulus interval of 1.25 sec, and may have been due to the effect of ageing on the recovery functions of these components rather than their absolute latencies. Beck et al (1975) found a more generalized latency increase in old age, together with a reduction in the amplitude of the late components.

Desmedt and Cheron (1980) found no increase in central sensory conduction time (separation between cervical and cortical SEP components following median nerve stimulation) in a group of octogenarians as compared with a group of subjects aged 20-25 years, although the peripheral sensory nerve action potentials were relatively delayed and of reduced amplitude. In this study the initial negative potential of the cortical SEP was slightly larger in the octogenarian group. Allison et al (1979) examined the relationship between age and latency for the early SEP components, incorporating data from other published accounts in addition to newly acquired data from subjects aged 10 to 80. There was found to be a marked increase in the latency of all components up to about 25 years of age but little consistent change thereafter.

SEPs IN RESPONSE TO LOWER LIMB STIMULATION

Spinal potentials

In response to stimulation of the posterior tibial nerve in the popliteal fossa, Cracco (1973) recorded a rostrally-moving 'travelling wave', triphasic in the manner of a nerve action potential, which had an apparent conduction velocity of 62-70 m/sec between lower thoracic and cervical recording electrodes. This observation was later confirmed by Jones and Small (1978), with the stimulus delivered at the ankle and the potentials recorded with a bipolar montage ascending the spine. Jones and Small (1978) also recorded a larger negative wave which was apparently of fixed latency in the lower thoracic and upper lumbar region, and was preceded and followed by 'travelling wave' activity in caudal and rostral leads respectively (see Figure 12.12).

In very similar independent studies Delbeke et al (1978) and Dimitrejevic et al (1978) investigated the properties of sacral, lumbar and lower thoracic potentials evoked by tibial nerve stimulation at the knee. At moderate stimulus intensities (optimal for elicitation of the monosynaptic H-reflex) two small negative waves with onset latencies of approximately 9 and 12 msec were recorded by an electrode at S1 vertebral level, while a large negativity of similar latency to the second sacral component was recorded between T11 and L2 (see also El-Negamy and Sedgwick, 1978). The latter wave and the earlier sacral potential showed a progressive increase in amplitude as the stimulus strength was increased to a level which produced a maximal direct motor response, while the second sacral component was diminished along with the H-reflex. The sacral potentials were thought to reflect afferent and efferent volleys in the roots of the cauda equina, connected via a monosynaptic reflex arc, while the more rostral negativity was thought to originate in the grey matter of the spinal cord. The recordings were remarkably similar to those obtained by Magladery et al (1951) using an intrathecal placement of electrodes, and were interpreted in a similar fashion. In the study of Dimitrejevic et al (1978) the relatively long refractory period of the rostral negativity (maximal over the T12 vertebra) was evidence in favour of a postsynaptic origin, perhaps equivalent to that of the N_1 potential recorded from the dorsum of the spinal cord in the cat by Gasser and Graham (1933) and Bernhard (1953). In the skin-surface recordings (Dimitrejevic et al, 1978; Delbeke et al, 1978) a late positive wave might, it was thought, have been due to synaptically mediated depolarization of primary sensory terminals, ('primary afferent depolarization', Wall, 1958; Eccles et al, 1962).

There are various similarities and lines of argument which suggest an analogy between the postsynaptic S or N_1 wave recorded from about T11 to L2 vertebral level in response to lower limb stimulation and the cervical $\overline{N13}$ potential following a median nerve stimulus. Both are of negative polarity and have a restricted distribution in the region of the appropriate root entry zone. $\overline{N13}$ has been shown to be bifid in some subjects (Jones, 1977), while Delbeke et al (1978) found that N_1 could also sometimes be resolved into two sub-components. These were thought to arise pre- and postsynaptically in the spinal cord, on account of a similarity with the animal recordings of Austin and McCouch (1955) in which the second subcomponent of N_1 was found to have a longer refractory period. Both subcomponents were more refractory than the preceding spike potential which was believed to originate in the dorsal columns. A human analogue of the latter may be present in the lumbar skin-surface recordings of Delbeke et al (1978) as a shoulder on the rising edge of N_1, while the cervical $\overline{N11}$ potential following median nerve stimulation has a similar relationship with $\overline{N13}$.

With regard to the 'travelling wave' recorded by Cracco (1973) and Jones and Small (1978), the significance of an apparent slight slowing of conduction in the lower thoracic region (Cracco, 1973) must be doubtful owing to the likelihood of distortion by overlap with the larger S or N_1 potential, distributed over several

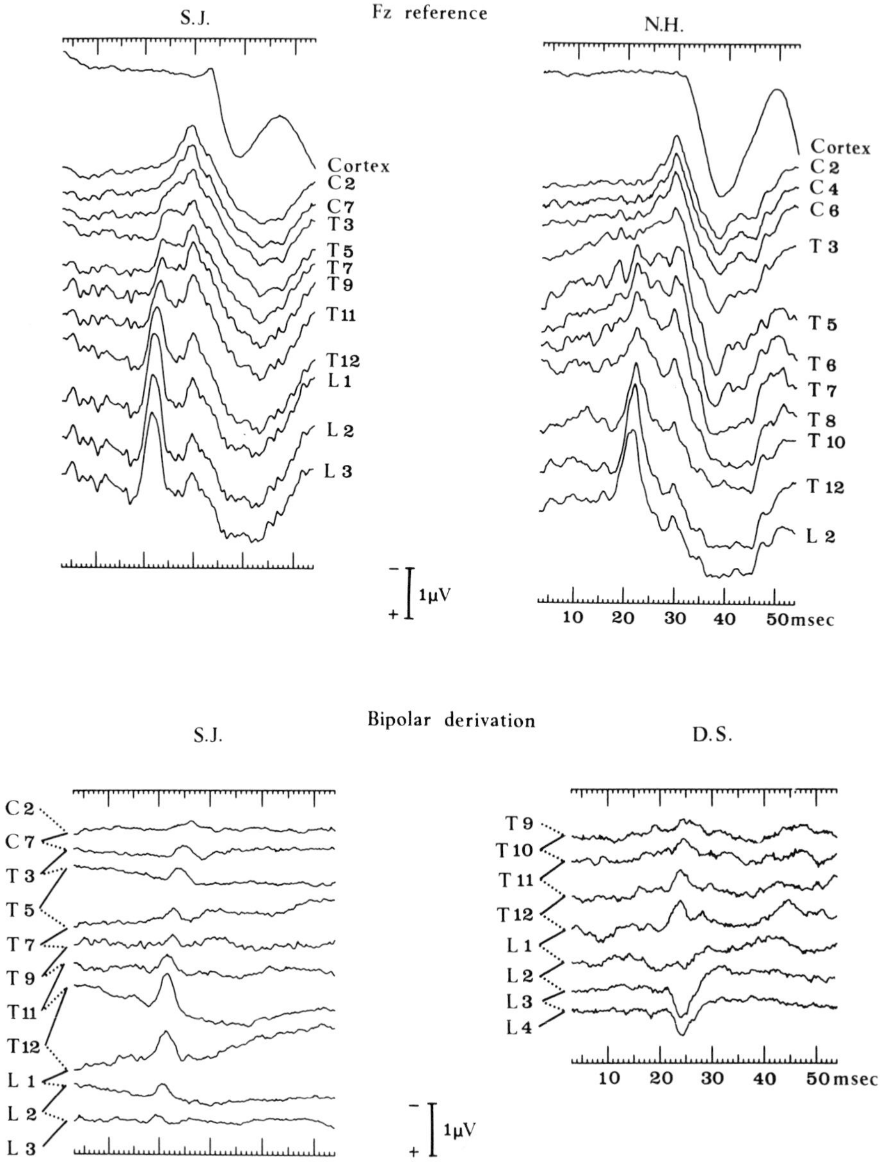

Figure 12.12 *Multi-channel recordings of spinal and cortical SEPs following posterior tibial nerve stimulation at the ankle. The mid-frontal (F$_z$) reference reveals two negative components, maximal in the lumbar and cervical regions respectively, both preceding the onset of the cortical response. The bipolar derivation in SJ (obtained by computer subtraction of adjacent channels in the common reference recording) shows a 'travelling wave' at all spinal levels. In DS the bipolar derivation shows phase reversal of the lumbar negativity (i.e. the point of maximal amplitude in referential recordings) at about L1-2. (From Jones and Small, 1978.)*

vertebrae with a constant latency. The apparent velocity of propagation over sacral and thoracic segments may be thought indicative of the conduction velocity of primary sensory axons in the cauda equina and dorsal columns respectively, but it should be noted that a much slower conduction velocity (30-50 m/sec) was obtained by Ertekin (1976b) from potentials recorded intrathecally. Direct electrical stimulation of the spinal cord has been shown to give rise to at least two distinct potentials recorded epidurally, having conduction velocities of about 75 and 50 m/sec (Tsuyama et al, 1978). Dorfman (1977) used the latency difference between cortical responses to median and posterior tibial nerve stimulation, together with F-wave latencies, to estimate conduction velocity in the human spinal cord. Briefly, the peripheral conduction times in the arm and the leg were estimated as half the corresponding F-wave latencies, and these values were subtracted from cortical response latencies (measured to the onset of the initial negativity for the arm and the initial positivity for the leg) to give measures of central conduction time. Conduction time in the central nervous system (cervical cord to cortex) was assumed to be the same for sensory input from the arm and the leg, and so spinal cord conduction time (over a length which was estimated to be the distance between the L1 and C7 vertebrae, plus half the distance between C7 and the inion) was derived from the difference in central conduction time from the arm and the leg. The conduction velocity arrived at was approximately 55 m/sec — somewhere between the values obtained from spinal skin surface (Cracco, 1973; Jones and Small, 1978) and intrathecal (Ertekin, 1976b) recordings. The indirect method contains several inherent sources of error (for example the approximation of spinal cord length and the use of motor-fibre mediated F-waves to estimate peripheral sensory conduction time) but has been adopted by some workers in the clinical field (Dorfman et al, 1978; Eisen and Nudleman, 1979).

Cracco and colleagues (Cracco et al, 1975, 1979), have examined the maturation of the spinal travelling wave from 34 weeks post-conception to adulthood. At birth the apparent sensory conduction velocities in the peripheral nerve and spinal cord were both about half the adult values, attaining maturity after 3-4 years and 5 years respectively (Cracco et al, 1979).

Dorfman and Bosley (1979) used the indirect method of Dorfman (1977) to study the effect of ageing on spinal cord conduction velocity in man. This was apparently fairly stable between 18 and 60 years, but was considerably reduced in subjects aged 60 to 86 years. Maturation of spinal cord conduction took place independently of the decline in peripheral nerve conduction velocity, which is a progressive change throughout adult life.

Subcortical and cortical potentials

In recordings obtained from the cervical spinal vertebrae with a mid-frontal reference, Jones and Small (1978) identified a negative-going potential following posterior tibial nerve stimulation, which was thought likely to be mainly due to activity of positive polarity at the reference site. The latency of approximately 30 msec was slightly longer than that of the travelling wave in the upper cervical region, suggesting an origin in the brainstem and a possible analogy with subcortical far-field potentials following median nerve stimulation. A similar subcortical positivity was recorded by Cracco (1973), although it was said to occur at roughly the same latency as the travelling wave in the cervical region. As yet there is little further evidence on the origin of this potential, although by analogy with the $\overline{P13}$ and $\overline{P15}$ components following median nerve stimulation it may be a manifestation of evoked activity in the brainstem lemniscal pathway.

Cortical responses evoked by stimulation of the major nerve trunks in the leg have been described by (amongst others) Tsumoto et al (1972), Cracco (1973), Fukushima and Mayanagi (1975), Dorfman (1977) and Jones and Small (1978). Tsumoto et al (1972) performed a thorough topographic analysis of the scalp response to stimulation of the lateral popliteal (common peroneal) nerve at the knee. Using an ear reference the initial recorded potential was a positivity ($\overline{P34}$), thought to be the primary response of the sensorimotor cortex. This and succeeding peaks ($\overline{N45}$, $\overline{P56}$, $\overline{N74}$, $\overline{P99}$, $\overline{N126}$, $\overline{P204}$) were all of near-maximal amplitude on the midline of the scalp approximately 2 cm posterior to the vertex, although the maximum of $\overline{N45}$ was slightly displaced towards the side ipsilateral to the stimulated leg, and the succeeding potentials had a slightly more anterior and sometimes contralateral distribution. In the study of Jones and Small (1978) the peak latency of the first cortical positivity was approximately 40 msec following stimulation at the ankle — clearly comparable with 34 msec from the knee. An initial negative deflection analogous to the median nerve $\overline{N20}$ is seldom present following lower limb stimulation, but has been reported in some subjects (Tsumoto et al, 1972; Jones and Small, 1978). This difference may, perhaps, be due to the location and orientation of the respective cortical generator areas, although the effect of electrical stimulation of the sensory cortex in man (see, for example, Penfield and Boldrey, 1937) suggests that the calf and foot region are most likely to be located on the medial surface of the hemisphere. One might therefore suppose that the dipoles which generate the primary response may be horizontally oriented in much the same manner as those of the primary hand area in the posterior wall of the central sulcus, with the result that an initial positive potential should be recorded over the inactive side and a negativity over the active hemisphere.

SEGMENTAL AND TRIGEMINAL NERVE RESPONSES

The cortical responses to segmental mechanical (Larsson and Prevec, 1970) and electrical (Blair, 1971; Baust and Jörg, 1977) stimulation are of interest mainly with regard to their possible clinical applications, and these are discussed in the next Chapter. Larsson and Prevec (1970), however, noted a progressive reduction in the latency of responses to a tap delivered at more proximal sites, and found that potentials evoked by tapping one side of the face had a bilateral scalp distribution. Cortical responses to segmental cutaneous stimulation are generally smaller and less well formed than median and digital nerve responses, but an early positive wave is reported to be a consistent feature, its latency related to the segmental level of spinal cord input (Schramm and Hashizume, 1977; Baust and Jörg, 1977).

Drechsler et al (1977) recorded a sequence of nine negative and positive potentials over the facial area of the somatosensory cortex following stimulation of the contralateral trigeminal nerve. The first potential ($\overline{N5}$) was believed to originate in the Gasserian ganglion and was abolished along with the succeeding $\overline{P9}$ after thermo-coagulation of that structure. Later potentials starting with $\overline{N13}$ and $\overline{P23}$ were thought to be generated in the cerebral cortex, and have since been described in more detail by Stöhr and Petruch (1979).

13

Somatosensory Evoked Potentials: The Abnormal Waveform

S.J. Jones

Reviewing the literature of the past 20 years it is sometimes difficult to draw a distinction between studies in which SEPs have been used as an aid to clinical investigation (diagnosis, prognosis, management, or pure research into pathological processes) and those in which clinical material has been used to throw light on aspects of the normal response. This reflects, no doubt, the attempt to develop a potentially powerful clinical tool before the underlying principles are fully understood. The author does not apologize for any overlap between this and the previous chapter, since it may serve to emphasize the need for mutual co-operation between neurologist and neurophysiologist if evoked potentials are to be of lasting value in clinical medicine.

Although it was soon established that the scalp-recorded SEP is susceptible to a wide variety of conditions affecting the peripheral and central nervous system, the waveform abnormalities generally lacked specificity in so far as the only variables which behaved independently to any marked degree were amplitude and latency. This situation has been greatly altered by the development of multi-channel recording techniques, and the realization that there are many suitable stimulation sites on the body. The immediate prospect, therefore, is one of renewed expansion as the potentiality of a revitalized technique is gradually explored.

PERIPHERAL NERVE DISORDERS

Although disorders of the peripheral nervous system have sometimes been regarded as the province of the electromyographer, there are many situations in which the SEP technique is both appropriate and of considerable value. Desmedt (1971) has stressed the importance of recording sensory nerve action potentials (SNAPs) from the fingers, wrist, elbow or axilla of the stimulated arm, in association with cortically-generated SEPs, and to this it need only be added that further vital information can often be provided by additional channels recording subcortically-generated SEP components.

Neuropathies, with and without CNS involvement

A typical finding in cases of peripheral sensory neuropathy is a marked attenuation or absence of SNAPs, even when large numbers of sweeps are averaged. The cortical SEP, however, is frequently preserved, albeit with fairly low amplitude and sometimes prolonged latency. Explanations one might advance for the greater robustness of cortically-generated potentials are largely speculative, but it seems reasonable to assume that integrative processes operating at central synapses might lead to an amplification and even a resynchronization of a weak and dispersed afferent volley. Even with SNAPs absent, therefore, it may be possible to obtain a value for peripheral sensory nerve conduction velocity in the surviving fibres from the change in SEP latency when the stimulus is delivered to two or more sites along the arm (see Desmedt, 1971).

Alajouanine et al (1958) reported the absence of cortical responses to stimulation of the foot in a case with a predominantly distal sensory neuropathy. This observation was later enlarged by Giblin (1964), who found SEPs to be absent in the most severe cases of mixed motor and sensory polyneuropathy, correlating with the degree of sensory impairment. However, for 3 patients in whom the sensory disturbance had largely or completely recovered SEPs were present with delayed onset and peak latencies. The difference in SEP latency with stimulation at the wrist compared with the fingers established that the delay could be entirely accounted for by reduced conduction velocity in the peripheral nerve.

In a further case of polyneuropathy documented by Giblin (1964) (sensory loss in the hands and feet with weakness of the arms, elevated motor thresholds and slowed sensory and motor conduction) the cortical response to median nerve stimulation was somewhat delayed at an intensity just sufficient to produce a thumb twitch, but became less so at higher intensities, to a degree much greater than is encountered in normal subjects. This may have been due to an elevation in the activation threshold of the largest (fastest conducting) sensory fibres. However, there was no increase in the amplitude of the SEP as the stimulus intensity was increased, and it is difficult to explain these findings fully with our present understanding of the mechanisms of peripheral neuropathy.

Bergamini et al (1965) investigated patients with a variety of peripheral nerve disorders, ranging from alcoholic neuropathy to a traumatic lesion of the ulnar nerve, and found the SEP latency and duration to be increased in all cases, consistent with a slowing of conduction and increase of temporal dispersion in the peripheral nerve. Delayed SEPs attributable to slowed peripheral nerve conduction have also been described by Desmedt (1971) in a case of infantile metachromatic leucodystrophy, and during recovery from Guillain-Barré polyneuritis.

Combining the evidence of SNAP and SEP recordings, Bergamini et al (1966) were able to demonstrate a distinction between degenerative diseases involving the peripheral nerves, the dorsal columns of the spinal cord or both. A reduction of SNAP amplitude was a consistent feature in cases of Charcot-Marie-Tooth (C-M-T) disease, although the cortical responses were said to be preserved, while only the cortical responses were affected in cases of tabes dorsalis. In Friedreich's ataxia, however, both potentials were of reduced amplitude, delayed and of prolonged duration.

Nine cases of the predominantly demyelinating form of C-M-T disease have recently been described by Noël and Desmedt (1980). Although SNAPs were severely degraded or absent, a slowing of peripheral sensory conduction (most marked in the distal segments) was demonstrated by the change in SEP latency when the stimulus was delivered to the fingers, wrist, elbow or axilla. The interval between subcortical and cortical SEP components was normal, suggesting the absence of CNS involvement.

A single case of Friedreich's ataxia was described by Desmedt and Noël (1973), in which SNAPs were absent while SEPs were of delayed onset latency. The difference in SEP latency with stimulation at the fingers and the axilla was 14-15 msec, which is markedly increased compared with normal subjects (6 msec approximately). Extrapolation of peripheral conduction time to the estimated point of spinal cord entry led the authors to conclude that the SEP delay could not be entirely accounted for by reduced peripheral conduction velocity, and therefore that central conduction must have been delayed also, either in the dorsal columns or elsewhere in the dorsal column/medial lemniscal pathway. In later investigations (Noël and Desmedt, 1976, 1980) the cortical responses of 6 patients were studied in detail by averaging large numbers of sweeps. Onset latency was found to be normal or near-normal, in keeping with a desynchronized SNAP in which the earliest deflection was of normal latency or only slightly delayed, but the initial cortical negativity ($\overline{N20}$) was split into 2 or 3 delayed subcomponents. Once again it was concluded that the pattern of SEP abnormality could not be entirely accounted for by the peripheral neuropathy, and the authors speculated that the apparent doubling or tripling of $\overline{N20}$ might be due to deafferentation followed by collateral re-innervation of thalamic relay neurones, resulting in the formation of reverberating thalamo-cortical circuits. A similar abnormality of the cortical SEP waveform, with SNAPs of very low amplitude, was reported for 6 cases of late spinocerebellar degeneration (Noël and Desmedt, 1980).

With the advent of subcortical SEP recording techniques the pattern of abnormality in Friedreich's ataxia becomes clearer. Both Sauer and Schenck (1977) and Mastaglia et al (1978) reported that the cervical responses to median nerve stimulation were of normal or near-normal latency (although absent in a large proportion of patients), while the cortical waveform was markedly broadened and delayed. We (Jones et al, 1980) have studied 22 Friedreich's cases, in whom it was found that broadened and delayed cortical SEPs (absent in only 2 cases) were mediated by peripheral nerve fibres with normal conduction velocity and no

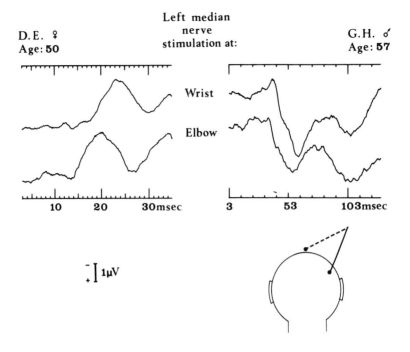

Figure 13.1 Cortical responses to wrist and elbow stimulation in 2 cases of Friedreich's ataxia, showing normal latency shift (less than 4 msec) and similarity of waveform. Note the much more delayed responses of GH, and the longer time base. (From Jones et al, 1980.)

marked temporal dispersion between stimulation sites at the wrist and the elbow (see Figure 13.1). This was consistent with the observation that potentials recorded over the brachial plexus and cervical vertebrae (absent in approximately 50% of cases) were undelayed in the great majority of those in whom they could be recorded (Figure 13.2). It may be possible to reconcile these findings with those of Desmedt and Noël (1973), since in the earlier study the more distal stimulus was delivered to the fingers rather than the wrist. If the degeneration of the peripheral nerve (primarily an axonal rather than a demyelinating process in this disease) involves the 'dying back' of axons from sensory receptors in the fingertips this may affect conduction velocity in the most distal segments of the nerve, while segments proximal to the wrist may be initially unaffected. Development of this idea might also account for the delay in central conduction, since a 'dying back' process affecting sensory axons in the dorsal columns might lead to slowed axonal conduction or to impaired synaptic processes in the brainstem cuneate nucleus. There are many other mechanisms which might be involved — for example secondary segmental or paranodal demyelination, shrinkage of fibres or drop-out of large axons — but it is difficult to see why these should induce a slowing of central

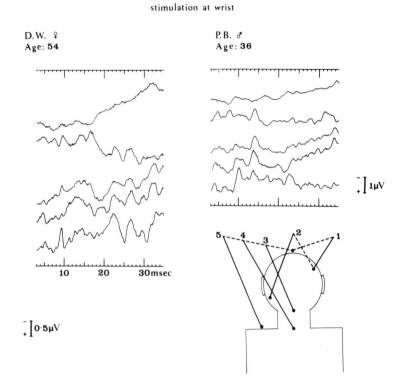

Figure 13.2 *Subcortical and early cortical SEPs in 2 cases of Friedreich's ataxia.*
$\overline{N9}$ *and* $\overline{N13}$ *are apparent in both cases, with very low amplitude but normal*
latency. $\overline{N14}$ *is present for DW (channel 2) but slightly delayed.* $\overline{N20}$ *shows a*
characteristically delayed peak (just visible at 34 msec for PB) although the onset
is much less delayed. (From Jones et al, 1980.)

conduction while causing no delay in the peripheral branch of the same neurones.
One possibility might be the different neuroglial environment of the central branch,
with myelin supplied by astrocytes and oligodendrocytes rather than by Schwann
cells.

Compressive and traumatic lesions of the peripheral nerves

Contrasting with the neuropathies, in which the SEP waveform is frequently
broadened as well as of prolonged latency, delayed responses with preserved waveform were described in 2 cases of carpal tunnel syndrome, the stimuli being
delivered to the distal phalanx of the third finger (Desmedt et al, 1966). Stimuli
delivered to the fifth finger or to the proximal phalanx of the third gave rise to SEPs
of normal latency, presumably mediated by fibres of the unaffected ulnar and radial
nerves. SNAPs recorded from the median nerve at the wrist were of reduced

amplitude and broadened waveform, but the delay of the initial peak was insufficient to account for the SEP delay. This was interpreted by Desmedt (1971) as implying a degree of temporal summation at cortical or subcortical synapses. As a further control in these cases stimulation of the median and ulnar nerves above the likely level of the lesion yielded SEPs of normal latency.

Desmedt and his colleagues have investigated a variety of compressive, ischaemic and traumatic lesions of the brachial nerves, reviewed by Desmedt (1971) and Desmedt and Noël (1973). In one case with a partial ulnar nerve lesion caused by a fracture of the elbow, a local region of slowed conduction was demonstrated, with a conduction velocity of 32 m/sec across the elbow compared with 57 m/sec below and 62 m/sec above. In this case no EMG abnormalities were apparent at the time of recording (10 months after the accident), and since no SNAPs could be recorded across the elbow the SEP delay was the only objective confirmation of the remaining dysfunction.

The presence of regenerating fibres in the hand following traumatic section of the median nerve at the wrist was demonstrated in 2 cases by the presence of delayed SEPs to digital nerve stimulation (Desmedt, 1971; Desmedt and Noël, 1973). In the first there were signs of returning sensation in the distal phalanges of the second and third fingers 5 months after surgical suture of the median nerve. This was reflected by a markedly delayed SEP (57.5 msec to the peak of $\overline{\text{N20}}$) of very small amplitude. Responses of normal latency were obtained to stimulation of the third finger at a more proximal site, presumably mediated by unaffected radial nerve fibres, and to median nerve stimulation above the level of the suture. No SNAPs could be recorded from the median nerve in response to distal stimulation of the third finger, and the cortical SEP therefore provided the sole confirmation of sensory fibre regeneration. The mean afferent conduction velocity in the hand was 5.4 m/sec, consistent with the early phase of regeneration in which the fibres are of very small diameter and thinly myelinated. In a second case (Desmedt and Noël 1973) there was complete recovery of sensation 6 years after a partial rupture of the median nerve, apart from a small hypoaesthetic area at the tips of the second and third fingers. SNAPs were of small amplitude, broadened and delayed by 1.6 msec compared with those recorded from the ulnar nerve. Comparison of SEP latencies following stimulation of the third and fifth fingers revealed a relative delay of 1.9 msec for the former, while the SEP waveform was fully normal apart from a slight reduction in $\overline{\text{N20}}$ amplitude. In this case the delay was almost identical to that of the fastest fibres contributing to the SNAP, in contrast to the findings for carpal tunnel syndrome.

Brachial plexus lesions

Desmedt and Noël (1973) described SEP findings for one case with an ischaemic lesion involving the distal part of the brachial plexus. The subclavian artery had been severed by a fracture of the clavicle and surgically repaired six months prior to the recording, but the arm was left completely paralysed and anaesthetic apart from evidence of a few surviving fibres in the radial nerve. From the intact arm SEPs were recorded following stimulation of the median nerve at the wrist, elbow and axilla, the afferent fibres concerned having a mean conduction velocity of 61 m/sec over these segments. From the injured arm (in which there was thought to be axonal regeneration) the cortical response to stimulation at the axilla was well-formed but delayed by 9 msec compared with the intact side. With elbow stimulation the SEP was severely degraded and delayed by approximately 25 msec, and no response could be obtained with stimulation at the wrist. The EMG showed only a few voluntary motor unit potentials in the triceps, and no SNAPs could be recorded. The derived sensory conduction velocity between the elbow and the axilla in the injured arm was 7.4 m/sec, consistent with the conduction velocity of axons in the early stage of regeneration. From the less delayed response to stimulation at the axilla it was concluded that ischaemic necrosis of the brachial plexus extended proximally by about 70 mm, this assuming the conduction velocity to be about the same throughout the length of regenerated axon. The SEP technique, therefore, provided a means of detecting axonal regeneration before neuromuscular connections had been re-established or sensory action potentials were recordable.

It has long been known that traction lesions of the brachial plexus can cause complete denervation of the lower arm (in the distribution of the C5 to T1 segments), accompanied by massive degeneration of motor axons. Sensory fibres, however, are frequently preserved, as can be demonstrated by the preservation of SNAPs although the arm may be completely anaesthetic (Bonney and Gilliatt, 1958). This is possible on account of the location of the sensory nerve cell bodies in the dorsal root ganglia just external to the spinal cord, such that the rupture may occur on their proximal (preganglionic) side. The recording of cortical SEPs in such cases may confirm the extent and severity of the lesion and, in conjunction with SNAP recordings, establish the major location of involvement proximal or distal to the dorsal root ganglia. Zalis et al (1970) found SEPs to be absent following median and ulnar nerve stimulation in one case where SNAPs were present and were propagated with normal velocity in the forearm. Myelography supported the diagnosis of root avulsion (lesion proximal to the dorsal root ganglia) by the presence of meningoceles at C7, C8 and T1 level on the damaged side.

Zverina and Kredba (1977) investigated seven cases of brachial plexus traction injury, mostly sustained in motor cycle accidents, by recording antidromic SNAPs from the first, second and fifth digits, and cortical SEPs in response to stimulation of the median nerve at the wrist, elbow and axilla. It was concluded that the preservation of SNAPs (with SEPs to wrist stimulation absent) was a reliable indicator of a root lesion proximal to the dorsal root ganglia (confirmed by myelography and surgical exploration) but that SNAPs might also be absent in such cases, presumably due to a double lesion involving the distal and proximal fibres. It was found that with stimulation at the axilla SEPs were present in a large proportion of cases with established root avulsions, this being explained by the possibility of mediation via the intercostobrachial nerve which by-passes the brachial plexus and enters the spinal cord at upper thoracic level. Small, delayed SEPs were still present following stimulation at the wrist when only a portion of a single root (C8) remained in continuity, and no SNAPs could be recorded.

One further case of a brachial plexus traction injury sustained in a motor cycle accident was described by Rosen et al (1977). In this study peripheral SNAPs were recorded in conjunction with cervical spinal cord potentials, the latter obtained with a bipolar montage at C5-C6 level with an inter-electrode distance of 30 mm. This technique necessitates the averaging of large numbers of sweeps, but provides a more immediate index of afferent activity reaching the central nervous system. The clinical picture 6 months after the accident was consistent with a lesion of the lower roots of the brachial plexus — atrophy and weakness of the hand muscles plus sensory loss in the ulnar part of the hand and forearm. SNAPs were of normal amplitude in the median and ulnar nerves at the wrist, but the spinal responses to ulnar nerve stimulation were grossly attenuated or absent. The diagnosis, therefore, was of a lesion proximal to the dorsal root ganglia at C8 and/or T1. The same authors reported a case in whom the spinal potentials were delayed compared with the intact arm, while SNAPs were entirely normal.

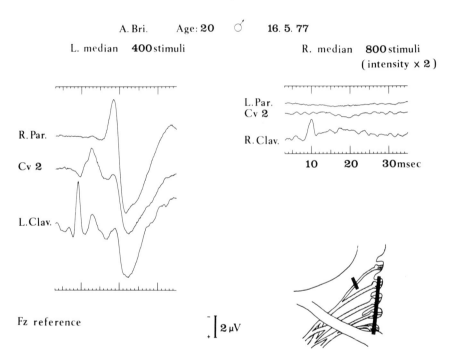

A. Bri. Age: 20 ♂ 16. 5. 77

L. median 400 stimuli

R. median 800 stimuli
(intensity × 2)

R. Par.

Cv 2

L. Clav.

Fz reference

L. Par.
Cv 2

R. Clav.

10 20 30 msec

2 μV

Figure 13.3 *Traction lesion of the right brachial plexus (C5 to T1) causing abolition of cervical and cortical potentials but with N̄9 preserved. At operation the C5 root was found to be ruptured distal to the dorsal root ganglion but C6 to T1 were avulsed from the spinal cord.*

Jones (1979) reported SEP findings for 26 patients with unilateral brachial plexus traction lesions, comparing clavicular, cervical and cortical potentials with those obtained from the intact arm. In about 40% of cases the locus of the lesion was subsequently established by surgical exploration. Since the clavicular N̄9 component is generated in the brachial plexus distal to the dorsal root ganglia (Jones, 1977), the relative attenuation of N̄9 compared with that of cervical (N̄13) and cortical (N̄20) potentials could be used to estimate the degree of preganglionic and postganglionic involvement. The findings in response to median nerve stimulation were found to reflect the integrity of the C6 and C7 roots, while the lower roots (C8 and T1) could be assessed by ulnar nerve stimulation (Jones et al, 1981). The first 26 cases were divided into three groups, according to whether there was clinical involvement of all 5 roots from C5 to T1, the upper roots from C5 to C7, or the C5 and C6 roots only. In the first group (13 cases) no cervical or cortical SEPs could be identified following median (or ulnar) nerve stimulation, but $\overline{N9}$ was preserved in approximately 40% of cases (see, for example, Figure 13.3). Surgical exploration of 5 cases confirmed that a preserved $\overline{N9}$ was invariably associated with a lesion of at least one root proximal to the dorsal root ganglion (more often 3 or 4 roots), but it also became apparent that a proximal root avulsion might be compounded by a distal lesion involving the same fibres. Such cases were indistinguishable (in pre-operative SEP recordings) from those in which the lesion was entirely post-ganglionic, and a myelogram might be necessary in order to detect the avulsed roots.

In patients with partial brachial plexus lesions involving the upper roots only the SEP technique (with median nerve stimulation) was more powerful. The relative degree of preservation of the $\overline{N9}$ and $\overline{N13}$ components compared with the intact arm was found to give an accurate indication of the major site of damage in the C6 and C7 roots in 4 out of 5 explored cases. In 2 of these $\overline{N9}$ was attenuated to an extent equal to or greater than $\overline{N13}$, suggesting a predominantly distal lesion which was confirmed at operation (see, for example, Figure 13.4). In another case $\overline{N13}$ and $\overline{N20}$ were markedly attenuated while $\overline{N9}$ was at least as large as from the intact side, suggesting a purely proximal lesion of at least one root. At operation the brachial plexus appeared to be intact, but by stimulating the exposed roots and recording SEPs from the somatosensory hand area of the contralateral scalp a failure of continuity was revealed between the C5 and C6 roots and the central nervous system, while the C7 and C8 roots were electrophysiologically intact. Nerve action potentials could be recorded in all 4 exposed roots, confirming the pre-operative impression that the lesion of the C5 and C6 roots was likely to be on the proximal side of the dorsal root ganglia (see Landi et al, 1980).

SEPs recorded at operation can also be of value during the grafting of ruptured nerves, since the preservation of a cortical response to stimulation of the proximal stump eliminates the possibility of a second, proximal lesion (Landi et al, 1980). Such stumps were shown to be capable of axonal regeneration, while the absence of cortical responses was usually associated with little or no recovery of function. In one further case described by Landi et al (1980) the suprascapular nerve appeared to be in continuity, although there had been no functional recovery many months after a traction injury. Since a small cortical response could be elicited the nerve was left intact. Some recovery of motor function occurred a few days post-operatively and full clinical recovery eventually ensued.

SPINAL CORD LESIONS

Cervical spondylosis

Since it has now been established that the afferent volley gives rise to recordable potentials on either side of the point of entry into the spinal cord (the transition probably occurring between $\overline{N9}$ and $\overline{N11}$) there has been considerable interest in the possibility of diagnosing cervical spondylotic conditions (radiculopathy and myelopathy) by the SEP technique. In this context studies of potentials recorded from within the epidural space (Matsukado et al, 1976; Caccia et al, 1976) appear to correspond well with conventional skin-surface recordings (Mastaglia et al, 1978; El-Negamy and Sedgwick, 1979; Small et al, 1980; Chiappa et al, 1980a). Caccia et al (1976), Mastaglia et al (1978) and Small et al (1980) simply observed a reduction or absence of potentials presumed to originate in the spinal cord. Matsukado et al (1976) demonstrated a dissociation between epidural P_1 ('spike') and N_1 potentials, which were thought to reflect activity in dorsal root fibres and the dorsal horn respectively. The N_1 and succeeding P_2 potentials were diminished or absent in a number of cases with cervical spondylotic myelopathy or disc protrusion, while P_1 was invariably preserved. The abnormality was thought to be due to ischaemia rather than to the direct effects of compression.

El-Negamy and Sedgwick (1979) and Chiappa et al (1980a) each described cases in which the latency separation between peripheral and cervical potentials recorded from the skin surface was increased beyond normal limits, suggesting a slowing of conduction across proximal segments of the dorsal roots. El-Negamy and Sedgwick

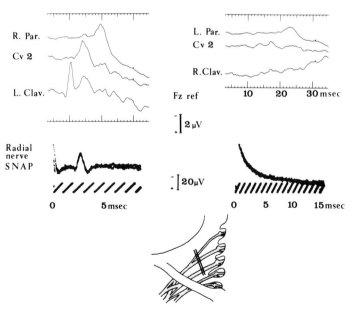

Figure 13.4 *Traction lesion of the right brachial plexus (C5 to C7) causing attenuation and delay of $\overline{N13}$ and $\overline{N20}$ but abolition of $\overline{N9}$ and the radial nerve SNAP. At operation the upper roots were found to be damaged distal to the dorsal root ganglia, although anatomical continuity was preserved. (From Jones et al, 1981.)*

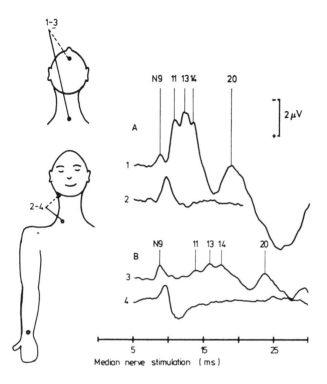

Figure 13.5 *Subcortical SEPs recorded in a normal adult (A) and a patient with cervical spondylosis (radiculopathy and myelopathy). (From El-Negamy and Sedgwick, 1979.)*

(1979) were able to divide their 14 cases into three groups: (1) 4 cases within normal limits; (2) 5 with increased $\overline{\text{N9-N13}}$ separation (see Figure 13.5); (3) 5 with $\overline{\text{N13}}$ absent. There was, however, no apparent correlation between the nature of the SEP abnormality and the severity of symptoms, or the existence of myelopathy (with clinical signs in the lower limbs) in addition to radiculopathy.

Noël and Desmedt (1980) studied 7 patients with extrinsic compression of the spinal cord at cervical level, causing loss of joint-position sense in the legs as well as pyramidal signs in all 4 limbs. Delayed cortical responses were obtained following stimulation of the sural nerve, although the responses to finger stimulation were of normal or near-normal latency. It was suggested that dorsal column axons may be more susceptible to compression when the locus of the lesion is remote from their cell body in the dorsal root ganglia, such that axons originating in lumbo-sacral segments are more affected by cervical compression than are axons arising more rostrally.

An alternative approach to the study of cervical spondylosis has been developed by Schramm (1980), using a segmental stimulation technique. In the majority of cases it was possible to distinguish between the effects of radiculopathy and myelopathy on the basis of the nature and severity of SEP abnormalities. Normal responses, and abnormalities confined to a single dermatome, were more often encountered in cases of radiculopathy, whereas a pattern in which SEPs were abnormal at several dermatomal levels was only found in the myelopathic group. In both groups, however, cases were recorded with abnormal SEPs from two adjacent segments, and it could not be established in these whether the cause was compression of the spinal cord or biradiculopathy.

Other spinal cord lesions

From a study of 14 cases with spinal cord lesions it was established by Halliday and Wakefield (1963) that the cortical SEP was affected only when there was clinical evidence of dorsal column involvement. In 3 patients with unilateral impairment of joint-position sense the SEP was delayed and/or of reduced amplitude following stimulation of the affected side, and SEPs were bilaterally abnormal in a further 3 patients with bilateral sensory loss. No SEP abnormalities were seen in 5 patients with impaired temperature and pain sensation but normal joint-position sense. In one case of Brown-Séquard syndrome the SEP was abnormal only on stimulation of the side with impairment of joint-position sense. These findings were supported by Giblin (1964), and by Larson et al (1966b) who found no change in the response to sciatic nerve stimulation after a spinal tractotomy which caused a loss of pain and temperature sensation below mid-thoracic level. Namerow (1969) showed that the SEP waveform was unaffected by cervical cordotomy when only the anterolateral columns were sectioned. The cortical SEP was thus shown to be mediated by the dorsal columns of the spinal cord, which are the tracts particularly concerned with the transmission of joint-position sense.

More recently the findings of Halliday and Wakefield (1963) were confirmed by Fukushima and Mayanagi (1975), using multiple stimulation sites in the upper and lower limbs. With criteria of normality derived from 50 normal subjects (including latency and amplitude limits, waveform characteristics and permissible differences between left and right limbs) abnormalities were present for each of 7 patients with impairment of vibration and joint-position sense, but not for 4 patients with exclusive pain and temperature loss. The regions from which abnormal SEPs were recorded did not always correspond precisely with the area of sensory loss.

Nakanishi et al (1974) recorded abnormal SEPs in response to mechanical stimulation of the fingers in 7 out of 8 cases with sensory impairment but preserved joint-position sense, the underlying pathologies including syringomyelia and intra-medullary tumour of the spinal cord. It was proposed that in these cases the SEP may be mediated by pathways other than the dorsal column/lemniscal system but, as suggested in the previous Chapter, an alternative explanation might be that an abnormal mechanically-evoked SEP is simply a more sensitive test of dorsal column involvement than the impairment of joint-position sense. From the clinical standpoint it is desirable to be able to demonstrate the existence of spinal cord lesions with and without dorsal column involvement, and it is possible (although supportive data is lacking) that this might be achieved by recording electrically- and mechanically-evoked SEPs respectively.

A further observation by Halliday and Wakefield (1963) was that SEP abnormalities attributable to a spinal cord lesion might persist during recovery, at a time when there was little or no sensory deficit revealed to clinical testing. In some diseases (particularly multiple sclerosis) it may be of diagnostic importance to demonstrate the existence of CNS lesions by electrophysiological or other means, although many years may have elapsed since the acute episode. In isolated cases there may have been virtually complete functional recovery, leaving minimal clinical signs, and in others the lesion may be genuinely clinically 'silent'. The extensive topic of the use of SEPs in the investigation and diagnosis of multiple sclerosis is covered later in this Chapter.

A question which has not yet been wholly answered by clinical or experimental evidence is whether the subcortical SEP components following median nerve stimulation are also generated exclusively in structures comprising the dorsal column/medial lemniscal pathway. It has been shown that all the major short latency SEP components from $\overline{N9}$ to $\overline{N20}$ depend on the activation of peripheral nerve fibres conducting at approximately 70 m/sec in the forearm (Jones, 1977). In the spectrum of nerve fibre conduction velocities this corresponds to the faster end of Group II, the axons being largely concerned with transmission of cutaneous and proprioceptive information. The majority pass directly into the dorsal columns to synapse in the dorsal column nuclei of the brainstem, but many also send off collaterals into the grey matter of the spinal cord. It now seems likely that the cervical $\overline{N13}$ potential may not reflect the propagation of the afferent volley in the dorsal columns, as was first thought, but may be mediated by the collateral projection to the dorsal horn (see previous Chapter). Under certain circumstances, therefore, $\overline{N13}$ may be susceptible to spinal cord lesions involving the grey matter only and sparing the dorsal columns. A dissociation between cervical and cortical SEP components, with $\overline{N13}$ abnormal and $\overline{N20}$ preserved, is sometimes observed in multiple sclerosis (Small et al, 1980, see below), and was reported by Mastaglia et al (1978) for a case of syringomyelia with cerebellar ectopia. Such a dissociation is clearly not compatible with the generation of $\overline{N13}$ in the dorsal columns or cuneate nucleus, since the preservation of $\overline{N20}$ presupposes the integrity of all the structures comprising the dorsal column/medial lemniscal system. As yet, however, there is no evidence that the dissociation between $\overline{N13}$ and $\overline{N20}$ can be related to any form of dissociated sensory loss.

The presence or absence of SEPs to upper and/or lower limb stimulation has been successfully used in the context of traumatic injury to the spinal cord, as an index of the completeness and approximate level of the lesion. Perot (1973, 1976) found that the cortical response to median nerve stimulation was abolished by a clinically complete spinal cord lesion in the mid or upper cervical region, but might be partially preserved with a lesion at C6 or C7. Partial involvement of the cervical cord caused prolongation of latency and abnormal waveform, but these features sometimes showed marked improvement alongside clinical recovery. Stimulation of the peroneal and sural nerves in the leg gave less consistent results, but successfully distinguished between complete (absent SEP) and partial lesions in the thoracic and lumbar region. There was no indication, however, as to whether the preservation of the response depended on preservation of the dorsal columns. It was found that with lesions below the cervical region there might be a transient effect on the median nerve response, which returned to normal after a few days.

Apart from the study of cervical spondylosis by Schramm (1980) there have been isolated attempts to use segmental stimulation of the body (including digital nerves and dermatomes of the skin) to locate the level of a spinal cord lesion by the segments which give rise to an abnormal SEP. Blair (1971) concluded that the responses to dermatomal stimulation were insufficiently reliable for the technique to be used as a method of sensory examination in young children, but Baust and Jörg (1977) reported more encouraging results in adults, the electrophysiological 'level' below which SEPs were abnormal or absent corresponding more exactly with the proven level of the lesion than did the results of routine clinical sensory testing. Schramm and Hashizume (1977) used similar techniques, and noted (cf Perot, 1973) that SEPs might be abnormal even when the level of input to the spinal cord was considerably above the level of sensory impairment. It was not established, however, whether this was a transient effect, perhaps due to spinal shock, or whether the SEP genuinely revealed the level of the lesion more accurately than clinical examination. Segmental SEPs so far published have not been of high technical quality, and further development is required if the technique is to fulfil the continuing need for a test capable of establishing the level of a spinal cord lesion.

Two investigations into the spinal potentials evoked by stimulation of the posterior tibial nerve include an account of a 'travelling wave', present at all levels of the spine and possibly reflecting the propagation of the afferent volley through the cauda equina and dorsal columns (Cracco, 1973; Jones and Small, 1978). Clearly this suggests a method for the objective localization of a spinal cord lesion, since Cracco (1973) found the travelling wave to be preserved in lower segments after complete or partial transection in the cervical or upper thoracic region. It should be stressed, however, that the travelling wave is hard to record even in normal adults, and the subsequent lack of published clinical findings may testify to this. Cracco et al (1975) recorded a spinal travelling wave more easily in very young children, suggesting that this method may be more successful as a means of sensory testing in the very young than the dermatomal stimulation technique tried and rejected by Blair (1971).

Spinal cord monitoring

As a consequence of recent advances in the surgical treatment of spinal scoliosis there has also been increased interest in the possibility of monitoring the function of the spinal cord during an operation (Harrington instrumentation) which carries a small but finite risk of post-operative paraplegia. Recording cortical responses to posterior tibial nerve stimulation, Nash et al (1977) reported that although there were transient abnormalities immediately after distraction of the spine in 5 out of 34 patients, all either resolved spontaneously (when the changes were mild) or improved following relaxation of the tensive force. When SEP recovery was complete there were found to be no post-operative neurological defects.

A complicating factor, however, is that cortical SEPs are subject to attenuation by anaesthesia (Clark and Rosner, 1973; Allison et al, 1963) and by hypotension (Nash et al, 1977), which is often artificially induced during scoliosis surgery. This increases the difficulty of obtaining good quality recordings in the operating theatre (never an ideal electrophysiological environment). The records so far published have not been of high quality, and in the author's experience a more sensitive and reliable method is to be found in the recording of spinal cord potentials, as practised by Tsuyama et al (1978), Tamaki (1977, 1979) and Axelgaard (1977, 1979). These can be recorded throughout the course of the operation using electrodes inserted into the epidural space (Tsuyama et al, 1978; Tamaki, 1979) or attached to the exposed vertebrae (Axelgaard, 1977). Relatively little averaging time is required (50 to 200 stimuli, delivered at 10 Hz or faster) and the waveform seems to be unaffected by fluctuations in blood pressure or anaesthetic level. The multiphasic responses recorded with an epidural electrode suggest that conduction might be monitored in more than one group of sensory afferent fibres (cord conduction velocity about 45-80 m/sec), and there is evidence that tracts other than the dorsal columns might be concerned (Tsuyama et al, 1978). Tamaki (1979) adopted the technique of direct spinal cord stimulation (cervical or lumbar) in preference to stimulation of a nerve trunk, and found that the ascending or descending volley was diminished or absent in cases with established spinal cord lesions, and might be transiently affected by minor trauma during surgery. A great deal of relevant experimental work in this area (although little human material) is described in '*Spine*', *Volume 4, No. 6 (1979)*.

BRAINSTEM AND THALAMIC LESIONS

In the pioneering study of Alajouanine et al (1958) 4 cases were described with lateral medullary infarction (Wallenberg syndrome) causing exclusive impairment of temperature and pain sensation. SEP findings were somewhat equivocal, in that although for 2 patients cortical responses were found to be of reduced amplitude at low stimulus intensities, this was not the case at higher levels. Later work has not confirmed these findings. Using mechanical tap and pin-prick stimuli Nakanishi et al (1974) recorded SEPs of normal configuration from all patients with brainstem lesions except those with impaired joint-position sense, contrasting with the same authors' findings in cases with spinal cord lesions, where SEPs were usually abnormal even when joint-position sense was preserved.

Noël and Desmedt (1975) examined 7 patients with vascular lesions of the brainstem or diencephalon. In 2 cases with Wallenberg syndrome there were no SEP abnormalities, nor were there in one case with a lesion of the lateral mesencephalon (Weber syndrome). In 2 cases with pontine infarction causing a 'locked in' syndrome it was possible to demonstrate involvement of the medial lemniscus by the delayed onset of the SEP (see Figure 13.6), although one patient was much less delayed when followed up 2 years later. SEPs were also abnormal (of delayed onset, with N20 reduced or absent) in 2 cases with thalamic infarction causing impairment of all sensory modalities. Abnormalities due to brainstem and thalamic lesions were distinguishable from those caused by cortical infarction, in that for the latter there was a reduction of amplitude but no delay.

Several reports concerning the effect on SEPs of vascular lesions involving the cerebral hemispheres include cases with thalamic as well as cortical involvement. Williamson et al (1970) found that abnormalities attributable to a thalamic lesion were invariably associated with the impairment of joint-position sense, although

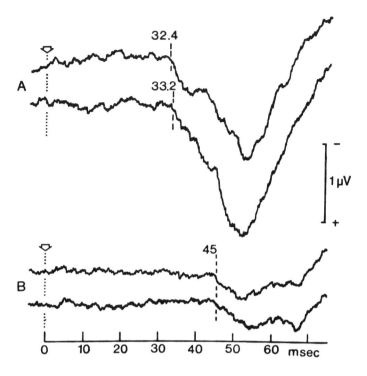

Figure 13.6 *Abnormal scalp-recorded SEPs (mid-forehead reference) to right (A) and left (B) median nerve stimulation in a patient with a pontine infarction causing a 'locked in' syndrome. (From Noël and Desmedt, 1975.)*

there were no cases with purely spinothalamic-type sensory loss. In a single patient with a left thalamic carcinoma (Tamura, 1972) the SEP was of normal waveform over each hemisphere following stimulation of the left hand, but no response was present on either side with stimulation on the right. Although Shibasaki et al (1977) found a high overall incidence of SEP abnormalities in patients with cerebrovascular lesions, the $\overline{N20}$ component was affected only when the thalamus or the internal capsule were involved. With thalamic infarction there was an increase in $\overline{N20}$ latency (as described by Noël and Desmedt, 1975), whereas with involvement of the internal capsule the response was simply attenuated or absent. One unexpected finding of this study, however, was that SEPs were abnormal in response to stimulation of either hand in 6 out of 8 cases with unilateral thalamic lesions.

The effect of brainstem and thalamic lesions on subcortical SEP components is relatively obscure at present, but Mastaglia et al (1978) noted that neither $\overline{N20}$ nor the $\overline{N13}$ potential recorded from the cervical region with a scalp reference was affected by a lateral medullary lesion causing exclusive impairment of pain and temperature sensation on the contralateral side. We have recently confirmed this finding in two cases (Jones and Halliday, unpublished). Mastaglia et al (1978) found cervical and cortical SEPs to be unaffected by a variety of midbrain and thalamic lesions, but surprisingly reported delayed or absent cervical potentials with lesions of the ventrolateral thalamus, sometimes causing enhancement rather than attenuation of the cortical response. This observation is in disagreement with those of Hume and Cant (1978), Small et al (1980) and Chiappa et al (1980a), all of whom found the cervical response to be unsusceptible to lesions of the brainstem or diencephalon, although there might be marked abnormalities of the cortical waveform. In particular Chiappa et al (1980a) noted the preservation of a cervical potential (albeit of small amplitude) following a vascular lesion of the brainstem causing abolition of the cortical response. The cervical wave was also preserved in a patient with a high brainstem (midbrain) haemorrhage, while the early cortical potentials were again absent. Finally, 2 patients who had survived a unilateral haemorrhage in the putaminal-thalamic region had normal cervical potentials with an absent cortical reponse.

Nakanishi et al (1978) studied the 'P15' component, recorded with a scalp-earlobe derivation, in 7 patients with thalamic lesions (6 vascular and one glioblastoma) and 2 with vascular lesions of the brainstem. In all the thalamic cases $\overline{P15}$ was preserved along with the cervical wave, while cortical potentials were present in one case only. $\overline{P15}$ was of reduced amplitude in both cases with brainstem involvement, but a negative-going cervical wave was again preserved. This supports experimental evidence that the positive-going potentials at 13-15 msec latency are likely to be generated caudal to the thalamus in the dorsal column nuclei or medial lemniscus.

In the previous chapter a number of studies were described in which SEPs recorded by electrodes directly implanted into the human thalamus were used as an aid to stereotaxic surgery (for example Ervin and Mark, 1964; Pagni, 1967; Fukushima et al, 1976). Thermocoagulation or cryogenic ablation of the thalamus for the relief of dyskinesia or intractable pain requires accurate location of individual nuclei, which cannot always be achieved simply by reference to stereotaxic coordinates. This application of the SEP technique has been less frequently practised in recent years (particularly since the development of effective drugs for the treatment of Parkinsonism) but may still be of value in certain circumstances.

LESIONS OF THE CEREBRAL CORTEX

In a wide-ranging study Alajouanine et al (1958) examined 10 patients who experienced sensory loss following a vascular lesion of the cerebral cortex. In 5 out of 7 cases with involvement confined to one parietal lobe, SEPs to median nerve stimulation were abolished over the affected hemisphere, and in the remaining 2 cases supra-normal stimuli were required to evoke a response. In a similar study Giblin (1964) found that not all cases with sensory impairment had demonstrably abnormal SEPs, or vice versa. There were 7 patients (out of a total of 17 with vascular or neoplastic lesions) in whom SEPs were of normal waveform despite sensory inattention or moderate to severe sensory loss. In the remainder SEPs were unilaterally abnormal over the damaged hemisphere, either absent or of greatly different waveform from those recorded from the intact side. In 13 out of 25 patients with no sensory loss there were no significant abnormalities, but in a further 11 there were marked amplitude asymmetries and in one (with the lesion sustained at birth) a marked attenuation of amplitude over the damaged hemisphere. Three of the patients with asymmetrical responses had *larger* potentials over the hemisphere from which a benign tumour had been removed. In the remainder extra components were observed unilaterally, sometimes over the damaged hemisphere. The possible significance of the last group has yet to be clarified by other workers.

Larson et al (1966a) studied the correlation between loss of SEP amplitude and the modality of sensory impairment in 22 patients with cerebrovascular disease. In 9 patients with normal joint-position and vibration sensitivity there was no loss of SEP amplitude or change in latency, but out of 13 cases with impairment of these modalities 12 had diminished or absent SEPs over the affected hemisphere. There was, therefore, only one patient with normal SEPs despite abnormal sensory testing, and none with normal sensation but abnormal SEPs. In a further 2 unconscious patients SEPs were severely attenuated. Clinical improvement was accompanied by a recovery of SEP amplitude in 4 out of 6 cases studied serially, but in the remaining 2 the SEP remained abnormal 1-10 months after the onset of the stroke, despite good clinical recovery. In 3 cases out of 13 with impaired joint-position or vibration sense SEPs recorded over the damaged hemisphere were also abnormal following stimulation of the ipsilateral (unaffected) arm.

A possible application for SEP studies following middle cerebral artery thrombosis was explored by Liberson (1966). Seventeen patients were examined, presenting with varying degrees of aphasia (later re-diagnosed as dysarthria in 2 cases) accompanying right hemiplegia. The degree of SEP abnormality over the left hemisphere was strongly correlated with the degree of aphasia. Only one patient out of 7 with well preserved SEPs was classified as being severely aphasic, whereas out of 10 patients with severely abnormal SEPs the aphasia was classified as severe in 8 cases and moderate in 2. Flash- or click-evoked cortical potentials showed no such correlation. It was suggested that SEP recordings might be of value as a prognostic index for speech therapy in such cases. The ipsilateral potentials (recorded over the unaffected hemisphere following stimulation of the right arm) were invariably abolished when contralateral SEPs were severely abnormal.

From a group of 20 patients with lesions of the parietal lobes (the majority neoplastic) Laget et al (1967) recorded SEPs of reduced amplitude but normal latency in 14, the attenuation being broadly related to the degree of sensory impairment. There was a suggestion that the degree of SEP attenuation might be even greater in patients with ischaemic cortical lesions, and that the recovery of SEP amplitude might not keep pace with the rate or extent of clinical recovery. The same authors noted that SEPs might be enhanced in association with an epileptic focus involving the appropriate limb.

The paper by Williamson et al (1970) was mentioned in the previous section. From a study of 17 patients with unilateral hemispheric lesions at or above thalamic level it was concluded that when SEPs were abnormal all components were affected to an equal degree, and that the abnormality was generally associated with impairment of joint-position sense. The majority of cases were of middle cerebral artery infarction and the results were generally compatible with those of previous studies, although, in contrast to the findings of Larson et al (1966a) and Laget et al

(1967), one patient was described in whom the recovery of sensory function 3 weeks after a stroke was mirrored by a return to normal SEP configuration.

In a much more detailed analysis of the relationship between SEP abnormalities and the sensory impairment caused by cerebrovascular lesions, Miyoshi et al (1971) rated sensory capacity on a five point scale for each of seven 'modalities' — touch, joint-position, vibration, temperature, pain, two-point discrimination and perception of the evoking stimulus delivered to the median nerve at the wrist. The SEPs were analysed for the peak latency of 5 early components ($\overline{N20}$ to $\overline{N55}$) the corresponding peak-to-peak amplitudes, and the amplitude and latency of a 'later component' of uncertain identification and up to 500 msec latency. Twenty-seven patients were compared with age-matched normal volunteers (data of Lueders, 1970). Normal SEPs, occurring in only 5 records out of 34 (some patients were seen on more than one occasion), were generally associated with no sensory impairment or only mild sensory loss in some or all modalities. There was a good correlation between the degree of SEP abnormality, which was classified as 'slight' in 11 records, 'moderate' in 4, 'severe' in 8 and 'flat' in 6, and the degree of sensory impairment across all modalities. In contrast to the findings of Williamson et al (1970) some SEP components were found to be less vulnerable than others. $\overline{N20}$ and $\overline{P30}$ were generally unaffected when sensory loss was confined to temperature and pain, but abnormalities of the later components were correlated with sensory impairment in any modality. In fact the first negativity was of normal amplitude and latency in 50% of records classified as severely abnormal by other criteria. The most sensitive component was that labelled P_2 ($\overline{P45}$, Goff et al, 1977), which was delayed in 6 out of 11 records classified as slightly abnormal and apparently of abnormally *short* latency in 3 others. Serial recordings revealed a gradual restoration of the SEP alongside clinical improvement, but even when clinical sensory recovery was complete there was frequently a residual delay of P_2 and later potentials. In 9 out of 34 recordings SEPs were also of abnormal waveform over the unaffected hemisphere, following stimulation of the contralateral arm. Although it is possible that the narrow criteria of normality employed ($\pm$ two standard deviations) and the large number of parameters analysed may have resulted in a number of 'false positives' (variants of the normal waveform wrongly classified as abnormal on account of perhaps one parameter more than two standard deviations from the normal mean), this study is the most comprehensive to date, and it is an important finding that later SEP components appear to be vulnerable to cortical lesions which do not affect earlier waves. This demonstrates fairly conclusively that some late components from $\overline{P45}$ on are not generated in the same cortical areas as are responsible for $\overline{N20}$ and $\overline{P30}$, but there is still doubt as to whether late waves depend exclusively on transcortical connections from a single 'primary' receiving area, or reflect the independent activation of other 'primary' areas by different afferent pathways.

Tsumoto et al (1973) studied the cortical response to median nerve stimulation in 23 cases of cerebrovascular disease, of which 15 were classified as infarctions and 8 as haemorrhages. Patients with sensory impairment in all modalities were found to have a reduction or absence of all SEP components, whereas in 5 out of 6 cases with loss of thermo-algesic sensation alone there was attenuation of the $\overline{N35}$ and $\overline{P45}$ components (see Figure 13.7). In cases with aphasia and paraparesis but no

A **B**

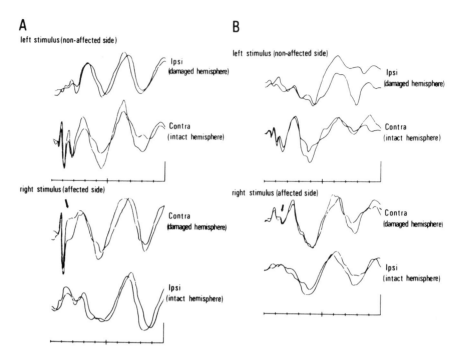

Figure 13.7 *Cortical SEPs in patients with cerebrovascular lesions causing impaired touch and pain/temperature sensation alone. A: The arrow indicates an absence of N_2 and P_2 waves from the contralateral response to right (affected side) stimulation. B: The arrow indicates reduced N_2 and P_2 waves of the contralateral response to the right (affected side) stimulation. Reference on earlobe contralateral to stimulus. (From Tsumoto et al, 1973.)*

sensory loss the late waves recorded from the damaged hemisphere might be selectively attenuated, leaving the early components (and both early and late potentials evoked from the undamaged hemisphere by stimulation of either arm) intact. In cases with hemiparesis alone no SEP abnormalities were found.

Using a mechanical (tap and pinprick) stimulation technique, Nakanishi et al (1974) recorded SEPs in 27 cases with unilateral cortical lesions. Out of 18 patients with sensory loss (10 vascular lesions, 8 tumours) the responses recorded over the damaged hemisphere were absent in 5, present but abnormal in 10 and normal in 3. Nine patients with no sensory impairment all had normal SEPs.

In a study of 15 patients with 'pure' motor hemiplegia, presumed to be due to a small infarction of the 'basis pontis', Chokroverty and Rubino (1975) found a moderate attenuation of SEP amplitude in 7 cases, suggesting a degree of medial lemniscal involvement also.

Shibasaki et al (1977) found SEPs to be abnormal in 61 out of 65 patients, mostly with vascular lesions of the cerebral hemispheres. Out of 56 unilateral cases abnormalities were seen exclusively over the damaged hemisphere in 64% and bilaterally in 30%. The fact that as many as 8 SEP parameters were studied with a

±2.38 standard deviation criterion for each may, however, have resulted in a certain proportion of "false positives". The likelihood of obtaining an abnormal record was not related to the location of the cortical lesion, although $\overline{N20}$ was affected only by lesions involving the thalamus and internal capsule. The third negativity ($\overline{N75}$), on the other hand, was abnormal in a large proportion of cases with a wide variety of cortical lesions, including those in which involvement was confined to the frontal lobes. In only three patients (with internal capsular lesions) was the SEP completely abolished over the affected hemisphere. $\overline{N20}$ and $\overline{N35}$ abnormalities (the latter even less frequent) were correlated with sensory loss in all modalities, particularly vibration and joint-position sense, but the overall incidence of SEP abnormality was almost as high among patients with no sensory impairment. The low incidence of $\overline{N35}$ abnormalities conflicts with the reported findings of Tsumoto et al (1973), but in the normative data of Shibasaki et al (1977) $\overline{N35}$ showed a wider range of variability than earlier or later potentials, which may have prevented the detection of abnormalities.

The latency separation between subcortical ($\overline{N13}$) and cortical ($\overline{N20}$) SEP components was examined by Symon et al (1979) in 16 cases admitted to a neurosurgical unit following subarachnoid haemorrhage. This measure ('central conduction time') was found to be increased uni- or bilaterally, before or after operation, in 5 out of 12 operated cases. Three of the 5 developed transient hemiplegia — in one instance 7 days after the increased SEP latency had been observed. The $\overline{N13}$-$\overline{N20}$ separation later returned to within normal limits in 2 cases, in keeping with a full clinical recovery. Although there were 2 other cases in which an increased central conduction time ($\overline{N20}$ recorded on the side of the original haemorrhage) was not followed by post-operative complications, it was concluded that the measure might be a sensitive index of hemispheric ischaemia, prior to the onset of clinical deficits. In one case of intraventricular haemorrhage central conduction time was seen to be prolonged before the development of a mild hemiparesis, although the electrophysiological recordings later returned to normal in parallel with the clinical symptoms.

Noël and Desmedt (1980) studied 7 patients, aged 8-22 years, with infantile hemiplegia due to unilateral cerebrovascular lesions sustained before the age of 2. In one case a subcortical $\overline{P17}$ was the only remaining scalp response to finger stimulation on the affected side, but in another with a lesion of the frontal cortex the postcentral cortical waveform ($\overline{N22}$ and $\overline{P44}$) was preserved over the damaged hemisphere although corresponding precentral components ($\overline{P22}$ and $\overline{N34}$) were absent (see Figure 13.8). From this and other evidence (see previous Chapter) it seems likely that the early cortically-generated components are of more complex aetiology and may originate in a wider area of the cerebral cortex than is supposed in the cortical dipole models of Broughton (1967) and Allison et al (1980). The possibility that some late waves evoked by thermal and painful stimuli may reflect the specific processing of small-fibre thermoalgesic input is more controversial, but may represent, if true, a considerable advance over previously held views, made possible by the development of sophisticated stimulation techniques and the derivation of more stringent criteria of SEP normality.

It is difficult to envisage a continuing application for SEP recordings in the diagnosis of cerebrovascular disease and cerebral tumours, particularly since the

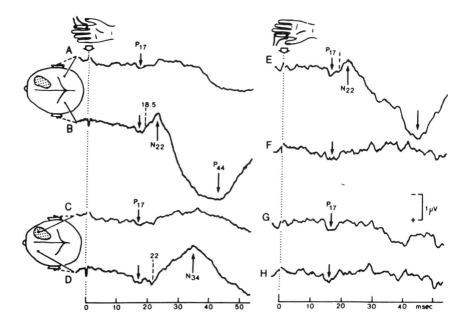

Figure 13.8 *Scalp recorded SEPs (ear reference) in a patient with a left infantile hemiplegia due to a prefrontal cortical lesion. The precentral $\overline{N34}$ component is abolished with stimulation on the left although the postcentral waveform is apparently unaffected. (From Noël and Desmedt, 1980.)*

advent of computerized brain tomography. However, the study on 'central conduction time' (Symon et al, 1979) suggests a possible rôle for SEPs in the management of neurosurgical cases.

MULTIPLE SCLEROSIS

Although multiple sclerosis (MS) usually follows a sporadic course, with acute relapses followed at first by periods of almost complete remission, the multiple areas of demyelination observed in the central nervous system at autopsy (particularly in the spinal cord, brainstem and optic nerves) are clearly likely to cause long-lasting interference with sensory conduction, and it is not surprising that EP abnormalities are seen in a high proportion of established cases. In the early stages, however, the diagnosis may be less than certain, and the finding of an abnormal evoked potential may be of considerable importance in confirming the nature of the lesion and, perhaps, in demonstrating the existence of 'clinically silent' plaques which have either appeared insidiously, giving rise to no neurological symptoms, or have recovered to the extent that symptoms and signs are no longer apparent. Several recent studies have shown that such lesions involving the somatosensory pathway may be revealed by SEP abnormalities, but in order to demonstrate the evolution of the technique some earlier accounts will first be described.

The 14 cases of spinal cord lesions documented by Halliday and Wakefield (1963) included 2 with the diagnosis of MS, and in both of these joint-position sense was bilaterally impaired in the fingers while pin-prick perception was preserved. Both patients had abnormal cortical SEPs of prolonged latency, and the amplitude of the response was smaller following stimulation of the more severely affected side.

Many more cases of clinically definite MS were described by Namerow (1968) and Baker et al (1968). Abnormal SEPs were found in 94% of cases where there was current impairment of joint-position and/or vibration sense in the appropriate limb (Namerow, 1968), but were also encountered in 29% of patients who denied any past or present disturbance of these modalities. The characteristic waveform change was absence of the initial $\overline{N20}$ component following median nerve stimulation at the wrist, and a broadening of $\overline{P30}$, which was of delayed onset and peak latency in most cases. A return to normal latency values was seen during remission of symptoms in 3 out of 5 cases studied serially (Namerow, 1968), although the SEP improvement generally lagged behind the clinical recovery. Similar findings were reported by Baker et al (1968) for 91 cases, of which 81 had clinical impairment of joint-position sense. SEPs were judged to be abnormal in 84% of this group (defined as a latency increase of at least 50%, a monophasic waveform or an absent response) and 5 out of 10 cases with no loss of joint-position sense also had abnormal SEPs. In 7 out of 8 cases recorded during and after an acute exacerbation, the response (initially abnormal) returned to within normal limits. Tamura and Kuroiwa (1972) reported a generally lower incidence of abnormality in 8 out of 16 patients studied and in 29% of cases without sensory disturbance in the hands.

Desmedt and Noël (1973) showed that the prolongation of cortical SEP latency in MS (see, for example, Figure 13.9) must be attributable to a slowing of conduction in the central somatosensory pathway, since peripheral nerve action potentials were of normal amplitude and latency even when cortical potentials were delayed by as much as 25 msec. Abnormal responses were recorded from all save 3 arms in 17 patients, and marked delays were more common when there was impairment of joint-position sense in the hand under investigation.

Fukushima and Mayanagi (1975) looked at cortical potentials evoked by stimulation of the lower as well as the upper limbs. The occasional finding of delayed responses from the leg when those from the arm were of normal latency was plainly suggestive of a dorsal column lesion caudal to the cervical region. The abnormalities were more marked than those caused by vascular, traumatic, radicular or space-occupying lesions, and were frequently encountered in spite of normal clinical findings.

Most studies since 1976 have concentrated on the potential diagnostic value of SEP recordings in MS, since it was discovered by Halliday et al (1973a) that clinically silent plaques in the optic nerves may be revealed by delayed visual evoked responses to a pattern reversal stimulus. In cases with, for example, spinal cord symptoms of uncertain aetiology the VEP is sometimes capable of establishing a diagnosis of MS by demonstrating the existence of a second demyelinating lesion which was not apparent on clinical examination, and a number of SEP studies have been undertaken with a similar aim in view. A second development made at about this time was the detection and characterization of subcortical SEP components, and it was soon established that these may also be abnormal in a large proportion of MS cases (see Figure 13.9).

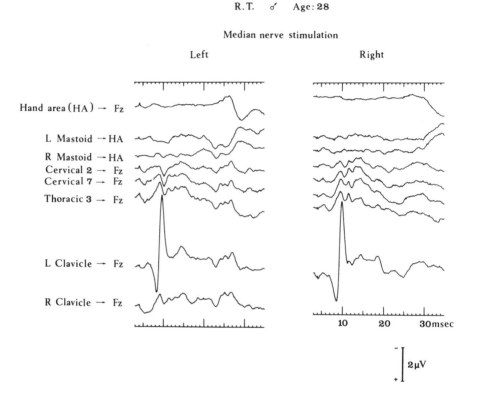

R.T.   ♂   **Age: 28**

Median nerve stimulation

Left   Right

Hand area (HA) → Fz
L Mastoid → HA
R Mastoid → HA
Cervical 2 → Fz
Cervical 7 → Fz
Thoracic 3 → Fz
L Clavicle → Fz
R Clavicle → Fz

10   20   30 msec

2 μV

Figure 13.9 *Subcortical and early cortical SEPs in multiple sclerosis, showing the preservation of $\overline{N9}$ and $\overline{N11}$, reduction but no delay of $\overline{N13}$ (almost within normal limits on the right), delay of $\overline{N14}$ (occurring at 20 msec latency on the left) and delay of $\overline{N20}$ (comparable to the delay of $\overline{N14}$ on the left.)*

Small and colleagues found the cervical SEP waveform (recorded with a mid-frontal reference) to be abnormal in a greater proportion of MS cases than was the initial component ($\overline{N20}$) of the cortical response (Small, 1976; Small et al, 1978, 1980). The original aim was to measure the sensory conduction velocity of the spinal cord between electrodes situated over the lower and upper cervical vertebrae, but latencies were found to be closely similar at the two sites, indicating that the major negative-going potential recorded at each was likely to originate in a nuclear structure (such as the dorsal horn in the appropriate root entry zone, or the cuneate nucleus of the brainstem) rather than an ascending tract such as the dorsal column.

In a large proportion of MS cases the amplitude of the major negative cervical potential ($\overline{N13}$) with reference to the scalp was below the normal minimum of approximately 1 μV, and in a smaller proportion the latency of the wave was more than 2.5 standard deviations from the regression line of latency against arm length in normal subjects. More subjectively, the cervical wave was also judged to be abnormal if the $\overline{N13}$ peak was reduced to below the level of the preceding and following negativities ($\overline{N11}$ and $\overline{N14}$). The initial cortical negativity ($\overline{N20}$) was assessed according to a similar latency criterion, although in amplitude terms, it could only be regarded as abnormal if completely absent.

In addition to the 'definite', 'probable' and 'possible' MS categories defined by McAlpine (1972), the patients examined by Small et al (1978) included cases of isolated optic neuritis as well as acute and chronic undiagnosed neurological complaints. The cervical wave was judged to be abnormal in 63 out of 132 examinations overall, due to a reduction of amplitude in 29 recordings but with 15 instances of increased peak latency and 19 of distorted waveform (attenuation of $\overline{N13}$ alone). Abnormalities were more frequent where there was clinically demonstrable sensory loss (59%, compared with 27% of cases with no sensory loss). Two cases out of 11 with 'isolated' optic neuritis had abnormal SEPs, perhaps reflecting the existence of a second lesion in the cervical cord or brainstem. Since SEPs were frequently bilaterally abnormal in cases with unilateral sensory loss, more than half of the abnormal records were in fact obtained from arms with no sensory impairment. Cervical SEP abnormalities were frequently associated with the presence of other spinal cord signs, but 9 out of 43 patients with no such signs (sensory or motor) had abnormal responses on one or both sides. The authors stressed, however, that abnormality of the cervical SEP was not in itself diagnostic of MS, since similar abnormalities were encountered in some cases of cervical spondylotic myelopathy or syringomyelia. In relation to the diagnostic category, $\overline{N13}$ was most often abnormal in clinically definite MS cases (69%) but the incidence was fairly high in probable (42%) and possible (52%) cases also. It was noted that the abnormality seen during a relapse might persist during complete clinical remission. In keeping with previous studies the cortical $\overline{N20}$ component was frequently abnormal, but in only 2 cases where $\overline{N13}$ was normal (both presenting with clinical signs of a brainstem lesion), whereas the converse pattern of abnormal N13 with normal $\overline{N20}$ was found in 18 cases (see, for example, Figure 13.10).

Mastaglia et al (1976) were among the first to try to exploit the diagnostic possibilities of EP recordings in MS to the full, by examining the 'yield' of abnormal visual and cervical somatosensory potentials in definite, probable and possible cases (categories of McAlpine, 1972). Abnormal cervical potentials were present in 94%, 50% and 30% respectively, although a high proportion of cases in each group also had clinical abnormalities of sensation, thereby rendering the abnormal SEP finding of lesser significance. Abnormal visual evoked potentials were found in a slightly smaller proportion of cases, but combining the results of both tests increased the 'hit rate' in the possible group to 59%.

In a second study (Mastaglia et al, 1977) a larger group of patients were classified according to the criteria of McDonald and Halliday (1977). Abnormal cervical and/or cortical SEPs were recorded in 74% of clinically definite cases, 58% of 'early probable or latent' (EP/L) MS and 33% of 'suspected' cases. The

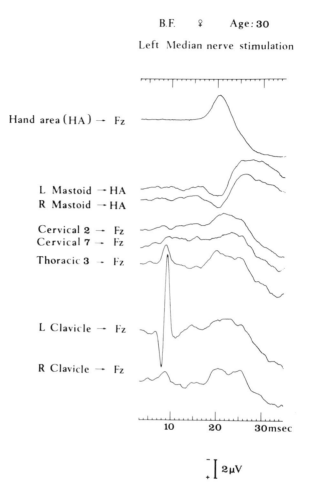

B.F.   ♀   Age: 30

Left Median nerve stimulation

Hand area (HA) → Fz

L Mastoid → HA
R Mastoid → HA

Cervical 2 → Fz
Cervical 7 → Fz

Thoracic 3 → Fz

L Clavicle → Fz

R Clavicle → Fz

10   20   30 msec

2 μV

Figure 13.10 *Subcortical and early cortical SEPs in MS, showing attenuated (or perhaps delayed) cervical potentials in conjunction with normal $\overline{N20}$.*

cervical wave was the more frequently abnormal, with a higher incidence of reduced amplitude than of prolonged latency. It was not clear how many of the suspected or EP/L patients had clinical evidence of spinal cord involvement, but out of 23 suspected MS cases with no sensory signs in the arms (the total group numbering 27), 5 had abnormal SEPs. If the technique can be relied upon, therefore, to detect lesions of the somatosensory pathway without producing an unacceptable proportion of 'false positives' (recordings at the limits of the normal range and incorrectly classified as abnormal) then there is clearly an application for SEPs in the diagnosis of MS by the detection of clinically silent plaques.

Matthews and Small (1979) have since reported that the waveform of the cervical SEP remains stable in MS patients who do not experience further relapse, but may change when the disease is active, even when the recent symptoms do not include sensory disturbance in the arms. A similar sensitivity to relapse, without the necessity of clinical involvement of the brainstem, has been reported for the brainstem auditory evoked response in MS patients (Robinson and Rudge, 1978). In the study of Matthews and Small (1979) the SEP waveform was particularly liable to deterioration following an acute exacerbation involving the spinal cord, although no improvements were seen during remission. The latter finding is in contrast with the return to normal latency and waveform which has been reported for the cortical SEP (Namerow, 1968; Baker et al, 1968).

Matthews et al (1979) looked at the changes in the cortical VEP and the cervical and cortical SEP waveform produced by raising the body temperature by 1°C. Normal subjects showed no significant SEP changes, apart from a slight reduction in latency. This could largely be attributed to an increase in peripheral nerve conduction velocity, since the interval between potentials recorded from the brachial plexus and the cortex remained relatively constant. In patients with MS the cervical response was abnormal at normal body temperature for 15 out of 32 arms tested, and underwent a further deterioration as a result of the 1°C increase. In 7 studies potentials which were initially within normal limits became statistically abnormal at the higher temperature, but for 2 arms a reduction of $\overline{N13}$ latency resulted in the opposite change of classification. Ten of the 32 arms tested gave cervical responses which were normal at both temperatures. No exacerbation of sensory symptoms was noticed, although many patients experienced a temporary worsening of other symptoms. At the higher temperature there was a general reduction of $\overline{N20}$ latency (initially abnormal for 9 arms), largely attributable to increased peripheral nerve conduction velocity. $\overline{N20}$ latency returned to within the normal range for 2 arms, but may have remained "abnormal" if the normal range had been redefined at the higher temperature. The effect of increasing body temperature on the visual evoked response was somewhat different, since both normals and patients showed a reduction of amplitude but no change in waveform or latency.

Changes in the cervical SEP waveform have also been reported after moderately successful treatment of MS symptoms by spinal cord stimulation (El-Negamy, 1978), the tendency being for the waveform to revert to a more normal configuration. In a study which attempted to confirm these findings (Hawkes and Jones, unpublished) the SEP changes were less marked, but there was a slight improvement in the cortical or cervical waveform in two cases (see Figure 13.11). Although spontaneous SEP recovery has been described during remission of acute symptoms (Namerow, 1968), for the patients receiving spinal cord stimulation the disease was stable or slowly progressing rather than relapsing and remitting, and the SEP changes and slight clinical improvement were therefore unlikely to have been a chance occurrence.

In the study of Eisen et al (1979) cervical responses were abnormal in 41% of suspected MS cases (increased to 50% when cortical potentials were taken into account), 79% of EP/L (increased to 89%) and 87% (no increase) of clinically definite. The cervical SEP abnormalities most frequently encountered were absence (in 43% of arms), attenuation and increased duration, with very few instances of increased latency. The cortical $\overline{N20}$ component was also frequently absent (in 31%

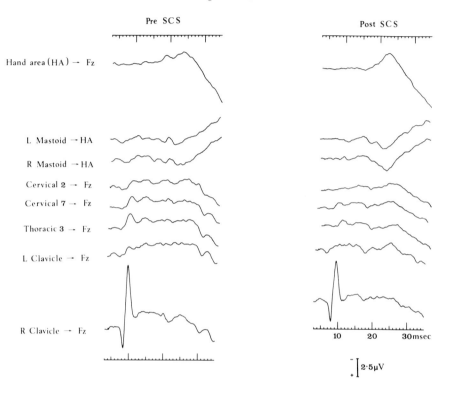

Figure 13.11 *Subcortical and early cortical SEPs in MS, showing a slight restoration of $\overline{N20}$ following 14 days of spinal cord stimulation. (Hawkes and Jones, unpublished.)*

of arms) and less often delayed. Peripheral nerve conduction was monitored by recording the sensory nerve action potential over the brachial plexus (Erb's point). The study is open to some criticism, since patients with apparently abnormal peripheral nerve conduction were excluded and an inadequate amplifier high frequency response (extending only to 200 Hz) may have been responsible for the very high incidence of absent potentials.

In recent years several groups have attempted slightly different approaches to the study of subcortical SEPs in MS. Anziska et al (1978) looked at the subcortical and early cortical potentials recorded from the surface of the scalp with reference to in electrode on the hand (contralateral to the stimulus), shoulder or knee. These responses are more likely to be contaminated by EMG and ECG interference than those recorded with a neck-scalp montage, and are in any case of smaller amplitude since the latter derivation summates negative potentials from the cervical region with simultaneous positive waves from the scalp. The neck-scalp montage may, however, result in cancellation or distortion of components generated simultaneously in different structures, whereas the more difficult method adopted by Anziska et al (1978) is theoretically sound. Only cases with clinically definite MS were included and 25 out of 26 had abnormal responses. The first positive peak (reflecting the approach of the afferent volley in the periphery) was invariably preserved, but subsequent components were frequently absent, reduced in amplitude compared with the other arm, or delayed in relation to preceding peaks. These abnormal features occurred almost as often in cases with no clinical sensory loss as in those with sensory impairment. The most frequent abnormalities were absent P3 and/or NI components, probably equivalent to the $\overline{P13}$ and $\overline{N20}$ waves recorded by other groups, but P2 (usually labelled $\overline{P11}$ or $\overline{P\,12}$) was also absent in a high proportion of cases. Arezzo et al (1979) have shown that $\overline{P11}$ is most likely to originate in the dorsal columns and $\overline{P13}$ in the brainstem lemniscal pathway.

Dorfman et al (1978) adopted the indirect method of recording upper and lower limb cortical SEPs in conjunction with M- and F-waves, in order to derive values for conduction velocity in the peripheral, spinal and supraspinal segments of the somatosensory pathway. The onset latency of the lower limb SEP (following stimulation of the posterior tibial nerve at the ankle) was therefore broken down into three components. Conduction time in the peripheral segment was calculated from M- and F-wave latencies, although these of course depend on efferent and antidromic afferent conduction in motor fibres, and were accordingly adjusted by a factor of 1.08 to allow for the slightly faster conduction of sensory fibres. Conduction time in the supraspinal segment was derived from the onset latency of the upper limb SEP when the corresponding peripheral component had been subtracted. The residual latency of the lower limb SEP after subtraction of peripheral and supraspinal conduction time was attributed to conduction time in the spinal cord. Out of 30 patients with definite, probable or possible MS, a depressed value for spinal cord conduction velocity (more than 2 standard deviations below the normal mean of 67 m/sec) was obtained unilaterally in 8 cases and bilaterally in 14. These 22 abnormal cases included 16 out of the 18 for which the likelihood of a spinal cord lesion was judged to be very high by clinical criteria. Conduction in the supraspinal segment was delayed bilaterally in 6 cases and unilaterally in 8. Slow conduction was correlated with sensory loss, particularly of vibration and joint-position sense, but there were some instances of delayed SEPs in spite of the absence of sensory symptoms and signs at the time of recording. One case was reported in which the SEP latency following lower limb stimulation returned to a normal value during remission of symptoms.

The same method was adopted by Eisen and Nudleman (1979) but apparently with a lesser degree of success in deriving a meaningful figure for spinal cord conduction velocity. As with Dorfman et al (1978) there was no significant difference in mean peripheral conduction time between normal and clinically definite MS groups, and no group difference was revealed in the derived spinal cord conduction velocity either, on account of the wide scatter of values in the patient group. In 10 out of 28 MS cases, however, cord conduction velocity was significantly reduced by more than 2.5 standard deviations from the normal mean (less than 39 m/sec). Conduction time in the cervical cord and cerebrum (following median nerve stimulation) was prolonged in 10 out of 16 cases with, and 4 out of 12 cases without, current sensory impairment in the arms, but just as many abnormalities were registered simply by comparing the latency of the cortical SEP with normative values. Following lower limb stimulation the subtraction of peripheral conduction time resulted in a very slight increase in the incidence of detected abnormalities (19 rather than 18 out of 28 cases). Conduction in the supraspinal segment following peroneal nerve stimulation was abnormal in 3 out of 7 patients with asymptomatic lower limbs, and in 16 out of the remaining 21 cases. The method was somewhat confounded by the occurrence (in 8 patients) of delayed upper limb responses where the responses from the lower limb on the same side were of normal or near-normal latency. This resulted in some clearly anomalous cases where the derived spinal cord conduction velocity was apparently abnormally fast. The likely explanation for this is that a small lesion involving the cervical spinal cord, the cuneate nucleus or the medial lemniscus may cause interference with sensory input from the arm, while nearby fibres deriving from the lower limb are unaffected. This highlights a major shortcoming of the indirect technique for assessing conduction velocity in the abnormal CNS, and the authors (Eisen and Nudleman, 1979) concluded that little was added to the conventional measurement of SEP latency values.

Conduction time in the central somatosensory pathway can be derived more directly from the separation between subcortical and cortical SEP components, provided it can be shown that a single afferent projection is concerned. Even if the latter is not the case, the inter-peak separation might still be useful as an empirical index related to the integrity of central conduction, and independent of peripheral conduction time. The method adopted by Eisen and Odusote (1980) involved calculation of the interval between cervical $\overline{N13}$ and cortical $\overline{N20}$ components following median nerve stimulation, and between lower thoracic $\overline{N21}$ and cortical $\overline{P40}$ components following stimulation of the posterior tibial nerve at the ankle. Peripheral nerve integrity was monitored by electrodes at Erb's point and in the popliteal fossa. $\overline{N13}$ was absent, however, in more than 35% of patients studied, and the $\overline{N13}$-$\overline{N20}$ separation was increased in only 16.7% of cases in which both components were identifiable. In 11 cases out of a total of 105 there was a significant left/right difference in $\overline{N13}$-$\overline{N20}$ separation, of more than 0.9 msec. In relation to the diagnostic classification (McDonald and Halliday, 1977) the frequency of abnormality (including cases with $\overline{N13}$ and/or $\overline{N20}$ of abnormally low amplitude) was as follows: 24 out of 29 clinically definite; 21 out of 24 EP/L; 15 out of 22 'spinal' (progressive, possible or probable) and 12 out of 30 suspected MS. Following lower limb stimulation $\overline{P40}$ was of prolonged latency or absent for 17 out of 20 limbs examined (at least one limb in all cases), and the $\overline{N21}$-$\overline{P40}$ separation was increased in 13 studies out of 15 where both were identifiable.

Trojaborg and Petersen (1979) examined only the latency of the cortical SEP, stimulating the common peroneal nerve at the head of the fibula as well as the median nerve at the wrist. Delays were more frequently encountered in patients with impaired vibration and/or joint-position sense (88%, 84% and 70% of cases classified as definite, probable or possible MS) but the incidence was fairly high in the remaining cases also (42%, 41% and 20%). In definite MS there was a higher overall incidence of SEP abnormality following peroneal than median nerve stimulation, but this was not the case in the other two categories, where median nerve responses were just as frequently abnormal. Combining the results of SEP and VEP studies resulted in a higher 'hit rate' than was achieved by either test alone, but this is of little diagnostic significance without more detailed information concerning the proportion of cases for which each technique revealed an extra lesion, not apparent on clinical examination.

Namerow (1970) studied the recovery cycle of the cortical SEP in MS cases, by subtracting the response to a single stimulus from that evoked by a doublet of variable interstimulus interval. It was found that, whereas in normals there was an increase in $\overline{P30}$ latency for the second of the paired stimuli when the interstimulus interval was less than 10 msec, in MS patients with impaired joint-position sense there was a latency *decrease* at interstimulus intervals below 60 msec, although the absolute values of $\overline{P30}$ latency were still above the normal range. The suggestion was made that the most severely affected (slowest conducting) fibres may have been more susceptible to conduction block at short interstimulus intervals, such that the second response came to be mediated by fibres with a lesser degree of demyelination and hence faster mean conduction velocity.

As a development of this approach Sclabassi et al (1974) measured the amplitude of the oscillatory potential recorded from the scalp in response to a train of impulses, total duration 250 msec, delivered to the median nerve with an intra-train frequency of 40 to 160 Hz. This enabled a discriminant function to be derived which correctly distinguished all clinically definite MS cases from normal subjects. In cases with severe impairment of vibration and joint-position sense the oscillatory potential was virtually absent at 40 Hz, whereas with no clinical sensory loss it might be of normal amplitude up to 100 Hz. Possible MS cases with no clinical evidence of somatosensory system involvement were generally indistinguishable from normals. It was concluded that the presence of a lesion in the somatosensory pathway was essential for any abnormality to be detected, and that the technique did not reveal any non-specific effect of MS at central synapses. In comparison with conventional SEP techniques this procedure is a complicated one, requiring a lengthy recording session and considerable off-line analysis, and did not apparently achieve greater success in detecting clinically 'silent' lesions.

The future of SEPs in MS diagnosis

It seems clear from a review of published work to date that the SEP technique is well able to demonstrate the existence of a demyelinating lesion in the central somatosensory pathway, particularly when subcortical potentials are examined in addition to the cortical waveform, norms are derived for the latency difference between left and right limb responses, and certain minor waveform abnormalities are recognized. The sensitivity of the technique depends to a large degree on detailed statistical criteria of normality, taking into account the correlation of latency with arm length (an alternative method of achieving this is to measure latencies from the peak of $\overline{N9}$) and the effects of maturation and ageing. This is sufficient for the technique to be of some value in the diagnosis of MS, when the clinical presentation is such that the neurologist requires objective confirmation of equivocal clinical signs, or the possible demonstration of 'clinically silent' plaques.

To evaluate the power of the SEP technique, however, it is not sufficient to classify the cases according to the criteria of McAlpine (1972) or McDonald and Halliday (1977) without taking into account the location as well as the number of lesions which are clearly defined by clinical criteria. For example a case falling into the 'early probable or latent' category is much more likely to have an abnormal SEP when there are symptoms suggesting a lesion of the cervical spinal cord or brainstem, than when the involvement is primarily of the visual pathways, and the significance of an attenuation of $\overline{N13}$ or an increase in the latency of $\overline{N20}$ is clearly much greater in the latter case. Some authors (notably Trojaborg and Petersen, 1979) subdivided the three diagnostic categories according to the presence or absence of sensory impairment in each case, but the majority have not recognized the importance of this and have limited themselves to a two-dimensional analysis. An alternative, and to some extent complementary, approach would be to assemble homogeneous groups with, for example, isolated optic neuritis, transverse myelitis or brainstem lesions, since in a proportion of these the lesion is likely to be a manifestation of MS in the very early stages, and some may already have subclinical lesions of other structures.

The published work to date has also done little to define the nature of the waveform changes which may be characteristic of MS and therefore diagnostically significant. It has been noted that peripheral nerve potentials are almost invariably normal, the cervical $\overline{N13}$ component is more often absent or attenuated than of prolonged latency, and the cortical response may be attenuated and/or delayed. In the present author's experience the most frequently encountered pattern is a normal peripheral response (the $\overline{N9}$ component recorded from the clavicle) followed by a cervical waveform in which $\overline{N11}$ may be preserved or absent, $\overline{N13}$ of low amplitude, fragmented or absent, and $\overline{N14}$ absent or delayed. In such cases the initial cortical negativity is generally delayed and of reduced amplitude. This pattern may not be unique to MS but it is different from that encountered in, for example, Friedreich's ataxia (Jones et al, 1980), where there is attenuation of the peripheral nerve component as well as other more subtle differences. The high incidence of significant left/right differences in MS may also distinguish this condition from others in which abnormalities are generally more symmetrical.

An important observation by Small and colleagues, and also implicit in the findings of others, was that $\overline{N13}$ might be abnormal in the presence of a normal $\overline{N20}$ (Small, 1976; Small et al, 1978). Small et al (1978) particularly remarked a waveform alteration in which $\overline{N13}$ was reduced to below the level of $\overline{N11}$ and $\overline{N14}$. A similar pattern has been observed several times in our laboratory (see Figure 13.12), and in other cases the cervical waveform may be virtually flat although $\overline{N20}$ is within normal amplitude and latency limits (see Figure 13.10). $\overline{N13}$, therefore, seems to be at least partially independent of the pathway which is responsible for mediating $\overline{N20}$, and is therefore unlikely to originate entirely in the dorsal columns, dorsal column nuclei or medial lemniscus as has often been suggested. A likely alternative is that $\overline{N13}$ reflects synaptic and postsynaptic activity in the spinal grey matter, and may therefore be susceptible to discrete lesions of the cervical cord which leave the dorsal columns intact.

The converse pattern of abnormality, with $\overline{N14}$ and $\overline{N20}$ delayed but $\overline{N13}$

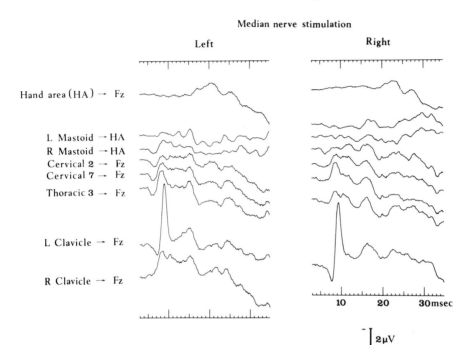

Figure 13.12 *Subcortical and early cortical SEPs in MS, showing attenuation of* $\overline{N13}$ *with* $\overline{N14}$ *and* $\overline{N20}$ *virtually normal (left) or slightly delayed (right).*

relatively well preserved, is also occasionally encountered (see Figures 13.9 and 13.13). This may be ascribed to a lesion of the medial lemniscus, cuneate nucleus or dorsal columns rostral to the C6 root entry zone. In mildly affected cases $\overline{N14}$ and $\overline{N20}$ may be delayed to a similar small degree (Figures 13.9, 13.13 and 13.14), suggesting that both are likely to be generated in or mediated by the dorsal column/medial lemniscal pathway, and that the lesion is likely to be caudal to the generator of $\overline{N14}$. Although one might expect to find evidence of dissociated sensory loss, with joint-position sense impaired but pain and temperature perception preserved, and perhaps the converse pattern in cases with isolated $\overline{N13}$ attenuation, so far no such effect has been reported.

In spite of the proliferation of papers, therefore, there are many further avenues to be explored in the application of SEPs to the investigation and diagnosis of MS. It is to be hoped that by the time diagnostic techniques have been fully refined an effective treatment for this disease may at last have been discovered.

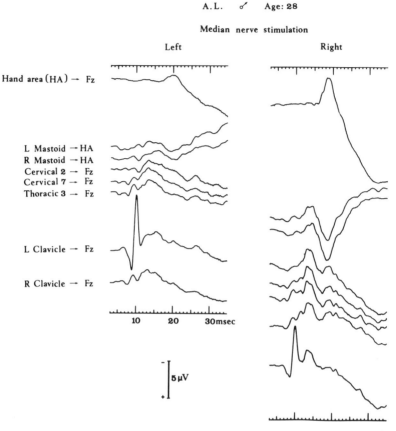

A.L. ♂ **Age: 28**

Median nerve stimulation

Left   Right

Hand area (HA) → Fz

L Mastoid → HA
R Mastoid → HA
Cervical 2 → Fz
Cervical 7 → Fz
Thoracic 3 → Fz

L Clavicle → Fz

R Clavicle → Fz

10   20   30msec

5 μV

Figure 13.13 Subcortical and early cortical SEPs in MS, showing unilateral attenuation of cervical and cortical potentials with slight delay of $\overline{N14}$ and $\overline{N20}$.

PATHOLOGICAL ENHANCEMENT OF CORTICAL SEP AMPLITUDE

Although the SEP abnormalities so far described have generally been a reduction of amplitude and/or prolongation of latency, the phenomenon of SEP enhancement by pathological processes (latency values usually remaining normal) has long been recognized — ever since this very curiosity first enabled Dawson (1947a, b) to record SEPs from the surface of the human scalp. The components most often affected lie in the 30-40 msec latency range, and in patients with progressive myoclonic epilepsy may assume amplitudes of up to ten times those of normal subjects (Halliday, 1967b), although a lesser degree of enhancement may be encountered in other conditions. It has been reported that the initial cortical negativity ($\overline{N20}$) is not similarly affected (Halliday, 1967d; Shibasaki et al, 1978b), but recent experience suggests that this may not invariably be the case (see, for example, Figure 13.15). No enhancement of subcortically generated potentials ($\overline{N9}$ to $\overline{P15}$) has yet been reported, and in our experience these are usually normal

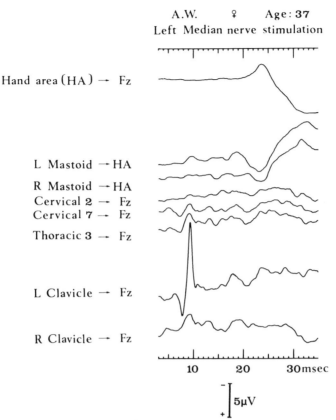

A.W.   ♀   Age: **37**
Left Median nerve stimulation

Hand area (HA) → Fz

L Mastoid → HA
R Mastoid → HA
Cervical 2 → Fz
Cervical 7 → Fz

Thoracic 3 → Fz

L Clavicle → Fz

R Clavicle → Fz

10   20   30 msec

5μV

Figure 13.14 *Subcortical and early cortical SEPs in MS, showing a characteristic preservation of $\overline{N9}$, attenuation or delay of $\overline{N11}$, attenuation of $\overline{N13}$, delay of $\overline{N14}$ and comparable delay of $\overline{N20}$.*

(Halliday and Jones, unpublished). The case illustrated in Figure 13.15 was interesting, however, in so far as $\overline{N14}$ and $\overline{N20}$ were both absent unilaterally, while the latter was abnormally large following stimulation of the arm for which $\overline{N14}$ was present. This patient had no sensory symptoms or signs, but had pyramidal weakness on the left (the side with $\overline{N14}$ and $\overline{N20}$ absent) as well as an action tremor involving both arms equally.

Shibasaki et al (1978b) found that, in addition to the enhanced early cortical potentials, later components might be of abnormal configuration due to absence of a negativity which is normally present at about 60 msec latency and enhancement of a negative slow wave peaking at approximately 150 msec. In any case the enhanced waveform cannot simply be regarded as a magnification of the normal response, since the second negativity ($\overline{N35}$ approximately) frequently exceeds the baseline level in myoclonic cases, although this is seldom seen in normals.

The most extreme SEP enhancement is suppressed when the myoclonic jerking is successfully controlled by drugs (Halliday, 1967b; Sutton and Mayer, 1974; Gath, 1969), or when the jerks are naturally contained for a period. It has also been observed (Halliday, 1967d; Sutton and Mayer, 1974) that the effect may be confined to one hemisphere when jerking is similarly confined to one (contralateral) side of the body, and there may be a close relationship between the degree of SEP enhancement and the severity of clinical involvement in each limb of a single patient (Halliday and Halliday, 1980). In this context it should be noted, perhaps, that the normal cortical response to stimulation of the lower limb may have a prominent negative component ($\overline{N45}$, Tsumoto et al, 1972) which exceeds the baseline in the same manner as the pathologically enhanced $\overline{N35}$ following median nerve stimulation.

Myoclonus arising at segmental (spinal cord or brainstem) level does not produce a marked enhancement of SEP amplitude, and the hereditary syndrome of benign essential myoclonus was found to be associated with responses of normal or just supra-normal amplitude (Halliday and Halliday, 1970). The SEP is therefore a useful tool in the diagnosis of myoclonic conditions, although there are reports of enhancement in cases of photosensitive epilepsy (Broughton et al, 1969), focal epilepsy (Bacia and Reid, l965) and cerebral tumour causing focal parietal epileptic attacks (Laget et al, 1967; Williamson et al, 1970). SEP enhancement of a lesser degree has been described in some non-epileptic cases with lesions of the spinal

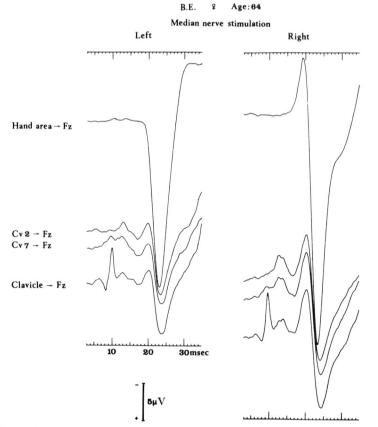

B.E. ♀ **Age:64**

Median nerve stimulation

Left   Right

Hand area → Fz

Cv 2 → Fz
Cv 7 → Fz

Clavicle → Fz

10   20   30msec

5μV

Figure 13.15 *Enhancement of cortical SEP amplitude in progressive myoclonic epilepsy, with normal $\overline{N9}$ to $\overline{N14}$ in association with enhanced $\overline{N20}$ (right arm), or normal $\overline{N9}$ to $\overline{N13}$ with absent $\overline{N14}$ and $\overline{N20}$ (left arm).*

cord, brainstem and cerebral hemispheres (Halliday and Wakefield, 1963; Giblin, 1964; Miyoshi et al, 1971; Tsumoto et al, 1973; Mastaglia et al, 1978), usually causing no sensory symptoms.

Shibasaki and colleagues developed a retrospective signal-averaging technique to record cerebral potentials preceding involuntary jerks of the arm (Shibasaki and Kuroiwa, 1975; Shibasaki et al, 1978b). In a group of patients with progressive myoclonic epilepsy the potentials were of very large amplitude and similar in waveform and distribution to the SEPs, which were enhanced in 13 out of 14 cases. It was also shown that, following unilateral median nerve stimulation, a latency difference of 8-15 msec between C-reflexes recorded from the ipsilateral and contralateral thenar muscles was similar to that between SEPs recorded over the contralateral and ipsilateral hemispheres. Furthermore, the latency from SEP onset to onset of the C-reflex was similar to the separation between the EEG potentials preceding a spontaneous jerk and the onset (EMG) of the jerk itself. It was suggested that in progressive myoclonic epilepsy the jerking may be mediated by the same cortico-spinal tracts as are responsible for the C-reflex, and may originate in a cortical discharge which can either occur spontaneously or can be evoked by peripheral nerve stimulation (Shibasaki et al, 1978b). It was also proposed that with local reflex myoclonus the jerking sometimes seen in the opposite limb may be induced via transcortical connections, with a delay of 8-15 msec attributable to interhemispheric conduction time. This was not greatly different from the 5-8 msec latency difference reported for contralateral and ipsilateral SEP components in normal subjects (Tamura, 1972). The origin of SEPs recorded over the ipsilateral hemisphere remains contentious, however, in myoclonic epileptics as in normals. It is possible that those described by Shibasaki et al (1978b) may have been partially due to activity at the reference electrode, which was on the earlobe contralateral to the stimulated arm and may not, therefore, have been entirely indifferent to the large responses generated in the adjacent sensorimotor cortex.

The processes which might give rise to myoclonic jerking and cause SEP enhancement have been discussed by Halliday (1974). Briefly, it is believed that epileptiform discharges arising in the reticular formation of the lower brainstem may influence sensory input to the cerebral cortex at the level of the thalamic relay nuclei or at the cortex itself. It is puzzling that the majority of studies should find little evidence for enhancement of N20, since this component is widely believed to be generated at suprathalamic level, but recent experience suggests that N20 may be affected more often than was previously thought. It is not clear what factors might be responsible for SEP enhancement in other neurological conditions, although one might presume the process to involve interference with tonic inhibitory mechanisms at brainstem, thalamic or cortical level.

CEREBRAL TRAUMA, COMA AND BRAIN DEATH

Clinical examination cannot always reveal the full extent of brain damage following cerebral trauma or asphyxia, nor even can scanning techniques, and a number of groups have looked at the possibility that EPs might be used as general or modality-specific indicators of brain function in such cases. Hrbek et al (1977a, b) concluded from their study that abnormal SEPs were a serious prognostic sign in infants with perinatal asphyxia, since the incidence of abnormality was found to be highly correlated with motor impairment, although the latter might only manifest itself several months later. SEP and VEP abnormalities were combined to give an overall 'risk score', which was found to be correlated with the degree of asphyxia and the ultimate severity of impaired cerebral function. In the milder cases pathological EPs might be the only early indicator of cerebral damage.

Lille et al (1967, 1968) used visual, auditory and somatosensory EPs to assess the depth of coma in 26 children aged 1-6 years. They concluded that EPs of all modalities became simpler, broader, flatter and of more prolonged latency as the coma deepened, and that EP changes occurred alongside the changing clinical picture. It was particularly noted that a convulsion might be immediately followed by a reduction of EP amplitude.

In recordings obtained from adults with head injuries Larson et al (1973) found no significant correlation between the waveform of the SEP and the clinical level of responsiveness. A reduction of amplitude was frequently encountered in cases with cortical ischaemia, whereas intracranial haematoma often resulted in an abnormal monophasic waveform.

Both Trojaborg and Jörgensen (1973) and Beck et al (1975) noted that SEPs might be elicited in deeply comatose patients with isoelectric EEGs. VEPs and SEPs were of simple waveform with late components absent (Trojaborg and Jörgensen, 1973), but the presence of early cortically-generated potentials was correlated with the preservation of cranial reflexes and the cerebral circulation (ascertained by angiography). The authors noted that, with somatosensory or visual stimulation, evoked cerebral potentials might be 'contaminated' by potentials of extracerebral origin which were more resistant to coma-induced changes. It is now, of course, widely recognized that SEP components arising in subcortical structures may be recorded over the scalp, but there is little likelihood of confusing these with cortically-generated potentials since the latter are of longer latency. It was concluded (Trojaborg and Jörgensen, 1973) that absent EPs provide reliable evidence of brain death, provided there is no local brain damage which might be responsible.

Hume et al (1979) recorded cervical and cortical SEPs in comatose patients, and used the separation in latency between '$\overline{N14}$' (here denoted $\overline{N13}$) and $\overline{N20}$ as a measure of central conduction time in the sensory pathway. This measure was abnormally large (more than 3 standard deviations above the normal mean) in 11 out of 24 patients with coma of traumatic or non-traumatic origin, but diminished with time in 13 out of 16 cases studied serially. In the most severe cases the $\overline{N13}$-$\overline{N20}$ separation might be double that of normal subjects (10-12 msec compared with a normal mean of 5.6 msec), and in 3 cases the cortical response was absent on one or both sides. The magnitude of the delay was predictive of the extent of eventual recovery, the correlation being better for recordings made 10-35 days after the onset of coma, but also significant for records obtained before 10 days. Of the 13 cases who did not make a good recovery 11 had delayed central conduction, whereas normal latency values were obtained from all 11 cases who made a good recovery. Central conduction time was not related to serum phenobarbital levels, and (it was suggested) might therefore be a particularly useful measure in patients under sedation where clinical examination is difficult or impossible. It was not established what mechanisms were responsible for the delayed onset of the cortical SEP, but the fact that findings were similar for groups of patients with coma of traumatic and non-traumatic origin suggested that physical force was not the major cause. It was thought, therefore, that ischaemia might be an important contributing factor. It is likely that a large proportion of the cervical wave recorded with a scalp reference is generated in the spinal grey matter rather than the brainstem, and is therefore independent of the dorsal column/medial lemniscal pathway, but even if the $\overline{N13}$-$\overline{N20}$ separation is not a rigorous measure of central sensory conduction time this does not invalidate the empirical usefulness of the technique.

In an ambitious and rewarding study of somatosensory, visual and auditory evoked potentials recorded from patients with severe head trauma, Greenberg and colleagues (1977a, 1977b) showed that there was a strong association between the degree of SEP abnormality and the duration of coma, the severity of residual disability and any focal motor deficits. Relatively mild abnormalities (absent late waves from approximately 50 msec after the stimulus) in records obtained less than 9 days after the trauma anticipated the recovery of responsiveness within 30 days with a success rate of more than 80%. A correlation was established for visual and auditory EPs also, but with a lower level of significance. Somatosensory (but not auditory or visual) EPs recorded only 3 days after the trauma were also found to be predictive of the eventual outcome, such that approximately 90% of patients with mildly abnormal responses might expect to have made a good recovery or to have only moderate disability 3 months later. EPs in other modalities were of some predictive value when recorded between 3 and 9 days after the trauma. SEP abnormalities were highly correlated with hemiparesis, recovering within 3 months in all cases where the electrophysiological abnormalities were mild. Hemiparesis was not seen to recover, however, in the group with more severely abnormal responses (only $\overline{P15}$ and possibly a negativity at about 23 msec remaining). SEP integrity was found to be a much better predictor of eventual outcome than were the results of clinical testing. As might be expected, abnormal visual and auditory EPs were associated with focal deficits in their respective modalities, as well as with established lesions of the occipital and temporal cortex. SEP abnormalities were associated with lesions of the parietal lobes, and also with brainstem and diencephalic lesions. Focal lesions of the frontal lobes, however, did not give rise to EP abnormalities, even at recording sites over the frontal cortex.

ARTIFICIALLY AND HYSTERICALLY INDUCED ANAESTHESIA

It is of obvious importance with regard to the possibility of recording SEPs routinely in the operating theatre that the effects of surgical anaesthesia be appreciated. Allison et al (1963) found the early components ($\overline{P15}$, $\overline{N20}$, $\overline{P30}$) to be unchanged by administration of barbiturates, although the later potentials were profoundly attenuated. Reviewing the results of earlier studies (Allison et al, 1963; Abrahamian et al, 1963), Clark and Rosner (1973) concluded that the 'specific' potentials of short latency and localized distribution were not attenuated under barbiturate anaesthesia, even at concentrations which caused short periods of suppressed EEG activity. Inhalational agents such as diethyl ether, nitrous oxide and cyclopropane, however, had a radically different effect, and might attenuate or abolish the specific SEP components in surgical concentrations (Clark et al, 1970; 1971). Another inhaled anaesthetic, enflurane, caused an apparent enhancement and delay of the initial negative component (Clark et al, 1971). This literature is well reviewed by Clark and Rosner (1973), and for the purposes of the present chapter it is sufficient to stress that a marked reduction of SEP amplitude, affecting early as well as late cortically-generated components, may be expected where a combination of inhaled and barbiturate anaesthetics is employed.

Other forms of anaesthesia have been less widely studied with regard to their effect on SEPs. Halliday and Mason (1964) were unable to demonstrate any significant effect of hypnotically-induced anaesthesia on the early part of the cortical waveform up to 180 msec latency. The subject was required to indicate when he could no longer feel the electrical evoking stimulus delivered regularly to the fingers, or a mechanical tap to the fingernail or pad, after it was suggested by the hypnotist that the intensity was gradually becoming less. A suggestion that the stimulus intensity had increased (although the voltage remained constant) also failed to induce any change in the amplitude of the SEP. The 'vertex' potential recorded in response to auditory stimulation was likewise found to be unaffected by hypnotically-induced deafness. It had previously been suggested by others that hypnotic anaesthesia might operate by attenuation of the afferent activity reaching the cortex, but the authors (Halliday and Mason, 1964) pointed out that this was unlikely to be the case since the perceptual block can be highly specific to the suggested stimulus. For example, under conditions of hypnotic deafness the hypnotist's voice will still be heard. It is therefore probable that the block (if it can be regarded as such) must be set up after a considerable amount of sensory processing, and that SEP changes, if any, might be found in the longer latency potentials not examined in this study.

A search of the literature has revealed only one abstract concerned with the effects of acupuncture on components of the SEP waveform. Arbus et al (1977) reported a concurrence between a flattening of the later part of the waveform (components of more than 200 msec latency) and the disappearance of pain sensitivity, with or without the passage of electrical current between the acupuncture needles. Blair et al (1975) had previously demonstrated a similar effect due to high frequency (25 or 100 Hz) epidural stimulation of the spinal cord (SCS) for the relief of chronic pain. The reduction of amplitude was particularly marked for a late negative wave (200-250 msec latency following stimulation at the ankle), but other components with a latency of more than 120 msec were also affected. At higher intensities of SCS all components were suppressed. The changes did not appear to be directly related to the relief of pain, since the SEP waveform returned to normal immediately after cessation of SCS, whereas the pain relief might persist for several hours.

In monkeys Larson et al (1965) studied the related phenomenon of electro-anaesthesia, whereby the passage of a small alternating current between electrodes at the nasion and the inion can produce unresponsiveness to electrical or mechanical stimulation of the body. Evoked potentials recorded directly from the medial lemniscus were unaffected under these conditions, but those recorded from the VPL nucleus of the thalamus were attenuated by approximately 50%. Cortical potentials directly recorded from the postcentral gyrus were abolished. It is doubtful whether this technique will ever be routinely applied to humans, but it is of interest since, unlike hypnosis and acupuncture, the anaesthetic effect does appear to be a consequence of the suppression of sensory input to the cerebral cortex.

An area in which the importance of sensory evoked potentials has been acknowledged for some time is that of hysterical disturbance of sensation, since the finding of an entirely normal EP may virtually eliminate the possibility of there being an organic cause for the complaint. Conversely it may be possible to establish the existence of an organic lesion when there is doubt concerning the aetiology of the symptoms, or clinical testing is confounded by a marked degree of 'hysterical overlay' (Halliday, 1972). Such positive evidence of organic disease is, of course, of greater diagnostic certainty than the finding of a response within normal limits, since the latter may simply be due to an insensitive technique. Alajouanine et al (1958) found SEPs to be normal in patients with hysterical anaesthesia of the hand and also recorded normal responses from one patient with congenital insensibility to pain. Hernandez-Peon et al (1963), on the other hand, reported cortical responses to be absent following cutaneous stimulation of the affected arm in a patient with glove and stocking anaesthesia but no impairment of joint-position sense. Levy and Behrman (1970) provided partial support for this observation, finding that the SEPs of an hysterically numb arm were of reduced amplitude compared with the unaffected side following cutaneous and low intensity nerve trunk stimulation, but normal for nerve trunk stimuli of higher intensity. These findings have never been disputed in the literature but are not universally accepted, and so the question as to whether SEPs can be affected by hysterical anaesthesia remains an open one for the present.

SEPs IN PSYCHIATRY

Intuitively, it does not seem likely that the recording of short latency SEP components could be of diagnostic importance in psychiatry, but Shagass and co-workers (1961, 1963, 1964, 1966, 1968) have devoted considerable effort to distinguishing between psychiatric patients according to differences in the SEP 'reactivity cycle'. A 'test' stimulus was delivered to the ulnar nerve a variable interval after a 'conditioning' shock, and the amplitude of the $\overline{P27}$ potential was plotted against the interstimulus interval (ISI). In normal subjects the recovery curve is polyphasic (see also Allison, 1962), with attenuation of the 'test' response at very short ISI, followed by a phase of full recovery or even enhancement when the ISI is between 5 and 20 msec. This is followed by a longer period of depressed responsiveness, with final recovery at 100 to 160 msec for this particular component (Schwartz and Shagass, 1964). In order to minimize contamination of the 'test' response by later potentials evoked by the 'conditioning' stimulus it was necessary to subtract an equal number of responses to single stimuli (regularly interspersed with the paired shocks) from the summated waveform. Comparing a group of psychotically depressed patients with age- and sex-matched normal controls, the early recovery phase was found to be significantly reduced or absent (Shagass and

Schwartz, 1966), which was not the case for a psychoneurotic group (Shagass and Schwartz, 1961, 1964). A return to a normal recovery cycle was observed after successful treatment by ECT or drugs. A similar depression of the early recovery phase was reported for patients with personality disorders or schizophrenia (Shagass and Schwartz, 1964), while in the latter group the corresponding curve showing the recovery of SEP latency (increased at short ISI) surprisingly revealed an enhancement of responsiveness (shortening of latency) compared with normal subjects. A more recent account suggests that certain SEP components including $\overline{P30}$ may have a more posterior scalp distribution in schizophrenic patients, compared with other patient groups and normal controls (Shagass et al, 1979).

The early peak in the SEP amplitude recovery cycle is reported to be depressed in normal volunteers receiving a regular oral dose of lithium carbonate, which is often prescribed as an antidepressant (Gartside et al, 1966). Although this and the effects described by Shagass and co-workers may be related to the pathological processes underlying mental disease, the precise connection is still unclear.

Remaining within the psychiatric field, SEPs have been employed to investigate the functioning of the cerebral hemispheres immediately before and after the administration of unilateral ECT (Kriss et al, 1980a). Two components ($\overline{N39}$ and $\overline{P49}$ following finger stimulation, equivalent to $\overline{N35}$ and $\overline{P45}$) were of significantly increased latency approximately 30 minutes after treatment compared with the immediate pre-treatment period, but this was likely to have been an effect of anaesthesia and was seen to an equal degree in recordings obtained from the untreated hemisphere (following stimulation of the contralateral hand). There were no consistent interhemispheric amplitude differences, but after ECT $\overline{P32}$ (equivalent to $\overline{P30}$) and $\overline{N39}$ were enhanced on both sides compared with the pre-treatment period. It was concluded that none of the observed SEP changes were likely to have been directly due to the effects of unilateral ECT, but that the general anaesthetic (intravenously administered barbiturate) was probably responsible for the slight enhancement of $\overline{P32}$ and the more marked alteration of later potentials. These are similar to anaesthetic effects described by Allison et al (1963).

To conclude, therefore, it appears that the SEP technique may at last have established a niche in clinical medicine, thanks to a more thoughtful and scientific approach, and to the identification of short latency subcortically-generated components. This chapter attempts to summarize and reconcile the significant (and in some cases not so significant) literature concerning the effects of disease and trauma on the SEP waveform, but there will inevitably be a few worthy studies which have escaped attention. To these authors I offer my apologies, but I hope that the ground that has been covered may give neurologists and clinical neurophysiologists a source of reference to what has already been achieved, and a point of departure for further investigations.

14

Movement-Related Cortical Potentials

H. Shibasaki

MOTOR POTENTIAL

Clinical, neurophysiological studies of central motor control have drawn much less attention from neurologists and neurophysiologists than those of the central sensory perception of various modalities. The electroencephalographic correlates of voluntary movements and of the conduction of impulses along the cortico-spinal tract have been of obvious interest, but still remain far from clinical application. Nonetheless, in this section the method of recording the cerebral potentials in association with voluntary movements (movement-related cortical potentials, MP) will be reviewed, together with findings in normal subjects, and some of the preliminary results of clinical studies.

History

It was Bates (1951) who first attempted to record cortical activity from the scalp in association with human voluntary movements. He used the photographic superimposition technique and demonstrated a small negative wave over the contralateral central area 20 to 40 msec after the beginning of the movement, but no activity before the movement. In 1965, Kornhuber and Deecke succeeded in recording potentials preceding voluntary movements by using reversed averaging. They registered a pulse at the onset of the electromyogram (EMG) and a second pulse 0.5 sec after the first pulse. They recorded all data on magnetic tape, and averaged it with a computer in a chronologically reversed way by playing the tape backwards and by using the second, delayed pulse as a trigger. By this method, they demonstrated a slow negative shift beginning as long as 1 sec before the onset of movement (*Bereitschaftspotential*, readiness potential) and a large positive complex after the movement onset (*reafferente Potentiale*). Later they found two more potentials just before the movement onset (pre-motion positivity and motor potential) (Deecke et al, 1969).

Vaughan et al have also studied movement-related potentials since 1965. Initially, they obtained the motor component of the cerebral activity in a reaction time paradigm by subtracting the cerebral potential changes recorded without a motor response (sensory component) from those associated with a motor response (sensory and motor components). Later, they also used reversed averaging and found a slow negative shift followed by a sharp negative wave preceding movements, maximal over the contralateral precentral region (Gilden et al, 1966). They too recognized 4 components of the MP and named them N_1, P_1, N_2 and P_2 (Vaughan et al, 1968). Since then, there have been many studies of the MP in normal subjects, but the physiological significance of each component, especially of the short-duration potentials immediately before and after the movement onset, has yet to be clarified.

Method of recording

The essential of the method is to average the electroencephalogram (EEG) preceding, and time-locked to, the movement onset. The time of movement onset has therefore to be determined as accurately as possible.

Recording can be performed by placing the subject either in a sitting, reclining or supine position. Eyes are usually kept open during the recording session. The subject is instructed to fixate his gaze upon some specific spot in front of him, and to avoid blinking in association with the movement. The same movement should be repeated voluntarily at a self-paced rate of once every 3 to 10 sec. Any kind of movement can be employed, but usually flexion or extension of a finger at the metacarpophalangeal joint, opposition or adduction of the thumb, flexion or extension of the wrist, fist-clenching, flexion or extension of the elbow, dorsiflexion of the foot, contraction of a facial muscle, and saccadic eye movements have been tried. Movements of finger or hand seem to be the easiest to perform and to show the best results. Movement of face or eyes are naturally associated with contamination of the EEG by artifacts from the EMG or the movement itself.

With regard to the movement onset, either the EMG onset or the onset of the mechanogram can serve as a trigger pulse. The EMG is recorded by a pair of surface electrodes placed over the contracting muscle. The time constant of the amplifier can be 0.03 to 0.1 sec, and the use of a high frequency cut should be avoided. The EMG is usually rectified and integrated, and a trigger pulse is obtained when the integrated EMG reaches a certain level. Deecke et al (1973a, 1976) use the onset of the discharge in the EMG recorded by a needle electrode as a trigger. Kato and Tanji (1972) trained their subjects to be able to produce a single motor unit potential repetitively and used it as a trigger. The mechanogram can be recorded with a potentiometer or accelerometer. The onset of the mechanogram usually lags behind the EMG onset by approximately 30 msec in a brisk voluntary contraction of hand muscles. For recording the MP associated with eye movements, the electro-oculogram (EOG) recorded from surface electrodes can be used as a trigger (Becker et al, 1972; Kurtzberg and Vaughan, 1973).

EEGs are recorded with non-polarizable electrodes, such as silver-silver chloride electrodes, fixed on the scalp with collodion. In the case of hand movements, the electrode location should include at least the vertex (C_z of the 10-20 International System) and the precentral hand motor area on both sides. The hand motor area electrodes can be replaced by C_3 and C_4 of the 10-20 system, but the author uses the point 2 cm in front of the somatosensory hand area. The latter is 7 cm lateral to the midline on a line connecting a point 2 cm posterior to the vertex to the external auditory meatus. It is desirable, if possible, to record from the frontal and parietal areas as well. Additional electrodes may be necessary for movements of eyes, face and foot. Electrode resistance should be less than 5 kilohms. Common monopolar derivations with reference to the linked ear electrodes are most often used, but bipolar derivations may also be employed. Deecke et al (1969, 1973a, 1976) claim that the bipolar derivation from both precentral motor areas is mandatory for recording the 'motor potential'. The time constant should be longer than 3.0 sec in order to record slow potentials.

An opisthochronic* averaging program is convenient for simultaneous on-line averaging of the EEG activity before and after movement onset during the recording session. With this program, data can be stored continuously, so that, when the trigger pulse occurs, data for a preset period before and after the triggering event can be automatically averaged. The window time should include at least 1.5 sec before, and 0.5 sec after, the trigger pulse, although this period can be modified as necessary. The sampling interval that the author is using is either 7.5 msec or 2.5 msec. The EOG and the rectified EMG can be averaged in the same way.

One recording session usually consists of 50 trials, and more than 2 sessions should be repeated for each movement. Demonstration of the short-duration potentials occurring in close association with the movement onset seems to require averaging of at least 200 samples in the author's experience.

Normal motor potential (MP)

At least 4 components have been recognized in the motor potential (MP), although some investigators report the presence of at least 8 components (Gerbrandt, 1977). There are 2 different terminologies; one by Deecke and Kornhuber (Figure 14.1) and the other by Vaughan et al (Figure 14.2). According to Deecke et al (1969, 1973a, 1976), the slow negative shift occurs approximately 1 sec before the movement onset, and is maximal at the vertex and symmetrically distributed, but becomes asymmetric at 400 to 500 msec before movement onset; it is larger contralaterally. This component is considered to reflect the preparatory events in the cerebral cortex for the forthcoming voluntary movement. Hence this is called *Bereitschaftspotential* or readiness potential. This might correspond to the changes in discharge rate of motor cortex neurons which were shown to occur several hundred milliseconds before the movement in monkeys (Schmidt et al, 1974; Tanji and Evarts, 1976) and cats (Neafsey et al, 1978).

* Literally, "backwards in time". The term was introduced by W. Grey Walter.

Vol. Rt Finger Movement

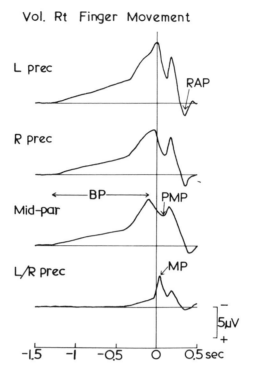

Figure 14.1 *Schematic illustration of the normal MP according to the terminology used by Deecke et al. Average of several hundred samples with right index finger movement. BP: Bereitschaftspotential, PMP: pre-motion positivity, MP: motor potential, RAP: reafferente Potentiale. The EMG onset is at time 0.*

The *Bereitschaftspotential* has been shown to be influenced by intention, motivation, effort and the muscle strength exerted in the movement; the greater these factors are, the larger the amplitude of the *Bereitschaftspotential*. It is also known that the faster the movement is performed, the later the *Bereitschaftspotential* begins and the smaller its amplitude (Deecke and Kornhuber, 1977).

The relationship between the *Bereitschaftspotential* and the contingent negative variation (CNV) has been discussed by many investigators. It is now generally believed that the CNV contains the *Bereitschaftspotential* as one of its components.

The author paid particular attention to the later negative slope, localized to the contralateral precentral region, beginning 400 to 500 msec before the movement onset and culminating in a negative peak at approximately 90 msec before the movement onset (Figure 14.3) (Shibasaki et al, 1980a). This negative slope might be more specifically related to the movement.

The 'pre-motion positivity' is not recorded in all subjects. Since it is localized over the anterior parietal region bilaterally and occurs 80 to 90 msec before the movement onset, Deecke et al (1973a, 1976) propose that this component is related to the initiation of voluntary movements. In monkeys trained to make voluntary movements of the forelimb, neurons in the dentate nucleus were shown to change their firing rate 90 msec before the motor cortex neurons change their discharge rate (Thach, 1970; 1975), and likewise those in the ventrolateral nucleus of the thalamus alter their discharge rate approximately 100 msec before (Strick, 1976). The pre-motion positivity has, therefore, been thought to correspond to the starting point of the cortico-cerebellar-motor cortex loop (Deecke et al 1973, 1976). But in the author's experience this positivity is lateralized to the ipsilateral hemisphere (P-50, Figures 14.3 and 14.4), and its significance remains unsettled.

The 'motor potential' is localized to the precentral region contralateral to the movement and begins 50 to 60 msec before the movement onset (Deecke et al, 1973a; 1976). This potential, therefore, is considered to reflect the activity of the cortico-spinal tract cells in the motor cortex. In monkeys trained to make voluntary movements of the forelimb, neurons in the precentral cortex were shown to increase their firing rate 60 to 100 msec before movement onset (Evarts, 1972). Arezzo and Vaughan (1975) demonstrated a negative wave by epidural recording over the contralateral precentral area, starting 85 to 110 msec before the monkey began moving his forelimb, and established the phase reversal of the potential within the cortex by laminar recording.

The large post-motor positive complex starts 30 to 90 msec after the movement onset (Kornhuber and Deecke, 1965). From its resemblance to a potential evoked by passive movements, they proposed that this complex might be related to kinesthetic feedback (*reafferente Potentiale*). Shibasaki et al (1980a) in a topographical study of the movement-related cortical potential, identified 4 post-

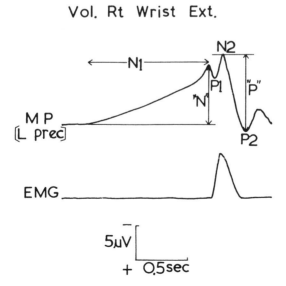

Figure 14.2 Schematic illustration of the normal MP according to the terminology used by Vaughan et al. Recorded from the left central area while movement was right wrist extension. The EMG is rectified and averaged.

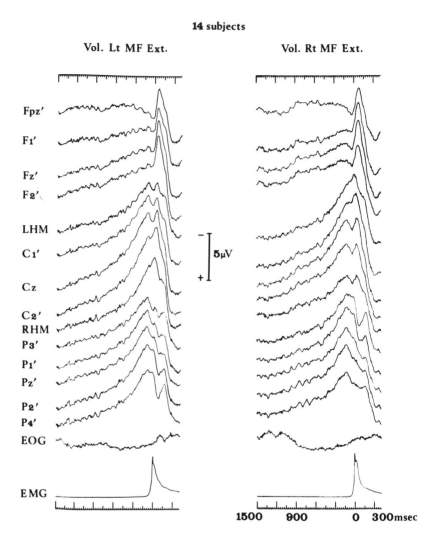

Figure 14.3 *Averaged cortical potentials associated with voluntary self-paced middle finger extensions. Grand average records from 14 normal subjects. 200 movements from each subject. LHM and RHM: left and right hand motor area, respectively. (From Shibasaki et al, 1980a.)*

motion components. These are a frontal negativity ($\overline{N50}$), a posteriorly located positivity ($\overline{P90}$), a contralateral parietal negativity ($\overline{N160}$) and a widespread positivity ($\overline{P300}$) (Figures 14.3 and 14.4).

Vaughan et al (1968) believe that all 4 components of the MP are generated in the precentral motor cortex (together making up the motor potential in its broader meaning). They divided the MP into the negative component before the movement onset ('N' of Figure 14.2) and the positive component after the movement onset ('P' of Figure 14.2), and they found that both 'N' and 'P' were maximal over the

14 subjects

Vol. Rt MF Ext.

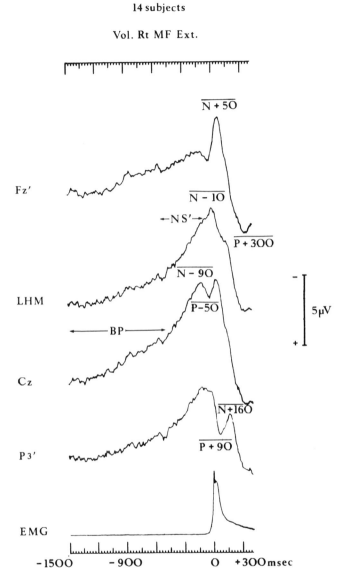

Figure 14.4 *Terminology of components proposed by Shibasaki et al (1980). Components other than two slow negativities were named according to the polarity and the mean time interval in msec between the peak and the initial peak of the averaged, rectified EMG. The interval is designated '-' if the peak occurs before the EMG peak, and '+' if it occurs after.*

precental area contralateral to the movement. They further demonstrated that the component 'N' showed its maximal distribution over the part of the precentral region corresponding to the movement; lateral with tongue movement, medial with foot movement and intermediate with hand movement. Although they also found P_1 only inconstantly, the time interval from the P_1 onset to the EMG onset was shown to be shortest with tongue movement, longest with foot movement and intermediate with hand movement. They treated P_1 and N_2 as a complex and related it to some processes closely associated with the initiation of movement. Although the component N_1 and P_2 by Vaughan et al seem to correspond to the *Bereitschaftspotential* and *reafferente Potentiale* of Kornhuber and Deecke, respectively, the relationship of P_1 and N_2 with the 'pre-motion positivity' and the 'motor potential' has not been clearly established. Some investigators, who studied the MP employing the terminology of Vaughan et al, found that the N_2 component occurred after the movement onset (Gerbrandt et al, 1973, Wilke and Lansing, 1973, Shibasaki and Kato, 1975).

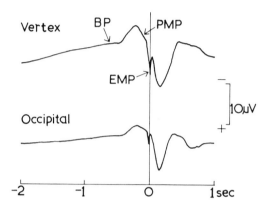

Figure 14.5 *Schematic illustration of the normal MP associated with saccadic lateral eye movements according to the method used by Becker et al (1972). BP: Bereitschaftspotential, PMP: pre-motion positivity, EMP: eye muscle potential. The onset of saccade is at time 0.*

These differences in the results of MP studies among investigators seem to result mainly from differences in the method of recording, as well as of identifying, each component. The N_2 component of Vaughan et al (1968) appears to be a composite of the two negativities $\overline{\text{N-10}}$ and $\overline{\text{N50}}$ found in the author's study (Shibasaki et al, 1980).

Only a few studies have been made on the MP associated with eye movements. Becker et al (1972) found a positive cortical potential 130 to 200 msec before the onset of saccades associated with lateral displacement of gaze, but no negative wave corresponding to the 'motor potential' associated with limb movements (Figure 14.5). They ascribed a very sharp positive deflection occurring simultaneously with the onset of the saccade to a muscle potential (eye muscle potential). Kurtzberg and Vaughan (1973) found two kinds of positive waves; one predominantly over the posterior frontal area, occurring 200 msec before the saccade onset, and the other over the parietal area 25 to 40 msec before. There seem to be great difficulties in recording MP associated with eye movements because of the inevitable artifacts. The same holds true for the MP associated with speech (Szirtes and Vaughan, 1977).

Clinical studies

The clinical application of the MP is still far from practical. Only a few studies have been made on the *Bereitschaftspotential* or the N_1 component in clinical material.

Shibasaki (1975) studied 20 patients with hemiparesis of varying severity due to unilateral cerebral hemisphere lesions and found an abnormality of the MP in 80% of the patients. The most frequent abnormality was a depressed amplitude of the N_1 component over the affected hemisphere. No correlation was found, however, between the abnormality of MP and the extent of the disability in the hand tested. In cases with a localized lesion near the cerebral convexity, the MP abnormality tended to be restricted to the affected hemisphere, but in cases showing diffuse cerebral dysfunction as a result of a deep-seated expanding lesion, the MP abnormality was extensive and bilateral.

Deecke et al (1973b, 1977) studied 33 patients with Parkinson's disease presenting especially with akinesia, and found that the *Bereitschaftspotential* was bilaterally abolished or even slightly positive in cases with bilateral akinesia, and that, in cases with hemiparkinsonism, the amplitude was reduced significantly over the affected hemisphere or on moving the akinetic hand. Shibasaki et al (1978a) also studied 20 patients with Parkinson's disease, of which MP was abnormal in 90%. The most frequent abnormalities included deformity or disorganization of the waveform and a depressed amplitude and earlier onset of the N_1 component. There was no correlation between the N_1 abnormality and the intensity of akinesia, rigidity or tremor.

Shibasaki et al (1978a) studied 20 patients with cerebellar ataxia of various aetiologies and found a MP abnormality in 55 percent. The most conspicuous finding was the inability to record the N_1 component, in spite of repeated examinations, in 5 patients with progressive myoclonic epilepsy and cerebellar ataxia. The motor potential (MP) was recorded in patients with cerebellar degeneration without intention myoclonus, although the amplitude of N_1 was depressed and its onset was earlier in some cases. In relation to these findings, 4 cases with a midbrain vascular lesion manifesting with ataxia of the contralateral hand and an ipsilateral partial oculomotor nerve palsy (Benedikt's syndrome) were studied. In 3 of these 4 cases, the N_1 amplitude was depressed on moving the affected hand as compared with the intact hand. The MP was studied serially in 4 patients with Parkinson's disease, who underwent a unilateral stereotaxic electrocoagulation of the ventral intermediolateral nucleus of the thalamus because of an intractable hand tremor. The N_1 component was recorded in all cases before surgery, but could not be recognized after surgery despite a satisfactory therapeutic effect on the tremor. These findings were interpreted as suggesting a possible influence of the dentato-thalamic pathway on the genesis of the N_1 component or *Bereitschaftspotential*.

Timsit-Berthier et al (1973) studied the MP in a large number of psychotic patients and found an abnormally prolonged pattern of the *Bereitschaftspotential* more frequently in patients with psychosis than in patients with neurosis or normal controls.

JERK-LOCKED AVERAGING

Since Grinker et al (1938) found an association between the myoclonic jerks and the spike discharges of the EEG spike-and-wave complexes in a family with myoclonic epilepsy, polygraphic studies of the spontaneously occurring myoclonus and the accompanying EEG have been the subject of many investigations using either the electroencephalogram or a cathode ray tube display (Dawson 1946; Halliday, 1967a, 1967b, 1967d, 1974; Halliday and Halliday, 1980). With the conventional polygraphic technique, however, it has often been difficult to determine whether there is a definite relationship between the myoclonic discharge and the EEG paroxysmal activities. By using a backward averaging program, Shibasaki and Kuroiwa (1975) were able to demonstrate an EEG spike preceding the myoclonic EMG discharge even where the conventional polygraph did not show any EEG spike in association with the myoclonus. Chadwick et al (1977) employed a similar technique in cases of post-hypoxic myoclonus and found similar EEG/EMG correlations. This technique appears to be useful for detecting cortical activity in association with involuntary jerks, when this is not recognizable on routine electroencephalography, and also for investigating the precise temporal and spatial relationship between the EEG and EMG activities.

Recording technique

The technique of jerk-locked averaging can be summarized as follows. Recording can be done either in the sitting, reclining or supine positions. Surface EMG electrodes are used to record the involuntary jerks. A pair of electrodes are placed approximately 3 cm apart on the skin overlying the muscle which contracts most frequently. The time constant of the amplifier is set to 0.03 or 0.1 sec, and the high frequency cut should not be used. The amplified EMG is preferably rectified and integrated to obtain a trigger pulse, but, in the absence of an integrator, the onset of the amplified EMG itself can also be used without integration.

To record the associated EEG spikes, electrodes should be placed along the central sulcus. When jerks are recorded from an upper extremity, electrodes are placed at the C_3 and C_4 locations of the 10-20 International System, or over the hand motor area on each side. A point 2 cm in front of the somatosensory hand area is used as the hand 'motor area', where the sensory area is taken as being 7 cm down from the midline on a line joining a point 2 cm posterior to the vertex and a point just in front of the external auditory meatus. It is better to include the vertex electrode (C_z) regardless of the site of EMG recording. Additional electrodes may be applied depending on the location of the jerks. The electrode impedance should be kept below 5 kilohms. Either common referential derivations with reference to the linked ear electrodes or bipolar derivations, or both, may be used. The frequency responses of the amplifier can be set to the same as for the routine EEG recording. The time constant employed is usually 0.1 to 0.3 sec and it is better not to use any high frequency cut. Electro-oculogram (EOG) should be recorded to detect any eye-movement or blink artifacts.

An opisthochronic averaging program is useful for averaging the EEGs both before and after the onset of the jerk. The EMG and EOG should be averaged at the same time as the EEG. Averaging can be done with various window times. To detect the myoclonus-related spike, a window time ranging, for example, from 400 msec before to 240 msec after the EMG onset, with an ordinate period of 2.5 msec, may be found adequate. It is convenient to record all the data on magnetic tape as it allows one to analyse the results in various different ways afterwards. Averaging 50 to 100 samples is generally adequate to demonstrate any jerk-related cortical activity which may be present.

Clinical application

In principle, jerk-locked averaging can be applied to the investigation of EEG-EMG correlations in any kind of involuntary movement, but slow involuntary movements, such as athetosis and dystonia, are not very suitable for this technique because of the difficulty of getting a precisely timed trigger point. Even when applied to jerking, the jerks have to involve the same muscle or the same group of muscles in a fairly repetitive way. Therefore, migratory involuntary movements such as chorea may not be a good candidate for this technique, although its use in this condition may not be impossible. It is obvious that the triggering movement must occur frequently in order to make the computer averaging practicable. For these reasons, this technique has in the past been applied exclusively to cases of myoclonus. Shibasaki et al (1978b) studied 15 patients with various kinds of myoclonus using jerk-locked averaging. In all 7 patients with progressive myoclonic epilepsy, in whom this technique was applied, a cortical spike or spike-and-wave was found to precede the myoclonus of the upper extremities by 7 to 15 msec and to be localized over the contralateral central region. Although the routine EEG tracings showed spike-and-wave bursts or complexes in most of the patients, a constant relationship between these paroxysmal discharges and the myoclonus was rare. Hallett et al (1979) reported similar findings in 2 patients with post-hypoxic myoclonus and 1 patient with post-traumatic myoclonus. In cases of essential myoclonus or of palatal myoclonus, no cortical activity associated with jerks was demonstrated by jerk-locked averaging.

In a patient with subacute spongiform encephalopathy or Creutzfeldt-Jakob disease, who had never shown periodic synchronous discharges on repeated EEG examinations, jerk-locked averaging demonstrated a slow sharp wave over the hemisphere contralateral to the upper extremity from which the myoclonus was recorded (Shibasaki and Kuroiwa, 1975; Shibasaki et al, 1981). An example of jerk-locked averaging in a patient with progressive myoclonic epilepsy is shown in Figure 14.6. This 23-year-old man had been progressively disabled by frequent intention myoclonus and occasional generalized convulsions since the age of 14.

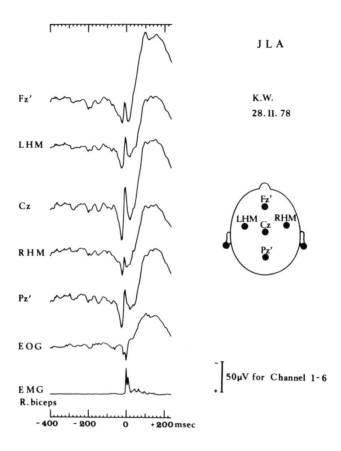

Figure 14.6 *EEGs, EOG and rectified EMG recorded by the jerk-locked averaging technique in a patient with progressive myoclonic epilepsy. EEGs are referred to linked ear electrodes. Average of 100 records.*

Myoclonus in this case characteristically affected the proximal muscles of upper or lower extremities bilaterally and simultaneously and frequently involved the trunk as well. The routine polygraphic recording of EEG and EMG did not show any constant temporal relationship between the EEG spikes and the myoclonus, but jerk-locked averaging demonstrated a positive/negative cortical spike preceding the jerks, which was maximal over the vertex and larger over the contralateral hemisphere.

15

Advanced Data Capture and Analysis Techniques for Clinical Evoked Potentials

G. Barrett

Earlier chapters of this book have described the basic methods required for evoked potential averaging and waveform measurement. This Chapter introduces some of the more advanced recording and analysis techniques which are already being used in research that will form the basis of future clinical testing. Two broad categories of activity can be identified with respect to evoked potential recording: data capture and data analysis. Data capture includes the basic technique of averaging and its alternatives, together with methods for averaging selected trials in a run. Data analysis can be divided into two sub-groups: data measurement and data representation. Measurement methods range from the analysis of single peaks to more sophisticated statistical procedures which compare entire evoked potential waveforms. Methods of data representation range from the standard waveform plot of amplitude against time to topographical maps showing waveform distributions across the scalp.

DATA CAPTURE

Dawson (1954a) first applied the averaging technique to the detection of small evoked potentials and the methods he described are still used, although the equipment on which the methods are implemented has advanced beyond recognition over the intervening years. The objective of averaging is the detection of a small constant signal occurring in relation to an event, masked by randomly occurring, high amplitude noise. This objective is achieved in most digital computers and averagers by adding together the digitized data occurring in relation to each stimulus. Dividing this sum by the number of trials in the average gives the mean. Both these averages have their advantages and disadvantages. The sum is a more precise measure of the evoked potential than the mean and this may be important where small differences between waveforms are concerned. Such comparisons, however, can be complicated if the number of trials contributing to each sum is different. In this case it is preferable to compare mean waveforms. Averaging has proved to be a powerful and efficient technique for extracting small signals from background noise. This is true to such an extent that the few alternatives which have been suggested have never gained widespread acceptance.

It is clear, however, that information about the electrical response related to an event can be lost when computing an average, because such a measure gives no information about the variability of the individual responses. The computation of amplitude variability for the points constituting an average waveform is similar to that of the average itself and can be performed concurrently. Computation of latency variability is more complicated because it involves detailed analysis of the response to each stimulus in an average.

Amplitude variability

Generally, in the clinical setting, measurement of amplitude variability has proved uninteresting with little or no differences being observed between peaks in the same waveform or between waveforms recorded under different conditions. However, the following two examples illustrate the utility of recording amplitude variability. Kriss (1976) recorded flash evoked potentials from patients undergoing a course of unilateral ECT treatment for depression. He recorded the amplitude variability of the potentials before ECT, during anaesthesia and during the recovery period after ECT. Figure 15.1 shows that the variability of the flash evoked potential is small before anaesthesia, increases during anaesthesia and the early recovery period after ECT and then returns to its original level during the late recovery period some 15-30 minutes after ECT. The figure also shows that although the ECT was administered unilaterally there is no corresponding asymmetry in the variability of the flash evoked potential (Kriss et al, 1980b).

Amplitude variability may also be of interest when the inter-subject consistency of evoked potentials is studied. Pattern reversal stimulation of the visual half-fields produces a consistent negative-positive-negative (NPN) complex which is recorded at electrodes in the midline and on the scalp ipsilateral to the stimulated half-field (Barrett et al, 1976 and Chapter 3). The response recorded over the contralateral scalp is less consistent, but on average a positive-negative-positive (PNP) complex is seen. The potential on the contralateral side is most variable between the midline and 5 cm lateral (Blumhardt and Halliday, 1979) and this inter-subject variability can be seen in Figure 3.15. In particular, the responses at the electrode 5 cm contralateral to the midline are more variable than those recorded at the 10 cm electrode on the same side.

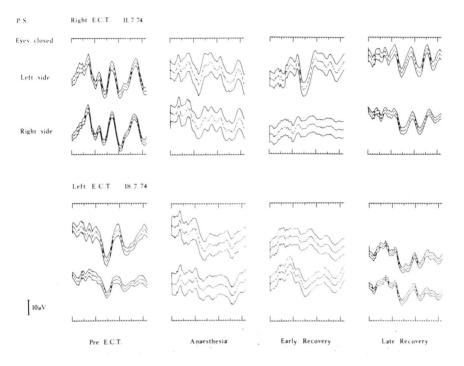

Figure 15.1 *Flash evoked potential and its variability in one depressed patient receiving unilateral ECT to the right and left hemisphere on separate occasions one week apart. The Figure shows the mean waveform as the dashed line with the values for one standard deviation above and below the mean plotted as solid lines. The variability of the response is clearly largest immediately after the administration of anaesthesia and during the early recovery period after the shock. There are no differences in variability referrable to the side of ECT administration, although the VEP itself is asymmetrical during the early recovery period in each case. Negativity of the active electrode is plotted as an upward deflection. Time scale marks at intervals of 10, 50 and 100 msec. (From Kriss, 1976.)*

Waveform variability

Although this illustration indicates the level of amplitude variability in the pattern evoked response to half-field stimulation, it does not provide information about the consistency of the waveform. It is clear from observing these responses from a group of individuals that the ipsilateral NPN complex occurs consistently despite large inter-individual differences in amplitude. The contralateral PNP complex, however, is not so consistent. One method of looking at waveform consistency in responses that have very little latency jitter across individuals is to make comparisons using normalized waveforms. Figure 15.2 shows a comparison between waveform variability computed from normalized data and amplitude variability computed from the same data before normalization. The raw seven-channel record for each of the 5 subjects in this illustration was normalized by finding the point of maximum excursion from a 25 msec post-stimulus baseline, assigning this point the value 100 and recomputing the amplitude of each ordinate as a percentage of this maximum value. Thus, for each subject the amplitude of the normalized responses is equated and direct comparisons of waveform can be made. Figure 15.2 shows clearly that the waveform of the ipsilateral NPN complex is comparatively invariant with respect to the contralateral complex, particularly for right half-field stimulation. This point is not made by the plot for the raw data which shows the same widespread distribution of amplitude variability as that seen for the 50 subjects depicted in Figure 3.15.

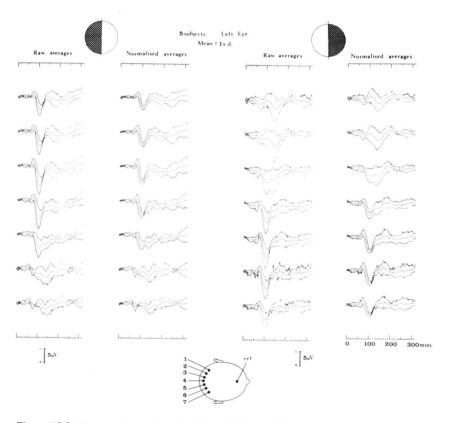

Figure 15.2 *A comparison of amplitude variability and waveform variability for the potentials evoked by pattern-reversal stimulation of the visual half-fields. The dashed line shows the mean value for 5 subjects and the solid lines are plotted one standard deviation above and below the mean. The raw averages indicate the amplitude variability of the response, whereas the normalized averages show the waveform variability (see text for method of computation). It can be seen for both half-fields that the amplitude variability is similar right across the scalp, whereas the waveform variability is smaller at the midline and ipsilateral electrodes than at the electrodes contralateral to the stimulated field.*

Latency variability and single trial analysis

Although amplitude variability can provide useful information, it is always possible that this variability is due to changes in the latency of the recorded potential peaks. This is particularly true for the later evoked potentials and slow potential shifts which are known to be related more to the experimental situation than to the stimulus *per se*. The computation of latency variability is far more complicated than for amplitude variability. This is because it is necessary first to identify the peak of interest in each trial of a recording and then to measure its latency from stimulus onset. The basic principle for identifying a response in a single trial is to match the single trial waveform to a template waveform representing all or part of the expected response. The matching is performed for successive points in time until the most similar match is found. Component latencies can then be measured from the single trial waveform. This procedure has to be repeated for every trial in order to compute latency variability. Different techniques for identifying single trial waveforms, many of which are based on a method described by Woody (1967), have been described by a number of authors (for examples see Otto, 1978 section IX; McGillem and Aunon, 1977; Wastell, 1977).

The procedure described by Woody was used by Kutas et al (1977) to study variations in the latency of the large positive component occurring 300 msec on average after the stimulus ($\overline{P300}$) in a reaction-time task. Three different series of visual stimuli were presented under three different response conditions. In the fixed name (FN) series the word 'Nancy' was presented to the subject on 20% of trials and the word 'David' appeared on the other 80% of trials. In the variable name series (VN) the subject was presented with one of several female names on 20% of occasions and one of several male names on the rest of the trials. In the synonym series (SYN) words with the same meaning as the word 'prod' were presented on 20% of trials while unrelated words were presented on the rest of the trials. The response conditions involved subvocal counting of the infrequent stimulus (count), a button press under conditions emphasizing accuracy of response (accurate RT) and a button press with the emphasis on speed of response (speed RT). Figure 15.3 shows the evoked potentials for each of the stimulus/response combinations for both the raw averages and the waveforms produced by summing individual trials aligned at the peak latency of the $\overline{P300}$ component (latency adjusted). It can be seen that the differences in response amplitude apparent in the raw average records are largely resolved in the latency adjusted waveforms. In fact there are no significant differences in amplitude between the different conditions for the latency adjusted data. Analysis of component latency for the individual trials suggested that $\overline{P300}$ latency corresponds to stimulus evaluation time and is independent of response selection.

The prospects for this type of analysis are enormous because it is self-evident that each individual waveform contributing to an average evoked potential is elicited under different circumstances. The waveform is altered by the subject's arousal, the direction of his attention, the background EEG and a variety of other factors, all of which are obscured in the average waveform. In the clinical setting the computation of latency variability will probably be of most use in recording the long latency cognitive evoked potentials from psychiatric patients. However, it is also

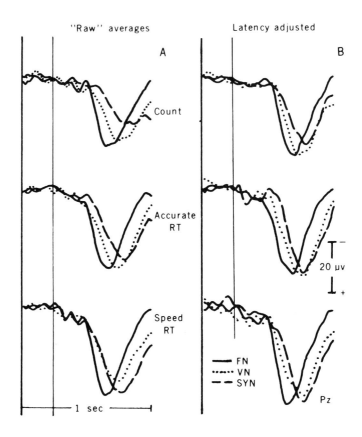

Figure 15.3 *A comparison of $\overline{P300}$ potentials recorded at the parietal electrode during a decision-making task. The waveforms were summed over 5 subjects and are shown before (A, 'raw' averages) and after peak alignment of the single trial waveforms using a template matching technique (B, latency adjusted). See text for a description of this technique and experimental details. It can be seen that the response amplitudes for the latency-adjusted waveforms are all similar, suggesting that the amplitude differences seen for the 'raw' averages are the result of trial-to-trial latency variability of the $\overline{P300}$ peak. (Reproduced from Kutas et al, 1977.)*

possible to envisage an application to shorter latency evoked potentials. Under normal averaging conditions, latency variability results in smearing or broadening of evoked potential components. Single trial analysis would indicate whether there was any periodicity underlying the variability. For example, latency shifts occurring in the response to the second of a pair of stimuli might suggest an effect on the refractoriness of the stimulated pathway which in turn might indicate the underlying pathophysiology in a particular group of patients. Similarly, under certain conditions, latency variability may occur for one component of an evoked response but not for another.

DATA ANALYSIS – MEASUREMENT

The variety of measurements of evoked potential waveforms extends from visual identification of peaks and their manual measurement to complicated statistical analyses of entire waveforms for the detection and separation of individual components. At present the former method is the most widely used, particularly in clinical testing, and the various techniques are described in Chapter 1.

Limits of normality for age-varying data

The method of determining the limits of normality for individual peak latencies or amplitudes needs careful consideration when the potentials being examined change with age. The usual practice is to set the limits of normality at 2.5 or 3 standard deviations above and below the mean value measured on a healthy control population for each particular component characteristic. However, it is clear that if a young control group is used for a component characteristic that increases with age, then the upper limit of normality will be too low for elderly patients tested and there will be a high proportion of false positives in this group. The inclusion of control subjects from a wide age range is no solution if the data are used to produce a single limit of normality, because the high variability of component values across age will produce a relatively insensitive test.

One method of dealing with age-varying evoked potential characteristics is to evaluate a healthy control group for each of a number of different age ranges. The problem with this method is that it requires a heavy recording commitment, particularly if a patient control group is also required. A second method, requiring fewer subjects, is to record potentials from individuals across a wide age range and compute the regression line and confidence limits relating the component characteristic of interest to age. The confidence limits can be set according to the level of statistical significance required, with decreasing probability of occurrence producing confidence limits at an increasing distance from the regression line. This method was used by Goodin et al (1978b) in their study relating an abnormally prolonged $\overline{P300}$ component in a simple auditory target detection task to dementia. In a previous study they established that for normal subjects the latency of $\overline{P300}$ in this detection task increased with age (Goodin et al, 1978a). The regression line and associated confidence limits computed from this normal data were used as a basis for testing the normality of $\overline{P300}$ latencies recorded from a group of demented patients and a group of non-demented patients performing the same task. As can be seen from Figure 15.4 a high proportion of the demented patients had $\overline{P300}$ latencies longer than the limit drawn two standard deviations above the regression line. Conversely, all but one of the latencies for the non-demented patients fell below this limit of normality.

The drawback of this method is that it cannot be used for data which show discontinuous changes related to age. For example, the pattern-evoked $\overline{P100}$ component for female subjects shows a sudden increase in latency during the sixth decade (see Figure 3.12 and Halliday et al, 1982). The regression line technique

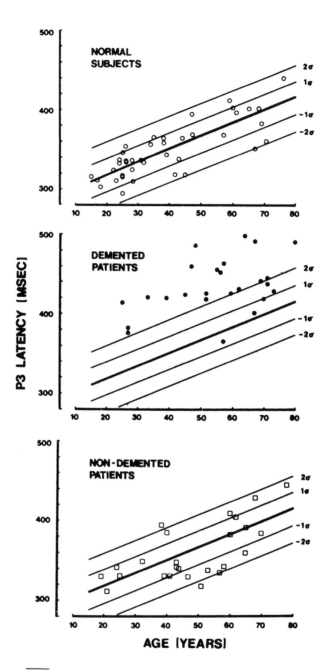

Figure 15.4 $\overline{P300}$ *latency plotted as a function of age for normal subjects, demented patients and non-demented patients. The regression line and confidence limits describing the normal data are reproduced for each group with the individual latency values superimposed. Only 5 of the demented patients had latencies shorter than the upper limit of two standard deviations above the regression line. Only one of the non-demented patients had a latency longer than this limit. (Reproduced from Goodin et al, 1978b.)*

could not be applied to data showing such changes, although it could possibly be applied on either side of the discontinuity.

The analysis of single waveforms is also important for the detection of trials containing artifacts and their exclusion from an average. This procedure is particularly necessary when recording slow potentials (e.g. CNV and readiness potential) and the late cognitive waves, as these potentials are disposed to contamination by potentials associated with eye-movements. By connecting one or more recording channels to monitor eye-movements, individual sweeps during a recording run can be accepted or rejected. This can be done either manually, by visual inspection of the activity on the monitoring channel, or by applying a decision-making rule implemented in computer hardware or software to this activity. Whichever method is chosen, it is important to note, particularly with eye-movement contamination of the slow waves, that the potentials recorded at electrodes on the scalp can be affected by activity which is not detected by the 'monitoring' electrodes. (See Chapter 2 and Hillyard, 1974, for a detailed discussion of eye-movement and other artifacts affecting slow potential shifts).

Artifacts due to the activity associated with muscle contraction can be detected with techniques similar to those used for the slower, large amplitude shifts associated with eye-movements. EMG bursts, due, for example, to swallowing, can be intrusive when recording slow potentials, such as the readiness potential preceding voluntary movement, even if they occur on only a small number of trials. Sweeps including muscle artifact can be excluded from the running average. Spikes due to muscle activity can also be eliminated from an average by digital filtering. In this procedure computer software is used to remove activity with defined frequency characteristics from the averaged waveform. This filtering can be used to produce smooth waveforms free from muscle artifact or mains interference. One particular smoothing procedure which is widely used on averaged responses involves computing the sliding mean amplitude value across a sequence of n points in the waveform starting at the first ordinate (where n is usually 3, 5 or 7). The resultant mean amplitude becomes the first point of the smoothed waveform and the n-point 'window' is advanced by one ordinate to compute the second point of the smoothed waveform and so on through the average.

The usefulness of single trial analysis has been extended from peak detection and artifact rejection to selection of trials fulfilling preset criteria for inclusion in an average. This technique of selective averaging has been used, for example, by Jones and Armington (1977) to compare visual evoked potentials elicited during periods of high background alpha activity with those elicited during low alpha activity.

The methods and applications described here give some idea of the potential of applying single trial analysis to evoked response recording. Indeed the success or failure of evoked potentials as an aid to diagnosis in psychiatry and movement disorders depends largely on the ability to recognize and reject artifactual trials which would otherwise confound the data. However, use of the described techniques should not be a substitute for care and attention to detail during a recording. In particular the exclusion of eye-movements and muscle spikes can largely be achieved by instructions to the subject. It will probably be more difficult for patients to comply with these instructions, due to anxiety or the nature of their disorder, and single trial analysis may therefore play a large part in the clinical recording of long latency evoked potentials and potential shifts.

Waveform comparisons

The measurement of single peaks ignores a great deal of information contained in the remainder of an evoked potential waveform and procedures have been developed to compare and contrast entire waveforms on an ordinate-by-ordinate basis. Comparisons can be made using a range of statistical procedures varying from correlation and *t*-test to multivariate analyses such as Principal Component Analysis and Discriminant Function Analysis. The decision regarding which statistic to use on a set of waveforms depends on the question being asked. The investigator usually wants to know whether waveforms are the same or different. If he is looking for similarity then he can use the cross-correlation method in which one waveform is compared with another for regular shifts in latency, with each latency providing a cross correlation coefficient and the plot of these coefficients producing a correlogram (see Section 8.7 in Cooper et al, 1974). The latency shift of the maximum positive peak of the correlogram is taken to represent the latency at which two waveforms are most similar. Figure 15.5 demonstrates an application of this technique in the quantification of component delays following unilateral optic neuritis. In a healthy individual the correlation between potential waveforms evoked from each eye by either flash or pattern reversal stimulation is almost perfect with zero time shift (see for example, Figure 3.6). Figure 15.5 shows the correlograms between the responses from each eye evoked by both flash and pattern stimulation in a patient who had recently suffered an episode of right optic neuritis. The correlogram peak for the flash responses is maximal at a delay of 3 msec, indicating no significant difference for this response, whereas the peak for the pattern response shows that the waveform for the right eye occurs 20 msec later than that for the left. This represents a significant latency difference between the two eyes and is abnormal. Unfortunately this technique can only be applied when the waveforms from the two eyes are similar, which is not always the case following optic nerve disease (see Chapter 6). Another major drawback of this technique is that the larger components in a response swamp the smaller components. The Burden group attempted to resolve this problem by computing correlation values for two separate components of a waveform and multiplying these together to give the Recognition Index (Weinberg and Cooper, 1972; Weinberg, 1978). Although this provides a definite improvement, it must always be remembered that correlation does not imply cause and effect. For example, a high correlation between two waveforms of opposite polarity recorded from different locations on the scalp is not conclusive evidence that both waveforms are produced by the same underlying event, such as the opposite ends of a generating dipole.

Differences between waveforms can be determined by applying *t*-tests to each corresponding ordinate. To do this for single average waveforms, such as those recorded from different electrodes for the same stimulus, it is necessary to know the amplitude variance for each ordinate so that *t* can be computed. If the difference between group data is being computed then it is necessary to treat each averaged waveform as a single observation and compute the mean and variance of each ordinate separately for the comparison groups. The major problem with this method is that so many *t*-tests have to be performed on a single waveform (one for each ordinate in the sweep) that it becomes necessary to set the level of statistical significance low enough to be able to attach functional significance to differences which can safely be assumed not to have occurred by chance. There is also the drawback that apparent differences in component amplitude may in fact be due to latency changes. An illustration of this method can be found in Shagass et al (1977). Where data from a number of different groups or experimental conditions have to be compared, it is possible to perform an analysis of variance on each ordinate to detect group differences (see for example Arnal et al, 1972b). Both this method and the application of multiple *t*-tests begin to identify differences between components rather than individual ordinates because the significant differences tend to cluster around particular points which prove to be the peaks and troughs of the evoked potentials. Clinical applications of these methods have not proved feasible, largely because of the amount of computing required, but also because of the statistical drawbacks and the possibility of misinterpretation of results.

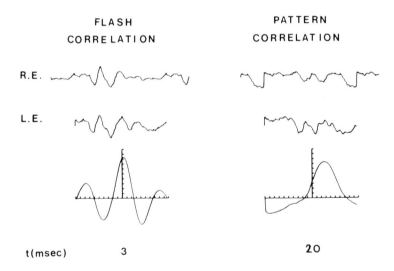

Figure 15.5 *Correlograms relating responses recorded for flash and pattern stimulation from the right and left eyes of a patient who had previously suffered an attack of right optic neuritis. See text for explanation. The vertical scale of the correlogram extends from 0 (no correlation) to 1 (perfect correlation) in steps of 0.1. (From Mushin, 1974.)*

Multivariate statistical analyses

More recently, multivariate statistical techniques have been applied to experimental data with considerable success. These statistics, notably Principal Component Analysis (PCA) and Discriminant Function Analysis (DA), enable the investigator to identify the major components in an evoked potential waveform (in the former case) and to identify those components which make one group of waveforms different from another group (in the latter case). An excellent tutorial review of the application of these techniques to evoked potential data is presented by Donchin and Heffley (1978). An attractive feature of multivariate analyses is that in some cases individual components may be identified by the analysis which are not clearly visible in the raw waveforms but may appear as points of inflexion on larger waves. The component is identified in relation to experimental parameters or clinical conditions according to the proportion of the total variance that can be allocated to it (PCA) or by the proportion of between-group variance (DA) that is explained by its presence. The application and usefulness of these techniques will be illustrated here by considering two examples from the literature. As with many of the analysis methods coming into vogue, both PCA and DA have primarily been used to analyse experiments studying the long latency event-related potentials.

Principal component analysis

Squires et al (1977) used PCA to analyse the evoked potentials obtained in an auditory detection task which manipulated both stimulus intensity and stimulus probability. Binaural tone bursts at either a loud (80 dB SPL) or soft (60 dB SPL) level were presented once every 1.3 seconds. In the first experiment subjects were required to count the loud tones (attend condition) which occurred with a probability of 0.1 in some blocks of trials and 0.9 in other blocks; the soft stimulus in each block occurred with the complementary probability. On some blocks of trials subjects were required to ignore the stimuli rather than count (ignore condition). The second experiment was identical except that additional blocks of trials were included in which the subjects were required to count the rare-soft stimuli. Recordings were made from 9 scalp electrodes. The experiments were concerned with the influence of task relevance and stimulus probability on the components of the auditory event-related potential.

The $\overline{\text{N100}}$ and $\overline{\text{P160}}$ components of this potential were prominent in the waveforms for all experimental conditions. Additionally, task-relevant rare stimuli elicited a $\overline{\text{N210}}$ component, a large $\overline{\text{P350}}$ and a 'slow wave' (SW) predominant from 500 msec onwards. For rare but irrelevant tones the $\overline{\text{N210}}$ wave remained prominent and was often followed by a $\overline{\text{P270}}$ peak, the $\overline{\text{P350}}$ component was comparatively attenuated and the SW was absent. These waveforms were compressed from 256 to 64 time points and then subjected to a Principal Component Analysis. Figure 15.6 shows plots of the factor loadings against time for the 6 main factors extracted by the analysis. PCA extracts factors in order of decreasing importance as measured by the variance attributable to their presence in the data set. Table I of Squires et al shows that in Experiment I, factor 1 accounted for 54.6 per cent of the total variance, factor 2 for 13.1 per cent and so on to factor 6 which accounted for 2.6 per cent. Additional factors accounted for 1 per cent or less of the variance and were therefore considered to be unimportant. It can be seen from the Figure that the time-courses of the maximum factor loadings for the different factors correspond closely to the component latencies defined above. Thus, factor 1 is related to the 'slow wave', factor 2 to $\overline{\text{P350}}$, factor 3 to $\overline{\text{N100}}$, factor 4 to $\overline{\text{N210}}$, factor 5 to $\overline{\text{P160}}$ (for experiment II only) and factor 6 to $\overline{\text{P270}}$. As Squires et al indicate, these data

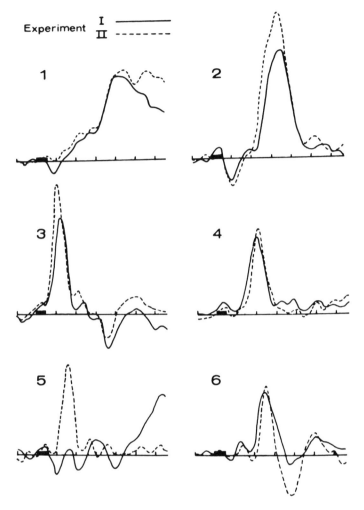

Figure 15.6 *Factor loadings for the six main factors extracted by the Principal Component Analysis of Experiment I (solid lines) and Experiment II (dashed lines). The time-scale extends from 100 msec before the stimulus to 668 msec after in 100 msec divisions. It can be seen that factor 1 is maximally loaded from 400 msec post-stimulus onwards, factor 2 is maximal around 300 msec, factor 3 around 100 msec, factor 4 around 200 msec, factor 5 around 150 msec (for Experiment II only) and factor 6 is maximal around 250 msec. See text for further details. (Reproduced from Squires et al, 1977.)*

simply suggest an identification between the factors and classical event-related potential components. Such interpretations need to be supported by examining the behaviour of the factors as a function of the experimental variables. This further analysis requires an analysis of variance relating the factor scores to the experimental variables for each factor. The results of this analysis are comprehensive and clearly show the complex relationships between the experimental variables and the factors (components). For example, the slow wave shows a dramatic interaction between electrode site and signal probability when tones are task-relevant. The factor scores are large and of opposite sign at F_z and P_z for relevant stimuli — suggesting a phase reversal in the antero-posterior direction for the slow wave in this condition. The scores are near zero for all frequent stimuli and for both rare and frequent tones when the tones are ignored — suggesting that stimuli have to be both rare and relevant to evoke the slow wave. The reader is referred to the original article for further details of the analysis and results of this study.

As stated earlier PCA can extract factors which appear only as points of inflexion in the raw waveforms. Equally, the full analysis of PCA followed by analysis of variance can extract relationships from the data which can be clearly seen in the raw waveforms in retrospect. Such relationships would be almost impossible to find by visual inspection alone because of the sheer volume of data requiring analysis.

Discriminant function analysis

Discriminant Function Analysis provides a method for distinguishing between both average and single trial waveforms. Squires and Donchin (1976) performed such an analysis on the data obtained by Squires et al (1977), already described above in the PCA section of this chapter. Their aim was to use discriminant functions to recognize and classify the responses evoked by single auditory stimuli. A discriminant function is a linear combination of variables (in the case of event-related potentials these are the amplitude values of individual ordinates in a waveform) which best separates two experimental sets of data. It is not necessary for all the variables (ordinates in a waveform) to be included in the linear combination. Stepwise Discriminant Analysis (SWDA) selects those variables which provide a discrimination almost as good as that obtained when all variables are included. It is seldom necessary for more than 6 variables to be included in the linear combination for optimal discriminating power (Donchin and Herning, 1975).

For each subject in their experiment, Squires and Donchin (1976) constructed discriminant functions designed to distinguish between waveforms associated with rare-loud stimuli and those associated with frequent-soft stimuli during the attend condition. A separate function was constructed to make the same discrimination during the ignore condition. A third function was designed to distinguish between waveforms associated with a rare-loud stimulus in the attend condition and wave-forms associated with the same stimulus in the ignore condition. The accuracy of waveform classification (defined according to presented stimulus, not according to the subject's responses) varied between 62 and 96 per cent correct across subjects with a mean accuracy of about 80 per cent. When the functions generated by this data set were applied to the waveforms obtained from seven separate individuals, the accuracy of classification ranged between 66 and 83 per cent. This indicates that the original functions were sufficiently general for accurate predictions to be made about waveforms from an independent group of subjects. The authors make the point that credence in this type of analysis is greatly enhanced if the ordinates used in the discriminant function correspond with recognizable event-related potential components and they demonstrate this to be the case in this experiment.

A further issue raised by the authors concerns the somewhat arbitrary definition of correctness of classification. 'Correctness' is defined according to the category of stimulus presentation. However, it is quite possible that a subject responds as if he had received a different stimulus category. This event would result in a mis-classification of the associated waveform. Squires and Donchin analysed the misclassified waveforms for the function discriminating rare-loud from frequent-soft stimuli in the attend condition. A comparison of these responses with those classified correctly is shown in Figure 15.7. The significant feature of the figure is that responses to the frequent-soft signal 'misclassified' as rare-loud show a clear $\overline{P300}$ component, whereas responses to the rare-loud signal 'misclassified' as frequent-soft show no such component. The suggestion, of course, is that subjects responded inappropriately on the 'misclassified' trials.

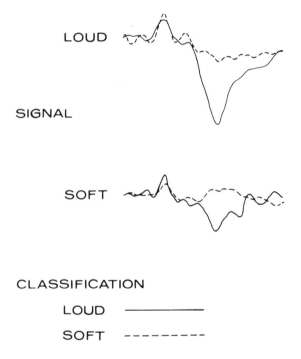

Figure 15.7 *Average event-related potential waveforms classified by a discriminant function according to the signal category. The subjects had to count the rarely occurring loud signals and ignore the frequent soft signals. The waveforms for the loud signals classified as loud have a large $\overline{P300}$ component reflecting the task relevance of this component. The waveform for the soft signals 'misclassified' as loud also shows a $\overline{P300}$ component suggesting that subjects mis-perceived the frequent-soft signal as the task relevant rare-loud signal on these trials. See text for further details. (Reproduced from Squires and Donchin, 1976.)*

These two multivariate statistical methods have obvious applications in clinical testing. For example, the presence of a particular component under certain experimental conditions may discriminate between different clinical categories. Indeed, the utility of cognitive components in psychiatric testing heralded by the paper of Goodin et al (1978b) (see Figure 15.4), coupled with the statistical procedures described here, will almost certainly play an increasingly important role in evoked potential research and clinical testing.

Another powerful statistical technique which has recently become popular in this field is Cluster Analysis (John et al, 1977). Using this method it is possible to observe the way in which individuals group together according to their scores on a variety of measures. If the clusters formed in this way correspond to nosological groups then this could be a useful technique for classifying patient material. The test data entered into the analysis program might include latencies and amplitudes of evoked potentials recorded for different modalities of stimulation together with data from other electrical investigations and even the results from psychological and other pencil and paper tests.

The statistical procedures described here require considerable computing power — usually more than can be provided by a laboratory computer. Thus it is likely that the basic rôle of these procedures will be in the research that leads to the application of evoked potential recording to clinical testing.

Frequency analysis

Although the preceding discussion has concentrated on the measurement of temporal characteristics of evoked potentials, other measures have been used in clinical work. In particular, Regan and his collaborators have looked at the frequency characteristics of potentials evoked by a sustained stimulus, such as a checkerboard pattern reversing six times a second or faster. The waveforms evoked in this way can be studied by separating the evoked potential into its constituent frequencies, each with its corresponding power or amplitude. This approach has been used for the rapid clinical assessment of amblyopia, astigmatism, colour vision, visual acuity, visual field defects and delays associated with optic nerve involvement in multiple sclerosis, as well as other defects of vision. An extensive review of these applications can be found in Regan (1977a).

DATA ANALYSIS – REPRESENTATION

The standard method of plotting evoked potential waveforms as ordinate amplitude (Y axis) against time (X axis) is generally sufficient to convey information about component latency and amplitude. When the number of recording channels is small this method also conveys adequate information about component distribution. When a large array of electrodes is used, covering a wide area of the head in both the coronal and sagittal plane, it is usually difficult to abstract information about component distribution and changes with time. A number of approaches have been made to this problem, some of which have resulted in a display that requires an even greater abstraction than the standard presentation!

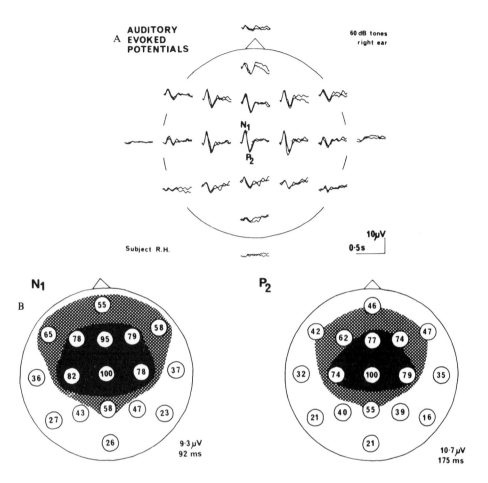

Figure 15.8 *Scalp distribution of the late components of the human auditory evoked potential, recorded with a chest reference. A. Each waveform is plotted at the corresponding electrode location on the scalp. The display gives a clear indication of component distribution in both the coronal and sagittal planes but cannot identify latency asymmetries if they exist. B. Mean amplitude distribution of the N_1 and P_2 components expressed as a percentage of maximum amplitude. The black area covers electrodes showing between 75 and 100% amplitude, whereas the hatched area covers the 50-75 percentage points. Both components have a very similar distribution with the N_1 component spreading slightly wider than the P_2. (Reproduced from Picton et al, 1974.)*

Picton and Hillyard and their collaborators have adopted the simple and sensible method of plotting individual waveforms at their corresponding electrode locations in an outline of the head. This method (see Figure 15.8) gives a clear indication of component localization and allows the observer to assess waveforms in the coronal and sagittal plane at the same time. This Figure also illustrates a

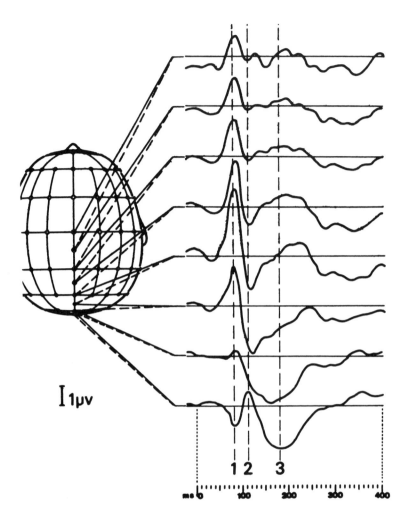

Figure 15.9 *Evoked potentials recorded from a bipolar chain of electrodes spaced 2 cm apart following the appearance of a 20° checkerboard pattern. Note that the polarity of each of the waves identified as 1, 2 and 3 reverses at some location in the chain. (Reproduced from Lesèvre, 1973.)*

method for representing amplitude distribution over the scalp. It is difficult, however, to extract information about asymmetries of component latency from these plots.

Another approach, which has been extensively utilized by Rémond and Lesèvre and their collaborators, is to represent differences in component amplitude at adjacent scalp locations as contour lines with the proximity of the lines indicating the gradient of potential change (see Figures 15.9 and 15.10). Time is plotted as the X axis and scalp location as the Y axis with amplitude being represented by the contour lines. One drawback of these chronotopograms is that each display can only represent a single spatial dimension on the head. Lehmann and his colleagues have also described a method of representation using contour lines. They recorded from 48 electrodes on the scalp and produced plots showing contours representing amplitude distribution across the scalp for successive points in time (see Lehmann and Skrandies, 1979, for examples). Another method using contour lines is that employed by Vaughan and Ritter (see Figure 15.11). The lines are drawn on an outline of the head joining points of equal percentage amplitude for one particular component. This type of display is particularly useful for component identification and comparison with the investigator's own data because it is usually constructed

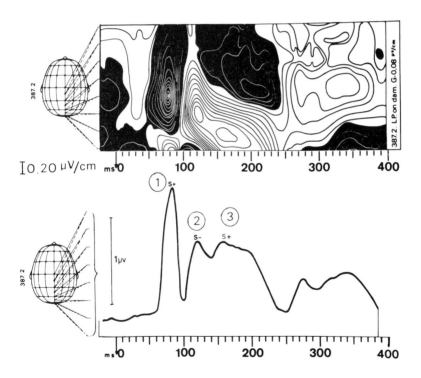

Figure 15.10 *Above. Spatio-temporal map representing the experimental data shown in Figure 15.9. The black areas on the map indicate regions of negative gradient, while the white areas indicate positive gradients. The amplitude is shown by the iso-gradient contours with each successive iso-gradient line corresponding to a difference in slope of 0.2 µV/cm for this particular map. The phase reversals of waves 1, 2 and 3 seen in Figure 15.9 are represented on this map as the locations in a vertical plane where white areas become black and black become white. This event occurs low down near the inion for waves 1 and 2 and more anteriorly for wave 3. Below. The integrated chronogram, as measured by the spatial root mean square amplitude shows the energy obtained at each moment on the whole montage. S+ and S- indicate surface positive and surface negative components. (Reproduced from Lesèvre, 1973.)*

from a large number of recordings. However, it does have the drawback, along with other methods using contours, that interpolation between adjacent recording electrodes can misrepresent the gradient of evoked potential change between these electrodes.

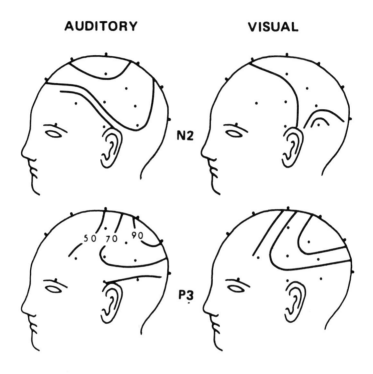

AUDITORY   **VISUAL**

Figure 15.11 *Scalp distributions of N_2 and P_3 components associated with omitted auditory and visual stimuli (grand mean of 8 subjects). Dots represent electrode placements, all referred to the nose. Successive isopotential curves depict areas in which response amplitude was 90, 70 and 50 per cent of maximum. (Reproduced from Ritter, 1978.)*

Our own method of representing evoked potential topography involves a three-dimensional display of activity on the scalp with the X and Z axes representing electrode locations in the coronal and sagittal planes and the Y axis representing the amplitude of activity at each electrode (Barrett et al, 1974; Halliday et al, 1977a, see Figure 15.12). Successive frames, which can either be displayed on an oscilloscope or plotted on paper, show the amplitude changes occurring at each electrode location with time. Thus it is possible to observe the changes in component amplitude and distribution across the scalp in a manner that is not possible with the standard method of presentation.

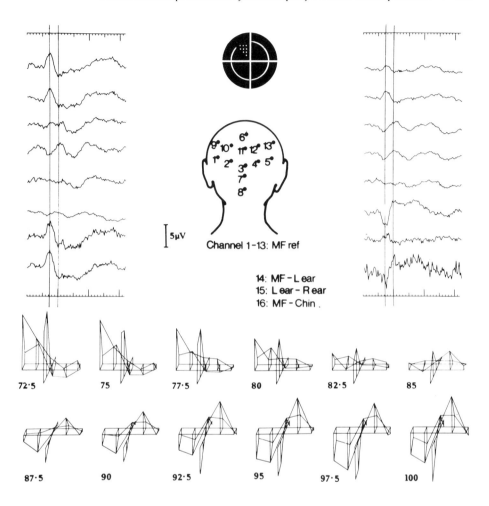

Figure 15.12 *Above. Standard waveform plot of amplitude against time showing the evoked potentials recorded to stimulation of the 0-8° left upper vertical octant of the visual field with a 50' checkerboard pattern. The responses were recorded from a widespread array of 13 scalp electrodes referred to a midfrontal electrode and from 3 inter-reference channels. The vertical lines are drawn between 72.5 and 100 msec. Negativity up. Time scale marks at 10, 50 and 100 msec. Below. The activity occurring between 72.5 and 100 msec represented as three-dimensional plots of the response amplitude at each scalp electrode for successive ordinates. For each time-point the montage is drawn in the X-Z plane and the amplitude, with respect to a baseline, of the response at each electrode is drawn in the Y direction. The Figure shows that at 72.5 msec the activity phase-reverses from negative to positive across the midline. There is also a reversal of polarity from negative to positive along the midline in the anterior direction. By 85 msec the response amplitudes at each electrode are comparatively similar. Between this latency and the 100 msec ordinate there is a systematic change to the opposite phase reversal from that seen at 72.5 msec. Such an interpretation would be almost impossible from visual inspection of the raw waveforms above. (Reproduced from Halliday et al, 1977.)*

The clinical application of such displays is limited at present because the response asymmetries that have proved useful clinically can generally be found using a suitable chain of a few electrodes. For example, asymmetries of the pattern evoked potential in hemianopic patients can be clearly seen in recordings from a transverse chain of five electrodes placed 5 cm above the inion (Blumhardt et al, 1977). Displays of component topography may be particularly useful when studying the motor potential in movement disorders because of the variety and differing localizations of the potentials associated with motor activity (Shibasaki et al, 1980a).

Derivation of electrode montages

The investigator studying evoked potential topography is often concerned about the indifference of his reference electrode and ideally wishes to record data from the same 'active' electrodes using a variety of reference sites. This can be done by including a number of inter-reference channels in the recording montage and deriving, by algebraic addition or subtraction, the waveforms that would have been recorded with the different references. For example, the visual evoked potential is often recorded using an ear reference. Figure 1.10 reproduced from Halliday et al (1979) shows that the use of such a reference for pattern stimulation of the visual half-field produces a different topographical distribution compared with a midfrontal reference. Indeed, as previous research has shown (Michael and Halliday, 1971), the ear is not indifferent for this type of stimulus. The waveforms depicted in Figure 1.10 were produced by recording from the 'active' electrodes referred to the common midfrontal electrode and including midfrontal to left ear and midfrontal to right ear connections in the montage (compare Channels 14-16 in Figure 15.12). The ear reference recordings were simply derived by adding the amplitude values of each ordinate of the midfrontal-to-ear waveform to the corresponding ordinates for each of the 'active' electrode waveforms. This procedure, which can be easily implemented on a digital computer, can also be used to derive bipolar connections from a chain of electrodes originally referred to a common reference. Although clinical applications of this practice are limited, it is useful for determining the relative indifference of a variety of electrodes and can also sometimes be used to rectify errors made when connecting electrodes at the start of a recording session!

EQUIPMENT CONSIDERATIONS

All the techniques described in this chapter require some level of computing power for their implementation. Most of them could be programmed to run on a laboratory micro- or mini-computer. The multivariate statistical techniques, however, require access to a large computer, such as those available at university computer centres.

Some manufacturers of averaging equipment are now providing software for data analysis combined with increasingly sophisticated special-purpose hardware. Indeed, the type of equipment purchased by laboratories specializing in evoked potential research could soon change. The existing general-purpose computers running data acquisition and analysis software written by the user may well be replaced by special-purpose hardware controlled by a computer running software written by the manufacturer. However, there will also be the facility for the user to write his own software so that the special-purpose equipment can be used as a general-purpose computer. The developments in this area are so rapid that it seems safe to predict that by 1986 manufacturers will be selling equipment with standard procedures for performing many of the advanced data acquisition and analysis techniques described in this chapter.

BIBLIOGRAPHY

ABBRUZZESE, G., ABBRUZZESE, M., FAVALE, E., IVALDI, M., LEANDRI, M. and RATTO, S. (1980) The effect of hand muscle vibration on the somatosensory evoked potential in man: an interaction between lemniscal and spinocerebellar inputs? J. Neurol., Neurosurg. Psychiat., 43: 433-437.

ABBRUZZESE, M., FAVALE, E., LEANDRI, M. and RATTO, S. (1978) New subcortical components of the cerebral somatosensory evoked potential in man. Acta Neurologica Scandinavica, 58: 325-332.

ABRAHAMIAN, H.A., ALLISON, T., GOFF, W.R. and ROSNER, B.S. (1963) Effect of thiopental in human cerebral evoked responses. Anaesthesiology, 24: 650-657.

ACHOR, L.J. and STARR, A. (1980a) Auditory brain stem responses in the cat. I. Intracranial and extracranial recordings. Electroenceph. clin. Neurophysiol., 48: 154-173.

ACHOR, L.J. and STARR, A. (1980b) Auditory brain stem responses in the cat. II. Effects of lesions. Electroenceph. clin. Neurophysiol., 48: 174-190.

ADAMS, W.L., ARDEN, G.B. and BEHRMAN, J. (1969) Responses of human visual cortex following excitation of peripheral retinal rods; some applications in the clinical diagnosis of functional and organic visual defects. Brit. J. Ophthal., 53: 439-452.

ADRIAN. E.D. (1926) The impulses produced by sensory nerve endings. J. Physiol., London, 61: 49-72.

AINSLIE, P.J., and BOSTON, J.R. (1980) Comparison of brainstem auditory evoked potentials for monaural and binaural stimuli. Electroenceph. clin. Neurophysiol., 49: 291-302.

ALAJOUANINE, T., SCHERRER, J., BARBIZET,J., CALVET, J. and VERLEY, R. (1958) Potentiels évoqués corticaux chez les sujets atteints de troubles somesthésiques. Rev. Neurol., 98: 757-762.

ALLEN, A.R. and STARR, A. (1978) Auditory brain stem potentials in monkey (M. Mulatta) and man. Electroenceph. clin. Neurophysiol., 45: 53-63.

ALLISON, T. (1962) Recovery functions of somatosensory evoked responses in man. Electroenceph. clin. Neurophysiol., 14: 331-343.

ALLISON, T. (1978) Calculated and empirical evoked potential distributions in human recordings. In: Otto D.A. (Ed.) *Multidisciplinary Perspectives in Event-Related Brain Potential Research.* Washington: US Environmental Protection Agency. 600/9-77-043. pp. 513-514.

ALLISON, T., GOFF, W.R., ABRAHAMIAN, H.A. and ROSNER, B.S. (1963) The effects of barbiturate anaesthesia upon human somatosensory evoked responses. Electroenceph. clin. Neurophysiol., Suppl. 24: 68-75.

ALLISON, T., GOFF, W.R. and WOOD, C.C. (1979) Auditory, somatosensory and visual evoked potentials in the diagnosis of neuropathology: recording considerations and normative data. In: Lehmann, D. and Callaway, E. (Eds.) *Human Evoked Potentials. Applications and Problems.* Plenum Press, New York. pp. 1-16.

ALLISON, T., GOFF, W.R., WILLIAMSON, P.D. and van GILDER, J.C. (1980) On the neural origin of early components of the somatosensory evoked potential. In: Desmedt, J.E. (Ed.) *Clinical Uses of Cerebral, Brainstem and Spinal Somatosensory Evoked Potentials. Progress in Clinical Neurophysiology.* Vol 7. Karger: Basel. pp 51-68.

ANDREEV, A.M., ARAPOVA, A.A. & GERSUNI, S.V. (1939) On the electrical potentials of the human cochlea. Journal of Physiology (USSR), 26: 205-212.

ANTINORO, F. and SKINNER, P. (1968) The effects of frequency on the auditory evoked response. Journal of Auditory Research, 8: 119-123.

ANTONELLI, A.R. (1976) Electrophysiological measures of auditory perception. Revue de Laryngologie, 97 supplementum: 613-621.

ANZISKA, B., CRACCO, R.W., COOK, A.W. and FELD, E.W. (1978) Somatosensory far-field potentials: studies in normal subjects and patients with multiple sclerosis. Electroenceph. clin. Neurophysiol., 45: 602-610.

APPLE, H. and BURGESS, R.C. (1976) An analysis of the use of active electrodes in electroencephalogram ambulatory monitoring. Postgraduate Medical Journal 52 (Suppl. 7): 78-84.

ARAN, J-M. (1971) L'Electro-cochléogramme, II Résultats. Les Cahiers de la Compagnie Française d'Audiologie, 13: 49-98.

ARAN, J.M. CAZALS, Y., CHARLET de SAUVAGE, R., GUILHAUME, A. and ERRE, J.P. (l980) Electrophysiological monitoring of the cochlea during and after total destruction of the organ of Corti. Acta Otolaryngologica, 89: 376-383.

ARAN, J.M. and LEBERT, G. (l968) Les résponses nerveuses cochléaires chez l'homme. Image du functionnement de l'oreille et nouveau test d'audiometrie objective. Revue de Laryngologie, 89: 361-378.

ARBUS, L., LAZORTHES, Y., ROUQUIE, P. and VERDIE, C. (1977) The study of soma-tosensory evoked responses: its interest with reference to analgesic surgery. Electroenceph. clin. Neurophysiol., 43: 554-555.

ARDEN, G.B. (1977) Abnormalities of the pattern EP in amblyopia. In: Spekreijse, H. and van der Tweel, H. (Eds.) *Spatial Contrast.* North Holland Publishing Company: Amsterdam. pp. 112-115.

ARDEN, G.B., BARNARD, W.M. and MUSHIN, A.S. (1974) Visually evoked responses in amblyopia. Brit. J. Ophthal., 58: 183-192.

ARDEN, G.B., BODIS-WOLLNER, I., HALLIDAY, A.M., JEFFREYS, A., KULIKOWSKI, J.J., SPEKREIJSE, H. and REGAN D. (1977a) Methodology of patterned visual stimulation. In: Desmedt, J.E. (Ed.) *Visual Evoked Potentials in Man: New Developments.* Clarendon Press: Oxford. pp. 3-15.

ARDEN, G.B., CARTER, R.M., HOGG, C., SIEGAL, I.M. and MARGOLIS, S. (1979) A gold foil electrode: extending the horizons for clinical electroretinography. Investigative Ophthalmology of Visual Science, 18: 421-426.

ARDEN, G.B., FAULKNER, D.J. and MAIR, C. (1977b) A versatile television pattern gener-ator for visual evoked potentials. In: Desmedt, J.E. (Ed.) *Visual Evoked Potentials in Man: New Developments.* Clarendon Press: Oxford.

ARDEN, G.B. and SHEOREY, U.B. (1977) The assessment of visual function in patients with opacities: a new evoked-potential method using a laser interferometer. In: Desmedt, J.E. (Ed.) *Visual Evoked Potentials in Man: New Developments.* Clarendon Press: Oxford. pp. 438-449.

ARDEN, G.B., VAEGEN, HOGG, C.R., POWELL, D.J. and CARTER, R.M. (1980) Pattern ERGs are abnormal in most amblyopes. Transactions of the Ophthalmological Society of United Kingdom.100: 453-460.

AREZZO, J. LEGATT, A.D. and VAUGHAN, H.G. Jr. (1979) Topography and intra-cranial sources of somatosensory evoked potentials in the monkey. I. Early components. Electroenceph. clin. Neurophysiol., 46: 155-173.

AREZZO, J. and VAUGHAN, H.G., Jr. (1975) Cortical potentials associated with voluntary movements in the monkey. Brain Res., 88: 99-104.

ARMINGTON, J.C. (1974) *The Electroretinogram.* Academic Press; New York.

ARMINGTON, J.C. (1980) Electroretinography. In: Aminoff, M.J. (Ed.) *Electrodiagnosis in Clinical Neurology.* Churchill Livingstone: London. pp. 305-347.

ARNAL, D., GERIN, P., SALMON, D., RAVAULT, M.P., MAGNARD, P. and HUGONNIER, R. (1972a) Intérêt des potentiels évoquées moyens visuels en ophtal-mologie. Electroenceph. clin. Neurophysiol., 32: 615-621.

ARNAL, D., GERIN, P., SALMON, D., RAVAULT, M.P., NAKACHE, J.P. and PERONNET, F. (1972b) Les diverses composantes des potentiels évoquées moyens visuels chez l'homme. Electroenceph. clin. Neurophysiol., 32: 499-511.

ASSELMAN, P., CHADWICK, D.W. and MARSDEN, C.D. (1975) Visual evoked responses in the diagnosis and management of patients suspected of multiple sclerosis. Brain, 98: 261-282.

AUNON, J.I. and CANTOR, F.K. (1977) VEP and AEP variability: interlaboratory vs. intra-laboratory and intersession vs. intrasession variability. Electroenceph. clin. Neurol., 42: 705-708.

AUSTIN, G.M. and McCOUCH, G.P. (1955) Presynaptic component of intermediary cord potential. J. Neurophysiol., 18: 441-451.

AXELGAARD, J. (1977) Spinal cord monitoring technique and equipment: a prospective view. In: Proceedings of a workshop on the clinical application of spinal cord monitoring for operative treatment of spinal diseases. Chairmen C.L. Nash and J.S. Brodkey, pp. 93-101 (unpublished).

AXELGAARD, J. (1979) Somatosensory evoked potentials (SSEP) recorded from vertebral bone: clinical. In: Proceedings of spinal cord monitoring workshop, data acquisition and analysis. Chairmen C.L. Nash and R.H. Brown, pp 115-128 (unpublished).

BABEL, J., STANGOS, N., KOROL, S. and SPIRITUS, M. (1977) *Ocular Electrophysiology: A Clinical and Experimental Study of Electroretinogram, Electro-oculogram and Visual Evoked Response.* Stuttgart. Georg Thieme Publishers. pp. 1-172.

BABLOUZIAN, B.L., NEURATH, P.W., SAMENT, S. and WATSON, C.W. (1969) Detection of photogenic epilepsy in man by summation of evoked scalp potentials. Electroenceph. clin. Neurophysiol., 26: 93-95.

BACIA, T. and REID, K. (1965) Visual and somatosensory evoked potentials in man, particularly in patients with focal epilepsy. Electroenceph. clin. Neurophysiol., 18: 718.

BAKER, J.B., LARSON, S.J., SANCES, A. and WHITE, P.T. (1968) Evoked potentials as an aid to the diagnosis of multiple sclerosis. Neurology (Minneapolis), 18: 286.

BALEN, A.T. van and HENKES, H.E. (1962) Attention and amblyopia. Brit. J. Ophthal., 46: 12-20.

BANCAUD, J., BLOCH, V. and PAILLARD, J. (1953) Contribution EEG á l'étude des potentiels évoquées chez l'homme au niveau du vertex. Rev. Neurol., 89: 382-399.

BARBER, C. and GALLOWAY, N.R. (1980) Adaptation effects in the transient visual evoked potential. In: Lehmann, D. and Callaway, E. (Eds.) *Human Evoked Potentials.* Plenum Press New York. pp. 17-30.

BARLOW, J.S. (1969) Some observations on the electrophysiology of timing in the nervous system. Electroenceph. clin. Neurophysiol., 27: 545.

BARNET, A.B., FRIEDMAN, S.L., WEISS, I.P. OHLRICH, E.S., SHANKS, B. and LODGE, A. (1980) VEP development in infancy and early childhood. A longitudinal study. Electroenceph. clin. Neurophysiol., 49: 476-489.

BARRETT, G., BLUMHARDT, L., HALLIDAY, A.M., HALLIDAY, E. and KRISS, A. (1976) A paradox in the lateralization of the visual evoked response. Nature (Lond.), 261: 253-255.

BARRETT, G., HALLIDAY, A.M., HALLIDAY, Elise and MICHAEL, W.F. (1974) A four-dimensional display of the potential field of evoked responses on the head. Electroenceph. clin. Neurophysiol. 37: 106.

BARTL, G., BENEDIKT, O., HITI, H. and MANDL, H. (1975) Das elektrophysiologische Verhalten gesunder und glaukomkranker menschlicher Augen bei kurzzeitiger intraocularer Druckbelastung. Graefes Arch. Ophth., 195, 201-206.

BARTL, G., VAN LITH, G.H.M. and VAN MARLE, G.W. (1978) Cortical potentials evoked by a TV pattern reversal stimulus with varying check sizes and stimulus field. Brit. J. Ophthal., 62: 216-219.

BARTLEY, S.H. and BISHOP, G.H. (1933) The cortical response to stimulation of the optic nerve in the rabbit. American Journal of Physiology, 103: 159-172.

BATES, J.A.V. (1951) Electrical activity of the cortex accompanying movement. J. Physiol., London 113: 240-257.

BAUST, W. and JORG, J. (1977) Clinical value of somatosensory cortical evoked potentials for the localisation and diagnosis of spinal transverse lesions. Electroenceph. clin. Neurophysiol., 43: 513.

BEAGLEY, H.A. (1979) *Auditory Investigation: The Scientific and Technological Basis.* Clarendon Press: Oxford.

BEAGLEY, H.A., FATEEN, A.M. and GORDON, A.G. (1972) Clinical experience of evoked response testing with sedation. Sound, 6: 8-13.

BEAGLEY, H.A. and GIBSON, W.P.R. (1976) Lesions mimicking acoustic neuroma using transtympanic electrocochleography. In: Stephens, S.D.G. (Ed.) *Disorders of Auditory Function II.* London, Academic Press. pp. 119-125.

BEAGLEY, H.A. and GIBSON, W.P.R. (1978) Electrocochleography in adults. In: Naunton, R.F. and Fernandez, C. (Eds.) *Evoked Electrical Activity in the Auditory Nervous System.* New York: Academic Press. pp. 259-272.

BEAGLEY, H.A., HUTTON, J.N.T. and HAYES, R.A. (1974) Clinical electrocochleography: a review of 106 cases. Journal of Laryngology and Otology, 88: 993-1000.

BEAGLEY, H.A. and SHELDRAKE, J.B. (1978) Differences in brainstem response latency with age and sex. British Journal of Audiology, 12: 69-77.

BEAUCHAMP, M., MATTHEWS, W.B., SMALLL, D. and STEIN, J.F. (1976) The topography of the visual evoked response to half-field stimulation. J. Physiol., London, 260: 46-47P.

BEAUMONT, G. and MAYES, A. (1977) Do task and sex differences influence the visual evoked potential? Psychophysiology, 14: 545-550.

BECK, E.C., DUSTMAN, R.E. and LEWIS, E.G. (1975) The use of the averaged evoked potential in the evaluation of central nervous system disorders. International Journal of Neurology, 9: 211-232.

BECKER, W., HOEHNE, O., IWASE, K. and KORNHUBER, H.H. (1972) Bereitschaftspotential, prämotorische Positivierung und andere Hirnpotentiale bei sakkadischen Augenbewegungen. Vision Res., 12: 421-436.

BEHRMAN, J., NISSIM, S. and ARDEN, G.B. (1972) A clinical method for obtaining pattern visual evoked responses. In: Arden, G.B. (Ed.) *Experimental Medicine and Biology.* Vol. 24: 199-206. Plenum Press.

BEKESY, G. von (1950) D-C potential and energy balance of the cochlear partition. Journal of the Acoustical Society of America, 22: 576-582.

BENDAT, J. and PIERSOL, A.G. (1971) *Random Data: Analysis and measurement procedures.* Wiley-Interscience.

BERGAMINI, L., BERGAMASCO, B., FRA, L., GANGDIGLIO, G., MOMBELLI, A.M. and MUTANI, R. (1965) Somatosensory evoked cortical potentials in subjects with peripheral nervous lesions. Electromyography, 5: 121-130.

BERGAMINI, L., BERGAMASCO, B., FRA, L., GANDIGLIO, G., MOMBELLI, A.M. and MUTANI, R. (1966) Réponses corticales et périphériques évoquées par stimulation du nerf dans la pathologie des cordons postérieurs. Rev. neurol., 115: 99-112.

BERLIN, C.I., GONDRA, M.I., CASEY, D.A., MARKS, H.W., CHICOLA, J.P., GARRETT, M.E. and LYONS, D.G. Jr. (1978) Bone conduction electrocochleography: clinical applications. Laryngoscope, 88: 756-763.

BERNHARD, C.G. (1953) The spinal cord potentials in leads from the cord dorsum in relation to the peripheral source of afferent stimulation. Acta Physiologica Scandinavica, 29, Suppl. 106: 1-29.

BERNHARD, C.G. and WIDEN, L. (1953) On the origin of the negative and positive spinal cord potentials evoked by stimulation of low threshold cutaneous fibres. Acta Physiologica Scandinavica, 29, Suppl. 106: 42-54.

BERRY, H., BLAIR, R.L., BILBAO, J. and BRIANT, T.D.R. (1976) Click evoked eighth nerve and brainstem responses (electrocochleogram) — experimental observations in the cat. Journal of Otolaryngology (Toronto), 5: 1, 64-73.

BERSON, E.L., GOURAS, P. and GUNKEL, R.D. (1968) Rod responses in retinitis pigmentosa. Dominantly inherited. Acta Ophthalmologica, 80: 58-67.

BERSON, E.L., GOURAS, P. and GUNKEL, R.D. (1969) Dominant retinitis pigmentosa with reduced penetrance. Arch. Ophthal. (Chicago), 81: 226-234.

BERSON, E.L. and HOWARD, J. (1971) Temporal aspects of the electroretinogram in sector retinitis pigmentosa. Archives of Ophthalmology, 86: 653-665.

BICKFORD, R.G. (1964) Properties of the photomoter response system. Electroenceph. clin. Neurophysiol., 17: 456.

BICKFORD, R.G. (1966) Human "microreflexes" revealed by computer-analysis. Neurology (Minneap.), 16: 302.

BICKFORD, R.G. (1972) Physiological and clinical studies of microreflexes. Electroenceph. clin. Neurophysiol., Suppl 31: 93-108.

BICKFORD, R.G., GALBRAITH, R.F. and JACOBSON, J.L. (1963a) The nature of averaged evoked potentials recorded from the human scalp. Electroenceph. clin. Neurophysiol., 15: 720.

BICKFORD, R.G., JACOBSON, J.L. and CODY, D.T.R. (1964) Nature of average evoked potentials to sound and other stimuli in man. Annals of the New York Academy of Sciences, 112: 204-223.

BICKFORD, R.G., JACOBSON, J.L. and GALBRAITH, R.F. (1963b) A new audiometer system in man. Electroenceph. clin. Neurophysiol., 15: 922.

BLACK, J.A., FARIELLO, R.G. and CHUN, R.W. (1979) Brainstem auditory evoked response in adrenoleukodystrophy. Ann. Neurol, 6: 269-270.

BLAIR, A.W. (1971) Sensory examinations using electrically induced somatosensory potentials. Develop. Med. Child. Neurol., 13: 447-455.

BLAIR, R.D.G., LEE, R.G. and VANDERLINDEN, G. (1975) Dorsal column stimulation. Its effect on the somatosensory evoked response. Archives of Neurology, 32: 826-829.

BLAKEMORE, C. (1969) Binocular depth discrimination and the nasotemporal division. J. Physiol., London, 205: 471-497.

BLAKEMORE, C. and COOPER, G.F. (1970) Development of the brain depends on the visual environment. Nature, 228: 477-478.

BLEGVAD, B. (1975) Binaural summation of surface-recorded electrocochleographic responses. Scandinavian Audiology, 4: 233-238.

BLOM, J.L., BARTH, P.G. and VISSER, S.L. (1980) The visual evoked potential in the first six years of life. Electroenceph. clin. Neurophysiol., 48: 395-405.

BLUMHARDT, L.D. (1980) *Topography of Normal and Abnormal Pattern Evoked Potentials in Man.* M.D. Thesis, University of Otago.

BLUMHARDT, L.D., BARRETT, G. and HALLLIDAY, A.M. (1977) The asymmetrical visual evoked potential to pattern reversal in one half-field and its significance for the analysis of visual field defects. British Journal of Ophthalmology, 61: 456-461.

BLUMHARDT, L.D., BARRETT, G. and HALLIDAY, A.M. (1982a) The pattern visual evoked potential in the clinical assessment of undiagnosed spinal cord disease. In: Courjon, J., Mauguiere, F. and Revol, M. (Eds.) *Clinical Applications of Evoked Potentials in Neurology.* New York: Raven Press. pp. 463-471.

BLUMHARDT, L.D., BARRETT, G., HALLIDAY, A.M. and KRISS, A. (1978) The effect of experimental "scotomata" on the ispilateral and contralateral responses to pattern-reversal in one half-field. Electroenceph. clin. Neurophysiol., 45: 376-392.

BLUMHARDT, L.D., BARRETT, G., KRISS, A. and HALLIDAY, A.M. (1982b) The pattern-evoked potential in lesions of the posterior visual pathways. Ann. N.Y. Acad. Sci. (In press)

BLUMHARDT, L.D. and HALLLIDAY, A.M. (1979) Hemisphere contributions to the composition of the pattern-evoked potential waveform. Exp. Brain Res., 36: 53-69.

BLUMHARDT, L.D. and HALLIDAY, A.M. (1980) The effect of lesions of the posterior visual pathways on the pattern-reversal response. Electroenceph. clin. Neurophysiol., 49.95P.

BLUMHARDT, L.D. and HALLIDAY, A.M. (1981) Cortical abnormalities and the visual evoked response. In: Spekreijse, H. and Apkarian, P. (Eds.) *Visual Pathways: Electrophysiology and Pathology.* Documenta Ophthalmologica. Proc. Ser., 27: 347-365. The Hague: Junk.

BODIS-WOLLNER, I. (1977) Recovery from cerebral blindness: evoked potential and psychophysical measurements. Electroenceph. clin. Neurophysiol., 42: 178-184.

BODIS-WOLLNER, I., ATKIN, A., RAAB, E. and WOLKSTEIN, M. (1977) Visual association cortex and vision in man: pattern-evoked occipital potentials in a blind boy. Science, 198: 629-631.

BODIS-WOLLNER, I., HENDLEY, C.D., MYLIN, A.T. and THORNTON, J. (1979) Visual evoked potentials and the visuogram in multiple sclerosis. Ann. Neurol., 5: 40-47.

BODIS-WOLLNER, I. and YAHR, M.D. (1978) Measurements of visual evoked potentials in Parkinson's Disease. Brain, 101: 661-671.

BONNEY, G. and GILLIATT, R.W. (1958) Sensory nerve conduction after traction lesion of the brachial plexus. Proceedings of the Royal Society of Medicine, 51: 365-367.

BORDA, R.P. (1977) Visual evoked potentials to flash in the clinical evaluation of the optic pathways. In: Desmedt, J.E. (Ed.) *Visual Evoked Potentials in Man: New Developments.* Clarendon Press, Oxford. pp. 481-489.

BORNSTEIN, M.B. and CRAIN, S.M. (1965) Functional studies of cultural brain tissue as related to "demyelinative disorders". Science, 148: 1242-1244.

BORNSTEIN, Y. (1975) The pattern evoked responses (VER) in optic neuritis. Arch. clin. exp. Ophthalmol., 197: 101-106.

BOSTON, H.R. and AINSLIE, P.J. (1980) Effects of analog and digital filtering on brainstem auditory evoked potentials. Electroenceph. clin. Neurophysiol., 48: 361-364.

BOYNTON, R.M. (1966) Vision. In Sidowski, J.B. (Ed.) *Experimental Methods and Instrumentation in Psychology.* McGraw Hill: New York. pp. 273-330.

BRAMSLEV, G.R., BRUUN, G., BUCHTHAL, F., GULD, G. and STEEN PETERSEN, H. (1967) Reduction of electrical interference in measurements of bioelectrical potentials in a hospital. Acta Polytechnica Scandinavica. Electrical Engineering Series No. 15.

BRINDLEY, G.S. (1972) The variability of the human striate cortex. J. Physiol., 225, 2, 1-3P.

BRINDLEY, G.S., GAUTIER-SMITH, P.C. and LEWIN, W. (1969) Cortical blindness and the functions of non-geniculate fibres of the optic tracts. J. Neurol. Neurosurg. Psychiat., 32: 259-264.

BRINDLEY, G.S. and LEWIN, W.S. (1968) The sensations produced by electrical stimulation of the visual cortex. J. Physiol., London, 196: 479-493.

BRODAL, A. (1981) *Neurological Anatomy in Relation to Clinical Medicine.* Oxford University Press: New York.

BROUGHTON, R.J. (1967) *Somatosensory Evoked Potentials in Man.* McGill University, Montreal. (Unpublished dissertation).

BROUGHTON, R., MEIER-EWERT, K.H. and EBE, M. (1969) Evoked visual somatosensory and retinal potentials in photosensitive epilepsy. Electroenceph. clin. Neurophysiol., 27: 373-386.

BROWN, K.T. (1968) The electroretinogram: its components and their origins. Vision Research, 8: 633-677.

BROWN, K.T. and MURAKAMI, M. (1964) A new receptor potential of the monkey retina with no detectable latency. Nature, 201: 626-628.

BROWN, K.T. and WATANABE, K. (1962) Isolation and identification of a receptor potential from pure cone fovea of the monkey retina. Nature, 193: 958-960.

BRUNETTE, J.R. and MOLOTCHNIKOFF, S. (1970) Calibration of flash tube photostimulators in electroretinography. Vision research, 10: 95-102.

BUCHSBAUM, M. and COPPOLA, R. (1974) Computer use in bioelectric data collection and analysis. In Thompson, R.F. and Patterson, M.M. (Eds.) *Bioelectric Recording Techniques,* New York: Academic Press.

BUCHSBAUM, M.S., HENKIN, R.I. and CHRISTIANSEN, R.L. (1974) Age and sex differences in averaged evoked responses in a normal population with observations on patients with gonadal dysgenesis. Electroenceph. clin. Neurophysiol. 37: 137-144.

BUCHWALD, J.S. and HUANG, C-M. (1975) Far field acoustic response: origins in the cat. Science, 189: 382-384.

BURIAN, K., GESTRING, G.F., GLONING, K. and HAIDER, M. (1972) Objective examination of verbal discrimination and comprehension in aphasia using contingent negative variation. Audiology, 11: 310-316.

BURIAN, K., GESTRING, G.F. and HAIDER, M. (1969) Objective speech audiometry. International Audiology, 8: 387-390.

BUTINAR, D., PREVEC, T.S. and RIBARIC, K. (1978) CNV audiometry in audiological patients with comments on P300. Unpublished paper read at International Evoked Potentials Symposium, Nottingham.

BYNKE, H., OLSSON, J.E. and ROSEN, I. (1977) Diagnostic value of visual evoked response, clinical eye examination and CSF analysis in chronic myelopathy. Acta Neurol. Scand., 56: 55-69.

CACCIA. M.R., UBIALI, E. and ANDREUSSI, L. (1976) Spinal evoked responses recorded from the epidural space in normal and diseased humans. J. Neurol. Neurosurg. Psychiat., 39: 962-972.

CALLAWAY, E. and HALLIDAY, R.A (1973) Evoked potential variability: effect of age, amplitude and methods of measurement. Electroenceph. clin. Neurophysiol, 4: 125-233.

CALMES, R.L., and CRACCO, R.Q. (1971) Comparison of somatosensory and somato-motor evoked responses to median nerve and digital nerve stimulation. Electroenceph. clin. Neurophysiol, 31: 547-562.

CAMACHO, L.M., WENZEL, W. and ASCHOFF, J.C. (1982) The pattern-reversal visual evoked potential in the clinical study of lesions of the optic chiasm and visual pathway. In: Courjon, J., Mauguiere and Revol, M. (Ed.) *Clinical Applications of Evoked Potentials in Neurology.* New York: Raven Press. pp. 49-59.

CAMPBELL, F.W. and MAFFEI, L. (1970) Electrophysiological evidence for the existence of orientation and size detectors in the human visual system. J. Physiol. Lond., 207: 635-652.

CANT, B.R., HUME, A.L. and SHAW, N.A. (1978) Effects of luminance on the pattern visual evoked potential in multiple sclerosis. Electroenceph. clin. Neurophysiol., 45: 496-504.

CAPPIN, J. and NISSIM, S. (1975) Visual evoked responses in the detection of field defects in glaucoma. Archives of Ophthalmology, N.Y., 93: 9-18.

CARELS, G. (1960) Etude physiopathologique d'un syndrome myoclonique chez deux enfants atteints d'une forme infantile tardive de l'idiotie amaurotique. Acta Neurol. Psychiat. Belg., 60: 435-464.

CARMON, A., MOR, J. and GOLDBERG, J. (1976) Evoked cerebral responses to noxious thermal stimuli in humans. Experimental Brain Research, 25: 103-107.

CARR, T.C., HOLT, A.L. and KATZ, P.N. (1974) Non-linear aspects of the bioelectrode-electrolyte interface. In: Miller H.A. and Harrison, D.C. (Eds.) *Biomedical Electrode Technology.* Academic Press.

CARROLL, W.M., JAY, B.S., McDONALD, W.I. and HALLIDAY, A.M. (1980a) Two distinct patterns of visual evoked response asymmetry in human albinism. Nature, 286: 604-606.

CARROLL, W.M., JAY, B., McDONALD, W.I. and HALLIDAY, A.M. (1980b) Pattern evoked potentials in human albinism. Evidence of two distinct topographical asymmetries reflecting abnormal retino-cortical projections. J. Neurol. Sci., 48: 265-287.

CARROLL, W.M., KRISS, A., BARAITSER, M., BARRETT, G. and HALLIDAY, A.M. (1980c) The incidence and nature of visual pathway involvement in Friedreich's ataxia. Brain, 103: 413-434.

CARROLL, W.M. and KRISS, A. (1981) Factors which alter or appear to alter the latency of pattern evoked potentials. (In preparation).

CARROLL, W.M. and MASTAGLIA, F.L. (1979) Leber's optic neuropathy: A clinical and visual evoked potential study of affected and asymptomatic members of a six generation family. Brain, 102: 559-580.

CASLER, J.A., HOFFMAN, R., BERGER, L., BILLINGER, T.W., SIMS, J.K. and BICKFORD, R.G.(1973) Use of photodiode stimulation in clinical and experimental electroencephalography and electroretinography. Electroenceph. clin. Neurophysiol., 34: 437-439.

CELESIA, G.G. (1979) Somatosensory evoked potentials recorded directly from the human thalamus and Sm1 cortical area. Archives of Neurology, 36: 399-405.

CELESIA, G.G., ARCHER, C.R., KUROIWA, Y. and GOLDFADER, P.R. (1980) Visual function of the extrageniculo-calcarine system in man. Arch. Neurol. (Chicago), 37: 704-706.

CELESIA, G.G. and DALY, R.F. (1977a) Effects of aging on visual evoked responses. Archives of Neurology, 34: 403-407.

CELESIA, G.G. and DALY, R.F. (1977b) Visual electroencephalographic computer analysis (VECA): A new electrophysiological test for the diagnosis of optic nerve lesions. Neurology (Minneapolis), 27: 637-641.

CELESIA, G.G., SONI, V.K. and RHODE, W.S. (1978) Visual evoked spectrum array and interhemispheric variations. Archives of Neurology, 35: 678-682.

CHADWICK, D., HALLETT, M., HARRIS, R., JENNER, P., REYNOLDS, E.H. and MARSDEN, C.D. (1977) Clinical, biochemical and physiological features distinguishing myoclonus responsive to 5-hydroxytryptophan, tryptophan with a monoamine oxidase inhibitor, and clonazepam. Brain, 100: 455-487.

CHAIN, F., MALLECOURT, J., LEBLANC, M. et LHERMITTE, F. (1977) Apport de l'enregistrement des potentiels évoqués visuels au diagnostic de la sclérose en plaques. Rev. Neurol., 133: 81-88.

CHATRIAN, G.E., CANFIELD, T.C., KNAUSS, T.A. and LETTICH, E. (1975) Cerebral responses to electrical tooth pulp stimulation in man: an objective correlate of acute experimental pain. Neurology (Minneap.), 25: 745-757.

CHATT, A.B. and KENSHALO, D.R. (1977) Cerebral evoked responses to skin warming recorded from the human scalp. Experimental Brain Research, 28: 449-455.

CHEN, A.C.N., CHAPMAN, C.R. and HARKINS, S.W. (1979) Brain evoked potentials are functional correlates of induced pain in man. Pain, 6: 365-374.

CHIAPPA, K.H. (1980) Pattern shift visual brainstem auditory and short latency somatosensory evoked potentials in multiple sclerosis. Neurology (Minneap.), 30: 110-123.

CHIAPPA, K.H. (1981) Brainstem auditory evoked potentials. In: Stälberg, E. and Young, R.R. (Eds) *Clinical Neurophysiology.* London: Butterworths, pp. 259-277.

CHIAPPA, K.H., CHOI, S.K. and YOUNG, R.R. (1980a) Short latency somatosensory evoked potentials following median nerve stimulation in patients with neurological lesions. In: Desmedt, J.E. (Ed.) *Clinical Uses of Cerebral, Brainstem and Spinal Somatosensory Evoked Potentials. Prog. in Clin. Neurophysiol., Vol. 7.* Karger: Basel. pp. 264-281.

CHIAPPA, K.H., HARRISON, J.L., BROOKS, E.B. and YOUNG, R.R. (1980b) Brainstem auditory evoked responses in 200 patients with multiple sclerosis. Ann. Neurol., 7: 135-143.

CHINN, I. and MILLER, J. (1975) Animal model of acoustic neuroma. Archives of Otolaryngology (Chicago), 101: 222-226.

CHOKROVERTY, S. and RUBINO, F.A. (1975) "Pure" motor hemiplegia. J. Neurol. Neurosurg. Psychiat., 38: 896-899.

CHRISTIE, M. and McCREARTY, E. (1977) Deep body temperature: Diurnal variation, sex and personality. J. Psychosom. Res., 21: 207-211.

CIGANEK, L. (1961a) *Die elektroencephalographische Lichtreizantwort der menschlichen Hirnrinde.* Thesis, Slovenskej Akademie Vied, Bratislava.

CIGANEK, L. (1961b) The EEG response (evoked potential) to light stimulus in man. Electroenceph. clin. Neurophysiol., 13: 163-172.

CIGANEK, L. (1969a) Visually evoked potential correlates of attention and distraction in man. Psychiat. clin., 2: 95-108.

CIGANEK, L. (1969b) Variability of the human visual evoked potential: normative data. Electroenceph. clin. Neurophysiol., 27: 35-42.

CIGANEK, L. (1975) Visual evoked responses. In: Storm van Leeuwen, W.S., Lopes da Silva, F.H. and Kamp, A. (Eds.) *Handbook of Electroencephalography and Clinical Neurophysiology. Vol. 8A.* Elsevier, Amsterdam. pp. 33-59.

CITRON, L., DIX, M.R., HALLPIKE, C.S. and HOOD, J.D. (1963) A recent clinicopathological study of cochlear nerve degeneration resulting from tumours and DS with particular reference to the finding of normal threshold sensitivity for pure tones. Acta Oto-Laryngologica (Stockholm), 56: 330-337.

CLARK, D.L., HOSICK, E.C. and ROSNER, B.S. (1971) Neurophysiological effects of different anaesthetics in unconscious man. J. Appl. Physiol., 31: 884-891.

CLARK, D.L. and ROSNER, B.S. (1973) Neurophysiological effects of general anaesthesia. I. The electroencephalogram and sensory evoked responses in man. Anaesthesiology, 38: 564-582.

CLARK, D.L., ROSNER, B.S. and BECK, C. (1970) Cerebral electrical activity during cyclopropane anaesthesia in man. J. Appl. Physiol., 28: 802-807.

CLEMIS, J.D. and MITCHELL, C. (1977) Electrocochleography and brain stem responses used in the diagnosis of acoustic tumours. J. Otolaryngol., 6: 447-459.

CLIFFORD-JONES, R.E., CLARKE, G.P. and MAYLES, P. (1979) Crossed acoustic response combined with visual and somato-sensory evoked responses in the diagnosis of multiple sclerosis. J. Neurol. Neurosurg. Psychiat., 42: 749-752.

CLYNES, M., KOHN, M. and LIFSHITZ, K. (1964) Dynamics and spatial behaviour of light evoked potentials, their modification under hypnosis and on-line correlation in relation to rhythmic components. Ann. N.Y. Acad. Sci., 112: 468-509.

COATS, A.C. (1981) The summating potential and Ménière's disease: 1. Summating potential amplitude in Ménière and non-Ménière ears. Arch. Otolaryngol; 107: 199-208.

COATS, A.C. and DICKEY, J.R. (1970) Non-surgical recording of the human auditory nerve potentials and cochlear microphonics. Annals of Otology, Rhinology and Laryngology, 79: 844-852.

COATS, A.C. and MARTIN, J.L. (1977) Human auditory nerve action potentials and brain-stem evoked responses. Archives of Otolaryngology (Chicago), 103: 605-622.

COBB, W.A. and DAWSON, G.D. (1960) The latency and form in man of the occipital potentials evoked by bright flashes. J. Physiol. (Lond.), 152: 108-121.

COBB, W.A. and MORTON, H.B. (1952) The human retinogram in response to high intensity flashes. Electroenceph. clin. Neurophysiol., 4: 547-556.

CODY, D.T.R. and BICKFORD, R.G. (1969) Averaged evoked myogenic responses in normal man. Laryngoscope, 79: 400-416.

CODY, D.T.R., JACOBSON, J.L., WALKER, J.C. and BICKFORD, R.G. (1964) Averaged evoked myogenic and cortical potentials to sound in man. Annals of Otology, Rhinology and Laryngology, 73: 763-777.

COHEN, J. (1969) Very slow brain potentials relating to expectancy: the CNV. In: Donchin, E. and Lindsley, D.B. (Eds.) *Average Evoked Potentials - Methods, Results and Evaluations.* NASA Symposium, 191. Washington D.C. U.S. Government Printing Office. pp. 143-198.

COHEN, S.N., SYNDULKO, K., TOURTELOTTE, W.W. and POTVIN, A.R. (1980) Critical frequency of photic driving in the diagnosis of multiple sclerosis. Arch. Neurol., 37: 80-83.

COHN, R. (1963) Evoked visual cortical responses in homonymous hemianopic defects in man. Electroenceph. clin. Neurophysiol., 15: 922P.

COHN, R. (1964) Rhythmic after-activity in visual evoked responses. Ann. N.Y. Acad. Sci., 112: 281-291.

COLEMAN, J., SYDNOR, C.F., WOLBARSHT, M.L. and BESSLER, M. (1979) Abnormal visual pathways in human albinos studied with visually evoked potentials. Experimental Neurology, 65: 667-679.

COLES, P.A. and BINNIE, C.D. (1968) An alternative method of chloriding EEG electrodes. Proceedings and Journal of the Electrophysiological Technologists Association, 15: 195-204.

COLLINS, D.W.K., BLACK, J.L. and MASTAGLIA, F.L. (1978) Pattern-reversal visual evoked potential method of analysis and results in multiple sclerosis. J. Neurol. Sci., 36: 83-95.

COLLINS, D.W.K., CARROLL, W.M., BLACK, J.L. and WALSH, M. (1979) The effect of refractive error on the visual evoked response. Brit. Med. J., 1: 231-232.

CONN, H.O, and NEIL, R.E. (1959) The prevention of the transmission of viral hepatitis by needle electrodes. Electroenceph. clin. Neurophysiol, 11: 476-677.

CONTAMIN, F. and CATHALA, H.P. (1961) Réponses électro-corticales de l'homme normal éveillé á des éclairs lumineux. Résultats obtenus a partir d'enregistrements sur le cuir chevelu, a l'aide d'un dispositif d'intégration. Electroenceph. clin. Neurophysiol., 13: 674-694.

COOPER, R. (1956) Storage of silver chloride electrodes. Electroenceph. clin. Neurophysiol., 8: 692.

COOPER, R., (1975) Detection of cerebral evoked responses. Journal of Electrophysiological Technology, 1: 108-122.

COOPER, R., OSSELTON, J.W. and SHAW, J.C. (1974) *EEG Technology*, 2nd Edition. Butterworths: London.

COOPER, R. and WALTER, W.J. (1957) Suction cup electrodes. Electroenceph. clin. Neurophysiol., 9: 733-734.

COPENHAVER, R.M. and PERRY, N.W. (1964) Factors affecting visually evoked cortical potentials such as impaired vision of varying etiology. Invest. Ophthalmol., 3: 665-675.

COWEY, A. (1964) Projection of the retina onto striate and pre-striate cortex in the squirrel monkey. J. Neurophysiol., 27: 366.

COWEY, A. (1973) Brain damage and seeing: a new look at some old problems. Trans. Ophthal. Soc. U.K., 93: 409-416.

CRACCO, J.B., CRACCO, R.Q. and GRAZIANI, L.J. (1975) The spinal evoked responses in infants and children. Neurology (Minneapolis), 25: 31-36.

CRACCO, J.B., CRACCO, R.Q. and STOLOVE, R. (1979) Spinal evoked potential in man: maturational study. Electroenceph. clin. Neurophysiol., 46: 58-64.

CRACCO, R.Q. (1973) Spinal evoked response: peripheral nerve stimulation in man. Electroenceph. clin. Neurophysiol., 35: 379-386.

CRACCO, R.Q. and BICKFORD, R.G. (1966) Comparison of evoked somatosensory and somatomotor responses in man. Electroenceph. clin. Neurophysiol., 21: 412P.

CRACCO, R.Q. and BICKFORD, R.G. (1968) Somatomotor and somatosensory evoked responses. Median nerve stimulation in man. Arch. Neurol. (Chicago), 18: 52-68.

CRACCO, R.Q. and CRACCO, J.B. (1976) Somatosensory evoked potential in man: far field potentials. Electroenceph. clin. Neurophysiol., 41: 460-466.

CREEL, D. (1979) Luminance-onset, pattern-onset and pattern-reversal evoked potentials in human albinos demonstrating visual system anomalies. J. Biomed. Eng., 1: 100-104.

CREEL, D., O'DONNELL, F.E. and WITKOP, C.J. (1978) Visual system anomalies in human ocular albinos. Science, 201: 931-933.

CREEL, D., WITKOP, C.J. and KING, R.A. (1974) Asymmetric visually evoked potentials in human albinos — evidence for visual system anomalies. Invest. Ophthalmol., 13: 430-440.

CREWS, S.J., THOMPSON, C.R.S. and HARDING, G.F.A. (1978) The ERG and VEP in patients with severe eye injury. Docum. Ophthal. Proc. Series, 15: 203-209.

CROWLEY, D.E., DAVIS, H. and BEAGLEY, H.A. (1975) Survey of the clinical use of electrocochleography. Annals of Otology, Rhinology and Laryngology, 84: 1-11.

CULLEN, J.K., Jr., ELLIS, M.S., BERLIN, C.I. and LOUSTEAU, R.J. (1972) Human acoustic nerve action potential recordings from the tympanic membrane without anaesthesia. Acta Oto-laryngologica, 74: 15-22.

DALLOS, P., SCHOENY, Z.G. and CHEATHAM, M.A. (1972) Cochlear summating potentials: descriptive aspects. Acta Oto-laryngologica, supplementum., 302: 1-46.

DANIEL, P.M. and WHITTERIDGE, D. (1961) The representation of the visual field in the cerebral cortex in monkeys. J. Physiol., London, 159: 203-221.

DAVIS, F.A. and SCHAUF, C.L. (1975) In: Davison, A.N., Humphrey, J.H., Liversedge, L.A., McDonald, W.I. and Porterfield, J.S. (Eds.) *Multiple Sclerosis Research* Proceedings of a joint conference held by the Medical Research Council and the Multiple Sclerosis Society of Great Britain and Northern Ireland, 17-18 October 1974). H.M. Stationery Office, London. pp. 102-131.

DAVIS, H. (1965) Sonomotor reflexes: myogenic evoked potentials. In: Davis, H. (Ed.) *The Young Deaf Child: Identification and Management.* Acta Oto-laryngologica, suppl. 206: 122-124.

DAVIS, H. (1976) Principles of electric response audiometry. Annals of Otology, Rhinology and Laryngology, Vol. 85, Supplement 28: 1-96.

DAVIS, H., DAVIS, P.A. LOOMIS, A.L. HARVEY, E.N. and HOBART G. (1939) Electrical reactions of the human brain to auditory stimuli during sleep. J. Neurophysiol., 2: 500-514.

DAVIS, H., FERNANDEZ, C. and McAULIFFE, D.R. (1950) The excitatory process in the cochlea. Proceedings of the National Academy of Sciences, USA, 36: 580-587.

DAVIS, H. and HIRSH, S.K. (1976) The audiometric utility of brain-stem responses to low-frequency sounds. Audiology, 15: 181-195.

DAVIS, H. and YOSHIE, N. (1963) Human evoked cortical responses to auditory stimuli. The Physiologist, 6: 164.

DAVIS, P.A. (1939) Effects of acoustic stimuli on the waking human brain. J. Neurophysiol., 2: 494-499.

DAWSON, G.D. (1946) The relation between the electroencephalogram and muscle action potentials in certain convulsive states. J. Neurol. Neurosurg. Psychiat., 9: 5-22.

DAWSON, G.D. (1947a) Cerebral responses to electrical stimulation of peripheral nerve in man. J. Neurol. Neurosurg. Psychiat., 10: 134-140.

DAWSON, G.D. (1947b) Investigations on a patient subject to myoclonic seizures after sensory stimulation. J. Neurol. Neurosurg. Psychiat., 10: 141-162.

DAWSON, G.D. (1951) A summation technique for the detection of small signals in a large irregular background. J. Physiol. (London), 115: 2-3P.

DAWSON, G.D. (1954a) A summation technique for the detection of small evoked potentials. Electroenceph. clin. Neurophysiol., 6: 65-84.

DAWSON, G.D. (1954b) A multiple scalp electrode for plotting evoked potentials. Electroenceph. clin. Neurophysiol., 6: 153-154.

DAWSON, G.D. and SCOTT, J.W. (1949) The recording of nerve action potentials through skin in man. J. Neurol. Neurosurg. Psychiat., 12: 259-267.

DAWSON, W.W. and DODDINGTON, H.W. (1973) Phase distortion of biological signals: extraction of signal from noise without phase error. Electroenceph. clin. Neurophysiol., 34: 207-211.

DEECKE, L., BECKER, W., GROZINGER, B., SCHEID, P. and KORNHUBER, H.H. (1973a) Human brain potentials preceding voluntary limb movements. Electroenceph. clin. Neurophysiol., Suppl. 33: 87-94.

DEECKE, L., ENGLITZ, H.G., KORNHUBER, H.H. and SCHMITT, G. (1977) Cerebral potentials preceding voluntary movement in patients with bilateral or unilateral Parkinson akinesia. In: Desmedt, J.E. (Ed.) *Attention, Voluntary Contraction and Event-related Cerebral Potentials. Progress in Clinical Neurophysiology, Vol. 1.* Basel: Karger. pp. 151-163.

DEECKE, L., GROZINGER, B. and KORNHUBER, H.H. (1976) Voluntary finger movement in man: Cerebral potentials and theory. Biol. Cybernetics, 23: 99-119.

DEECKE, L. and KORNHUBER, H.H. (1977) Cerebral potentials and the initiation of voluntary movement. In: Desmedt, J.E. (Ed.) *Attention, Voluntary Contraction and Event-related Cerebral Potentials. Progress in Clinical Neurophysiology, Vol. 1.* Basel: Karger. pp. 132-150.

DEECKE, L., KORNHUBER, H.H. and SCHMITT, G. (1973b) Bereitschaftspotential in Parkinson patients. Pflügers Arch., 343 (Suppl.), R75, (Abstract).

DEECKE, L., SCHEID, P. and KORNHUBER, H.H. (1969) Distribution of readiness potential, pre-motion positivity, and motor potential of the human cerebral cortex preceding voluntary finger movements. Exp. Brain Res., 7, 158-168.

DE HAAS, J.P. (1972) Electrophysiological examination of central scotomata due to pathological changes in the optic nerve. In: Cant, J.S. (Ed.). *The Optic Nerve.* Henry Kempton, London. pp. 79-87.

DELBEKE, J., McCOMAS, A.J. and KOPEC, S.J. (1978) Analysis of evoked lumbosacral potentials in man. J. Neurol. Neurosurg. Psychiat., 41: 293-302.

DELTENRE, P., VAN NECHEL, C., VERCRUYSSE, A., STRUL, S., CAPON, A. and KETELAER, P. (1982) Results of a prospective study on the value of combined visual, somatosensory, brainstem auditory evoked potentials and blink reflex measurements for disclosing subclinical lesions in suspected multiple sclerosis. In: Courjon, J., Mauguiere, F. and Revol, M. (Eds.) *Clinical Applications of Evoked Potentials in Neurology.* New York: Raven Press. pp. 473-479.

DESMEDT, J.E. (1971) Somatosensory cerebral evoked potentials in man. In: Cobb, W.A. (Ed.) *Somatic Sensation. Handbook of Electroencephalography and clinical Neurophysiology, Vol. 9.* Elsevier, Amsterdam. pp. 55-82.

DESMEDT, J.E. (1977a) (Ed.) *Visual Evoked Potentials in Man: New Developments.* Clarendon Press, Oxford.

DESMEDT, J.E. (1977b) Some observations on the methodology of cerebral evoked potentials in man. In: Desmedt, J.E. (Ed.) *Attention, Voluntary Contraction and Event-Related Cerebral Potentials. Progress in Clinical Neurophysiology.* Vol. 1. Karger: Basel. pp. 12-29.

DESMEDT, J.E. and BRUNKO, E. (1980) Functional organisation of far-field and cortical components of somatosensory evoked potentials in normal adults. In: Desmedt, J.E. (Ed.) *Clinical Uses of Cerebral, Brainstem and Spinal Somatosensory Evoked Potentials. Progress in Clinical Neurophysiology, Vol. 7.* Karger: Basel. pp. 27-50.

DESMEDT, J.E., BRUNKO, E. and DEBECKER, J. (1976) Maturation of the somatosensory evoked potentials in normal infants and children, with special reference to the early N1 component. Electroenceph. clin. Neurophysiol., 40: 43-58.

DESMEDT, J.E., BRUNKO, E., DEBECKER, J. and CARMELIET, J. (1974) The system band pass required to avoid distortion of early components when averaging somatosensory evoked potentials. Electroenceph. clin. Neurophysiol., 37: 407-410.

DESMEDT, J.E. and CHERON, G. (1980) Somatosensory pathway and evoked potential in normal human aging. In: Desmedt. J.E. (Ed.) *Clinical Uses of Cerebral, Brainstem and Spinal Somatosensory Evoked Potentials. Progress in Clinical Neurophysiology, Vol. 7.* Karger: Basel. pp. 162-169.

DESMEDT, J.E., MANIL, J., BORENSTEIN, S., DEBECKER, J., LAMBERT, C., FRANKEN, L. and DANIS, A. (1966) Evaluation of sensory nerve conduction from averaged cerebral evoked potentials in neuropathies. Electromyography, 6: 263-269.

DESMEDT, J.E. and NOEL, P. (1973) Average cerebral evoked potentials in the evaluation of lesions of the sensory nerves and the central somatosensory pathway. In: Desmedt, J.E. (Ed.) *New Developments in Electromyography and Clinical Neurophysiology, Vol 2.* Karger, Basel pp. 352-371.

DIAMOND, S.P. (1964) Input - output relations. Ann. N.Y. Acad. Sci., 112: 160-171.

DICK, E. and MILLER, R. (1978) Light-evoked potassium activity in mud puppy retina: its relationship to the b-wave of the electroretinogram. Brain Research, 154: 388-394.

DIENER, H.C. and SCHIEBLER, H. (1980) Follow-up studies of visual potentials in multiple sclerosis evoked by checkerboard and foveal stimulation. Electroenceph. clin. Neurophysiol., 49: 490-496.

DIMITREJEVIC, M.R., LARSSON, L.E., LEHMKUHL, D. and SHERWOOD, A. (1978) Evoked spinal cord and nerve root potentials in humans using a noninvasive recording technique. Electroenceph. clin. Neurophysiol., 45: 331-340.

DIX, M.R. (1965) Observations upon the nerve fibre deafness of MS with particular reference to the phenomenon of loudness recruitment. Journal of Laryngology and Otology (London), 79: 695-706.

DOBBIE, A.K. (1965) Electrical interference in hospitals. Proceedings of the Electrophysiological Technicians Association, 12: 21-24.

DOBIE, R.A., and BERLIN, C.I. (1979) Binaural interaction in brainstem-evoked responses. Arch. Otolarynogol., 105: 391-398.

DOBIE, R.A., and NORTON, S.J. (1980) Binaural interaction in human auditory evoked potentials. Electroenceph. clin. Neurophysiol., 49: 303-313.

DOMINO, E.F., MATSUOKA, S., WALTZ, J. and COOPER, I.S. (1965) Effects of cryogenic thalamic lesions on the somesthetic evoked response in man. Electroenceph. clin. Neurophysiol., 19: 127-138.

DON, M., ALLEN, A.R. and STARR, A. (1977) The effect of click rate on the latency of auditory brainstem responses in humans. Annals of Otology, Rhinology and Laryngology, 86: 186-195.

DON, M. and EGGERMONT, J.J. (1978) Analysis of the click-evoked brainstem potentials in man using high-pass noise masking. Journal of the Acoustical Society of America, 63:1084-1092.

DONALD, M.W. and GOFF, W.R. (1971) Attention-related increases in cortical responsivity dissociated from CNV. Science, 172: 1163-1166.

DONCHIN, E. (1969) Discriminant analysis in average evoked response studies: The study of single trials data. Electroenceph. clin. Neurophysiol., 27: 311-314.

DONCHIN, E. and HEFFLEY, E.F., III (1978) Multivariate analysis of event-related potential data: a tutorial review. In: Otto, D.A. (Ed.) *Multidisciplinary Perspectives in Event-Related Brain Potential Research.* U.S. Environmental Protection Agency: Washington DC. pp. 555-572.

DONCHIN, E. and HERNING, R.I. (1975) A simulation study of the efficacy of stepwise discriminant analysis in the detection and comparison of event related potentials. Electroenceph. clin. Neurophysiol., 38: 51-68.

DORFMAN, L.J. (1977) Indirect estimation of spinal cord conduction velocity in man. Electroenceph. clin. Neurophysiol., 42: 26-34.

DORFMAN, L.J. and BOSLEY, T.M. (1979) Age-related changes in peripheral and central nerve conduction in man. Neurology (Minneap.), 29: 38-44.

DORFMAN, L.J., BOSLEY, T.M. and CUMMINS, K.L. (1978) Electrophysiological localisation of central somatosensory lesions in patients with multiple sclerosis. Electroenceph. clin. Neurophysiol., 44: 742-753.

DORFMAN, L.J., NIKOSKELAINEN, E., ROSENTHAL, A.R. and SOGG, R.L. (1977) Visual evoked potentials in Leber's optic neuropathy. Annals of Neurology, 1: 565-568.

DOUEK, E.E. (1981) Auditory myogenic responses. In: Beagley, H.A. (Ed.) *Audiology and audiological Medicine*. Oxford: Oxford University Press. pp. 769-780.

DOUEK, E.E., GIBSON, W.P.R. and HUMPHRIES, K.N. (1973) The "crossed" acoustic response. Journal of Laryngology and Otology, 87: 711-726.

DOWLING, J.E. (1970) Organisation of vertebrate retinae. Investigative Ophthalmology, 9: 655-680.

DOWLING, J.E. and RIPPS, H. (1976) From sea to sight. Oceanus, 19: 28-33.

DRECHSLER, F., WICKBOLD, T.J., NEUHAUSER, B. and MILTNER, F. (1977) Somatosensory trigeminal evoked potentials in normal subjects and in patients with trigeminal neuralgia before and after thermocoagulation of the ganglion gasseri. Electroenceph. clin. Neurophysiol., 43: 496.

DUCLAUX, R., FRANZEN, O., CHATT, A.B., KENSHALO, D.R. and STOWELL, H. (1974) Responses recorded from human scalp evoked by cutaneous thermal stimulation. Brain Research, 78: 279-290.

DUFFY, F.H., ROBB, R.M. and LOMBROSO, C.T. (1967) Visual evoked response to plain and patterned light in amblyopia ex-anopsia. Electroenceph. clin. Neurophysiol., 23: 492.

DURRANT, J.D. (1977) Study of a combined non-invasive ECochG and BSER recording technique. Journal of the Acoustical Society of America, 62, supplement 1: S87.

DUS, V. and WILSON, S.J. (1975) The click-evoked post-auricular myogenic response in normal subjects. Electroenceph. clin. Neurophysiol., 39: 523-525.

DUSTMAN, R.E. and BECK, E.C. (1969) The effects of maturation and aging on the waveform of visually evoked potentials. Electroenceph. clin. Neurophysiol., 26: 2-11.

DUSTMAN, R.E., SCHENKENBERG, T., LEWIS, E.G. and BECK, E.C. (1977) The cerebral evoked potential: life-span changes and twin studies. In: Desmedt, J.E. (Ed.) *Visual Evoked Potentials in Man: New Developments*. Clarendon Press, Oxford. pp. 363-377.

DUWAER, A.L. and SPEKREIJSE, H. (1978) Latency of luminance and contrast evoked potentials in multiple sclerosis patients. Electroenceph. clin. Neurophysiol., 45: 244-258.

EBE, M., MEIER-EWERT, K.-H. and BROUGHTON, R. (1969) Effects of intravenous diazepam (Valium) upon evoked potentials of photosensitive epileptic and normal subjects. Electroenceph. clin. Neurophysio., 27: 429-435.

EBE, M., MIKAMI, T. and ITO, H. (1964) Clinical evaluation of electrical responses of retina and visual cortex in photic stimulation in ophthalmic diseases. Tohoku J. exp. med., 84: 92-103.

ECCLES, J.C., KOSTYUK, P.G. and SCHMIDT, R.F. (1962) Central pathways responsible for depolarisation of primary afferent fibres. J. Physiol., London, 161: 237-257.

EFRON, R. (1964) Artificial synthesis of evoked responses to light flash. Ann. N.Y. Sci., 112: 292-304.

EGGERMONT, J.J. (1976) Electrocochleography. In: Keidel, W.D. and Neff, W.D. (Eds.). *Handbook of Sensory Physiology: Vol. 5 Auditory System*. Springer-Verlag, Berlin. pp. 625-705.

EGGERMONT, J.J., DON, M., and BRACKMANN, D.E. (1980) Electrocochleography and auditory brainstem electric responses in patients with pontine angle tumours. Arch. Otolaryngol., 89, supplement 75: 1-19.

EGGERMONT, J.J. and ODENTHAL, D.W. (1974a) Frequency selective masking in electrocochleography. Revue de Laryngologie, 95: 489-495.

EGGERMONT, J.J. and ODENTHAL, D.W. (1974b) Electrophysiological investigation of the human cochlea. Audiology, 13: 1-22.

EISEN, A. and NUDLEMAN, K. (1979) Cord to cortex conduction in multiple sclerosis. Neurology (Minneapolis), 29: 189-193.

EISEN, A. and ODUSOTE, K. (1980) Central and peripheral conduction times in multiple sclerosis. Electroenceph. clin. Neurophysiol., 48: 253-265.

EISEN, A., STEWART, J., NUDLEMAN, K. and COSGROVE, J.B.R. (1979) Short latency somatosensory responses in multiple sclerosis. Neurology (Minneap.), 29: 827-834.

EISENGART, M.A. and SYMMES, D. (1971) Effect of eye blink on the visual evoked response in children. Electroenceph. clin. Neurophysiol., 31: 71-75.

ELBERLING, C. (1974) Action potentials along the cochlear partition recorded from the ear canal in man. Scandinavian Audiology (Copenhagen), 3: 13-19.

ELBERLING, C. and SALOMON, G. (1971) Electrical potentials from the inner ear in man in response to transient sounds generated in a closed acoustic system. Revue de Laryngologie, supplementum, 691-707.

ELBERLING, C. and SALOMON, G. (1973) Cochlear microphonics recorded from the ear canal in man. Acta Oto-laryngologica, 75: 489-495.

ELLENBERGER, C., PETRO, D.J. and ZIEGLER, S.B. (1978) The visually evoked potential in Huntington's disease. Neurology (Minneap.), 28: 95-97.

ELLENBERGER, C. and ZIEGLER, S.B. (1977) Visual evoked potentials and quantititave perimetry in multiple sclerosis. Annals of Neurology, 1: 561-564.

ELLINGSON, J.R. (1958) Electroencephalograms of normal full-term infants immediately after birth with observations on arousal and visual evoked responses. Electroenceph. clin. Neurophysiol., 10: 31-50.

ELLINGSON, R.J. (1964) Cerebral electrical responses to auditory and visual stimuli in the infant (human and subhuman studies). In: Kellaway, P. and Petersen, I. (Eds.). *Neurological and Electroencephalographic Correlative Studies in Infancy.* Grune and Stratton: New York. pp. 78-114.

ELLINGSON, R.J. (1968) Clinical application of evoked potential techniques in infant children. Electroenceph. clin. Neurophysiol., 24: 293.

ELLINGSON, R.J. (1970) Variability of visual evoked responses in the human newborn. Electroenceph. clin. Neurophysiol., 29: 10-19.

ELLINGSON, R.J., LATHROP, G.H., DANAHY, T. and NELSON, B. (1973) Variability of visual evoked potentials in human infants and adults. Electroenceph. clin. Neurophysiol, 34: 113-124.

EL-NEGAMY, E.H.M. (1978) *Subcortical Somatosensory Evoked Potentials Studied in Man.* Thesis: University of Southampton.

EL-NEGAMY, E. and SEDGWICK, E.M. (1978) Properties of a spinal somatosensory evoked potential recorded in man. J. Neurol. Neurosurg. Psychiat., 41: 762-768.

EL-NEGAMY, E. and SEDGWICK, E.M. (1979) Delayed cervical somatosensory potentials in cervical spondylosis. J. Neurol. Neurosurg. Psychiat., 42: 238-241.

EMDE, J.W. (1964) A time locked, low level calibrator. Electroenceph. clin. Neurophysiol., 16: 616-618.

EMDE, J.W. and SHIPTON, H.W. (1970) A digitally controlled constant current stimulator. Electroenceph. clin. Neurophysiol., 29: 310-313.

ENGEL, R. (1971) Early waves of the electroencephalic auditory response in neonates. Neuropediatrie, 3: 147-154.

ERTEKIN, C. (1973) Human evoked electrospinogram. In: Desmedt. J.E. (Ed.) *New Developments in Electromyography and Clinical Neurophysiology, Vol 2.* Karger, Basel. pp. 344-351.

ERTEKIN, C. (1976a) Studies on the human evoked electrospinogram; 1) The origin of the segmental evoked potentials. Acta Neurol. Scandinav., 53: 3-20.

ERTEKIN, C. (1976b) Studies on the human evoked electrospinogram; 2) The conduction velocity along the dorsal funiculus. Acta Neurol. Scandinav., 53: 21-38.

ERVIN, F. and MARK, V. (1964) Studies of the human thalamus. IV Evoked responses. Ann. N.Y. Acad. Sci., 112: 81-92.

ESTEVEZ, O. and SPEKREIJSE, H. (1974) Relationship between pattern appearance-disappearance and pattern reversal responses. Exp. Brain Res., 19: 233-238.

EVANS, B.T., BINNIE, C.D. and LLOYD, D.S.L. (1974) A simple visual pattern stimulator. Electroenceph. clin. Neurophysiol., 37: 403-406.

EVANS, E.F. (1975) The sharpening of cochlear frequency selectivity in the normal and abnormal cochlea. Audiology, 14: 419-442.

EVARTS, E.V. (1972) Contrasts between activity of precentral and post-central neurons of cerebral cortex during movement in the monkey. Brain Res., 40: 25-31.

FAINGOLD, C.L. and CASPARY, D.M. (1979) Frequency-following responses in primary auditory and reticular formation structures. Electroenceph. clin. Neurophysiol., 47: 12-20.

FAUST, V., HEINTEL, H. and HOEK, R. (1978) Altersabhängigkeit der P2-Latenz-zeiten schachbrettmusterevozierter Potentiale. Z. EEG-EMG, 9: 219-221.

FEINSOD, M., ABRAMSKY, O. and AUERBACH, E. (1973) Electrophysiological examination of the visual system in multiple sclerosis. J. Neurol. Sci., 20 (2): 161-175.

FEINSOD, M. and HOYT, W.F. (1975) Subclinical optic neuropathy in multiple sclerosis. J. Neurol. Neurosurg. Psychiat., 38: 1109-1114.

FEINSOD, M., HOYT, W.F. and WILSON, W.B. (1974) Suprastriate hemianopia. Lancet i: 1225-1226.

FEINSOD, M., HOYT, W.F., WILSON, W.B. and SPIRE, J.P. (1975a) Electrophysiological parameters in the evaluation of occipital apoplexy. Europ. Neurol., 13, 451-460.

FEINSOD, M., HOYT, W.F., WILSON, B.W. and SPIRE, J.P.(1977) The use of visual evoked potential in patients with multiple sclerosis. In: Desmedt, J.E. (Ed.) *Visual Evoked Potentials in Man: New Developments.* Clarendon, Oxford. pp. 458-460.

FEINSOD, M., MADEY, J.M.J. and SUSAL, A.L. (1975b) A new photostimulator for continuous recording of the visual evoked potential. Electroenceph. clin. Neurophysiol., 38: 641-642.

FERRIS, G.S., DAVIS, G.D., DORSEN, M.McF. and HACKETT, E.R. (1967) Changes in latency and form of the photically induced average evoked responses in human infants. Electroenceph. clin. Neurophysiol., 22: 305-312.

FINE, E.J. and HALLETT, M. (1980) Neurophysiological study of subacute combined degeneration. J. Neurol. Sci., 45: 331-336.

FIORENTINI, A. and MAFFEI, L. (1974) Evoked potentials in astigmatic subjects. Vision Research, 13: 1781-1783.

FISHMAN, R.S. and COPENHAVER, R.M. (1967) Macular disease and amblyopia. Arch. Ophthalmol., 77: 718-725.

FOULDS, W. (1979) The retinal pigment epithelial interface. Brit. J. Ophthalmol., 63: 71-84.

FOX, R., BLAKE, R. and BOURNE, J.R. (1973) VECP during pressure-blinding. Vis. Res., 13: 501-503.

FRANZEN, O. and OFFENLOCH, K. (1965) Evoked response correlates of psychophysical magnitude. Estimates for tactile stimulation in man. Exp. Brain Res., 8: 1-18.

FRASER, J.G., CONWAY, M.J., KEENE, M.H. and HAZELL, J.W.P. (1978) The post-auricular response: a new instrument which simplifies its detection by machine scoring. Journal of Laryngology and Otology, 92: 293-303.

FREEMAN, J.A. (1971) An electronic stimulus artifact suppressor. Electroenceph. clin. Neurophysiol., 31: 170-172.

FREEMAN, R.D. and THIBOS, L.N. (1973) Electrophysiological evidence that abnormal early visual experience can modify the human brain. Science, 180: 876-878.

FRICKER, S.J. (1971) Analysis of the visual evoked response by synchronous detector techniques. Invest. Ophthalmol., 10: 340-7.

FROMM, B., NYLEN, C.D. and ZOTTERMAN, Y. (1935) Studies in the mechanism of Wever-Bray effect. Acta Oto-laryngologica, 22: 477-486.

FRUHSTORFER, H., GUTH, H. and PFAFF, U. (1976) Cortical responses evoked by thermal stimuli in man. In: McCallum, W.C, and Knott, J.R. (Eds.) *The Responsive Brain.* John Wright, Bristol. pp. 30-33.

FUKUSHIMA, T. and MAYANAGI, Y. (1975) Neurophysiological examination (SEP) for the objective diagnosis of spinal lesions. In: Klug, W., Brock, M., Klager, M. and Spoerri, O. (Eds.) *Advances in Neurosurgery, Vol 2.* Springer-Verlag, Berlin. pp. 158-168.

FUKUSHIMA, T., MAYANAGI, Y. and BOUCHARD, G. (1976) Thalamic evoked potentials in somatosensory stimulation in man. Electroenceph. clin. Neurophysiol., 40: 481-490.

GADJUSEK, D.C., GIBBS, C.J., ASHER, D.M., BROWN, P., DIWAN, A., HOFFMAN, P., NEMO, G., ROHWER, R. and WHITE, L. (1977) Precautions in medical care of, and in handling materials from, patients with transmissable virus dementia (Creutzfeldt-Jakob disease). New England Journal of Medicine, 297: 1253-1258.

GALAMBOS, R.G. and HECOX, K. (1978) Clinical applications of the auditory brain stem response. Otolaryngologic Clinics of North America (Philadelphia), 11: 709-722.

GALAMBOS, R.G., SCHWARTZHOPET, J. and RUPERT, A. (1959) Microelectrode study of superior olivary nuclei. American Journal of Physiology (Bethesda), 197: 527-536.

GALE, A. and SMITH, D. (1980) On setting up a psychophysiological laboratory. In: Martin, I. and Venables, P. (Eds.) *Techniques in Psychophysiology.* Wiley: New York. pp. 565-582.

GALVIN, R., EBIED, D. and SMALL, D. (1980) Pattern reversal visual evoked responses generated by a television stimulator. Electroenceph. clin. Neurophysiol., 49: 98P.

GAMBI, D., ROSSINI, P.M., ALBERTINI, G., SOLLAZO, D., TORRIOLI, M.G. and POLIDORI, G.C. (1980) Follow-up of visual evoked potential in full-term and pre-term control newborns and in subjects who suffered from perinatal respiratory distress. Electroenceph. clin. Neurophysiol., 48: 509-516.

GARDI, J.N., MERZENICH, M. and McKEAN, C. (1979) Origins of brainstem frequency following response in the cat. Audiology, 18, 353-381.

GARDI, J.N., SALAMY, A. and MENDELSON, T. (1979) Scalp-recorded frequency-following responses in neonates. Audiology, 18: 494-506.

GARTSIDE, I.B., LIPPOLD, O.C.J. and MELDRUM, B.S. (1966) The evoked cortical somatosensory response in normal man and its modification by oral lithium carbonate. Electroenceph. clin. Neurophysiol., 20: 382-390.

GASSER, H.S. and GRAHAM, H.T. (1933) Potentials recorded in the spinal cord by stimulation of the dorsal roots. Am. J. Physiol., 103: 303-320.

GASTAUT, H., BOSTEM, F., POIRE, R., WALTREGNY, A. and REGIS, H. (Eds.) (1967a) *Les activités électriques cérébrales spontanées et évoquées chez l'homme.* Gauthier-Villars, Paris, 236.

GASTAUT, H., ORFANOS, A., POIRE, R., REGIS, H., SAIER, J. and TASSINARI, C.A. (1966) Effects de l'adaptation á l'obscurité sur les potentiels évoquées visuels de l'homme. Rev. Neurol., 34: 63-72.

GASTAUT, H. and REGIS, H. (1965) Visually evoked potentials recorded transcranially in man. In: Proctor, L.D. and Adey, W.R. (Eds.) *The Analysis of Central Nervous System and Cardiovascular Data Using Computer Methods.* NASA: Washington. pp. 7-34.

GASTAUT, H., REGIS, H., LYAGOUBI, S., MANO, T. and SIMON, L. (1967b) Comparison of the potentials recorded from the occipital, temporal and central regions of the human scalp, evoked by visual, auditory and somato-sensory stimuli. Electroenceph. clin. Neurophysiol., Suppl. 26: 19-28.

GASTAUT, Y. (1953) Les points negatives évoquées sur le vertex. Leur signification psycho-physiologique. Revue Neurologique, 89: 382-399.

GATH, I. (1969) Effect of drugs on the somatosensory evoked potentials in myoclonic epilepsy. Arch. Neurol. (Chic.), 20: 354-357.

GATZKE, R.D. (1974) The electrode: a measurement systems viewpoint. In: Miller H.A. and Harrison, D.C. (Eds.) *Biomedical Electrode Technology.* Academic Press: New York. pp. 99-116.

GAWEL, M.J., DAS, P.K., VINCENT, S. and CLIFFORD ROSE, F. (1980a) Visual and auditory evoked responses in Parkinson's syndrome. Electroenceph. clin. Neurophysiol., 50: 531P.

GAWEL, M.J., KENNARD, C., CLIFFORD ROSE, F. and RUDOLF, N. de M. (1980b) Visual evoked potentials in migraine patients. Electroenceph. clin. Neurophysiol., 49: 98P.

GAWEL, M.J., KENNARD, C., RUDOLF, N. de M. and ROSE, F.C. (1979) Pattern reversal VEP in migraine. Proc. 2nd European Congress of EEG clin. Neurophysiol. Salzburg, Excerpta Medica ICS, 506: 75.

GEDDES, L.A. (1972) *Electrodes and the Measurement of Bioelectric Events.* Wiley. Interscience.

GEDDES, L.A. and BAKER, L.E. (1968) *Principles of Applied Biomedical Instrumentation.* Wiley: New York.

GEISLER, C.D., FRISHKOPF, L.S. and ROSENBLITH, W.A. (1958) Extracranial responses to acoustic clicks in man. Science, 128: 1210-1211.

GEORGE, G. (1968) An experiment to determine the life span of a set of stick-on electrodes. The Proceedings and Journal of the Electrophysiological Technologists Association, 15: 269-272.

GERBRANDT, L.D. (1977) Analysis of movement potential components. In: Desmedt, J.E. (Ed.), *Progress in Clinical Neurophysiology, Vol. 1, Attention, Voluntary Contraction and Event-related Cerebral Potentials.* Karger, Basel, pp. 174-188.

GERBRANDT, L.K., GOFF, W.R. and SMITH, D.B. (1973) Distribution of the human average movement potential. Electroenceph. clin. Neurophysiol., 34: 461-474.

GERKEN, G.M., MOUSHEGIAN, G., STILLMAN, R. and RUPERT, A.L. (1975) Human frequency following responses to monaural and binaural stimuli. Electroenceph. clin. Neurophysiol., 38: 379-386.

GIBLIN, D.R. (1964) Somatosensory evoked potentials in healthy subjects and in patients with lesions of the nervous system. Ann. N.Y. Acad. Sci., 112: 93-142.

GIBSON, W.P.R. (1974) *Investigations of the Post-auricular Myogenic Responses.* Unpublished M.D. thesis: University of London.

GIBSON, W.P.R. (1978) *Essentials of Clinical Electric Response Audiometry.* Churchill Livingstone, Edinburgh, London and New York. pp. 1-232.

GIBSON, W.P.R. (1980) Clinical electrocochleography; the significance of the summating potential in Ménière's disorder. In: Barber, C. (Ed.) *Evoked Potentials.* MTP Press Ltd., Lancaster. pp 347-352.

GIBSON, W.P.R. and BEAGLEY, H.A. (1976) Electrocochleography in the diagnosis of acoustic neuroma. Journal of Laryngology and Otology, 90: 127-140.

GIBSON, W.P.R., MOFFAT, D.A. and RAMSDEN, R.T. (1977) Clinical electrocochleography in the diagnosis and management of Ménière's disorder. Audiology, 16: 389-401.

GIBSON, W.P.R. and WALLACE, D. (1975) Basilar artery ectasia (an unusual cause of a cerebello-pontine angle lesion and hemifacial spasm). Journal of Laryngology and Otology, 89: 721-731.

GILDEN, L., VAUGHAN, H.G., Jr. and COSTA, L.D. (1966) Summated human EEG potentials with voluntary movement. Electroenceph. clin. Neurophysiol., 20: 433-438.

GIRTON, D.G. and KAMIYA, J. (1974) A very stable electrode system for recording human scalp potentials with direct coupled amplifiers. Electroenceph. clin. Neurophysiol., 37: 85-88.

GLASS, J.D., CROWDER, J.V., KENNERDELL, J.S. and MERIKANGAS, J.R. (1977) Visual evoked potentials from occipital and precentral cortex in visually deprived humans. Electroenceph. clin. Neurophysiol., 43: 207-217.

GOFF. G.D., MATSUMIYA, Y., ALLISON, T. and GOFF, W.R. (1977) The scalp topography of human somatosensory and auditory evoked potentials. Electroenceph. clin. Neurophysiol., 42: 57-76.

GOFF, W.R. (1974) Human average evoked potentials: procedures for stimulating and recording. In: Thompson, R.F. and Patterson, M.M. (Eds.) *Methods in Physiological Psychology, Part B. Electroencephalography and Human Brain Potentials.* Academic Press: New York. pp. 102-156.

GOFF, W.R., ALLISON, T. and VAUGHAN, H.G. Jr. (1978) The functional neuroanatomy of event related potentials. In: Callaway, E., Tueting, P. and Koslow, S.H. (Eds.) *Event Related Brain Potentials in Man.* Academic Press: New York. pp. 1-79.

GOFF, W.R., MATSUMIYA, Y., ALLISON, T. and GOFF, G.D. (1969) Cross modality comparisons of averaged evoked potentials. In: Donchin, E. and Lindsley, D.B. (Eds.) *Average Evoked Potentials.* NASA SP-191. pp. 95-141.

GOFF. W.R., ROSNER, B.S. and ALLISON, T. (1962) Distribution of cerebral somatosensory evoked responses in normal man. Electroenceph. clin. Neurophysiol., 14: 697-713.

GOLDSTEIN, M.H. and KIANG, N.Y-S (1958) Synchrony of neural activity in electrical responses evoked by transient acoustic stimuli. Journal of the Acoustical Society of America, 30: 107-114.

GOLDSTEIN, R. (1965) Early components of the AER. Acta Oto-laryngologica, Suppl. 206: 127-128.

GOLDSTEIN, R. and RODMAN, L.B. (1967) Early components of averaged evoked responses to rapidly repeated auditory stimuli. Journal of Speech and Hearing Research, 10: 697-705.

GOODIN, D.S., SQUIRES, K.C., HENDERSON, B.H. and STARR, A. (1978a) Age-related variations in evoked potentials to auditory stimuli in normal human subjects. Electro-enceph., clin. Neurophysiol., 44: 447-458.

GOODIN, D.S., SQUIRES, D.C. and STARR, A. (1978b) Long latency event-related components of the auditory evoked potential in dementia. Brain, 101: 635-648.

GORDON, D.H. (1975) Triboelectric interference in the ECG. I.E.E.E. Transactions on Biomedical Engineering, 22: 252-255.

GOTT, P.,S., WEISS, M.H., APUZZO, M. and VAN DER MEULEN, J.P. (1979) Checker-board visual evoked response in evaluation and management of pituitary tumors. Neuro-surgery, 5: 553-558.

GRADER, J. and HELLER, G.L. (1964) Photic stimulation and the EEG in macular disease. Arch. Ophthal. N.Y., 72: 763.

GRAHAM, C.H. (1965) Color: Data and theories. In: Graham, C.H. (Ed.) *Vision and Visual Perception.* Wiley. pp. 414-451.

GRAHAM, J.M., RAMSDEN, R.T., MOFFATT, D.A. and GIBSON, W.P.R. (1978) Sudden sensorineural hearing loss: electrocochleographic findings in 70 patients. Journal of Laryngology and Otology, 92: 581-589.

GRANIT, R. (1933) The components of the retinal action potential in mammals and their relation to the discharge in the optic nerve. Journal of Physiology, 77: 207-239.

GREEN, D.G. (1970) Testing the vision of cataract patients by means of laser-generated interference fringes. Science, 168: 1240-1242.

GREEN, J.B. (1971) Neurophysiological studies in Batten's disease. Dev. Med. Child Neurol., 13: 477-489.

GREENBERG, R.P., BECKER, D.P., MILLER, J.D. and MAYER, D.J. (1977b) Evaluation of brain function in severe human head trauma with multimodality evoked potentials. Part 2: Localisation of brain dysfunction and correlation with post-traumatic neurological conditions. J. Neurosurg., 47: 163-177.

GREENBERG, R.P., MAYER, D.J., BECKER, D.P. and MILLER, J.D. (1977a) Evaluation of brain function in severe human head trauma with multimodality evoked potentials. Part I: Evoked brain injury potentials, methods and analysis. J. Neurosurg., 47: 150-162.

GRINKER, R.R., SEROTA, H. and STEIN, S.I. (1938) Myoclonic epilepsy. Arch. Neurol. Psychiat. (Chicago), 40: 968-980.

GUILLERY, R.W., OKORO, A.N. and WITKOP, C.J. (1975) Abnormal visual pathways in the brain of a human albino. Brain Res., 96: 373-377.

GUTIN, P.H., KLEMME, W.M., LAGGER, R.L., MACKAY, A.R., PITTS, L.H. and HOROBUCHI, Y. (1980) Management of the unresectable cystic craniopharyngioma by aspiration through an Ommaya reservoir drainage system. J. Neurosurg., 52: 36-40.

HALLETT, M., CHADWICK, D. and MARSDEN, C.D. (1979) Cortical reflex myoclonus. Neurology (Minneap.), 29: 1107-1125.

HALLIDAY, A.M. (1967a) Changes in the form of cerebral evoked responses in man associated with various lesions of the nervous system. In: Widén, L. (Ed.) *Recent Advances in Clinical Neurophysiology.* Electroenceph. clin. Neurophysiol., Suppl. 25, 178-192.

HALLIDAY, A.M. (1967b) Cerebral evoked potentials in familial progressive myoclonic epilepsy. Journal of the Royal College of Physicians, London, 1: 123-134.

HALLIDAY, A.M. (1967c) The clinical incidence of myoclonus. In: Williams D. (Ed.) *Modern Trends in Neurology* 4th edition. Butterworths, London, pp. 69-105.

HALLIDAY, A.M. (1967d) The electrophysiological study of myoclonus in man. Brain, 90: 241-284.

HALLIDAY, A.M. (1972) Evoked responses in organic and functional sensory loss. In: Fessard, A. and Lelord, G. (Eds.) *Activités évoquées et leur conditionnement chez l'homme normal et en pathologie mentale.* Editions Inserm, Paris. pp. 189-212.

HALLIDAY, A.M. (1974) The neurophysiology of myoclonic jerking: a re-appraisal. In: Charlton, M.H. (Ed.) *Myoclonic Seizures.* Excerpta Medica, Amsterdam. pp. 1-32.

HALLIDAY, A.M. (1975a) Somatosensory evoked responses. In: Storm van Leeuwen, W.S., Lopes da Silva, F.H. and Kamp, A. (Eds.) *Evoked Potentials. Handbook of Electroencephalography and Clinical Neurophysiology* Vol. 8A. Amsterdam: Elsevier. pp. 60-67.

HALLIDAY, A.M. (1975b) The effect of lesions of the visual pathway and cerebrum on the visual evoked response. In: Storm van Leeuwen, W.S., Lopes da Silva, F.H. and Kamp, A. (Eds.) *Evoked Potentials. Handbook of Electroencephalography and Clinical Neurophysiology, Vol. 8A.* Amsterdam: Elsevier. pp. 119-129.

HALLIDAY, A.M. (1976) Visually evoked response in optic nerve disease. Transactions of the Ophthalmological Societies of the United Kingdom. 96: 372-376.

HALLIDAY, A.M. (1978a) Clinical applications of evoked potentials. In: Matthews, W.B. and Glaser, G.M. (Eds.). *Recent Advances in Clinical Neurology, 2.* Edinburgh: Churchill Livingstone. pp 47-73.

HALLIDAY, A.M. (1978b) New developments in the clinical appplication of evoked potentials. In: Cobb, W.A. and van Duijn, H. (Eds.) *Contemporary Clinical Neurophysiology.* Amsterdam: Elsevier. pp. 105-121.

HALLIDAY, A.M. (1978c) Commentary: Evoked potentials in neurological diagnosis. In: Callaway, E., Tueting, P. and Koslow, S.H. (Eds.) *Event-Related Brain Potentials in Man.* New York: Academic Press. pp. 197-213.

HALLIDAY, A.M. (1980a) Evoked brain potentials: how far have we come since 1875? In: Barber, C. (Ed.) *Evoked Potentials* MTP Press, Lancaster. pp. 3-18

HALLIDAY, A.M. (1980b) Discussion of paper by G.E. Holder. Abnormalities of the pattern visual evoked potential in patients with homonymous visual field defects. In: Barber, C. (Ed.) *Evoked Potentials.* MTP Press, Lancaster. pp. 292-298.

HALLIDAY, A.M. (1980c) Event-related potentials and their diagnostic usefulness. In: Deecke, L. and Kornhuber, H.H. (Eds.) *Motivation, Motor and Sensory Processes of the Brain: Electrical Potentials, Behaviour and Clinical Use.* Progress in Brain Research, Vol. 54. Amsterdam: Elsevier/North Holland. pp. 469-485.

HALLIDAY, A.M. (1981) Visual evoked potentials in demyelinating disease. In: Waxman, S.G. and Ritchie, J.M. (Eds.) *Demyelinating Disease: Basic and Clinical Electrophysiology.* New York: Raven Press. pp. 201-215.

HALLIDAY, A.M., BARRETT, G., BLUMHARDT, L.D. and KRISS, A. (1979a) The macular and paramacular subcomponents of the pattern evoked response. In: Lehmann, D. and Callaway, E. (Eds.) *Human Evoked Potentials: Applications and Problems.* Plenum Press: New York. pp. 135-151.

HALLIDAY, A.M., BARRETT, G., CARROLL, W.M. and KRISS, A. (1982a) Problems in defining the normal limits of the VEP. In: Courjon, J., Mauguiere, F. and Revol, M. (Eds.) *Clinical Applications of Evoked Potentials in Neurology.* Raven Press: New York. pp. 1-9.

HALLIDAY, A.M., BARRETT, G., HALLIDAY, E., KRISS, A. and MUSHIN, J. (1982b) The relative sensitivity of the flash and pattern evoked potentials in the detection of demyelinating lesions. Electroenceph. clin. Neurophysiol. (In press).

HALLIDAY, A.M., BARRETT, G., HALLIDAY, Elise and MICHAEL W.F. (1977a) The topography of the pattern evoked potential. In: Desmedt, J.E. (Ed.) *New Developments in Visual Evoked Responses in the Human Brain.* Oxford University Press: London. pp. 121-133.

HALLIDAY, A.M., BARRETT, G., HALLIDAY, E. and MUSHIN, J. (1979b) A comparison of the flash and pattern-evoked potential in unilateral optic neuritis. Wissenschaftliche Zeitschrift der Ernst-Moritz-Arndt-Universitat. Greifswald, 28: 89-95.

HALLIDAY, A.M., CARROLL, W.M., and JONES, S.J. (1981) Visual and somatosensory evoked potential studies in Charcot-Marie-Tooth disease (CMTD). Electroenceph. clin. Neurophysiol., 52: S84.

HALLIDAY, A.M. and HALLIDAY, E. (1970) Cortical evoked potentials in patients with benign essential myoclonus and progressive myoclonic epilepsy. Electroenceph. clin. Neurophysiol., 29: 106-107.

HALLIDAY, A.M. and HALLIDAY, E. (l980) Cerebral somatosensory and visual evoked potentials in different clinical forms of myoclonus. In: Desmedt, J.E. (Ed.) *Clinical Uses of Cerebral, Brainstem and Spinal Somatosensory Evoked Potentials. Prog. clin. Neurophysiol., Vol. 7.* Karger: Basel, pp. 292-310.

HALLIDAY, A.M., HALLIDAY, E., KRISS, A., McDONALD, W.I. and MUSHIN, J. (1976) The pattern-evoked potential in compression of the anterior visual pathways. Brain, 99: 357-374.

HALLIDAY, A.M. and McDONALD, W.I. (1977) Pathophysiology of demyelinating disease. British Medical Bulletin, 33: 21-27.

HALLIDAY, A.M., McDONALD, W.I. and MUSHIN, J. (1972) Delayed visual evoked response in optic neuritis. Lancet (i): 982-985.

HALLIDAY, A.M., McDONALD, W.I. and MUSHIN, J. (1973a) Visual evoked responses in the diagnosis of multiple sclerosis. British Medical Journal, 4: 661-664.

HALLIDAY, A.M., McDONALD, W.I. and MUSHIN, J. (1973b) Delayed pattern-evoked responses in optic neuritis in relation to visual acuity. Transactions of the Ophthalmological Society, U.K., 93: 315-324.

HALLIDAY, A.M., McDONALD, W.I. and MUSHIN, J. (1977b) Visual evoked potentials in patients with demyelinating disease. In: Desmedt, J.E. (Ed.). *New Developments in Visual Evoked Potentials in the Human Brain.* London: Oxford University Press. pp. 438-449.

HALLIDAY, A.M. and MASON, A.A. (1964) The effect of hypnotic anaesthesia on cortical responses. J. Neurol. Neurosurg. Psychiat., 27: 300-312.

HALLIDAY, A.M. and MICHAEL, W.F. (1970) Changes in pattern-evoked responses in man associated with the vertical and horizontal meridians of the visual field. J. Physiol., 208: 499-513.

HALLIDAY, A.M. and MUSHIN, J. (1980) The visual evoked potential in neuro-opthalmology. In: Sokol, S. (Ed.). *International Ophthalmology Clinics, 20, 1: Electrophysiology and Psychophysics: Their Use in Ophthalmic Diagnosis.* Boston: Little Brown. pp. 155-183.

HALLIDAY, A.M. and WAKEFIELD, G.S. (1963) Cerebral evoked potentials in patients with dissociated sensory loss. J. Neurol. Neurosurg. Psychiat., 26: 211-219.

HANLEY, J., HAHN, P.M. and ADEY, W.R. (1974) Electrode for recording the EEG in active subjects. In: Miller, H.A. and Harrison, D.C. (Eds.) *Biomedical Electrode Technology.* Academic Press: New York. pp. 283-313.

HAPPEL, L.T., ROTHSCHILD, H. and GARCIA, C. (1980) Visual evoked potentials in two forms of hereditary spastic paraplegia. Electroenceph. clin. Neurophysiol., 48: 233-236.

HARDEN, Ann and PAMPIGLIONE, G. (1972) ERG, VER and EEG In twelve children with late infantile neuronal lipidosis. In: Arden, G.B. (Ed.) *The Visual System: Neurophysiology, Biophysics and their Clinical Applications.* Plenum Press: New York. pp. 287-293.

HARDEN, A. and PAMPIGLIONE, G. (1977) Visual evoked potentials, electroretinogram, and electroencephalogram studies in progressive neurometabolic storage diseases of childhood. In: Desmedt, J.E. (Ed.). *Visual Evoked Potentials in Man: New Developments.* Clarendon Press: Oxford. pp. 470-480.

HARDEN, Ann, PAMPIGLIONE, G. and PICTON-ROBINSON, N. (1973) Electroretinogram and visual evoked response in a form of 'neuronal lipidosis' with diagnostic EEG features. Journal of Neurology, Neurosurgery and Psychiatry, 36: 61-67.

HARDING, G.F.A. (1977) The use of the visual evoked potential to flash stimuli in the diagnosis of visual defects. In: Desmedt, J.E. (Ed.). *Visual Evoked Potentials in Man: New Developments.* Clarendon Press, London. pp. 500-508.

HARDING, G.F.A. and CREWS, S.J. (1982) The VER in hereditary optic atrophy of the dominant type. In: Courjon, J., Mauguiere, F., and Revol, M. (Eds.) *Clinical Applications of Evoked Potentials in Neurology.* New York: Raven Press. pp. 21-30.

HARDING, G.F.A., CREWS, S.J. and GOOD, P.A. (1980a) VEP in neuro-ophthalmic disease. In: Barber, C. (Ed.). *Evoked Potentials.* MTP Press, Lancaster. pp. 235-241.

HARDING, G.F.A., SMITH, G.P. and SMITH, P.A. (1980b) The effect of various stimulus parameters on the lateralization of the VEP. In: Barber, C. (Ed.) *Evoked Potentials.* MTP Press: Lancaster. pp. 213-218.

HARDING, G.F.A., THOMSON, C.R.S. and PANAYIOTOPOULOS, C. (1969) Evoked response diagnosis in visual field defects. Proc. Electrophysiol. Techn. Assoc., 16: 159-163.

HARTER, M.R. and WHITE, C.T. (1968) Effects of contour sharpness and check-size on visually evoked cortical potentials. Vision Res., 8: 701-711.

HARTER, M.R. and WHITE, C.T. (1969) Evoked cortical responses to checkerboard patterns: effect of check-size as a function of visual acuity. Electroenceph. clin. Neurophysiol., 28: 48-54.

HASHIMOTO, I., ISHIYAMA, Y., TOTSUKA, G., ARUGER, J., JOSHITA, H. and MIZUTANI, M. (1980) Monitoring brainstem function during posterior fossa surgery with brainstem auditory evoked potentials. In: Barber, C. (Ed.) *Evoked Potentials.* MTP Press, Lancaster. pp. 377-390.

HASHIMOTO, I., ISHIYAMA, Y., YOSHIMOTO, T., and NEMOTO, S. (1981) Brainstem auditory evoked potentials recorded directly from human brainstem and thalamus. Brain, 104: 841-859.

HAWKINS, J.E. Jr, and ENGSTROM, H. (1964) Effect of kanamycin on cochlear cytoarchitecture. Acta Oto-laryngologica, supplementum 188: 100-103.

HAYWARD, M. and MILLS, I.M. (1980) Design effects of video pattern generators on the visual evoked potential. In: Barber, C. (Ed.) *Evoked Potentials.* MTP Press: Lancaster. pp. 87-9

HAZEMANN, P., OLIVIER, L. and DUPONT, E. (1969) Potentiels évoqués somesthésiques recuellis sur le scalp chez 6 hémisphérectomisés. Rev. Neurol., 121: 246-257.

HECOX, K. (1975) Electrophysiological correlates of human auditory development. In: Cohen, L.B. and Salapatek, P. (Eds.) *Infant Perception: From Sensation to Cognition, Vol. II.* New York Academic Press. pp.151-191.

HECOX, K. and GALAMBOS, R. (1974) Brainstem auditory evoked responses in human infants and adults. Archives of Otolaryngology, 99: 30-33.

HECOX, K., SQUIRES, N. and GALAMBOS, R. (1976) Brainstem auditory evoked responses in man. I. Effect of stimulus rise-fall time and duration. Journal of the Acoustical Society of America (Lancaster PA), 60: 1187-1192.

HENNERICI, M., WENZEL, D. and FREUND, H.J. (1977) The comparison of small-size rectangle and checkerboard stimulations for the evaluation of delayed visual evoked responses in patients suspected of multiple sclerosis. Brain, 100: 119-136.

HENNERICI, M. and WIST, E.R. (1982) A modification of the VEP method involving small luminance decrements for the diagnosis of demyelinating diseases. In: Courjon, J., Mauguiere, F. and Revol, M. (Eds.) *Clinical Applications of Evoked Potentials in Neurology.* New York: Raven Press. pp. 433-441.

HERNANDEZ-PEON, R., CHAVEZ-IBARRA, G. and AGUILAR-FIGUEROA, E. (1963) Somatic evoked potentials in one case of hysterical anaesthesia. Electroenceph. clin. Neurophysiol., 15: 889-892.

HILLYARD, S.A. (1974) Methodological issues in CNV research. In: Thompson, R.F. and Patterson, M. (Eds.) *Bioelectric Recording Techniques. Part B, Electroencephalography and Human Brain Potentials.* Chapter 8. New York: Academic Press. pp. 281-304.

HILLYARD, S. and GALAMBOS, R. (1970) Eye movement artifact in the CNV. Electroenceph. clin. Neurophysiol., 28: 173-182.

HILLYARD, S.A. and PICTON, T.W. (1978) Event related brain potentials and selective information processing. In: Desmedt, J.E. (Ed.) *Cognitive Components in Cerebral Event-Related Potentials and Selective Attention. Progress in Clinical Neurophysiology, Vol. 6.* Karger: Basel. pp. 1-50.

HILLYARD, S.A., PICTON, T.W. and REGAN, D. (1978) Sensation, perception and attention: analysis using ERPs. In: Callaway, E., Tueting, P. and Koslow, S.H. (Eds.) *Event-Related Brain Potentials in Man.* Academic Press: New York. pp. 223-321.

HIRASUGI, Y., YATOMI, T. and MIZUKOSHI, O. (1979) Prognosis of sudden deafness by electrocochleography. Nippon Jibinkoko Gokkai Kain, 82: 869-878.

HIRSCH, J.F., PERTUISET, B., CALVET, J., BUISSON-FEREY, J., FISCHGOLD, H. and SCHERRER, J. (1961) Etude des réponses électrocorticales obtenues chez l'homme par des stimulations somesthésiques et visuelles. Electroenceph. clin. Neurophysiol., 13: 411-424.

HIRSH, I.J. (1966) Audition. In: Sidowski, J.B. (Ed.) *Experimental Methods and Instrumentation in Psychology*. McGraw-Hill: New York.

HISHIKAWA, Y., YAMAMOTO, J., FURUYA, E., YAMADA, Y., MIYAZAKI, K. and KANEKO, Z. (1967) Photosensitive epilepsy: relationship between the visual evoked responses and the epileptiform discharges induced by intermittent photic stimulation. Electroenceph. clin. Neurophysiol., 23: 320-334.

HOFFMAN, R.F. (1978) Developmental changes in human infant visual evoked potentials to patterned stimuli recorded at different scalp locations. Child Dev., 49: 110-118.

HOLMES, G. (1918) Disturbance of vision by cerebral lesions. Brit. J. Ophthalmol., 2: 353-384.

HOLMES, G. (1945) The organisation of the visual cortex in man. Proc. Roy. Soc. B, 132: 348-361.

HOLMGREN, F. (1865) Method att objectivera effecten av ljusinstryck pa retina. Upsula läkareforenings Førhandlingar, 1: 177-191.

HOROWITZ, S.F., LARSON, S.J. and SANCES, A. Jr. (1966) Evoked potentials as an adjunct to auditory evaluation of patients. In: Proceedings of the Symposium on Biomedical Engineering 1: 49-52. Milwaukee, Marquette University.

HOSPITAL TECHNICAL MEMORANDUM No. 14 (1965) *Abatement of Electrical Interference*. H.M. Stationery Office, London. pp. 1-26.

HOU, S.M. and LIPSCOMB, D.M. (1979) An investigation of the auditory frequency following responses as compared to cochlear potentials. Archives of Otolaryngology, 222: 235-240.

HOUSE, J.W. and BRACKMANN, D.E. (1979) Brainstem audiometry in neuro-otologic diagnosis. Arch. Otolaryngol., 105: 305-309.

HOWE, J.W. and MITCHELL, K.W. (1980) Visual evoked potentials from quadrantic field stimulation in the investigation of homonymous field defects. In: Barber, C. (Ed.). *Evoked Potentials*. MTP Press, Lancaster. pp. 279-283.

HRBEK, A., HRBKOVA, M. and LENARD. H.G. (1968) Somatosensory evoked responses in newborn infants. Electroenceph. clin. Neurophysiol., 25: 443-448.

HRBEK, A., KARLBERG, P., KIELLER, J., OLSSON, T. and RIHA, M. (1977a) Clinical application of evoked electroencephalographic responses in newborn infants. I. Perinatal asphyxia. Develop. Med. Child Neurol., 19: 34-44.

HRBEK, A., KARLBERG, P., KIELLER, I., OLSSON, T. and RIHA, M. (1977b) Clinical application of evoked responses in newborn infants with perinatal asphyxia. Electroenceph. clin. Neurophysiol., 43: 456.

HRBEK, A., KARLBERG, P. and OLSSON, T. (1973) Development of visual and somatosensory evoked responses in pre-term newborn infants. Electroenceph. clin. Neurophysiol., 34: 225-232.

HRBEK, A. and MARES, P. (1964) Cortical evoked responses to visual stimulation in full-term and premature newborns. Electroenceph. clin. Neurophysiol., 16: 575-581.

HUANG, C-M. and BUCHWALD, J.S. (1977) Interpretation of the vertex short latency acoustic response. A study of single neurons in the brainstem. Brain Research, 137: 219-303.

HUANG, C-M. and BUCHWALD, J.S. (1978) Factors that affect the amplitudes and latencies of the vertex short latency acoustic responses in the cat. Electroenceph. clin. Neurophysiol., 44: 179-186.

HUBEL, D.H. and WIESEL, T.N. (1965) Binocular interaction in striate cortex of kittens reared with artificial squint. J. Neurophysiol., 29: 1041-1059.

HUBEL, D.H. and WIESEL, T.N. (1967) Cortical and callosal connections concerned with the vertical meridian of visual fields in the cat. J. Neurophysiol., 30: 1561-1573.

HUBEL, D.H., and WIESEL, T.N. (1971) Aberrant visual projections in the Siamese cat. J. Physiol., (London), 218: 33-62.

HUBER, C. (1981) Pattern-evoked cortical potentials and automated perimetry in chronic glaucoma. In: Spekreijse, H., and Apkarian, P. (Eds.) *Visual Pathways : Electrophysiology and Pathology.* Documenta Ophthalmologica Proc. Ser. 27: 87-94. The Hague, Junk.

HUBER, C. and WAGNER, T. (1978) Electrophysiological evidence for glaucomatous lesions in the optic nerve. Ophthal. Res., 10: 22-29.

HUGHES, J.R. and FINO, J. (1980) Usefulness of piezoelectric earphones in recording the brainstem auditory evoked potentials: a new early deflection. Electroenceph. clin. Neurophysiol., 48: 357-360.

HUHTA, J.C. and WEBSTER, J.G. (1974) Interference in biopotential recording. In: Miller, H.A. and HARRISON, D.C. (Eds.) *Biomedical Electrode Technology.* Academic Press: New York. pp. 129-142.

HUME, A.L. and CANT, B.R. (1976) Pattern visual evoked potentials in the diagnosis of multiple sclerosis and other disorders. Proc. Aust. Assoc. Neurol., 13: 7-13.

HUME, A.L. and CANT, B.R. (1978) Conduction time in central somatosensory pathways in man. Electroenceph. clin. Neurophysiol., 45: 361-375.

HUME, A.L., CANT, B.R. and SHAW, N.A. (1979) Central somatosensory conduction time in comatose patients. Annals of Neurology, 5: 379-384.

HUMPHRIES, K.N., ASHCROFT, P.B. and DOUEK, E.E (1977) Extra-tympanic electrocochleography. Acta Oto-laryngologica, 83: 303-309.

HUMPHRIES, K.N., ASHCROFT, P.B., DOUEK, E. and CLARKE, G. (1976) Delayed auditory evoked potentials in brainstem lesions. I.E.R.E. Conference Proceedings No. 34, Institute of Electronic and Radio Engineers, London. pp. 311-318.

HUTTON, J.N.T. (1976) Anaesthesia for electrocochleography. Clinical Otolaryngology, 1:39-44.

IGGO, A. (1966) Cutaneous receptors with a high sensitivity to mechanical displacement. In: de Reuck, A.V.S. and Knight, J. (Eds.) *Touch, Heat and Pain, Ciba Foundation Symposium.* J. and A. Churchill Ltd., London. pp. 237-256.

IKEDA, H. (1976) Electrophysiology of the retina and visual pathway. In: Clifford Rose, F. (Ed.) *Medical Ophthalmology.* Chapman and Hall, London. pp. 38-55.

IKEDA, H. (1980) Visual acuity, its development and amblyopia. Journal of the Royal Society of Medicine, 73: 546-555.

IKEDA, H., TREMAIN, K.E. and SANDERS, M.D. (1978) Neurophysiological investigation in optic nerve disease: combined assessment of the visual evoked response and electroretinogram. British Journal of Ophthalmology, 62: 227-239.

INANAGA, K. and YAMAGUSHI, E. (1969) The averaged photo-palpebral reflex in man. Electroenceph. clin. Neurophysiol., 27: 665P.

IRIG (1969) Inter-Range Instrumentation Group. Telemetry Standards. New Mexico: Secretariat, Range Commanders Council, White Sands Missile Range.

JACOBSON, J.H., HIROSE, T. and SUZUKI, T.A. (1968) Simultaneous ERG and VER in lesions of the optic pathway. Invest. Ophthal., 7: 279-292.

JANZ, G.J. and IVES, D.J.G. (1968) Silver, silver chloride electrodes. Annals of New York Academy of Sciences, 148: 210-221.

JASPER, H.H. (1958) Report to the Committee on Methods of Clinical Examination in Electroencephalography. Electroenceph. clin. Neurophysiol., 10: 370-375.

JASPER, H.H. (1974) Traditional methods of examination in clinical EEG. In: Remond, A. (Ed.) *Handbook of Electroencephalography and Clinical Neurophysiology.* Vol. 3, Part C. Appendix. Elsevier: Amsterdam.

JEAVONS, P.M. and HARDING, G.F.A. (1975) *Photosensitive Epilepsy.* Clinics in Developmental Medicine No. 56. Heinemann, London. pp. 121.

JEAVONS, P., HARDING, G.F.A. , PANAYIOTOPOULOS, C.P. and DRASDO, N. (1972) The effect of geometric patterns combined with intermittent photic stimulation in photosensitive epilepsy. Electroenceph. clin. Neurophysiol., 33: 221-224.

JEFFREYS, D.A. (1968) Separable components of human evoked responses to spatially patterned visual fields. Electroenceph. clin. Neurophysiol., 24: 596P.

JEFFREYS, D. A. (1977) The physiological significance of pattern visual evoked potentials. In: Desmedt, J.E. (Ed.) *Visual Evoked Potentials in Man: New Developments.* Clarendon Press: Oxford. pp. 134-167.

JEFFREYS, D.A. and AXFORD, J.G. (1972a) Source locations of pattern-specific components of human visual evoked potentials I. Components of striate cortical origin. Experimental Brain Research, 16: 1-21.

JEFFREYS, D.A. and AXFORD, J.G. (1972b) Source location of pattern-specific components of human visual evoked potentials. II. Components of extrastriate cortical origin. Experimental Brain Research, 16: 22-40.

JEWETT, D.L. (1970a) An average response technique for recording potentials relative to a distant point without EKG interference. Electroenceph. clin. Neurophysiol., 28: 414-416.

JEWETT, D.L. (1970b) Volume-conducted potentials in response to auditory stimuli as detected by averaging in the cat. Electroenceph. clin. Neurophysiol., 28: 609-618.

JEWETT, D.L. and ROMANO, M.N. (1972) Neonatal development of auditory system potentials averaged from the scalp of rat and cat. Brain Research, 36: 101-115.

JEWETT, D.L. and WILLISTON, J.S. (1971) Auditory-evoked far-fields averaged from the scalp of humans. Brain, 94: 681-696.

JOHN, E.R., KARMEL, B.Z., CORNING, W.C., EASTON, P., BROWN, D., AHN, H., JOHN, M., HARMONY, T., PRICHEP, L., TORO, A., GIERSON, I., BARTLETT, F., THATCHER, R., KAYE, H., VALDES, P. and SCHWARTZ, E. (1977) Neurometrics. Science, 196: 1393-1410.

JOHNSTON, T.B. and WHILLIS, J. (1938) *Gray's Anatomy*. Longman's Green and Co. London.

JONES, E.G. and POWELL, T.P.S. (1970) Connections of the somatic sensory cortex of the rhesus monkey. III. Thalamic Connections. Brain, 93: 37-56.

JONES, K.G. and ARMINGTON, J.C. (1977) The removal of alpha from the VECP by means of selective averaging. Vision Res., 17: 949-956.

JONES, L.A., HARDING, G.F.A. and SMITH, P.A. (1980) Comparison of auditory cortical evoked potentials, brainstem evoked potentials and post-auricular myogenic potentials in normals and patients with known auditory defects. In: Barber, C. (Ed.) *Evoked Potentials*. MTP Press, Lancaster. pp. 337-344.

JONES, S.J. (1977) Short latency potentials recorded from the neck and scalp following median nerve stimulation in man. Electroencep. clin. Neurophysiol., 43: 853-863.

JONES, S.J. (1979) Investigation of brachial plexus traction lesion by peripheral and spinal somatosensory evoked potentials. J. Neurol. Neurosurg. Psychiat., 42: 107-116.

JONES, S.J. (1980) The effect of simultaneous interfering somatosensory stimulation on cortical and subcortical SEPs. Electroenceph. clin. Neurophysiol., 50: 233P.

JONES, S.J., BARAITSER, M. and HALLIDAY, A.M. (1980) Peripheral and central somatosensory nerve conduction defects in Friedreich's ataxia. J. Neurol. Neurosurg. Psychiat., 43: 495-503.

JONES, S.J. and SMALL, D.G. (1978) Spinal and subcortical evoked potentials following stimulation of the posterior tibial nerve in man. Electroenceph. clin. Neurophysiol., 44: 299-306.

JONES, S.J., WYNN PARRY, C.B. and LANDI, A (1981) Diagnosis of brachial plexus traction lesions by sensory nerve action potentials and somatosensory evoked potentials. Injury, 12: 376-382.

JONES. T.A., STOCKARD, J.J., ROSSITER, V.S. and BICKFORD, R.G. (1976) Application of cryogenic techniques in the evaluation of afferent pathways and coma mechanisms. Proceedings San Diego Biomedical Symposium. 15: 249-255

KAAS, J.H. and GUILLERY, R.W. (1973) The transfer of abnormal visual field representations from the dorsal lateral geniculate nucleus to the visual cortex in Siamese cats. Brain Res., 59: 61-65.

KAMP, A. (1975) Stimulus parameters. In: Remond, A. (Ed.) *Evoked Potentials. Handbook of Electroencephalography and Clinical Neurophysiology*. Volume 8, Part A. Elsevier: Amsterdam. pp. 12-19.

KAMP, A., SEM-JACOBSEN, C.W., STORM VAN LEEUWEN, W. and VAN DER TWEEL, L.H. (1960) Cortical responses to modulated light in human subjects. Acta Physiologica Scandinavica, 48: 1-12.

KARPE, G. (1945) The basis of clinical electroretinography. Acta Ophthalmologica, Supplement 24: 1-118.

KATO, M. and TANJI, J. (1972) Cortical motor potentials accompanying volitionally controlled single motor unit discharges in human finger muscles. Brain Res., 47: 103-111.

KAYED, K. ROSJO, O. and KASS, B. (1978) Practical application of patterned visual evoked responses in multiple sclerosis. Acta neurol. Scandinav., 57: 317-324.

KEIDEL, W.D. (1971) DC potentials in auditory evoked response in man. Acta Oto-laryngologica, 71: 242-248.

KELLY, D.L., GOLDRING, S. and O'LEARY, J.L. (1965) Average evoked somatosensory responses from exposed cortex in man. Arch. Neurol. (Chic.), 13: 1-9.

KENDALL, J.P. and LAWES, I.N.C. (1978) The clinical reliability of brainstem auditory evoked response. British Journal of Audiology, 12: 23-30.

KHECHINASHVILI, S.N. and KEVANISHVILI, Z.S. (1974) Experiences in computer audiology (ECOG and ERA). Audiology, 13: 391-402.

KIANG, N.Y-S. (1965) Discharge patterns of single fibres in the cat's auditory nerve. MIT Research Monograph, No. 35, MIT Press, Cambridge, Massachusetts.

KIANG, N.Y-S., CHRIST, A.H., FRENCH, M.A. and EDWARDS, A.G. (1963) Post-auricular electrical response to acoustic stimuli in humans. Quarterly Progress Report, No. 68. Research Laboratory of Electronics, Massachusetts Institute of Technology, Cambridge, Massachusetts: MIT press, 68: 218-225.

KIANG, N.Y-S. and PEAKE, W.T. (1960) Components of electrical responses recorded from the cochlea. Annals of Otology, Rhinology and Laryngology, 69: 448-458.

KIMURA, J. (1975) Electrically elicited blink reflex in diagnosis of multiple sclerosis. Brain, 98: 413-426.

KING, J.O. (1975) Progressive myoclonic epilepsy due to Gaucher's disease in an adult. J. Neurol. Neurosurg. Psychiat., 38: 849-854.

KJAER, M. (1982) The value of a multimodal evoked potential approach in the diagnosis of multiple sclerosis. In: Courjon, J., Mauguiere, F. and Revol, M. (Eds.) *Clinical Applications of Evoked Potentials in Neurology.* New York: Raven Press. 507-512.

KLASS, D. and BICKFORD, R.G. (1960) Glossokinetic potentials in the electroencephalo-gram. Electroenceph. clin. Neurophysiol., 12: 239.

KLINE, R.P., RIPPS, H. and DOWLING, J.E. (1978) Generation of b-wave currents in the skate retina. Proceedings of National Academy of Science, USA, 75: 5727-5731.

KLORMAN, R., THOMPSON, L.W. and ELLINGSON, R.J. (1978) Event related potentials across the life span. In: Callaway, E., Tueting, P. and Koslow, S.H. (Eds.) *Event Related Brain Potentials in Man.* Academic Press: New York. pp. 511-583.

KNOTT, J.R. and IRWIN, D.A. (1968) Anxiety, stress and contingent negative variation. Electroenceph. clin. Neurophysiol, 24: 286-287.

KO, W.H. and HYNECEK, J. (1974) Dry electrodes and electrode amplifiers. In: Miller, H.A. and Harrison, D.C. (Eds.) *Biomedical Electrode Technology.* Academic Press: New York. pp. 169-181.

KOHLER, W. and WEGENER, J. (1955) Currents of the human auditory cortex. Journal of Cellular and Comparative Physiology, 45, Suppl. 1: 25-54.

KOOI, K.A., GUVENER, A.M. and BAGCHI, B.K. (1965) Visual evoked responses in lesions of the higher visual pathways. Neurology, 15: 841-854.

KOOI, K.A. and SHARBROUGH, F.W. (1966) Electrophysiological findings in cortical blindness. Report of a case. Electroenceph. clin. Neurophysiol., 20: 260-263.

KOOI, K.A., TIPTON, A.C. and MARSHALL, R.E. (1971) Polarities and field configuration of the vertex components of the human evoked response: a reinterpretation. Electroenceph. clin. Neurophysiol., 31: 166-169.

KORNHUBER, H.H. and DEECKE, L. (1964) Hirnpotentialänderungen beim Menschen vor und nach Wilkürbewegungen, dargestellt mit Magnetbandspeicherung und Rückwärtsanalyse. Plügers Arch. ges. Physiol., 281: 52.

KORNHUBER, H.H. und DEECKE, L. (1965) Hirnpotentialänderungen bei Willkürbe-wegungen und passiven Bewegungen des Menschen: Bereitschaftspotential und reafferente Potentiale. Pflügers Arch. ges. Physiol., 284: 1-17.

KOROL, S. and STANGOS, N. (1972) Les potentiels évoquées corticaux dans les affections du nerf optique. Rev. Oto-neuro-ophthal., 44: 387-394.

KRISS, A. (1976) *A Neurophysiological Study of Unilateral ECT.* Unpublished Ph.D. thesis. University of Aston in Birmingham.

KRISS, A., CARROLL, W.M., BLUMHARDT, L.D. and HALLIDAY, A.M. (1982) Pattern- and flash-evoked potential changes in toxic (nutritional) optic neuropathy. In: Courjon, J., Mauguiere, F. and Revol, M. (Eds.) *Clinical Applications of Evoked Potentials in Neurology.* New York: Raven Press. pp. 11-19.

KRISS, A. and HALLIDAY, A.M. (1980) A comparison of occipital potentials evoked by pattern onset, offset and reversal by movement. In: Barber, C. (Ed.) *Evoked Potentials.* MTP Press: Lancaster. pp. 205-212.

KRISS, A., HALLIDAY, A.M., HALLIDAY, E. and PRATT, R.T.C. (1980a) Evoked potentials following unilateral ECT. I. The somatosensory evoked potential. Electroenceph. clin. Neurophysiol., 48: 481-489.

KRISS, A., HALLIDAY, A.M., HALLIDAY, Elise, and PRATT, R.T.C. (1980b) Evoked potentials following unilateral ECT. II. The flash evoked potential. Electroenceph. clin. Neurophysiol., 48: 490-501.

KRITCHEVSKY, M. and WIEDERHOLT, W.C. (1978) Short latency somatosensory evoked responses in man. Arch. Neurol., 35: 706-711.

KUROIWA, Y. and CELESIA, G.G. (1981) Visual evoked potentials with hemifield pattern stimulation. Their use in the diagnosis of retro-chiasmatic lesions. Archives of Neurology (Chicago), 38: 86-90.

KURTZBERG, D. and VAUGAN, H.G., Jr. (1973) Electrocortical potentials associated with eye movements. In: Zikmund, V. (Ed.) *The Oculomotor System and Brain Functions.* Butterworths, London. pp. 135-145.

KUTAS, M., McCARTHY, G. and DONCHIN, E. (1977) Augmenting mental chronometry: the P300 as a measure of stimulus evaluation time. Science, 197: 792-795.

LAGET, P., FLORES-GUEVARA, R., d'ALLEST, A.M., OSTRE, C., RAIMBAULT, J. et MARIANI, J. (1977) La maturation des potentiels évoqués visuels chez l'enfant normal. Electroenceph. clin. Neurophysiol. 43: 732-744.

LAGET, P., FLORES-GUEVARA, R., MARIANI, J. and RAIMBAULT, J. (1978) Etude des reponses évoquées visuelles chez le grand enfant normal ou presentant des reponses paroxystiques á la stimulation lumineuse intermittente. Electroenceph. clin. Neurophysiol., 44: 626-640.

LAGET, P., MAMO, H. and HOUDART, R. (1967) De l'interêt de potentiels évoqués somesthésique dans l'étude des lésions du lobe parietal de l'homme. Neuro-chirurgie, 13: 841-853.

LANDI, A., COPELAND, S., WYNN PARRY, C. and JONES, S.J. (1980) The role of somatosensory evoked potentials and nerve conduction studies in the surgical management of brachial plexus injuries. Journal of Bone and Joint Surgery, 62: 492-496.

LANE, J.F. (1970) Electrical impedances of superficial limb tissues: epidermis, dermis and muscle sheath. Annals of the New York Academy of Sciences, 170: 812-825.

LARSON, S.J. and SANCES, A. (1968) Averaged evoked potentials in stereotactic surgery. J. Neurosurg., 28: 227-232.

LARSON, S.J., SANCES, A. Jr., ACKMANN, J.J. and REIGEL, D.H. (1973) Non-invasive evaluation of head trauma patients. Surgery, 74: 34-40.

LARSON, S.J., SANCES, A. and BAKER, J.B. (1966a) Evoked cortical potentials in patients with stroke. Circulation, 33, Suppl. 2: 15-19.

LARSON, S.J., SANCES, A., and CHRISTENSON, P.C. (1966b) Evoked somatosensory potentials in man. Arch. Neurol. (Chicago), 15: 88-93.

LARSON, S.J., SANCES, A. Jnr. and JACOB, J.E. (1965) Electroanesthesia and conduction over corticopetal pathways. Arch. Neurol. (Chic.), 13: 10-14.

LARSSON, L.E. and PREVEC, T.S.(1970) Somatosensory response to mechanical stimulation as recorded in the human EEG. Electroenceph. clin. Neurophysiol. 28: 162-172.

LAWSON, E.A., BARRETT, G., KRISS, A. and HALLIDAY, A.M. (1981) P3 and VEPs in Huntington's Chorea. Proc. EPIC VI: 6th International Conference on Event-Related Slow Potentials of the Brain. Lake Forest, Illinois. June 21-27, 1981. (In press).

LEADBITTER, A.C.F. (1963) Screening against electrical interference. World Medical Electronics, 2: 17-20.

LEE, B. (1967) A shielded, sound-attenuating chamber. Psychophysiology, 3: 255-257.

Le GRAND, Y. (1968) *Light, Colour and Vision.* Chapman and Hall: London.

LEHMANN, D., KAVANAGH, R.N. and FENDER, D.H. (1969) Field studies of averaged visually evoked EEG potentials in a patient with a split chiasm. Electroenceph. clin. Neurophysiol., 26: 193-199.

LEHMANN, D. and SKRANDIES, W. (1979) Multichannel mapping of spatial distributions of scalp potential fields evoked by checkerboard reversal to different retinal areas. In: Lehmann, D. and Callaway, E. (Eds.) *Human Evoked Potentials: Applications and Problems.* Plenum Press: New York. pp. 201-214.

LEHTINEN, L. and BERGSTROM, L. (1970) Naso-ethmoidal electrode for recording the electrical activity of the inferior surface of the frontal lobe. 28: 303-305.

LEHTONEN, J.B. and KOIVIKKO, M.J. (1971) The use of a non-reference electrode in recording cerebral evoked potentials in man. Electroenceph. clin. Neurophysiol, 31: 154-156.

LEMPERT, J., MELTZER, P.E., WEVER, E.G. and LAWRENCE, M. (1950) The cochleogram and its clinical application. Archives of Otolaryngology, 51: 307-311.

LESEVRE, N. (1973) Potentiels évoqués par des patterns chez l'homme: influence de variables caractérisant le stimulus et sa position dans le champ visuel. In: Fessard, A. and Lelord, G. (Eds.) *Activités évoquées et leur conditionnement chez l'homme normal et en pathologie mentale.* Editions INSERM: Paris. pp. 1-22.

LEV, A. and SOHMER, H. (1972) Sources of averaged neural responses recorded in animal and human subjects during cochlear audiometry (electro-cochleogram). Arch. Klin. Exp. Ohr., 201: 79-90.

LEVINE, R.A. (1981) Binaural interaction in brainstem potentials of human subjects. Ann. Neurol., 9: 384-393.

LEVY, R. and BEHRMAN, J. (1970) Cortical evoked responses in hysterical hemianaesthesia. Electroenceph. clin. Neurophysiol., 29: 400-402.

LEWIS, E.G., DUSTMAN, R.E. and BECK, E.C. (1978) Visual and somatosensory evoked potential characteristics of patients undergoing hemodialysis and kidney transplantation. Electroenceph. clin. Neurophysiol., 44: 223-231.

LIBERSON, W.T. (1966) Study of evoked potentials in aphasics. Amer. J. Phys. Med., 45: 135-142.

LIBERSON, W.T. and KIM, K.C. (1963) The mapping out of evoked potentials elicited by stimulation of the median and peroneal nerves. Electroenceph. clin. Neurophysiol., 15: 721.

LIBERSON, W.T., VORIS, H.C. and UEMATSU, S. (1970) Recording of somatosensory evoked potentials during mesencephalotomy for intractable pain. Confin. Neurol. (Basel), 32: 185-194.

LILLE, F., BORLONE, M., LERIQUE, A., SCHERRER, J. and THIEFFRY, S. (1967) Evaluation de la profondeur du coma chez l'enfant par la technique des potentiels évoqués. Rev. neurol., 117: 216-217.

LILLE, F., LERIQUE, A., POTTIER, M., SCHERRER, J. and THIEFFRY (1968) Evoked cortical responses during coma in childhood. Presse med., 76: 1411-1414.

LINDBLOM. U.F. and OTTOSSON, J.O. (1953) Localisation of the structure generating the negative cord dorsum potential evoked by stimulation of low threshold cutaneous fibres. Acta Physiol. Scand., 29, Suppl. 106: 180-190.

LINDLEY, W.J. and HARDING, G.F.A. (1974) A simple on-line calibrator for use in averaging evoked potentials. The Proceedings and Journal of the Electrophysiological Technologists Association, 21: 20-28.

LINDSLEY, D.B. and WICKE, J.D. (1974) The electroencephalogram. Autonomous-electrical activity in man and animals. In: Thompson, R.I. and Patterson, M.M. (Eds.) *Bioelectrical Recording Techniques, Part B. Electroencephalography and Human Brain Potentials.* Academic Press: New York. pp. 3-83

LOMBROSO, C.T., DUFFY, H.F. and ROBB, R.M. (1969) Selective suppression of cerebral evoked potentials to patterned light in amblyopia ex anopsia. Electroenceph. clin. Neurophysiol., 27: 238-247.

LOW, M.D., COATS, A.C., RETTIG, G.M. and McSHERRY, J.W. (1967) Anxiety, attentiveness - alertness. A phenomenological study of the CNV genesis. Neuropsychologica, 5: 379-384.

LOWITZSCH, K. (1980) Pattern evoked visual potentials in 251 MS patients in relation to ophthalmological findings and diagnostic classification. In: Bauer, H.J., Poser, S. and Ritter, G. (Eds.). *Progress in Multiple Sclerosis Research.* Springer Verlag, Berlin. pp. 571-577.

LOWITZSCH, K., KUHNT, U., SAKMANN, C., MAURER, K., HOPF, H.C., SCHOTT, D. and THATER, K. (1976) Visual pattern evoked responses and blink reflexes in assessment of MS diagnosis. J. Neurol., 213: 17-32.

LOWITZSCH, K. and MAURER, K. (1982) Pattern-reversal visual evoked potentials in reclassification of 472 MS patients. In: Courjon, J., Mauguiere, F. and Revol, M. (Eds.) *Clinical Application of Evoked Potentials in Neurology.* Raven Press, New York. pp. 487-491.

LOWITZSCH, K., RUDOLPH, H.D., TRINCKER, D. and MULLER, E. (1980) Flash and pattern-reversal visual evoked responses in retrobulbar-neuritis and controls: a comparison of conventional and TV stimulation techniques. In: Lechner, H. and Aranibar, A. (Eds.). *EEG and Clinical Neurophysiology.* Excerpta Medica: Amsterdam. pp. 451-463.

LUEDERS, H. (1970) The effects of ageing on the waveform of the somatosensory cortical evoked potentials. Electroenceph. clin. Neurophysiol., 29: 450-460.

LUEDERS, H., LESSER, P. and KLEM, G. (1980) Pattern evoked potentials. In: Henry, C.E. (Ed.). *Current Clinical Neurophysiology.* Elsevier, Amsterdam. pp. 467-525.

LUDLAM, W.M. and MEYERS, R.R. (1972) The use of visual evoked responses in objective refraction. Trans. N.Y. Acad. Sci. 34: 154-170.

LUXON, L.M. (1980) Hearing loss in brainstem disorders. J. Neurol. Neurosurg. Psychiat., 43: 510-515.

McALPINE, D. (1972) In: McAlpine, D., Lumsden, C.E. and Acheson, E.D. (Eds.) *Multiple Sclerosis: A reappraisal.* 2nd edition. p . 202. Churchill Livingstone, Edinburgh.

McCALLUM, W.C. and WALTER, W.G. (1968) The effects of attention and distraction on the contingent negative variation in normal and neurotic subjects. Electroenceph, clin. Neurophysiol., 25: 319-332.

McCLELLAND, R.J., CHEUNG, P. and FENTON, G.N. (1980) Intersubject variability of the auditory evoked brain stem potential. Electroenceph. clin. Neurophysiol., 49: 92P.

McCLELLAND, R.J. and McCREA, R.S. (1979) Intersubject variability of the auditory evoked brain stem potentials. Audiology, 18(6): 455-546.

McCOMAS, A.J., WILSON, P., MARTIN-RODRIGUEZ, C., WALLACE, C. and HANKINSON, J. (1970) Properties of somatosensory neurones in the human thalamus. J. Neurol. Neurosurg. Psychiat., 33: 716-717.

McCORMACK, G. and MARG, E. (1973) Computer-assisted eye examination. II. Visual evoked response meridional refractometry. Am. J. Optom., 50: 889-902.

McDONALD, W.I. (1977) Pathophysiology of conduction in central nerve fibres. In: Desmedt, J.E. (Ed.) *Visual Evoked Potentials in Man: New Developments.* Clarendon Press, Oxford. pp. 427-437.

McDONALD, W.I. and HALLIDAY, A.M. (1977) Diagnosis and classification of multiple sclerosis. Brit. Med. Bull, 33: 4-8.

McDONALD, W.I. and SEARS, T.A. (1970) The effects of experimental demyelination on conduction in the central nervous system. Brain, 93: 583-598.

McGILLEM, C.D. and AUNON, J.I. (1977) Measurements of signal components in single visually evoked brain potentials. I.E.E.E. Transactions on Biomedical Engineering. BME-24, 232-241.

MacGILLIVRAY, B.B. (Ed.) (1974) *Traditional Methods of Examination in Clinical EEG. Handbook of Electroencephalography and Clinical Neurophysiology, Vol. 3C.* Elsevier, Amsterdam. pp. 1-126.

McINNES, A. (1980) Evoked potentials in hydrocephalus. Electroenceph. clin. Neurophysiol, 50: 233-234P.

McLEOD, J.G., LOW, P.A. and MORGAN, J.A. (1978) Charcot-Marie-Tooth disease with Leber optic atrophy. Neurology (Minneap.), 28: 179-184.

McNIE, E.M. (1967) An experiment to determine the life span of stick-on electrodes. The Proceedings and Journal of the Electrophysiological Technologists Association, 14: 163-166.

MAGLADERY, J.W., PORTER, W.E., PARK, A.M. and TEASDALL, R.D. (1951) Electrophysiological studies of nerve and reflex activity in normal man. IV The two-neurone reflex and identification of certain action potentials from spinal roots and cord. Bull. Johns Hopkins Hosp., 88: 499-519.

MANIL, J., DESMEDT, J.E., DEBECKER, J. and CHORAZYNA, H. (1967) Les potentiels cérébraux évoqués par la stimulation de la main chez le nouveau-né normal. Rev. neurol., 117: 53;61.

MARCUS, N.M. (1977) Visual evoked potentials to flash and pattern in normal and high risk infants. In: Desmedt, J.E. (Ed.) *Visual Evoked Potentials in Man: New Developments.* Clarendon Press, London. pp. 480-499.

MARKAND, O.N., OCHS, R., WORTH, R.M. and DEMYER, W.E. (1980) Brainstem auditory evoked potentials in chronic degenerative central nervous system disorders. In: Barber, C. (Ed.). *Evoked Potentials.* MTP Press Ltd.: Lancaster. pp. 367-375.

MARSH, J., BROWN, W.S. and SMITH, J.C. (1975) Far field recorded frequency following responses; correlates of low pitch auditory perception in humans. Electroenceph. clin. Neurophysiol., 38: 113-119.

MARTIN, J.L. and COATS, A.C. (1973) Short latency auditory evoked responses recorded from human nasopharynx. Brain Research, 60: 496-502.

MARTIN, M.E. and MOORE, E.J. (1977) Scalp distribution of early (0-10 msec) auditory evoked responses. Archives of Otolaryngology (Chicago) 103: 326-328.

MAST, T.E. (1963) Muscular vs cerebral sources for the short latency human evoked responses to clicks. Physiologist, 6: 229.

MAST, T.E. (1965) Short latency human evoked responses to clicks. Journal of Applied Physiology, 20: 725-730.

MASTAGLIA, F.L., BLACK, J.L., CALA, L.A. and COLLINS, D.W.K. (1977) Evoked potentials, saccadic velocities and computerised tomography in diagnosis of multiple sclerosis. British Medical Journal, i: 1315-1317.

MASTAGLIA, F.L., BLACK, J.L., CALA, L.A.and COLLINS, D.W.K. (1980) The contribution of visual and somatosensory evoked potentials and quantitative electro-oculography in the diagnosis of multiple sclerosis. In: Barber, C. (Ed.) *Evoked Potentials.* MTP Press, Lancaster. pp. 559-565.

MASTAGLIA, F.L., BLACK, J.L. and COLLINS, D.W.K. (1976) Visual and spinal evoked potentials in diagnosis of multiple sclerosis. British Medical Journal, iii: 732.

MASTAGLIA, F.L., BLACK, J.L., EDIS, R. and COLLINS, D.W.K. (1978) The contribution of evoked potentials in the functional assessment of the somatosensory pathway. In: Tyrer, J.H. and Eadie, M.J. (Eds.) *Clinical and Experimental Neurology (Proceedings of the Australasian Association of Neurologists), Vol. 15.* Adis Press, Sydney. pp. 279-298.

MATHEWS, G., BERTRAND, G. and BROUGHTON, R. (1970) Thalamic somatosensory evoked potential in Parkinsonian patients correlation with unit responses and thalamic stimulation. Electroenceph. clin. Neurophysiol., 28: 98-99.

MATSUKADO, Y., YOSHIDA, M., GOYA, T. and SHIMOJI, K. (1976) Classification of cervical spondylosis or disc protrusion by pre-operative evoked spinal electrogram. J. Neurosurg., 44: 435-441.

MATSUMITA, Y., GENNARELLI, T.A. and LOMBROSO, C.T. (1971) Somatosensory evoked responses in the hemispherectomised man. Electroenceph. clin. Neurophysiol., 31:289.

MATTHEWS, W.B., BEAUCHAMP, M. and SMALL, D.G. (1974) Cervical somatosensory evoked responses in man. Nature, 252: 230-232.

MATTHEWS, W.B., READ, D.J. and POUNTNEY, E. (1979) Effect of raising body temperature on visual and somatosensory evoked potentials in patients with multiple sclerosis. J. Neurol. Neurosurg. Psychiat., 42: 250-255.

MATTHEWS, W.B. and SMALL, D.G. (1979) Serial recording of visual and somatosensory evoked potentials in multiple sclerosis. Journal of Neurological Sciences (Amsterdam), 40: 11-21.

MATTHEWS, W.B., SMALL, D.G., SMALL, M. and POUNTNEY, E. (1977) The pattern reversal evoked visual potential in the diagnosis of multiple sclerosis. J. Neurol. Neurosurg. Psychiat., 40: 1009-1014.

MAUGUIERE, F., MITROU, H., CHALET, E., POURCHER, E. and COURJON, J. (1979) Intérêt des potentiels évoqués visuels dans la sclérose multiloculaire (SM): Étude comparative des résultats, obtenus en stimulation par éclair lumineux et inversion de damier. Revue EEG Neurophysiologie, 9: 209-220.

MAURER, K. and LOWITZSCH, K. (1982) Brainstem auditory evoked potentials in reclassification of 143 MS patients. In: Courjon, J., Mauguiere, F. and Revol, M. (Eds.) *Clinical Appplications of Evoked Potentials in Neurology.* New York: Raven Press. pp. 481-486.

MAURER, K., SCHAFER, E. and LEITNER, H. (1980) The effect of varying stimulus polarity (rarefaction vs condensation) on early auditory evoked potentials (EAEPs). Electroenceph. clin. Neurophysiol., 50: 332-334.

MEDICAL ROYAL COLLEGES (1976) Diagnosis of brain death. Brit. Med. Journal, 2: 1187-1188.

MEIER-EWERT, K. and BROUGHTON, R.J. (1967) Photomyoclonic response of epileptic and non-epileptic subjects during wakefulness, sleep and arousal. Electroenceph. clin. Neurophysiol., 23: 142-151.

MEIER-EWERT, K., GLEITSMANN, K. and REITER, F. (1974) Acoustic jaw reflex in man; its relationship to other brainstem and microreflexes. Electroenceph. clin. Neurophysiol., 36: 629-637.

MENDEL, M.I. (1974) Influence of stimulus level and sleep stage on the early components of the averaged electroencephalic response to clicks during all-night sleep. Journal of Speech and Hearing Research, 17: 5-17.

MENDEL, M.I., ADKINSON, C. and HARKER, L. (1977) Middle components of the auditory evoked potentials in infants. Annals of Otology, Rhinology and Laryngology, 86: 293-299.

MICHAEL, W.F. and HALLIDAY, A.M. (1971) Differences between the occipital distribution of upper and lower field pattern-evoked responses in man. Brain Research, 32: 311-324.

MICHALEWSKI, H.J., THOMPSON, L.W., PATTERSON, J.V., BOWMAN, T.E. and LITZELMAN, D. (1980) Sex differences in the amplitudes and latencies of the human auditory brainstem potential. Electroenceph. clin. Neurophysiol., 48: 351-356.

MILLER, R.F. and DOWLING, J.E. (1970) Intracellular responses of the Muller (glial) cells of mudpuppy retina: their relation to the b-wave of the electroretinogram. Journal of Neurophysiology, 33: 323-341.

MILLODOT, M. (1977) The use of visual evoked potentials in optometry. In: Desmedt, J.E. (Ed.) *Visual Evoked Potentials in Man: New Developments.* Clarendon Press: Oxford. pp. 401-409.

MILLODOT, M. and RIGGS, L.A. (1970) Refraction determined electrophysiologically. Archs. Ophthal., N.Y., 84: 272-278.

MILNARCH, R.F., TOURNEY, G. and BECKETT, P.G.S. (1957) Electroencephalographic artifact arising from dental restorations. Electroenceph. clin. Neurophysiol., 9: 337-339.

MILNER, B.A., REGAN, D. and HERON, J.R. (1974) Differential diagnosis of multiple sclerosis by visual evoked potential recording. Brain, 97: 755-772.

MITCHELL, D.E. and BLAKEMORE, C. (1970) Binocular depth perception and the corpus callosum. Vision Research, 10: 49-54.

MIYOSHI, S., LUEDERS, H., KATO, M. and KUROIWA, Y. (1971) The somatosensory evoked potential in patients with cerebrovascular diseases. Folia Psychiat. neurol. jap., 25: 9-25.

MOFFAT, D.A., GIBSON, W.P.R., RAMSDEN, R.T., MORRISON, A.W. and BOOTH, J.B. (1978) Transtympanic electrocochleography during glycerol dehydration. Acta Otolaryngologica, 85: 158-l66.

MOFFAT, D.A. and RAMSDEN, R.T. (1977) Profound bilateral sensorineural hearing loss during gentamicin therapy. Journal of Laryngology and Otology, 9l: 511-516.

MONTAGU, J.D. and COLES, E.M. (1966) Mechanism and measurement of the galvanic skin response. Psychological Bulletin, 65: 261-269.

MONTANDON, P.B., MEGILL, N.D., KAHN, A.R., PEAKE, W.T. and KIANG, N.Y-S (1975a) Recording auditory-nerve potentials as an office procedure. Annals of Otology, Rhinology and Laryngology, 84: 2-10.

MONTANDON, P.B., SHEPARD, N.T., MARR, E.M., PEAKE, W.T. and KIANG, N.Y-S. (1975b) Auditory-nerve potentials from ear canals of patients with otologic problems. Annals of Otology, Rhinology and Laryngology, 84: 164-174.

MORRISON, A.W., GIBSON, W.P.R. and BEAGLEY, H.A. (1976) Trans-tympanic electrocochleography in the diagnosis of retro-cochlear tumours. Clinical Otolaryngology, 1: 153-167.

MOWERY, G.L. and BENNETT, A.E. (1957) Some technical notes on monopolar and bipolar recording. Electroenceph. clin. Neurophysiol. 9: 377.

MULLER, W. (1962) Untersuchungen über das Verhalten der Corticalzeit bei bitemporaler Hemianopsie. Albrecht v. Graefes Archiv für Ophthalmologie, 165: 214-218.

MULLER, W. (1963) Die corticale Antwort bei ausgelöschtem Elektroretinogramm. V. Graefes Archiv für Ophthalmologie, 166: 383-386.

MUSHIN, J.C. (1974) *The Visual Evoked Response as a Measure of Optic Nerve Conduction in Patients with Demyelinating Disease.* Thesis. London.

MYERS, R.E. (1962) Commissural connections between occipital lobes of the monkey. J. comp. Neurol., 118: 1-16.

NAKANISHI, T., SHIMADA, Y., SAKUTA, M. and TOYOKURA, Y. (1978) The initial positive component of the scalp-recorded somatosensory evoked potential in normal subjects and in patients with neurological disorders. Electroenceph. clin. Neurophysiol., 45: 26-34.

NAKANISHI, T., SHIMADA, Y. and TOYOKURA, Y. (1974) Somatosensory evoked responses to mechanical stimulation in normal subjects and in patients with neurological disorders. J. Neurol. Sci., 21: 289-298.

NAKANISHI, T., TAKITA, K. and TOYOKURA, Y. (1973) Somatosensory evoked responses to tactile tap in man. Electroenceph. clin. Neurophysiol., 34: 1-6.

NAMEROW, N.S. (1968) Somatosensory evoked responses in multiple sclerosis patients with varying sensory loss. Neurology (Minneap.), 18: 1197-1204.

NAMEROW, N.S. (1969) Somatosensory evoked responses following cervical cordotomy. Bull. Los Angeles Neurol. Soc., 34: 184-188.

NAMEROW, N.S. (1970) Somatosensory recovery functions in multiple sclerosis patients. Neurology (Minneap.), 20: 813-817.

NAMEROW, N.S. (1971) Temperature effect on critical flicker fusion in multiple sclerosis. Arch. Neurol. (Chicago), 25: 269-275.

NAMEROW, N.S. and ENNS, N. (1972) Visual evoked responses in patients with multiple sclerosis. J. Neurol. Neurosurg. Psychiat., 35: 829-833.

NAMEROW, N.S., SCLABASSI, R.J. and ENNS, N.F. (1974) Somatosensory responses to stimulus trains: normative data. Electroenceph. clin. Neurophysiol., 37: 11-21.

NASH, C.L., LORIG, R.A., SCHATZINGER, L.A. and BROWN, R.H. (1977) Spinal cord monitoring during operative treatment of the spine. Clinical Orthopaedics and Related Research, 126: 100-105.

NEAFSEY, E.J., HULL, C.D. and BUCHWALD, N.A. (1978) Preparation for movement in the cat. I. Unit activity in the cerebral cortex. Electroenceph. clin. Neurophysiol., 44: 706-713.

NEUMAN, M.R. (1978) Biopotential electrodes. In: Webster, J.G. (Ed.) *Medical Instrumentation: Application and Design.* Houghton-Mifflin: Boston. pp. 215-272.

NILSSON, B.Y. (1978) Visual evoked responses in MS: comparison of two methods for pattern reversal. J. Neurol. Neurosurg. Psychiat., 41: 499-504.

NISHIDA, H. and KUMAGAMI, H. (1978) Electrocochleographic study of sudden deafness. Annals of Otology, Rhinology and Laryngology, 87: 571-578.

NOEL, P. and DESMEDT, J.E. (1975) Somatosensory cerebral evoked potentials after vascular lesions of the brainstem and diencephalon. Brain, 98: 113-128.

NOEL, P. and DESMEDT, J.E. (1976) The somatosensory pathway in Friedreich's ataxia. Acta Neurologica Belgica, 76: 271.

NOEL, P. and DESMEDT, J.E. (1980) Cerebral and far-field somatosensory evoked potentials in neurological disorders involving the cervical spinal cord, brainstem, thalamus and cortex. In: Desmedt, J.E. (Ed.) *Clinical Uses of Cerebral, Brainstem and Spinal Somatosensory Evoked Potentials. Progress in Clinical Neurophysiology Vol 7.* Karger: Basel, pp. 205-230.

NOGAWA, T., KATAYAMA, K., TABATA, Y., KAWAHARA, T. and OHSHIO, T. (1973) Visual evoked potentials estimated by "Wiener filtering". Electroenceph. clin. Neurophysiol., 35: 375-378.

OAKLEY, B. and GREEN, D.C. (1976) Correlation of light-induced changes in retinal extracellular potassium concentration with c-wave of the electroretinogram. J. Neurophysiol., 39: 1117-1133.

OCHS, A.L. and AMINOFF, M.J. (1981) Pattern-reversal and pattern-onset visual evoked potentials in normal subjects and patients with possible multiple sclerosis. Electroenceph. clin. Neurophysiol., 51: 27P.

OEPEN, G., BRAUNER, C., DOERR, M. and THODEN, U. (1982a) Visual evoked potentials by central foveal and checkerboard reversal stimulation in multiple sclerosis. In: Courjon, J., Mauguiere, F. and Revol, M. (Eds.). *Clinical Appplication of Evoked Potentials in Neurology.* Raven Press, New York. pp. 427-431.

OEPEN, G., DOERR, M. and THODEN, U. (1982b) Huntington's Disease: alterations of visual and somatosensory cortical evoked potentials in patients and offspring. In: Courjon, J., Mauguiere, F. and Revol, M. (Eds.). *Clinical Applications of Evoked Potentials in Neurology.* Raven Press, New York. pp. 141-147.

OOSTERHUIS, H.J.G.H., PONSEN, L., JONKMAN, E.J. and MAGNUS, O. (1969) The average visual response in patients with cerebrovascular disease. Electroenceph. clin. Neurophysiol. 27: 23-34.

OSSELTON, J.W. (1966) Bipolar, unipolar and average reference recording methods. I. Mainly theoretical considerations. The Proceedings and Journal of the Electrophysiological Technologists Assocation, 13: 99-110.

OSSELTON, J.W. (1970) Bipolar, unipolar and average reference recording methods. II. Mainly practical considerations. The Proceedings and Journal of the Electrophysiological Technologists Association, 17: 45-63.

OTTO, D.A. (Ed.) (1978) *Multidisciplinary Perspectives in Event-related Brain Potential Research.* U.S. Environmental Protection Agency: Washington. pp. 1-670.

PAGNI, C.A. (1967) Somatosensory evoked potentials in thalamus and cortex of man. Electroenceph. clin. Neurophysiol., Suppl. 26: 147-155.

PAMPIGLIONE, G. and HARDEN, Ann (1973) Neurophysiological identification of a late infantile form of 'neuronal lipidosis'. J. Neurol. Neurosurg. Psychiat., 36: 68-74.

PANAYIOTOPOULOS, C.P., JEAVONS, P.M. and HARDING, G.F.A. (1970) Relation of occipital spikes evoked by intermittent photic stimulation to visual evoked responses in photosensitive epilepsy. Nature, 228: 566-567.

PANAYIOTOPOULOS, C.P., JEAVONS, P.M. and HARDING, G.F.A. (1972) Occipital spikes and their relation to visual evoked responses in epilepsy, with particular reference to photosensitive epilepsy. Electroenceph. clin. Neurophysiol., 32: 179-190.

PAPAKOSTOPOULOS, D. and CROW, H.J. (1980) Direct recording of the somatosensory evoked potentials from the cerebral cortex of man and the difference between precentral and postcentral potentials. In: Desmedt, J.E. (Ed.) *Clinical Uses of Cerebral, Brainstem and Spinal Somatosensory Evoked Potentials. Progress in Clinical Neurophysiology, Vol. 7.* Karger: Basel. pp. 15-26.

PAPAKOSTOPOULOS, D., WINTER, A. and NEWTON, P. (1973) New techniques for the control of eye potential artifacts in multichannel CNV recordings. Electroenceph. clin. Neurophysiol., 34: 651-653.

PARKER, D.J. and THORNTON, A.R.D. (1978a) The validity of the derived cochlear nerve and brainstem evoked responses of the human auditory system. Scandinavian Audiology (Copenhagen), 7: 45-52.

PARKER, D.J. and THORNTON, A.R.D. (1978b) Frequency specific components of the cochlear nerve and brainstem evoked responses of the human auditory system. Scandinavian Audiology (Copenhagen) 7: 53-60.

PARSONS, F.G. and KEENE, L. (1919) Sexual differences in the skull. J. Anat. Physiol., 54: 58-65.

PARSONS, O.A. and MILLER, P.N. (1957) Flicker fusion thresholds in multiple sclerosis. Arch. Neurol. Psychiat. (Chicago), 77: 134-139.

PATY, D.W., BLUME, W.T., BROWN, W.F., JAATOUL, N., KERTESZ, A. and McINNES, W. (1978) Chronic progressive myelopathy: Investigation with CSF electrophoresis, evoked potentials, and CAT scan. Trans. Amer. Neurol. Assoc., 103: 110-112.

PATY, J., BRENAUT, P., HENRY, P. and FAURE, J.M.A. (1976) Potentiels évoqués visuels et sclérose en plaques. Revue Neurologique, 132: 605-621.

PATY, J., DELIAC, Ph., GIOUX, M. and FRANQUI-ZANNETTACCI, M. (1980) An approach to diagnosis of multiple sclerosis with cerebral evoked potentials (visual, auditory, somatosensory). In: Barber, C. (Ed.). *Evoked Potentials.* MTP Press, Lancaster. pp 593-603.

PATY, J., NAVARTE, M-M, BENSCH, C. and FAURE, J.M.A. (1974) Diagnostic electrophysiologique de cécités corticales. Bordeaux Med. 8: 1143-1155.

PEDERSEN, L. and TROJABORG, W. (1981) Visual, auditory and somatosensory pathway involvement in hereditary cerebellar ataxia. Friedreich's ataxia and familial spastic paraplegia. Electroenceph. clin. Neurophysiol., 52: 283-297.

PENFIELD, W.G. and BOLDREY, E. (1937) Somatosensory and motor representation in the cerebral cortex of man as studied by electrical stimulation. Brain, 60: 389-443.

PERKIN, G.D. and ROSE, F.C. (1976) Uhthoff's syndrome. Brit. J. Ophthal., 60: 60.

PERLMAN, H.B. and CASE, T.J. (1941) Electrical phenomena of the cochlea in man. Archives of Otolaryngology, 34: 710-718.

PEROT, P.L. (1973) The clinical use of somatosensory evoked potentials in spinal cord injury. Clin. Neurosurg., 20: 367-381.

PEROT, P.L. (1976) Somatosensory evoked potentials in the evaluation of patients with spinal cord injury. In: Morley, T.P. (Ed.) *Current Controversies in Neurosurgery.* W.B. Saunders, Philadelphia. pp. 160-167.

PERRY, N.W. and CHILDERS, D.G. (1968) Cortical potentials in normal and amblyopic binocular vision. In: *Advances in Electrophysiology and Pathology of the Visual System.* Georgge Thieme, Leipzig.

PERRY, N.W. and CHILDERS, D.G. (1969) *The Human Visual Evoked Response: Method and Theory.* Springfield: Thomas. pp. 1-187.

PERSSON, H.E. and SACHS, Ch. (1978) Provoked visual impairment in multiple sclerosis studied by visual evoked responses. Electroenceph. clin. Neurophysiol., 44: 664-668.

PERSSON, H.E. and SACHS, Ch. (1980) Visual evoked potentials during provoked visual impairment in multiple sclerosis. In: Barber, C. (Ed.). *Evoked Potentials.* MTP Press, Lancaster. pp 575-579.

PICTON, T.W. (1979) Human visual evoked potentials. American EEG Society, September 18th, Atlanta, Georgia.

PICTON, T.W. and DURIEUX SMITH, A. (1978) The practice of evoked potential audiometry. Otolaryngologic Clinics of North America (Philadelphia), 11: 263-281.

PICTON, T.W. and HILLYARD, S.A. (1972) Cephalic skin potentials in electroencephalography. Electroenceph. clin. Neurophysiol., 33: 419-424.

PICTON, T.W. and HILLYARD, S.A. (1974) Human auditory evoked potentials. II. Effects of attention. Electroenceph. clin. Neurophysiol., 36: 191-200.

PICTON, T.W., HILLYARD, S.A., KRAUSZ, H.I. and GALAMBOS, R. (1974) Human auditory evoked potentials I: Evaluation of components. Electroenceph. clin. Neurophysiol., 36: 179-190.

PICTON, T.W. and HINK, R.F. (1974) Evoked potentials: How? What? Why? American Journal of EEG Technology, 14: 9-44.

PICTON, T.W., OVELLETEE, J., HAMEL, G. and DURREUX SMITH, A. (1979) Brainstem evoked potentials to tone pips in notched noise. Journal of Otolaryngology, 8: 289-313.

PICTON, T.W., WOODS, D.L., BARIBEAU-BRAUN, A.B.J. and HEALEY, T.M.G. (1977) Evoked potential audiometry. Journal of Otolaryngology, (Toronto), 6: 90-119.

PICTON, T.W., WOODS, D.L. and PROULX, G.B. (1978a) Human auditory sustained potentials. I. The nature of the response. Electroenceph. clin. Neurophysiol., 45: 186-197.

PICTON, T.W., WOODS, D.L. and PROULX, G.B. (1978b) Human auditory sustained potentials. II. Stimulus relationships. Electroenceph. clin. Neurophysiol., 45: 198-210.

PICTON, T.W., WOODS, D., STUSS, D. and CAMPBELL, K. (1978c) Methodology and meaning of human evoked potential scalp distribution studies. In: Otto, D.A. (Ed.) *Multidisciplinary Perspectives in Event-Related Brain Potential Research.* U.S. Environmental Protection Agency 600/9-77-043. pp. 515-522.

PITMAN, J.R. and WHITESIDE, T.C.D. (1955) A clip-on electrode for recording action potentials from the scalp. Electroenceph. clin. Neurophysiol., 7: 653-654.

PLANTZ, R.G., WILLISTON, J.S. and JEWETT, D.L. (1974) Spatio-temporal distribution of auditory evoked far field potentials in rat and cat. Brain Research, 68: 55-71.

POLYAK, S.W. (1957) *The Vertebrate Visual System.* Chicago: University of Chicago Press.

PORTMANN, M., ARAN, J-M. and LEBERT, G. (1968) Electro-cochleogramme humain en dehors de toute intervention chirurgicale. Acta Oto-Laryngologica, 71: 253-261.

POSTHUMUS MEYJES, F.E. Jr. (1969) Some characteristics of the early components of the somatosensory evoked response to mechanical stimulus in man. Psychiatrica, Neurologica, Neurochirurgia, 72: 263-268.

POTTS, A.M., MODRELL, K.W. and KINGSBURY, C. (1960) Permanent fractionation of the electroretinogram by sodium glutamate. American Journal of Ophthalmology, 50: 900-907.

PRASHER, D.K. and GIBSON, W.P.R. (1980a) Brainstem auditory evoked potentials: significant latency differences between ipsilateral and contralateral stimulation. Electroenceph. clin. Neurophysiol., 50: 240-246.

PRASHER, D.K. and GIBSON, W.P.R. (1980b) Brainstem auditory evoked potentials: A comparative study of monaural versus binaural stimulation in the detection of multiple sclerosis. Electroenceph. clin. Neurophysiol., 50(3): 247-253.

PRATT, H., AMLIE, R.N. and STARR, A. (1979) Short latency mechanically evoked somatosensory potentials in humans. Electroenceph. clin. Neurophysiol., 47: 524-531.

PREVEC, T.S. and BUTINAR, D. (1977) Changes in somatosensory evoked potentials in multiple sclerosis patients. Electroenceph. clin. Neurophysiol., 43: 574-575.

PREVEC, T.S., LOKAR, J. and CERNELC, S. (1974) The use of CNV audiometry. Audiology, 13: 447-457.

PURVES, S.J. and LOW, M.D. (1976) Visual evoked potentials to a reversing-pattern light-emitting diode stimulator in normal subjects and patients with demyelinating disease. Electroenceph. clin. Neurophysiol., 41: 651-652.

QUY, R.J. (1978) A miniature preamplifier for ambulatory monitoring of the electroencephalogram. Journal of Physiology (London), 284: 23-24P.

RADINOVA, E.A. (1971) Two types of neurons in the cat cochlear nucleus and their role in audition. In: Gusani, G.V. (Ed.) *Sensory Processes at the Neuronal and Behavioural levels.* Academic Press: New York. pp 135-155.

RAMSDEN, R.T., GIBSON, W.P.R. and MOFFAT, D.A. (1977a) Anaesthesia of the tympanic membrane using iontophoresis. Journal of Laryngology and Otology, 91: 779-785.

RAMSDEN, R.T., MOFFAT, D.A. and GIBSON, W.P.R. (1977b) Transtympanic electro-cochleography in patients with syphilis and hearing loss. Annals of Otology, Rhinology and Laryngology, 86: 827-834.

RAPIN, I. and SCHIMMEL, H. (1977) Assessment of auditory sensitivity in infants and in uncooperative handicapped children by using the late components of the average auditory evoked potential. In: Desmedt, J.E. (Ed.). *Auditory Evoked Potentials in Man. Psychopharmacology Correlates of Evoked Potentials.* S. Karger, Basel. pp. 79-92.

RASMINSKY, M. and SEARS, T.A. (1972) Internodal conduction in undissected demyelinated nerve fibres. Journal of Physiology, 227: 323-350.

REGAN, D. (1972a) *Evoked Potentials in Psychology, Sensory Physiology and Clinical Medicine.* Chapman and Hall, London.

REGAN, D. (1972b) Evoked potentials to changes in the chromatic contrast and luminance contrast of checkerboard stimulus patterns. Adv. exp. Med. Biol., 24: 171-187.

REGAN D. (1973) Objective refraction using evoked brain potentials. Invest. Ophthal., 12: 669-679.

REGAN, D. (1977a) Steady-state evoked potentials. J. Opt. Soc. Am., 67: 1475-1489.

REGAN, D. (1977b) Rapid methods for refracting the eye and for assessing visual acuity in amblyopia using steady-state visual evoked potentials. In: Desmedt, J.E. (Ed.). *Visual Evoked Potentials in Man: New Developments.* Clarendon Press, Oxford. pp. 418-426.

REGAN, D. and CARTWRIGHT, R.F. (1970) A method of measuring the potentials evoked by simultaneous stimulation of different retinal regions. Electroenceph. clin. Neurophysiol. 28: 314-319.

REGAN, D. and HERON, J.R. (1969) Clinical investigation of lesions of the visual pathway: a new objective technique. J. Neurol. Neurosurg. Psychiat., 32: 479-483.

REGAN, D. and HERON, J.R. (1970) Simultaneous recording of visual evoked potentials from the left and right hemispheres in migraine. In: Cochrane, A.L. (Ed.). *Background to Migraine.* Heinemann, London. pp. 66-77.

REGAN, D., MILNER, B.A. and HERON, J.R. (1976) Delayed visual perception and delayed visual evoked potential in the spinal form of multiple sclerosis and in retrobulbar neuritis. Brain, 99: 43-63.

REGAN, D., MILNER, B.A. and HERON, J.R. (1977) Slowing of visual signals in multiple sclerosis, measured psychophysically and by steady-state evoked potentials. In: Desmedt, J.E. (Ed.) *Visual Evoked Potentials in Man: New Developments.* Oxford University Press, London. pp. 461-469.

REGAN, D. and RICHARDS, W.A. (1971) Independence of evoked potentials and apparent size. Vision Res., 11: 679-684.

REGAN, D. and RICHARDS, W. (1973) Brightness contrast and evoked potentials. J. Opt. Soc. Am., 63: 606-611.

REILLY, E.L., KONDO, C., BRUNBERG, J.A. and DOTY, D.B. (1978) Visual evoked potentials during hypothermia and prolonged circulatory arrest. Electroenceph. clin. Neurophysiol., 45: 100-106.

REMOND, A. (1964) Level of organization of evoked responses in man. Annals of the New York Academy of Sciences, 112: 143-159.

RICHEY, E.T, KOOI, K.A. and TOURTELLOTTE, W.W. (1971) Visually evoked responses in multiple sclerosis. J. Neurol. Neurosurg. Psychiat., 34: 275-280.

RIEMSLAG, F.C.C., SPEKREIJSE, H. and van WALBEEK, H. (1982) Pattern evoked potential diagnosis of multiple sclerosis: a comparison of various contrast stimuli. In: Courjon, J., Mauguiere, F. and Revol, M. (Eds.) *Clinical Applications of Evoked Potentials in Neurology.* New York: Raven Press. pp. 417-426.

RIETVELD, W.J., TORDOIR, W.E.M., HAGENOUW, J.R.B., LUBBERS, J.A. and SPOOR, Th.A.C. (1967) Visual evoked responses to blank and to checkerboard patterned flashes. Acta Physiol. Pharmacol. Neerl., 14: 259-285.

RIGGS, L.A. (1941) Continuous and reproducible records of the electrical activity of the human retina. Proceedings of the Society of Experimental Biology, 48: 204-207.

RIGGS, L.A. (1965) Light as a stimulus for vision. In: Graham, C.H. (Ed.) *Vision and Visual Perception.* New York: Wiley. pp. 321-349.

RIGOLET, M.H., MALLECOURT, J., LEBLANC, M. and CHAIN, F. (1979) Étude de la vision des couleurs et des potentiels évoqués visuels dans le diagnostic de la sclérose en plaques. J. Fr. Ophthalmol., 2, 10: 553-560.

RIPPS, H. (1978) Electrophysiology of the visual system (1928-1978). Investigative Opthalmology, 17, Suppl., pp. 46-54.

RITTER, W. (1978) Intracranial sources of event-related potentials. In: Otto, D.A. (Ed.) *Multidisciplinary Perspectives in Event-Related Brain Potential Research.* U.S. Environmental Protection Agency, Washington D.C. pp. 523-525.

ROBERTS, J.R., HICKS, B., PIPER, R. and BINNIE, C.D. (1974) An improved apparatus for slow chloriding of EEG electrodes. The Proceedings and Journal of the Electrophysiological Technologists Association, 21: 62-65.

ROBINSON, K. and RUDGE, P. (1975) Auditory evoked responses in multiple sclerosis. Lancet, (i), 1164-1166.

ROBINSON, K. and RUDGE, P. (1977a) The early components of the auditory evoked potential in multiple sclerosis. In: Desmedt, J.E. (Ed.) *Auditory evoked potentials in man. Psychopharmacology Correlates of EPs. Progress in Clinical Neurophysiology, Vol. 2.* Karger: Basel. pp. 58-67.

ROBINSON, K. and RUDGE, P. (1977b) Abnormalities of the auditory evoked potentials in patients with multiple sclerosis. Brain, 100: 19-40.

ROBINSON, K. and RUDGE, P. (1978) The stability of the auditory evoked potentials in normal man and patients with multiple sclerosis. Journal of Neurological Sciences, 36: 147-156.

ROBINSON, K. and RUDGE, P. (1980) The use of the auditory evoked potential in the diagnosis of multiple sclerosis. J. Neurol. Sci., 45: 235-244.

ROBINSON, K. and RUDGE, P. (1981) Waveform analysis of the brainstem evoked response. Electroenceph. clin. Neurophysiol., 52: 583-594.

ROBY, R. and LETTICH, E. (1975) A simplified circuit for stimulus artifact suppression. Electroenceph. clin. Neurophysiol., 39: 85-87.

RODIECK, R.W. (1973) Field potentials. In: *The Vertebrate Retina.* W.H. Freeman and Co., San Francisco. pp. 525-558.

RODIN, E.A., GRISELL, J.L., GUDOBBA, R.D. and ZACHARY, G. (1965) Relationship of EEG background rhythms to photic evoked responses. Electroenceph. clin. Neurophysiol., 19: 301-304.

RONIS, B.J. (1966) Cochlear potentials in otosclerosis. Laryngoscope, 76: 212-231.

ROSEN, I., BYNKE, H. and SANDBERG, M. (1980) Pattern-reversal visual evoked potentials after unilateral optic neuritis. In: Barber C. (Ed.). *Evoked Potentials.* MTP Press, Lancaster. pp. 567-574.

ROSEN, I., SORNAS, R. and ELMQVIST, D. (1977) Cervical root avulsion: electrophysiological analysis with electrospinogram. Scand. J. Plast. Reconstr. Surg., 11: 247-250.

ROSENHAMER, H.J. and SILFVERSKIOLD, B.P. (1980) Slow tremor and delayed brainstem auditory evoked responses in alcoholics. Arch. Neurol., 37: 293-296.

ROUHER, F., PLANE, C. and SOLE, P. (1969) Intérêt des potentiels évoqués visuels dans les affections du nerf optique. Arch. Ophthal. (Paris), 29: 555-564.

ROUHER, F., SOLE, P., ALFIERI, R., RIGAL, J.P. and PLANE, C. (1968) Intérêt pratique de l'étude des potentiels evoqués visuels. Bull. Soc. Ophthalmol. France, 4: 1-12.

ROWE, M.J. (1981) A sequential technique for half-field pattern visual evoked potential testing. Electroenceph. clin. Neurophysiol., 51: 463-469.

RUBEN, R.J., BORDLEY, J.E. and LIEBERMAN, A.T. (1961) Cochlear potentials in man. Laryngoscope, 71: 1141-1164.

RUBEN, R.J., SEKULA, J., BORDLEY, J.E., KNICKERBOCKER, G.G., NAGER, G.T. and FISCH, U. (1960) Human cochlear responses to sound stimuli. Annals of Otology, Rhinology and Laryngology, 69: 459-476.

RUBEN, R.J. and WALKER, A.E. (1963) The VIIIth nerve action potential in Ménière's disease. Laryngoscope, II: 1456-1464.

RUCHKIN, D.S., SUTTON, S. and STEGA, M. (1980) Emitted P300 and slow wave event-related potentials in guessing and detection tasks. Electroenceph. clin. Neurophysiol., 49: 1-14.

RYERSON, S.G., and BEAGLEY, H.A. (1981) Brainstem electric responses and electrocochleography: a comparison of threshold sensitivities in children. Brit. J. Audiol., 15: 41-48.

SAEZ, R.J., ONOFRIO, B.M. and YANAGIMARA, T. (1976) Experience with Arnold Chiari malformation, 1960-1970. J. Neurosurg., 45: 416-422.

SALAMY, A. (1978) Commissural transmission: maturational changes in humans. Science, 200: 1409-1411.

SANCES, A. Jr., LARSON, S.J., CUSICK, J.F., MYKLEBUST, J., EWING, C.L., JODAT, R., ACKMANN, J.J. and WALSH, P. (1978) Early somatosensory evoked potentials. Electroenceph. clin. Neurophysiol., 45: 505-514.

SANDBERG, M.A. and ARIEL, M. (1977) A hand-held two channel stimulator ophthalmosope. Archives of Ophthalmology, 95: 1881-1882.

SATYA-MURTI, S., CACACE, A.T. and HANSON, P.A. (1978) Abnormal auditory evoked potentials in hereditary motor-sensory neuropathy. Ann. Neurol., 5: 445-448.

SAUER, M. and SCHENCK, E. (1977) Electrophysiologic investigations in Friedreich's heredoataxia and in hereditary motor and sensory neuropathy. Electroenceph. clin. Neurophysiol., 43: 623.

SAUL, L.J. and DAVIS, H.A. (1932) Action currents in the central nervous system. I. Action currents of the auditory tracts. Archives of Neurology and Psychiatry, 28: 481-483.

SCHAUF, C.L. and DAVIS, F.A. (1974) Impulse conduction in multiple sclerosis: A theoretical basis for modification by temperature and pharmacological agents. J. Neurol. Neurosurg. Psychiat., 37: 152-161.

SCHMIDT, E.M., JOST, R.G. and DAVIS, K.K. (1974) Cortical cell discharge patterns in anticipation of a trained movement. Brain Res., 75: 309-311.

SCHRAMM, J. (1980) Clinical experience with objective localisation of the lesion in cervical myelopathy. In: Grote, W., Brock, M., Clar, H-E., Klinger, M. and Nau, H-E. (Eds.) *Advances in Neurosurgery, Vol. 8.* Springer-Verlag: Berlin. pp. 26-32.

SCHRAMM, J. and HASHIZUME, K. (1977) Somatosensory evoked potentials (SEP) in patients with peripheral, spinal and supraspinal lesions of the sensory system. In: Wullenburger, R., Wenker, H., Brock, M. and Klinger, M. (Eds.) *Advances in Neurosurgery, Vol. 4.* Springer: Berlin pp.250-256.

SCHULMAN-GALAMBOS, C. and GALAMBOS, R. (1975) Brainstem auditory evoked responses in premature infants. Journal of Speech and Hearing Research, 18: 456-465.

SCHWARTZ, M., EMDE, J.W. and SHAGASS, C. (1964) Comparison of constant current and constant voltage stimulators for scalp-recorded somatosensory responses. Electroenceph. clin. Neurophysiol., 17: 81-83.

SCHWARTZ, M. and SHAGASS, C. (1964) Recovery functions of human somatosensory and visually evoked potential. Ann. N.Y. Acad. Sci., 112: 510-525.

SCLABASSI, R.J., NAMEROW, N.S. and ENNS, N.F. (1974) Somatosensory response to stimulus trains in patients with multiple sclerosis. Electroenceph. clin. Neurophysiol., 37: 23-33.

SELTERS, W.A. and BRACKMANN, D.E. (1977) Acoustic tumour detection with brainstem electric response audiometry. Archives of Otolaryngology, 103: 181-187.

SEM-JACOBSEN, C.W. (1979) Clinical applications of auditory brainstem potentials to operational diving in the North Sea. J. Biomed. Eng., 1, 105.

SHACKEL, B. (1959) A rubber suction cup surface electrode with high electrical stability. Journal of Aplied Physiology, 13: 153-158.

SHAGASS, C. (1968) Cerebral evoked responses in schizophrenia. Condit. Reflex, 3: 205-216.

SHAGASS, C. (1972) *Evoked Brain Potentials in Psychiatry.* Plenum Press: New York. pp. 87-106.

SHAGASS, C., ROEMER, R.A., STRAUMANIS, J.J. and AMADEO, M. (1979) Deviant topography of somatosensory evoked potentials in schizophrenia. Electroenceph. clin. Neurophysiol., 46: 11.

SHAGASS, C. and SCHWARTZ, M. (1961) Reactivity cycle of somatosensory cortex in humans with and without psychiatric disorder. Science, 134: 1757-1759.

SHAGASS, C. and SCHWARTZ, M. (1963) Psychiatric correlates of evoked cerebral cortical potentials. Amer. J. Psychiat., 119: 1055-1061.

SHAGASS, C. and SCHWARTZ, M. (1964) Evoked potential studies in psychiatric patients. Ann. N.Y. Acad. Sci., 112: 526-542.

SHAGASS, C. and SCHWARTZ, M. (1965) Age, personality and somatosensory evoked responses. Science, 148: 1359-1361.

SHAGASS, C. and SCHWARTZ, M. (1966) Somatosensory cerebral evoked responses in psychotic depression. Brit. J. Psychiat., 112: 799-807.

SHAGASS, C., STRAUMANIS, J.J. Jr., ROEMER, R.A. and AMADEO, M. (1977) Evoked potentials of schizophrenics in several sensory modalities. Biol. Psychiat., 12: 221-235.

SHAHROKHI, F., CHIAPPA, K.H. and YOUNG, R.R. (1978) Pattern shift visual evoked responses in two hundred patients with optic neuritis and/or multiple sclerosis. Arch. Neurol., 35: 65-71.

SHAW, N.A. and CANT, B.R. (1980) Age dependent changes in the latency of the pattern visual evoked potential. Electroenceph. clin. Neurophysiol., 48: 237-241.

SHEPHERD, G.M. (1974) Retina. In: *The Synaptic Organisation of the Brain.* Oxford University Press. pp. 145-178.

SHIBASAKI, H. (1975) Movement-associated cortical potentials in unilateral cerebral lesions. J. Neurol., 209: 189-198.

SHIBASAKI, H., BARRETT, G., HALLIDAY, Elise and HALLIDAY, A.M. (1980a) Components of the movement-related cortical potential and their scalp topography. Electroenceph. clin. Neurophysiol., 49: 211-226.

SHIBASAKI, H., BARRETT, G., HALLIDAY, A.M. and HALLIDAY, E. (1980b) Scalp topography of the movement-related cortical potentials. In: Kornhuber, H.H. and Deecke, L. (Eds.). *Motivation, Motor and Sensory Processes, Behavior and Clinical Use.* Progr. in Brain Res., 54: 237-242. Elsevier/North Holland, Amsterdam.

SHIBASAKI, H. and KATO, M. (1975) Movement-associated cortical potentials with unilateral and bilateral simultaneous hand movement. J. Neurol., 208: 191-199.

SHIBASAKI, H. and KUROIWA, Y. (1975) Electroencephalographic correlates of myoclonus. Electroenceph. clin. Neurophysiol., 39: 455-463.

SHIBASAKI, H., MOTOMURA, S., YAMASHITA, Y., SHII, H. and KUROIWA, Y. (1981) Periodic synchronous discharge and myoclonus in Creutzfeldt-Jakob disease. Diagnostic application of jerk-locked averaging method. Ann. Neurol., 9: 150-156.

SHIBASAKI, H., SHIMA, F. and KUROIWA, Y. (1978a) Clinical studies of the movement-related cortical potential (MP) and the relationship between the dentatorubrothalamic pathway and readiness potential (RP). J. Neurol., 219: 15-25.

SHIBASAKI, H., YAMASHITA, Y. and KUROIWA, Y. (1978b) Electroencephalographic studies of myoclonus. Myoclonus-related cortical spikes and high amplitude somatosensory evoked potentials. Brain, 101: 447-460.

SHIBASAKI, H., YAMASHITA, Y. and TSUJI, S. (1977) Somatosensory evoked potentials. Diagnostic criteria and abnormalities in cerebral lesions. J. Neurol. Sci, 34: 427-439.

SHIMOJI, K., HIGASHI, H. and KANO, T. (1971) Epidural recording of spinal electrogram in man. Electroenceph. clin. Neurophysiol., 30: 236-239.

SHIMOJI, K., KANO, T., HIGASHI, H., MORIOKA, T. and HENSCHEL, E.O. (1972) Evoked spinal electrograms recorded from epidural space in man. J. Appl. Physiol., 33: 468-471.

SHIMOJI, K., MATSUKI, M., ITO, Y., MASUKO, K., MARUYAMA, M., IWANE, T. and AIDA, S. (1976) Interactions of human cord dorsum potential. J. Appl. Physiol, 40: 79-84.

SHIMOJI, K., MATSUKI, M., SHIMIZU, H. (1977) Waveform characteristics and spatial distribution of evoked spinal electrograms. J. Neurosurg., 46: 304-313.

SHIMOJI, K., SHIMIZU, H. and MARUYAMA, Y. (1978) Origin of somatosensory evoked responses recorded from the cervical skin surface. J. Neurosurg., 48: 980-984.

SIEGEL, L.G. (1975) Symposium on fluctuant hearing loss. Otolaryngologic Clinics of North America (Philadelphia). 8: 2-17. New York: W.B. Saunders Co.

SIEGEL, S. (1956) *Non-parametric Statistics for the Behavioural Sciences.* McGraw Hill, New York.

SIMSON, R., VAUGHAN, H.G. and RITTER, W. (1976) The scalp topography of potentials associated with missing visual or auditory stimuli. Electroenceph. clin. Neurophysiol., 40: 33-42.

SKINNER, P. and GLATTKE, T.J. (1977) Electrophysiologic response audiometry: state of the art. Journal of Speech and Hearing Disorders, 42: 179-198.

SMALL, D.G. (1976) Peripherally evoked spinal cord potentials in neurological diagnosis. In: Nicholson, J.P. (Ed.) *Scientific Aids in Hospital Diagnosis.* Plenum Press, New York. pp. 155-163.

SMALL, D.G., BEAUCHAMP, M. and MATTHEWS, W.B. (1980) Subcortical somatosensory evoked responses in normal man and in patients with central nervous system lesions. In: Desmedt, J.E. (Ed.) *Clinical Uses of Cerebral, Brainstem and Spinal Somatosensory Evoked Potentials. Progress in Clinical Neurophysiology. Vol. 7.* Basel: Karger. pp. 190-204.

SMALL, D.G., MATTHEWS, W.B. and SMALL, M. (1978) The cervical somatosensory evoked potential in the diagnosis of multiple sclerosis. J. Neurol. Sci., 35: 211-224.

SMITH, D.B., LELL, M.E., SIDMAN, R.D. and MAVOR, H. (1973) Nasopharyngeal phase reversal of cerebral evoked potentials and theoretical dipole implications. Electroenceph. clin. Neurophysiol., 34: 654-658.

SMITH, J.C., MARSH, J.T. and BROWN, W.S. (1975) Far-field recorded frequency-following responses: evidence for the locus of brainstem sources. Electroenceph. clin. Neurophysiol., 39: 465-472.

SMITH, K.J., BLAKEMORE, W.F. and McDONALD, W.I. (1979) Central remyelination restores secure conduction. Nature, 280: 395-396.

SOHMER, H. and FEINMESSER, M. (1967) Cochlear action potentials recorded from the external ear in man. Annals of Otology, Rhinology and Laryngology, 76: 427-435.

SOHMER, H. and FEINMESSER, M. (1970) Cochlear and cortical audiometry. Israel Journal of Medical Sciences (Jerusalem), 6: 219-223.

SOHMER, H., FEINMESSER, M. and SZABO, G. (1974) Sources of electrocochleographic responses as studied in patients with brain damage. Electroenceph. clin. Neurophysiol., 37: 663-669.

SOKOL, S. (1977) Visual evoked potentials to checkerboard pattern stimuli in strabismic amblyopia. In: Desmedt, J.E. (Ed.) *Visual Evoked Potentials in Man: New Developments.* Clarendon Press, Oxford. pp. 410-417.

SOKOL, S. (Ed.) (1980) *Electrophysiology and Psychophysics: their use in Ophthalmic Diagnosis. International Ophthalmology Clinics 20, 1.* Little Brown, Boston.

SOKOL, S., DOMAR, A., MOSKOWITZ, A. and SCHWARTZ, B. (1981) Pattern evoked potential latency and contrast sensitivity in glaucoma and ocular hypertension. In: Spekreijse, H. and Apkarian, P. (Eds.) *Visual Pathways: Electrophysiology and Pathology.* Documenta Ophthalmologica. Proc. Ser. 27: 79-86. Junk, The Hague.

SPALDING, J.M.K. (1952) Wounds of the visual pathway, Part II: The striate cortex. J. Neurol. Neurosurg. Psychiat. 15: 169-183.

SPEHLMANN, R. (1965) The averaged electrical responses to diffuse and to patterned light in the human. Electroenceph. clin. Neurophysiol., 19: 560-569.

SPEHLMANN, R., GROSS, R.A., HO, S.U., LEESTMA, J.E. and NORCROSS, K.A. (1977) Visual evoked potentials and post-mortem findings in a case of cortical blindness. Ann. Neurol., 2: 531-534.

SPEHLMANN, R. and SMATHERS, C.C. (1968) A small photic stimulator with fibre optical guides. Electroenceph. clin. Neurophysiol., 25: 282-283.

SPEKREIJSE, H. (1966) *Analysis of Responses to Sine Wave Modulated Light.* Ph.D. Thesis. University of Amsterdam. Dr. W. Junk. The Hague.

SPEKREIJSE, H., DUWAER, A.L. and POSTHUMUS MEYJES, F.E. (1979) Contrast evoked potentials and psychophysics in multiple sclerosis patients. In: Lehmann, D. and Callaway, E. (Eds.) *Human Evoked Potentials: Applications and Problems.* Plenum, New York. pp. 363-381.

SPEKREIJSE, H. and ESTEVEZ, O. (1972) The pattern appearance-disappearance response. Trace, 6: 13-19.

SPEKREIJSE, H., ESTEVEZ, O. and REITZ, D. (1977) Visual evoked potentials and the physiological analysis of visual processes in man. In: Desmedt, J.E. (Ed.) *Visual Evoked Potentials in Man: New Developments.* Clarendon Press: Oxford. pp. 16-89.

SPEKREIJSE, H., KHOE, L.H. and van der TWEEL, L.H. (1972) A case of amblyopia: electrophysiology and psychophysics of luminance and contrast. In: Arden, G.B. (Ed.) *The Visual System.* Plenum Press, New York. pp. 141-156.

SPEKREIJSE, H., van der TWEEL, L.H. and ZUIDEMA, Th. (1973) Contrast evoked responses in man. Vision Research, 13: 1577-1601.

SPRAKER, T.E. and ARNETT, D.W. (1977) An electronic checkerboard pattern generator for vision research. Electroenceph. clin. Neurophysiol., 42: 259-263.

SPRENG, M. and KEIDEL, W.D. (1967) Separierung von Cerebroaudiogram (CAG), Neuroaudiogram (NAG) und Otoaudiogram (OAG) in der objektiven Audiometrie. Archiv für klinische und experimentelle Ohren - Nasen und Kehlkopfheilkunde, 189: 225-246.

SQUIRES, K.C. and DONCHIN, E. (1976) Beyond averaging: the use of discriminant functions to recognize event related potentials elicited by single auditory stimuli. Electroenceph. clin. Neurophysiol., 41: 449-459.

SQUIRES, K.C., DONCHIN, E., HERNING, R.I. and McCARTHY, G. (1977) On the influence of task relevance and stimulus probability on event-related potential components. Electroenceph. clin. Neurophysiol., 42: 1-14.

SQUIRES, N.K., SQUIRES, K.C. and HILLYARD, S.A. (1975) Two varieties of long-latency positive waves evoked by unpredictable auditory stimuli in man. Electroenceph. clin. Neurophysiol., 38: 387-401.

STARR, A. (1976) Auditory brainstem responses in brain death. Brain 99: 543-554.

STARR, A. and ACHOR, L.J. (1975) Auditory brainstem responses in neurological disease. Archives of Neurology (Chicago), 32: 761-768.

STARR, A. and HAMILTON, A.E. (1976) Correlation between confirmed sites of neurological lesions and abnormalities of far field auditory brainstem responses. Electroenceph. clin. Neurophysiol., 41: 595-608.

STARR, A., SOHMER, H. and CELESIA, G.G. (1978) Some applications of evoked potentials to patients with neurological and sensory impairment. In: Callaway, E., Tueting, P. and Koslow, S.H. (Eds.). *Event-Related Brain Potentials in Man.* Academic Press, New York. pp. 155-196.

STENSAAS, S.S., EDDINGTON, D.K. and DOBELLE, W.H. (1974) The topography and variability of the primary visual cortex in man. J. Neurosurg., 40: 747-755.

STEPHENSON, W.A. and GIBBS, F.A. (1951) A balanced non-cephalic reference electrode. Electroenceph. clin. Neurophysiol., 3: 237-240.

STEVENS, J.R. (1974) The electroencephalogram: human recordings. In: Thompson, R.F. and Patterson, M.M. (Eds.) *Bioelectric Recording Technique, Part B.* Academic Press: New York. pp. 85-98.

STILLMAN, R.D., CROW, G. and MOUSHEGIAN, G. (1978) Components of the frequency following potential in man. Electroenceph. clin. Neurophysiol., 44: 438-446.

STILLMAN, R.D., MOUSHEGIAN, G. and RUPERT, A.L. (1976) Early tone-evoked responses in normal and hearing impaired subjects. Audiology, 15: 10-22.

STOCKARD, J.J., HUGHES, J.F. and SHARBROUGH, F.W. (1979) Visually evoked potentials to electronic pattern reversal: latency variations with gender, age and technical factors. Amer. J. EEG Technol, 19: 171-204.

STOCKARD, J.J. and ROSSITER, V.S. (1977) Clinical and pathologic correlates of brainstem auditory response abnormalities. Neurology (Minneap.), 27: 316-325.

STOCKARD, J.J., ROSSITER, V.S., WIEDERHOLT, W.C. and KOBAYASHI, R.M. (1976) Brain stem auditory-evoked responses in suspected central pontine myelinolysis. Arch. Neurol. (Chicago), 33: 726-728.

STOCKARD, J.J., STOCKARD, J.E. and SHARBROUGH, F.W. (1977) Detection and localization of occult lesions with brainstem auditory responses. Mayo Clinic Proceedings (Rochester MN), 52: 761-769.

STOCKARD, J.J., STOCKARD, J.E. and SHARBROUGH, F.W. (1978) Nonpathologic factors influencing brainstem auditory evoked potentials. Amer. J. EEG. Technol., 18: 177-209.

STOCKARD, J.J., STOCKARD, Janet E. and SHARBROUGH, F.W. (1980) Brainstem auditory evoked potentials in neurology: methodology, interpretation, clinical application. In: Aminoff, M.J. (Ed.) *Electrodiagnosis in Clinical Neurology.* Churchill Livingstone: Edinburgh. pp. 370-453.

STOHR, M. and PETRUCH, F. (1979) Somatosensory evoked potentials following stimulation of the trigeminal nerve in man. Journal of Neurology, 220: 95-98.

STOHR, P.E. and GOLDRING, S. (1969) Origin of somatosensory evoked scalp responses in man. J. Neurosurg., 31: 117-127.

STOWELL, H. (1977) Cerebral slow waves related to the perception of pain in man. Brain Res. Bulletin, 2: 23-30.

STRAUMANIS, J., SHAGASS, C. and OVERTON, D.A. (1969) Problems associated with application of the contingent negative variation to psychiatric research. Journal of Nervous and Mental Disease, 148: 170-179.

STRELETZ, L.J., KATZ, L., HOHENBERGER, M. and CRACCO, R.G. (1977) Scalp recorded auditory evoked potentials and sonomotor responses: an evaluation of components and recording techniques. Electroenceph. clin. Neurophysiol., 27: 316-325.

STRICK, P.L. (1976) Activity of ventrolateral thalamic neurons during arm movement. J. Neurophysiol., 39: 1032-1044.

SUTTON, G.G. and MAYER, R.F. (1974) Focal reflex myoclonus. J. Neurol. Neurosurg. Psychiat., 37: 207-217.

SUTTON, S., TUETING, P. and ZUBIN, J. (1967) Information delivery and the sensory evoked potential. Science, 155: 1436-1439.

SUZUKI, T., HIRAI, Y. and HORIUCHI, R. (1977) Auditory brainstem responses to pure tone stimuli. Scandinavian Audiology, 6: 51-56.

SWALLOW, D.M., EVANS, L., STEWART, G., THOMAS, P.K. and ABRAMS, J.D. (1979) Sialidosis Type l: cherry red spot-myoclonus syndrome with sialidase deficiency and altered electrophoretic mobility of some enzymes known to be glycoproteins. II. Enzyme studies. Ann. Hum. Genet. Lond., 43: 27-35.

SWANSON, D.K. and WEBSTER, J.G. (1974) A model for skin-electrode impedance. In: Miller, H.A. and Harrison, D.C. (Eds.) *Biomedical Electrode Technology.* Academic Press. pp. 117-128.

SYMON, L. HARGADINE, J., ZAWIRSKI, M. and BRANSTON, N. (1979) Central conduction time as an index of ischaemia in subarachnoid haemorrhage. J. Neurol. Sci., 44: 95-l03.

SZIRTES, J. and VAUGHAN, H.G., Jr. (1977) Characteristics of cranial and facial potentials associated with speech production. Electroenceph. clin. Neurophysiol., 43: 386-396.

TACKMANN, W. and KUHLENDAHL, D. (1979) Evoked potentials in neuronal ceroid lipofuscinosis. Eur. Neurol., 18: 234-242.

TACKMANN, W., STRENGE, H., BARTH, H. and SOJKA-RAYTSCHEFF, A. (1979) Diagnostic validity for different components of pattern shift visual evoked potentials in multiple sclerosis. Eur. Neurol., 18: 243-248.

TACKMANN, W. and RADU, E.W. (1980) Pattern shift visual evoked potentials in Charcot-Marie-Tooth Disease, HMSN Type I. J. Neurol., 224: 71-74.

TAMAKI, T. (1977) Clinical application of spinal cord action potentials. In: Proceedings of a Workshop on the Clinical Application of Spinal Cord Monitoring for Operative Treatment of Spinal Diseases. Chairman C.L. Nash and J.S. Brodkey, pp. 21-26 (unpublished).

TAMAKI, T. (1979) Clinical experiences in the recording of spinal evoked potentials during surgery. In: Proceedings of Spinal Cord Monitoring Workshop, data acquisition and analysis. Chairmen C.L. Nash and R.H. Brown, pp. 83-94 (unpublished).

TAMURA, K. (1972) Ipsilateral somatosensory evoked responses in man. Folia Psychiat. Neurol. Jap., 26: 83-94.

TAMURA, K. and KUROIWA, Y. (1972) Somatosensory evoked responses in patients with multiple sclerosis. Folia Psychiat. Neurol. Jap., 26: 269-274.

TANJI, J. and EVARTS, E.V. (1976) Anticipatory activity of motor cortex neurons in relation to direction of an intended movement. J. Neurophysiol., 39: 1062-1068.

TAYLOR, F.M. and ABRAHAM, P. (1969) A search for a safe Bentonite paste. The Proceedings and Journal of the Electrophysiological Technologists Association, 16: 80-83.

TEAS, D.C., ELDREDGE, D.H. and DAVIS, H. (1962) Cochlear responses to acoustic transients: an interpretation of the whole-nerve action potentials. Journal of the Acoustical Society of America, 34: 1438-1459.

TERKILDSEN, K., OSTERHAMMEL, P. and VELD, F.H. (1974) Far field electro-cochleography, electrode positions. Scandinavian Audiology, 3: 123-129.

TERKILDSEN, K., OSTERHAMMEL, P. and VELD, F.H. (1975) Far field electro-cochleography. Frequency specificity of the response. Scandinavian Audiology, 4: 167-172.

THACH, W.T. (1970) Discharge of cerebellar neurons related to two maintained postures and two prompt movements. I. Nuclear cell output. J. Neurophysiol., 33: 527-536.

THACH, W.T. (1975) Timing of activity in cerebellar dentate nucleus and cerebral motor cortex during prompt volitional movement. Brain Res., 88: 233-241.

THOMAS, P.K., ABRAMS, J.D., SWALLOW, D. and STEWART, G. (1979) Sialidosis Type l: Cherry red spot-myoclonus syndrome with sialidase deficiency and altered electrophoretic mobilities of some enzymes known to be glycoproteins. J. Neurol. Neurosurg. Psychiat., 42: 873-888.

THOMPSON, C.R.S. and HARDING, G.F.A. (1978) The visual evoked potential in patients with cataracts. Docum. Ophthal. Proc. Series, 15: 193-201.

THOMPSON, N.P. and YARBROUGH R.B. (1967) The shielding of electroencephalographic laboratories. Psychophysiology, 4: 244-248.

THORNTON, A.R.D. (1975a) Bilaterally recorded early acoustic responses. Scandinavian Audiology, 4: 173-181.

THORNTON, A.R.D. (1975b) The diagnostic potential of surface recorded electrocochleography. British Journal of Audiology (London), 9: 7-13.

THORNTON, A.R.D. (1976) Properties of auditory brainstem evoked responses. Revue de Laryngologie 97: 593-601.

THORNTON, A.R.D. and COLEMAN, M.J. (1975) The adaptation of cochlear and brainstem auditory evoked potentials in humans. Electroenceph. clin. Neurophysiol., 39: 399-406.

TIMSIT-BERTHIER, M., DELAUNOY, J. AND ROUSSEAU, J.C. (1973) Slow potential changes in psychiatry. II. Motor potential. Electroenceph. clin. Neurophysiol., 35: 363-367.

TITCOMBE, A.F. and WILLISON, R.G. (1961) Flicker fusion in multiple sclerosis. J. Neurol. Neurosurg. Psychiat., 24: 260-265.

TOWLE, V.L. and HARTER, M.R. (1977) Objective determination of human visual acuity: pattern evoked potentials. Invest. Ophthal. Visual Sci., 16: 1073-1076.

TOWNSEND, R.E. (1973) A device for generation and presentation of modulated light stimuli. Electroenceph. clin. Neurophysiol., 34: 97-99.

TROJABORG, W. and JORGENSEN, E.O. (1973) Evoked cortical potentials in patients with 'isoelectric' EEGs. Electroenceph. clin. Neurophysiol., 35: 301-309.

TROJABORG, W. and PETERSEN, E. (1979) Visual and somatosensory evoked cortical potentials in multiple sclerosis. J. Neurol. Neurosurg. Psychiat., 42: 323-330.

TRONCOSO, J., MANCALL, E.L. and SCHATZ, N.J. (1979) Visual evoked responses in pernicious anaemia. Archives of Neurology, 36: 168-169.

TSOBOKAWA, T. NISHIMOTO, H., YAMAMOTO, T., KITAMURA, M. KATAYAMA, Y. and MORIYASU, N. (1980) Assessment of brainstem damage by auditory brainstem response in acute severe head injury. J. Neurol. Neurosurg. Psychiat., 43: 1005-1011.

TSUMOTO, T., HIROSE, N., NONAKA, S. and TAKAHASHI, M. (1972) Analysis of somatosensory evoked potentials to lateral popliteal nerve stimulation in man. Electroenceph. clin. Neurophysiol., 33: 379-388.

TSUMOTO, T., HIROSE, N., NONAKA, S. and TAKAHASHI, M. (1973) Cerebrovascular disease: changes in somatosensory evoked potentials associated with unilateral lesions, Electroenceph. clin. Neurophysiol., 35: 463-473.

TSUTSUI, J., NAKANURA, Y., TAKENAKA, J. and FUKAI, S. (1973) Abnormality of the visual evoked response in various types of amblyopia. Jap. J. Ophthalmol., 17: 83-93.

TSUYAMA, N., TSUZUKI, N., KUROKAWA, T. and IMAI, T. (1978) Clinical application of spinal cord action potential measurement. International Orthopaedics (SIGOT), 2: 39-46.

UHTHOFF, W. (1889) Untersuchungen über die bei der multiplen Herdsklerose vorkommenden Augenstörungen. Arch. Psychiat. Nervenkr., 21: 303-410.

ULRICH, W.D., BOHNE, B.D., REIMANN, J. and WERNECKE, K.D. (1980) VEP and intraocular pressure. In: Barber, C. (Ed.) *Evoked Potentials.* MTP Press. Lancaster. pp. 251-255.

UNGAN, P. and BASAR, E. (1976) Comparison of Wiener filtering and selective averaging of evoked potentials. Electroencpeh. clin. Neurophysiol., 40: 516-520.

UZIEL, A. and BENEZECH, J. (1978) Auditory brainstem responses in comatose patients: relationship with brainstem reflexes and levels of coma. Electroenceph. clin. Neurophysiol. 45: 515-524.

VAN DER TWEEL, L.H. and VERDUYN LUNEL, H.F.E. (1965) Human visual responses to sinusoidally modulated light. Electroenceph. clin. Neurophysiol. 18: 587-598.

VAN LITH, G.H.M., VAN MARLE, G.W. and VAN DOK-MAK, G.T.M. (1978) Variation in latency times of visually evoked cortical potentials. British Journal of Ophthalmology, 62: 220-222.

VAUGHAN, H.G. (1969) The relationship of brain activity to scalp recording of event related potentials. In: Donchin, E. and Lindsley, D.B. (Eds.) *Average Evoked Potentials.* NASA SP-191. pp. 45-94.

VAUGHAN, H.G. (1974) The analysis of scalp-recorded brain potentials. In: Thompson, R.F. and Patterson, M.M. (Eds.) *Methods in Physiological Psychology. Vol. 1 Bioelectric Recording Techniques.* Academic Press, New York. pp. 157-207.

VAUGHAN, H.G., Jr., COSTA, L.D., GILDEN, L. and SCHIMMEL, H. (1965) Identification of sensory and motor components of cerebral activity in simple reaction-time tasks. Proc. 73rd Conv. Amer. Psychol. Assoc., 1: 179-180.

VAUGHAN, H.G., Jr., COSTA, L.D. and RITTER, W. (1968) Topography of the human motor potential. Electroenceph. clin. Neurophysiol., 25: 1-10.

VAUGHAN, H.G. and KATZMAN, R. (1964) Evoked response in visual disorders. Ann. N.Y. Acad. Sci., 112: 305-319.

VAUGHAN, H.G., KATZMAN, R. and TAYLOR, J. (1963) Alterations of visual evoked responses in the presence of homonymous field defects. Electroenceph. clin. Neurophysiol., 15: 737-746.

VAUGHAN, H.G. and RITTER, W. (1970) The sources of auditory evoked response recorded from the human scalp. Electroenceph. clin. Neurophysiol., 28: 360-367.

VENABLES, P.H. and MARTIN, I. (1967) *A Manual of Psychophysiological Methods.* North Holland: Amsterdam.

WACHTMEISTER, L. and DOWLING, J.E. (1978) The oscillatory potentials of the mud puppy retina. Investigative Ophthalmology, Visual Science, 17: 1176-1788.

WALL, P.D. (1958) Excitability changes in afferent fibre terminations and their relation to slow potentials. J. Physiol., (London), 142: 1-21.

WALTER, W.G. (1966) Electrophysiologic contributions to psychiatric therapy. Current Psychiatric Therapeutics, 6: 13-25.

WALTER, W.G., COOPER, R., ALDRIDGE, V.J., McCALLUM, W.C. and WINTER A.L. (1964) Contingent negative variation: an electric sign of sensorimotor association and expectancy in the human brain. Nature, 203: 380-384.

WANGER, P. and NILSSON, B.Y. (1978) Visual evoked responses to pattern-reversal stimulation in patients with amblyopia and/or defective binocular functions. Acta Ophthalmol., 56: 617-627.

WASTELL, D.G. (1977) Statistical detection of individual evoked responses: an evaluation of Woody's adaptive filter. Electroenceph. clin. Neurophysiol., 42: 835-839.

WASTELL, D.G. (1979) The application of low-pass linear filters to potential data: filtering without phase distortion. Electroenceph. clin. Neurophysiol., 46: 355-356.

WATANABE, K., IWASE, K. and HARA, K. (1972) Maturation of visual evoked responses in low-birthweight infants. Dev. Med. Child Neurol., 14: 425-435.

WATANABE, K., IWASE, K. and HARA, K. (1973) Visual evoked responses during sleep and wakefulness in pre-term infants. Electroenceph. clin. Neurophysiol., 34: 571-579.

WATSON, C.W. and DENNY-BROWN, D. (1955) Studies of the mechanism of stimulus-sensitive myoclonus in man. Electroenceph. clin. Neurophysiol., 7: 341-356.

WEINBERG, H. (1978) Comments on methods of signal analysis and signal detection. In: Otto, D.A. (Ed.) *Multidisciplinary Perspectives in Event-Related Brain Potential Research.* U.S. Environmental Protection Agency: Washington D.C. pp. 593-600.

WEINBERG, H. and COOPER, R. (1972) The recognition index: a pattern recognition technique for noisy signals. Electroenceph. clin. Neurophysiol., 33: 608-613.

WEINBERG, H., GREY WALTER, W., COOPER, R. and ALDRIDGE, V.J. (1974) Emitted cerebral events. Electroenceph. clin. Neurophysiol., 36: 449-456.

WEINMANN, H., CREUTZFELDT, O. and HEYDE, G. (1965) Die Entwicklung der visuellen Reizantwort bei Kindern. Neurologie, 207: 323-341.

WENZEL, W., CAMACHO, L., CLAUS, D. and ASCHOFF, J. (1982) Visually evoked potentials in Friedreich's ataxia. In: Courjon, J., Mauguiere, F. and Revol, M. (Eds.) *Clinical Applications of Evoked Potentials in Neurology.* New York: Raven Press. pp. 131-139.

WERBLIN, F.S. (1977) Regenerative amacrine cell depolarisation and formation of on-off ganglion cell response. J. Physiol., 264: 767-785.

WESTHEIMER, G. (1966) The Maxwellian View. Vision Research, 6: 669-682.

WEVER, E.G. and BRAY, C.W. (1930) Action currents in the auditory nerve in response to acoustic stimulation. Proceedings of the National Academy of Science, USA, 16: 344-350.

WHITFIELD, I.C. (1960) *An Introduction to Electronics for Physiological Workers.* Macmillan: London.

WHITFIELD, I.C. (1967) *The Auditory Pathway.* Camelot Press Ltd., London and Southampton.

WHITFIELD, I.C. and ROSS, H.F. (1965) Cochlear-microphonic and summating potentials and the outputs of individual hair-cell generators. Journal of the Acoustical Society of America, 38: 126-131.

WIESEL, T.N. and HUBEL, D.H. (1965a) Comparison of the effects of unilateral and bilateral eye closure on cortical unit responses in kittens. J. Neurophysiol., 28: 1029-1040.

WIESEL, T.N. and HUBEL, D.H. (1965b) Extent of recovery from the effects of visual deprivation in kittens. J. Neurophysiol., 28: 1060-1072.

WILDBERGER, H.G.H. and van LITH, G.H.M. (1976) Color vision and visually evoked response (VECP) in the recovery period of optic neuritis. Colour Vision Deficiencies. III Int. Symp. Amsterdam, 1975. Mod. Probl. Ophthal., 17. Karger, Basel. pp. 320-324.

WILDBERGER, G., van LITH, G. and MAK, G. (1976a) Comparative study of flash and pattern evoked VECPs in optic neuritis. Ophthal. Res., 8: 179-185.

WILDBERGER, H.G.H., van LITH, G.H.M., WIJNGAARDE, R. and MAK, G.T.M. (1976b) Visually evoked cortical potentials in the evaluation of homonymous and bitemporal visual field defects. Brit. J. Ophthal., 60: 273-278.

WILKE, J.T. and LANSING, R.W. (1973) Variations in the motor potential with force exerted during voluntary arm movements in man. Electroenceph. clin. Neurophysiol., 35: 259-265.

WILLIAMSON, P.D., GOFF, W.R. and ALLISON, T. (1970) Somatosensory evoked responses in patients with unilateral cerebral lesions. Electroenceph. clin. Neurophysiol., 28: 566-575.

WILSON, P. and RAMSDEN, R.T. (1977) Immediate effects of tobramycin on the human cochlea and correlation with serum tobramycin levels. British Medical Journal, I: 259-261.

WILSON, W.B. (1978) Visual-evoked response differentiation of ischaemic optic neuritis from the optic neuritis of multiple sclerosis. American Journal of Ophthalmology, 86: 530-535.

WILSON, W.B. and KEYSER, R.B. (1980) Comparison of the pattern and diffuse-light visual evoked responses in definite multiple sclerosis. Arch. Neurol., 37: 30-34.

WILSON, W.B., KIRSCH, W.M., NEVILLE, H., STEARS, J., FEINSOD, M. and LEHMAN, R.A.W. (1976) Monitoring of visual function during parasellar surgery. Surg. Neurol., 5: 323-329.

WOLBARSHT, M. (1964) Interference and its elimination. In: Nastuk, W.L. (Ed.) *Physical Techniques in Biological Research.* Academic Press. pp. 353-372.

WOLBARSHT, M.L. and SPEKREIJSE, H. (1968) Interference and noise in biological instrumentation. In: Levine, S.N. (Ed.) *Advances in Biomedical Engineering and Medical Physics.* Vol. 2. Wiley. pp. 205-242.

WOLIN, L.R., MASSOPUST, L.C. and MEDER, J. (1964) Electroretinogram and cortical evoked potentials under hypothermia. Arch. Ophthal., 72: 521-524.

WOODBURY, J.W. (1960) Potentials in a volume conductor. In: Ruch, T.C. and Fulton, J.F. (Eds.) *Medical Physiology and Biophysics.* Saunders, London. pp. 83-95.

WOODS, D.L., HILLYARD, S.A., COURCHESNE, E. and GALAMBOS, R. (1980) Electrophysiological signs of split-second decision-making. Science, 207: 655-657.

WOODY, C.D. (1967) Characterization of an adaptive filter for the analysis of variable latency neuroelectric signals. Med. biol. Engineering, 5: 539-553.

WORDEN, F.G. and MARSH, J.T. (1968) Frequency-following (microphonic-like) neural responses evoked by sound. Electroenceph. clin. Neurophysiol., 25: 42-52.

YAMADA, T., McKEE, J. and KIMURA, J. (1977) The effect of peripheral ischaemia on somatosensory evoked potentials. Electroenceph. clin. Neurophysiol., 43: 505.

YONEMURA, D. and KAWASAKI, K. (1978) Electrophysiological study on activities of neuronal and non-neuronal retinal elements in man with reference to its clinical application. Japanese Journal of Ophthalmology, 22: 195-213.

YOSHIE, N. (1968) Auditory nerve action potential responses to clicks in man. Laryngoscope, 178: 198-215.

YOSHIE, N. (1973) Diagnostic significance of the electrocochleogram in clinical audiometry. Audiology, 12: 504-539.

YOSHIE, N., OHASHI, T. and SUZUKI, T. (1967) Non-surgical recordings of auditory nerve action potentials in man. Laryngoscope, 77: 76-85.

YOSHIE, N. and OKUDAIRA, T. (1969) Myogenic evoked potential responses to clicks in man. Acta Oto-laryngologica, suppl. 252: 89-103.

ZABLOW, L. and GOLDENSOHN, E.S. (1969) A comparison between scalp and needle electrodes for the EEG. Electroenceph. clin. Neurophysiol., 26: 530-533.

ZALIS, A.W., OESTER, Y.T. and RODRIQUEZ, A.A. (1970) Electrophysiologic diagnosis of cervical nerve root avulsion. Archives of Physical Medicine and Rehabilitation, 51: 708-710.

ZEESE, J.A. (1977) Pattern visual evoked responses in multiple sclerosis. Archives of Neurology (Chicago), 34: 314-316.

ZERLIN, S. (1969) Travelling wave velocity in the human cochlea. Journal of the Acoustical Society of America, 46: 1011-1015.

ZVERINA, E. and KREDBA, J. (1977) Somatosensory cerebral evoked potentials in diagnosing brachial plexus injuries. Scand. J. Rehabil. Med., 9: 47-54.

ZWICKER, E. and FASTL, H. (1972) On the development of the critical band. Journal of the Acoustical Society of America, 52: 699-702.

Index